MEDICAL RADIOLOGY

Diagnostic Imaging and Radiation Oncology

Springer
Berlin
Heidelberg
New York
Barcelona
Hong Kong
London
Milan
Paris
Singapore
Tokyo

P. Van Houtte · J. Klastersky · P. Rocmans (Eds.)

Progress and Perspective in the Treatment of Lung Cancer

With Contributions by

K.S. Albain · J.J. Aristu · P. Armstrong · P. Baldeyrou · D. Ball · T. Berghmans
L.J. Boersma · H. Buenemann · F.A. Calvo · M. Cappello · F. Cappuzzo · C. Castaigne
J.D. Cox · L. Crino · A. Cull · J.E. Dancey · S. Danhier · D. Devriendt · B. Emami
S.A. Fisher · P. DeFrancquen · M.R. Green · A. Gregor · J.A. Hanson · H.-P. Heilmann
J. Klastersky · R. Komaki · Y. Lalami · E. Lartigau · T. Le Chevalier · S.S. Leong · S. Luce
F. Macbeth · H. Marsiglia · R.O. Mirimanoff · M. Moreno · F. Mornex · K. Østerlind
M. Paesmans · C.M.S. Rocha Lima · P. Rocmans · M. Santos · M.I. Saunders · P. Scalliet
C. Schiepers · J.P. Sculier · F.A. Shepherd · J.B. Sørensen · C. Sotiriou · P. Van Houtte
P. Vermylen · H. Wagner · F. Wuerschmidt · A. Zappala

Foreword by

L.W. Brady and H.-P. Heilmann

Springer

P. van Houtte, MD
Professor, Department of Radiation Oncology
Service de Radiothérapie
Institut Jules Bordet
1, rue Héger-Bordet, B-1000 Bruxelles, Belgium

J. Klastersky, MD
Professor, Service de Médecine Interne
et Laboratoire d'Investigation Clinique H.J. Tagnon
Centre des Tumeurs de l'Université Libre de Bruxelles
Institut Jules Bordet
1, rue Héger-Bordet, B-1000 Bruxelles, Belgium

P. Rocmans, MD
Professor, Service de Chirurgie Thoracique
Hôpital Erasme
808, route de Lennik, B-1070 Bruxelles, Belgium

MEDICAL RADIOLOGY · Diagnostic Imaging and Radiation Oncology

Continuation of
Handbuch der medizinischen Radiologie
Encyclopedia of Medical Radiology

With 56 Figures and 79 Tables

ISSN 0942-5373
ISBN 3-540-62548-8 Springer-Verlag Berlin Heidelberg New York

Library of Congress Cataloging-in-Publication Data
Progress and perspectives in the treatment of lung cancer / P. van Houtte, J. Klastersky, P. Rocmans (eds.); with contributions by K.S. Albain . . . [et al.]; foreword by L.W. Brady and H.-P. Heilmann. p. cm. – (Medical radiology) Includes bibliographical references and index. ISBN 3-540-62548-8 (alk. paper). 1. Lungs – Cancer – Treatment. I. Houtte, Paul van, 1949– . II. Klastersky, J. (Jean) III. Rocmans, P., 1937– . IV. Albain, K.S. (Kathy S.) V. Series. [DNLM: 1. Lung Neoplasms – radiotherapy. 2. Lung Neoplasms – drug therapy. 3. Combined Modality Therapy. WF 658P964 1999] RC280.L8P76 1999 616.99′42406 – dc21 DNLM/DLC for Library of Congress 98-35108

Cover design: de'blik, Berlin
Typesetting: Best-set Typesetter Ltd., Hong Kong

SPIN 10559881 21/3135 – 5 4 3 2 1 0 – Printed on acid-free paper

Foreword

Lung cancer is not a single disease process but is a group of biologically variable diseases. Therefore, accurate and complete diagnosis along with complete workup of the patient prior to decision-making in treatment is essential to devise the most appropriate treatment strategy. In North America adenocarcinoma of the lung now accounts for about 40% of all lung cancers and stage for stage these tumors have a poorer prognosis than squamous cell cancers of the lung.

Many prognostic indicators have been identified such as genetic markers and neuroendocrine differentiation, which have important roles to play in identifying the patients who would benefit most from active treatment.

Screening and early detection have been thought to be sine qua non in early diagnosis of lung cancer. However, a number of control led trials assessing the value of annual screening for lung cancer have demonstrated in some studies that chest X-rays and/or cytology screening may improve stage distribution, resectability, survival, and fatality but has not shown an impact on disease-specific mortality rates. The Mayo Clinic lung project comparing quarterly chest X-rays and sputum cytology with routine care in more than 10 000 male smokers indicated that 5-year survival following treatment in the screened patients was better than rates in contemporary clinical practice. However, arguments have been advanced as to factors that might have biased the clinical benefits. Other trials are currently under way to deal with this issue along with new molecular markers that may enhance sputum sensitivity.

In large measure, cancer of the lung is already advanced at the time of the original diagnosis. However, advances in staging and classification of tumours coupled with identification of potential new prognostic factors, enhance our ability to make sound and scientifically based treatment decisions for patients. Even though the prognosis remains poor for many of these patients because of the advanced stage at the time of presentation, the ability to prolong survival has been enhanced by new treatment regimens along with a better understanding of how these treatment regimems may best be used. Not only surgery, but also radiotherapy today gives a moderate chance of survival to patients who are inoperable or suffer from advanced stages.

Clearly, active treatment is cost-effective and is a viable option for patients regardless of the stage of disease. Even in late stage patients, modest survival advantages can be gained through aggressive multimodal integrated programs of management, if the individual tolerance of the patient is taken into consideration.

The present volume edited by Dr. Paul Van Houtte clearly identifies the problems in screening, staging, and histologic typing of lung cancer, and the appropriate treatment regimens for management.

Philadelphia
Hamburg

Luther W. Brady
Hans-Peter Heilmann

Preface

Lung cancer remains a major challenge owing to its low cure rate but also due to its very high incidence in most countries. Facing this enemy, the medical community has only two possible approaches: prevention and treatment. Despite the many information campaigns and the greater public awareness of the health risks, tobacco smoking is certainly not declining worldwide, even if some progress has been made, mainly in North America and in the countries of northern Europe. Tobacco smoking remains very fashionable in many countries of southern and eastern Europe and in Asia and South America. So, for the next few decades, improving our treatments remains a major health issue: any small step forward will immediately translate into a large number of patients cured.

The management of lung cancer remains the task of a team involving chest physicians, radiologists, pathologists, surgeons, medical oncologists, radiation oncologists ... and of course general practitioners. This book is a perfect illustration of such teamwork and follows the spirit of our meetings and workshops organized during the past 20 years. The first meeting was held in Brussels in 1979 with the collaboration and support of the European Organization for the Research and Treatment of Cancer (EORTC). A series of workshops were held in Le Havre, Fontainebleau and Bruges under the sponsorship of the International Association for the Study of Lung Cancer (IASLC). Lectures and papers including consensus reports were published in the *International Journal of Radiation Oncology, Biology and Physics* and in *Lung Cancer*.

Following our last workshop in Bruges in 1996, L. Brady and S. Heilman asked us to edit this book, retaining the philosophy of multidisciplinarity with experts from all parts of the world. The different aspects of the management of lung cancer are reviewed: prognostic factors, imaging techniques, combined treatments for small cell and non-small cell lung cancers, new drugs and best supportive care, among other topics. Several chapters are dedicated to aspects of radiotherapy such as the problems of fractionation, biological modifiers, prophylactic cranial irradiation and palliative treatment. This book is also the story of a long-standing friendship leading not only to workshops but also helping us in our daily life.

Over the years, we have had successful partnerships not only with all our colleagues at our institutions in Brussels (Institut Bordet and Erasme Hospital) but also with those from the Institut Gustave Roussy (Paris): R. Arriagada, D. Grunenwald, T. Le Chevalier. The last meeting in Bruges was a perfect illustration of real teamwork. Workshops were designed to share information, to challenge aspects of our current practice, to raise questions and to develop new strategies. The support of the IASLC and its secretary H. Hansen was very helpful in preparing and organizing our meetings.

The principal credit for this book must go to all the authors, whose papers remind us of the atmosphere and spirit of our meetings: arguments, science, discussions and friendship. Last but not least, we also wish to acknowledge the great help, support and enduring work of Ursula Davis and Anna Deus in completing our task and the many hours spent by Carine Vandevelde in preparing manuscripts.

Finally we wish to dedicate this book to our families: they have supported and encouraged us for many years during our daily work with our patients and with the preparation of our meetings.

Brussels

For the editors
P. Van Houtte

Contents

1 Prognostic Factors: From Clinical Parameters to New Biological Markers

J.B. SØRENSEN and K. ØSTERLIND

CONTENTS

1.1 Introduction

The current treatment results for lung cancer clearly call for improved therapy and also for careful selection of patients for the treatment options from which they are most likely to benefit. A detailed knowledge of prognostic factors, meaning variables with a well established relation to the prognosis, is important for achieving these goals. Any clinical trial must therefore include an assessment of the possible influence of such prognostic factors on the therapeutic result.

The ideal prognostic test divides the patients into two or more groups with very different outlooks and, accordingly, with no overlaps. However, this situation is relatively uncommon in clinical practice and a more likely situation is using a prognostic test, which is able to divide patients into "high-risk" and "low-risk" subgroups with significant differences in outlook. However, a high degree of uncertainty remains, since not all the "high-risk" patients will recur and not all the "low-risk" patients escape the poor outcome. If such test results were used to decide the treatment, many patients would receive the appropiate therapy, but not without the occurrence of some overtreatment and some undertreatment.

One way to overcome this obstacle and make a more accurate prediction of the outcome is to consider a number of predictors simultaneously. Thus, a multivariate model is necessary if the influence of several concurrent factors is to be investigated. The most common method is the Cox proportional hazards regression model (Cox 1972):

$$H(t) = H_0(t) \times \exp(z_1\beta_1 + z_2\beta_2 + z_3\beta_3 + \ldots + z_n\beta_n)$$

This model postulates that the death hazard $H(t)$ for any patient is proportional to an imperical base line hazard $H_0(t)$, which is the death hazard function for patients in whom all the regression variables (z) are zero. In a stepwise computer analysis, a set of best fitting coefficients (β), with a significant contribution in the equation, are obtained. This stepwise process is called forward, if the variables are included one by one (and discarded again if the influence is insignificant); the reverse process is called the backward procedure. Interactions among variables may result in minor differences between final models obtained with the two procedures; thus both procedures are often carried out, combined with tests for interactions, for proportionality, and for variation with time. For interpretation of the model, it is important that all $z = 0$ codes are related to clinical and meaningful attributes, e.g. normal laboratory tests and normal findings at imaging procedures.

The Cox model assumes the same influence of each variable (i.e., a fixed β value) throughout the data and constant interaction between two variables, if interaction occurs. However, unanticipated biological peculiarities may be overlooked. If peculiari-

J.B. SØRENSEN, The Finsen Center, Department of Oncology, Copenhagen University Hospital, 9 Blegdamsvej, DK-2100 Copenhagen Ø, Denmark
K. ØSTERLIND, Department of Internal Medicine F, Hillerød County Hospital, DK-3400 Hillerød, Denmark

ties are suspected, other statistical models are optional, e.g. the recursive partition and amalgamation methods (RECPAM) (CIAMPI et al. 1988). RECPAM is based on statistical clustering theories. For example, the patient material is split, step by step, like a branching tree, into a minimum of 30 patients in a branch; every branch ends in a terminal node. Survival data from different terminal nodes are compared, and if differences are small, relative to predefined criteria, nodes are merged (or amalgamated) to form final prognostic classes. The resulting tree thus has a similarity to the stepwise order of a clinical examination program. Specific variables may be influential in some, but not in other, parts of the tree, which may inspire new biological hypotheses; the risk of overfitting should always be kept in mind, however.

Even when combining the variables with an independent significant prediction of prognosis as established by a multivariate analysis, in a prognostic index, the current variables describing anatomic stages and clinical, histological, and clinical chemistry features do not completely predict the prognosis and a large fraction of the varibility remains unexplained. One possible explanation for this phenomenon is that the most frequently used prognostic variables are in reality epiphenomena of the true cellular and molecular characteristics of the disease, and relatively little is known about the biological model of the disease itself, even though the impact of a variety of biological phenomena have recently been evaluated. Thus, more knowledge on these cellular and molecular characteristics is still needed.

The objective of the following is to provide an update on the current knowledge of prognostic variables in lung cancer, which have been established through multivariate analysis, or RECPAM analysis, and which have a documented impact on prognosis.

1.2 Prognostic Factors in Non-Small Cell Lung Cancer

An update on the current knowledge of prognostic variables in non-small cell lung cancer (NSCLC), which has been established through multivariate analysis, is given in the following. Studies are reviewed provided that they describe prognostic factors for survival solely in NSCLC patients and provide clear descriptions of the variables included in a multivariate analysis. No abstracts have been included. The studies are divided according to whether the study populations consisted of resectable patients or of non-resectable patients treated with either chemotherapy with or without radiotherapy or with radiotherapy alone. In addition, a number of studies including NSCLC patients in all stages of disease have been included.

1.2.1 Clinical and Laboratory (Clinical Chemistry) Variables

A recent review on prognostic factors in NSCLC (SØRENSEN 1994) revealed 20 studies (GAIL et al. 1984; LIPFORD et al. 1984; CHASTANG et al. 1985; SØRENSEN and BADSBERG 1990; DELAURIER et al. 1989; LITTLE et al. 1990; HARADA et al. 1992; FONTANINI et al. 1992; MACCHIARINI et al. 1992; STIPA et al. 1993; MØRKVE et al. 1993; HORIO et al. 1993; PENA et al. 1992; BATTIFORA et al. 1992; LIEWALD et al. 1992; TARTTER et al. 1984; ZIMMERMANN et al. 1987; ALAMA et al. 1990; VAN BODEGOM et al. 1989; ISCHINOSE et al. 1993) including a total of 3500 patients with resected NSCLC, 14 studies (MILLER et al. 1986; FINKELSTEIN et al. 1986; EINHORN et al. 1986; EVANS et al. 1987; O'CONNELL et al. 1986; RAPP et al. 1988; SUKURAI et al. 1987; SØRENSEN et al. 1989; ALBAIN et al. 1991; SHINKAI et al. 1992; KOJIMA et al. 1991; KAWAHARA et al. 1991; BONOMI et al. 1991; PUJOL et al. 1993) including a total of 5875 patients with inoperable disease including in chemotherapy trials with or without radiotherapy, and 1 study (GRAHAM et al. 1992) including 1565 patients treated with radiotherapy alone. Also 6 studies (VOLM et al. 1988; HILSENBECK et al. 1993; STEVENSON et al. 1990; HANNISDAL and ENGAN 1991; BUCCHERI et al. 1993; MITSUDOMI et al. 1993) including a total of 1701 patients with NSCLC of all stages and treated with either surgery, irradiation, or chemotherapy were included in the review. The results from this review, together with a comprehensive review of the more recent literature on independent prognostic variables, are as shown in the tables. Table 1.1 highlights the impact of clinical and laboratory (clinical chemistry) variables, which have been attributed independent prognostic impact on survival.

Variables which have been evaluated in less than three multivariate studies have not been included in the tables. When a variable has been attributed a independent prognostic impact in more than half of the studies in which it has been evaluated, it has been attributed a definite prognostic impact in the tables.

Table 1.1. Clinical and laboratory (clinical chemistry) variables attributed prognostic impact on survival in multivariate analysis of NSCLC

Variable	Resected pts.			Chemotherapy +/− radiotherapy			Radiotherapy alone			All stages		
	Definite	Possible	Minor importance	Definite	Possible	Minor importance	Definite	Possible	Minor importance	Definite	Possible	Minor importance
Performance status	+			+			+			+		
Age			+			+	+					+
Gender			+	+			+				+	
Stage	+			+						+		
T-stage		+										+
N-stage	+									+		
Tumour size		+										
Weight loss					+		+					
Smoking index			+									
Operation type			+									
Limited/ extensive disease				+								
Metastases to												
Liver					+							
Bone					+							
Perioperative blood transfusion	+											
Albumin				+								
Hemoglobin					+							
WBC					+							
LDH					+						+	

LDH, lactate dehydrogenase; WBC, with blood cell count.

Variables which were of prognostic significance in less than half but more than one-third of the studies are called possible prognostic predictors, and variables which were of prognostic significance in less than one-third of the studies are attributed a minor or no importance in the tables. It is apparent that none of the variables were evaluated in all studies.

A large number of studies have evaluated prognostic variables among resected patients. Besides 20 studies included in a recent review (Sørensen 1994), a further 22 studies have recently been published (Buhr et al. 1997; Higashiyama et al. 1997a,b; Ogawa et al. 1997; Dosaka-Akita et al. 1997; Koukourakis et al. 1997; Esposito et al. 1997; Kessler et al. 1996; Cangemi et al. 1996; Yamashita et al. 1996; Harpole et al. 1995, 1996; Dalquen et al. 1996; Fujino et al. 1995; Ischinose et al. 1995; Lee et al. 1995; Kolodziejski et al. 1997; Nishio et al. 1997; Apolinario et al. 1997; Pastorino et al. 1997; Gasinska et al. 1997; Pappot et al. 1996; Giatromanolaki et al. 1996). Definite prognostic factors for long survival include good performance status, low stage and low lymph node category (N) and lack of need for perioperative blood transfusion (Table 1.1). Also, low tumour category (T) and tumour size in itself has been a major predictor of survival in many trials, but the variables describing T and N were not independent significant predictors of survival in all studies evaluating these factors. This observation might be explained by the phenomenon that T and N categories may be less important in Cox multivariate regression analysis when stage of disease is included in the analysis as well.

Effect of perioperative blood transfusions was a significant prognostic variable in two studies (Little et al. 1990; Tartter et al. 1984) while it was not significant in a third study (Kolodziejski et al. 1997). The observation that perioperative transfusion significantly worsened the patients' prognosis may be due to an adverse effect of the transfusion itself, but may rather serve as a marker of another, still undetermined, risk factor.

Minor importance was observed for age and gender (Table 1.1). A smoking index, defined as number of pack-years, was without prognostic significance in three studies (Fujino et al. 1995; Harpole et al. 1995; Kolodziejski et al. 1997). Also the operation type, divided into pneumonectomia, lobectomia or smaller resections, was of prognostic significance in only 3 out of 14 studies (Sørensen 1994; Buhr et al. 1997; Cangemi et al. 1996; Harpole et al. 1995; Apolinario et al. 1997; Gasinska et al. 1997).

The prognostic variables for patients in advanced disease receiving chemotherapy with or without radiotherapy have been reported in 14 studies including a total of 5875 patients in a recent review (Sørensen 1994), and subsequently also in a further 4 studies (Sculier et al. 1994; Espinosa et al. 1995; Hespanhol et al. 1995; Takigawa et al. 1996). The results are summarized in Table 1.1 with respect to clinical and laboratory variables. Performance status has been evaluated in 18 studies and was significant in 16 of these, indicating that performance status is still the best documented prognostic variable in NSCLC patients with advanced disease.

The new international staging system, as described by Mountain in 1986, has also been a definite prognostic factor. Other established prognostic variables include gender, with a worse survival outlook for males, and a poor survival outlook has also been observed with patients having limited disease or low pretreatment plasma albumin level (Table 1.1).

Other variables which may be possible predictors of poor prognosis include high weight loss, metastases to liver or bones, low pretreatment hemoglobin level, high white blood cell count or high LDH (Table 1.1). Age has been of only minor importance, as indicated by lack of significant influence in the majority of studies.

Patients treated with radiotherapy alone were included in 3 multivariate studies, including a total of 3326 patients, out of which 2 studies were multivariate Cox regression analyses (Volm et al. 1988; Jeremic and Shibamoto 1996) while 1 study was a RECPAM analysis (Scott et al. 1997). Definite prognostic variables include performance status and age, which were both major prognostic variables in all three studies, while gender and weight loss were of prognostic influence in two out of these three trials (Table 1.1).

Ten studies (Volm et al. 1988; Hilsenbeck et al. 1993; Stevenson et al. 1990; Hannisdal and Engan 1991; Buccheri et al. 1993; Mitsudomi et al. 1993; Thiberville et al. 1995; Visakorpi et al. 1995; Weiskopf et al. 1995; Goto et al. 1996) including patients with NSCLC of all stages and treated with either surgery, irradiation, or chemotherapy, have reported data in multivariate analysis of variables predicting survival. Again, not all variables have been included in all analyses, which somewhat limits the conclusions. Only performance status has been an important predictor of prognosis in all the studies in which it was evaluated, while other definite prognostic variables include stage and lymph node status (N). Possible prognostic factors include gender and LDH, while a minor or no influence was observed for tumour size or localization (T), age or histologic type.

1.2.2 Histopathologic Variables

Although 29 studies have evaluated the histologic type for possible prognostic impact among resectable NSCLC patients in multivariate analysis, only five studies revealed a prognostic impact (Gail et al. 1984; Lipford et al. 1984; Delaurier et al. 1989; Cangemi et al. 1996; Fujino et al. 1995). Both Gail et al. (1984) and Delaurier et al. (1989) observed an independent and significant prediction for long-term survival among patients with squamous cell carcinoma compared with patients with non-squamous histology, although these observations were not confirmed in a study by Lipford et al. (1984). However, the latter study revealed a significantly worse prognosis for patients having large cell carcinoma. Fujino et al. reported that patients with large and adenosquamous cell carcinomas had a shorter survival than those with adenocarcinoma and squamous cell carcinoma, while Cangemi et al. observed that squamous cell carcinomas predicted a poor survival expectancy in elderly patients above 70 years of age, while no significant influence was observed in the younger patient population. Thus, the results with respect to histologic types are conflicting in the studies in which a statistical influence was observed. Taken together with the fact that the majority of studies have not observed any prognostic influence, it seems fair to conclude that histologic type is of only minor or no importance for prediction of survival among resected patients.

The degree of differentiation or intratumour necroses also proved to be of minor importance (Table 1.2). The proliferative activity of the tumour cells was of prognostic importance in three out of nine studies. Only intratumoural blood vessel invasion seems at this point to be considered a definite prognostic variable among resectable NSCLC patients, being a significant predictor in five out of six studies (Sørensen 1994; Kessler et al. 1996; Ischinose et al. 1995; Harpole et al. 1995, 1996).

Among patients with non-resectable disease, only histologic type was evaluated in three or more multivariate studies and was also attributed minor importance in these patients (Table 1.2). The same lack of prognostic information was attributed to histologic type in studies including all stages of NSCLC treated with either surgery, radiotherapy or chemotherapy (Table 1.2). Histologic type has not been sufficiently evaluated in radiotherapy studies, but was without significant prognostic impact in one multivariate study including 1592 patients (Scott et al. 1997).

Table 1.2. Histopathologic variables attributed prognostic impact on survival in multivariate analysis of NSCLC

Variable	Resected pts.			Chemotherapy +/− radiotherapy			Radiotherapy alone			All stages		
	Definite	Possible	Minor importance	Definite	Possible	Minor importance	Definite	Possible	Minor importance	Definite	Possible	Minor Importance
Histologic type			+			+						+
Differentiation			+									
Proliferative activity		+										
Necrosis intratumoral			+									
Intratumoral blood vessel invasion	+											

1.2.3 Biological Features

In addition to clinical chemistry, and histopathologic variables attributed a prognostic impact as shown in Tables 1.1 and 1.2, many other factors are important for predicting the prognosis in NSCLC. These factors include the biological properties inherent in the tumour cells themselves. The relative imprecision of the previously mentioned criteria in estimating prognosis has led to a re-examination of the tumours themselves. Technological advances in molecular biology offer important opportunities to study the molecular characteristics of NSCLC and to discover important pathophysiologic and prognostic data. Thus, the literature is rapidly expanding in this field. Biological variables which have been evaluated in multivariate analysis in NSCLC are shown in Table 1.3, and will be discussed in the following.

1.2.3.1 Genetic Features

1.2.3.1.1 DNA ANEUPLOIDY

DNA aneuploidy (abnormal chromosomal number) has been investigated for the influence on prognosis in seven studies (Mørkve et al. 1993; Liewald et al. 1992; Zimmermann et al. 1987; van Bodegom et al. 1989; Ischinose et al. 1993; Visakorpi et al. 1995; Kolodziejski et al. 1997). Three studies (Kern et al. 1990; Ogawa et al. 1992; Kolodziejski et al. 1997) observed that patients with diploid tumours had longer survival times than patients with aneuploid tumours. The first two studies (Kern et al. 1990; Ogawa et al. 1992) included patients with both NSCLC and SCLC tumours, while the latter study (Kolodziejski et al. 1997) included solely patients with squamous cell lung cancer. Another study by Isobe et al. (1990) included 130 patients with NSCLC and similarly observed a more favourable survival for patients with a diploid DNA pattern compared with patients with aneuploid patterns. Also an earlier study by Volm et al. (1988) showed an independent and significant impact of DNA diploidy on survival, while two more recent studies (Muers et al. 1996; Visakorpi et al. 1995) reported DNA aneuploidy to be without prognostic information.

1.2.3.1.2 CHROMOSOME ABNORMALITY

Analyses of chromosome abnormalities show that non-random deletions of the short arm of chromosom 3 are frequent in NSCLC, occurring in 40%–60% of cases (Thiberville et al. 1995). Even though univariate analyses previously have pointed towards a prognostic impact of 3p 21–22 allelic loss as a predictor of prognosis, a multivariate analysis by Thiberville et al. (1995) observed no influence of chromosome 3p deletion on survival.

1.2.3.1.3 ONCOGENES

Proto-oncogenes will induce autonomous cellular proliferation when activated to oncogenes. Activation will occur by point mutation, overexpression or deletion of genetic material. Proto-oncogenes are usually dominant. Oncogenes evaluated for prognostic impact in NSCLC include the *ras* oncogenes, c-*erb*B-1 oncogene, c-*erbB*-2 oncogene, also called HER-2 and *neu* oncogene, and *Bcl*-2 oncogene.

ras Oncogene. The *ras* protooncogene family includes the genes k-, h- and n-*ras*, of which k-*ras* has been evaluated for prognostic impact in NSCLC (Szabo and Mulshine 1993; Dosaka-Akita et al. 1997; Fujino et al. 1995). Point mutations at codons 12, 13 or 61 change *ras* genes to oncogenic forms.

Table 1.3. Biological variables evaluated for prognostic impact on survival in multivariate analysis in NSCLC

Variables	References
Genetic features	
DNA aneuploidy	Mørkve et al. 1993; Liewald et al. 1992; Zimmermann et al. 1987; van Bodegom et al. 1989; Ischinose et al. 1993; Kolodziejski et al. 1997; Visakorpi et al. 1995
Chromosome abnormality (3p 21–22 allelic loss)	Thiberville et al. 1995
Oncogenes	
K-*ras*	Szabo and Mulshine 1993; Dosaka-Akita et al. 1997; Fujino et al. 1995
c-*erb*B2 (= HER2, = *neu*)	Harpole et al. 1996
Bcl-2	Higashiyama et al. 1997
Tumour suppressor genes	
p53	Dosaka-Akita et al. 1997; Dalquen et al. 1996; Fujino et al. 1995; Lee et al. 1995; Nishio et al. 1996; Apolinario et al. 1997; Pastorino et al. 1997; Pappot et al. 1996; Giatromanolaki et al. 1996; Horio et al. 1993; Ebina et al. 1994
Retinoblastoma (Rb gene)	Dosaka-Akita et al. 1997
Other genes	
CYP1A1	Goto et al. 1996
GLUT1 and GLUT3	Ogawa et al. 1997
Markers of differentiation	
EGF-R (epidermal growth factor receptor, c-*erb*B1)	Pastorino et al. 1997; Giatromanolaki et al. 1996
Cyfra 21-1 (cytokeratin – 19 fragment)	Weiskopf et al. 1995
Tumour cell proteases	
Plasminogen activator system	Pappot et al. 1996
Polymorphonuclear leukocyte elastase (PMN-E)	Yamashita et al. 1996
Tumour associated antigenes	
Blood-group carbohydrate antigenes	Lee et al. 1991; Miyake et al. 1992
CA 242	Pujol et al. 1993
Antigen 43-9F	Battifora et al. 1992
Tumour cell proliferation	
Proliferative index	Kessler et al. 1996; Harpole et al. 1995, 1996; Lee et al. 1995; Kolodziejski et al. 1997; Gasinska et al. 1997; Visakorpi et al. 1995; Sørensen 1994
Ki-67 proliferation-associated nuclear antigen	Harpole et al. 1996; Giatromanolaki et al. 1996
Other biological markers	
Monomeric lamina receptor (67LR)	Pastorino et al. 1997
Motility-related protein-1 (MRP-1/CD9)	Higashiyama et al. 1997

This results in continuous stimulation of cellular growth. The activated *ras* genes are among the most dominant identified oncogenes in human tumours (Kanters et al. 1995). k-*ras* is the most frequent genetic mutation primary and metastatic in NSCLC, with an incidence of 20%–30% among resected NSCLC specimens (Moore and Lee 1996). Slebos et al. (1990) examined the prognostic impact of k-*ras* mutation among 69 patients with completely resected adenocarcinoma. Patients with tumours having the k-*ras* mutation at codon 12 had a significantly reduced survival outlook. Dosaka-Akita et al. (1997) reported that *ras* mutation was a significant prognostic factor in multivariate analysis among 44 patients with adenocarcinoma, but not in a cohort of 41 patients with squamous cell carcinoma. All patients were curatively resected.

Also Fujino et al. (1995) examined 96 patients with NSCLC, who underwent surgical resection, 63 of whom also received postoperative combination chemotherapy. Expression of *ras*-oncogen product was not statistically significant in multivariate analysis, but a combined analysis of mutated p-53 and *ras* p-21 expression in the same tumour specimens revealed that patients with p-53 and *ras* p-21-negative tumours survived longest compared to patients with other p-53 and *ras* p-21 features (Fujino et al. 1995). Further studies with larger patient cohorts have to reveal whether *ras* mutation is a definite and independent prognostic variable in NSCLC.

c-erbB-2. c-*erb*B-2 oncogene is also known as HER-2 or *neu* and codes for a membrane growth factor receptor. An immunohistochemical study of 203 primary NSCLC tumours detected c-*erb*B-2 expression in 18% of stage I and 60% of stage 4 tumours (TATEISHI et al. 1991). A subsequent multivariate survival analysis by HARPOLE et al. (1996) among 275 consecutive patients resected for stage I NSCLC revealed no prognostic impact in the Cox analysis for c-*erb*B-2.

Bcl-2. *Bcl*-2 is a proto-oncogene that inhibits programmed cell death (apoptosis). Lower expression of *Bcl*-2 oncoprotein probably plays a role in tumorigenesis and tumour development. Im-munostaining for *Bcl*-2 oncoprotein was performed by HIGASHIYAMA et al. (1997a) on 182 patients with resectable NSCLC. Thirty-six patients (19.8%) showed a positive immunostaining for *Bcl*-2 oncoprotein, and in a multivariate analysis, a positive *Bcl*-2 oncoprotein status was confirmed with improved survival for patients with squamous cell carcinoma, but not in other cell types. The mechanism by which mutation of a known oncogene carries a favourable prognosis is still unclear. It has been questioned whether *Bcl*-2 oncoprotein biologically participates in the hemotogenous metastatic process and reduces the incidence of distant metastases (HIGASHIYAMA et al. 1997a), but this remains to be elucidated.

1.2.3.1.4 TUMOUR SUPPRESSOR GENES

Inactivation of genes that normally regulate cellular growth and thereby have a restraining effect of tumorigenesis (tumour suppressor genes) can lead to uncontrolled cell proliferation. In many cases, inactivation occurs by a point mutation of one allele and, subsequently, loss of an amount of genetic material in the other allele. For many types of cancer, multiple mutations in both tumour suppressor genes and oncogenes are ultimately required to achieve full malignant transformation.

p53-Suppressor Genes. The p53 gene is thought to regulate transcription of deoxyrebonuclic acid (DNA). The wild-type p53 protein blocks the progression of cells through the cell cycle late in the G1 phase of replication. The mutant protein does not have this function and may even promote cellular proliferation (KANTERS et al. 1995). Alterations in this gene are among the most common genes associated with cancer. p53 is very frequently abnormal in lung cancer, with mutation in >50% of NSCLC (KANTERS et al 1995; CHIBA et al. 1990). The prognostic impact of p53 alterations has been evaluated in 11 multivariate studies out of which 6 studies (DOSAKA-AKITA et al. 1997; NISHIO et al. 1996; APOLINARIO et al. 1997; PASTORINO et al. 1997; PAPPOT et al. 1996; GIATROMANOLAKI et al. 1996) did not report any significant prognostic impact, while 5 studies (DALQUEN et al. 1996; FUJINO et al. 1995; LEE et al. 1995; HORIO et al. 1993; EBINA et al. 1994) pointed towards independent prognostic information among NSCLC patients. Thus, the prognostic significance of p53 is as yet unclear.

Retinoblastoma Genes. The retinoblastoma gene (Rb) is a prototype tumour suppressor gene, producing a nuclear phosphoprotein involved in cell cycle regulation located in chromosome 13q. The Rb protein is thought to bind and sequester transcription factors, which promotes cell cycling. Originally described in retinoblastomas, abnormalities of the Rb gene have subsequently been described in many other tumours, including leukaemias, sarcomas and carcinomas. It is mostly SCLCs (>95%), which have absent or abnormal Rb protein, whereas only a modest fraction of NSCLCs are affected, ranging from 20% for stage I and II to 60% for stages III and IV (XU et al. 1991)

In a study including 91 patients with curatively resected NSCLC stages I to IIIA, DOSAKA-AKITA et al. (1997) observed that 21% of the tumours showed negative Rb-protein expression. When evaluated in multivariate analysis, Rb-protein expression was not statistically correlated with survival in this cohort of NSCLC patients, neither alone nor when combined with *ras* mutation or with p53 protein expression. However, in a separate analysis including 19 patients with pulmonary adenocarcinoma, patients having Rb-protein expression together with *ras*-p21 protein expression had a 5-year survival rate of 82% in contrast to patients without Rb-protein expression together with *ras*-p21-protein expression, who had a 5-year survival rate of only 13%. This difference was significant in a multivariate analysis, but neither Rb-protein expression nor *ras*-p21-protein expression alone were significant predictors of survival.

1.2.3.1.5 OTHER GENES

CYP 1A1. The CYP 1A1 gene is responsible for the metabolic activation of benzopyrene in cigarette smoke and a high susceptibility to smoking related lung cancer has been associated with polymorphism of the CYP 1A1 gene. In a study of 232 patients with

NSCLC of all stages who received treatment with either chemotherapy, radiotherapy, or surgery, GOTO et al. (1996) examined the prognostic impact of CYP 1A1 gene polymorphism on survival. Patients with at least one susceptible allele of polymorphism of the CYP 1A1 gene had shortened survival ($n = 131$; median survival time 24.2 months) compared with those with non-susceptible homozygous alleles ($n = 101$; median survival time 65.2 months) ($P = 0.005$, log rank test). A multivariate analysis also revealed that CYP 1A1 polymorphism was an independent prognostic factor among 98 patients with non-resectable advanced stage NSCLC, while CYP 1A1 gene types were without prognostic information among the patients with early stage resectable disease (GOTO et al. 1996).

GLUT1 and GLUT3. Increased glucose transport is a common characteristic of most tumours. The molecules responsible for increased glucose metabolism are membrane glucoprotein carriers that depend on the glucose concentration gradient and do not require cellular energy. Among seven glucose transporter type genes (GLUT) identified, GLUT1 and GLUT3 are responsible for basal glucose uptake. The rule of elevated glucose uptake in lung cancer was examined by OGAWA et al. (1997), who performed PCR amplification of GLUT1 and GLUT3 in 312 surgically resected NSCLC tumours. The survival of patients whose tumour showed GLUT1 amplification was significantly shorter than that of patients whose tumours did not ($P < 0.001$), and in multivariate analysis, GLUT1 remained a statistically significant prognostic factor. GLUT3 was without prognostic information.

The observation of higher glucose metabolism in cancer cells forms a basis for the use of positron emission tomography (PET scan) with labelled glucose analogues for the diagnosis of a variety of cancers. Accordingly, the current studies suggest that PET imaging may be a tool for estimating the prognosis of patients with lung cancer, which, however, requires further investigation.

1.2.3.2 Markers of Differentiation

EGF-R. The c-*erb*B1 gene encodes for the epidermal growth factor receptor (EGF-R). EGF-R are found predominantly in the NSCLC.The production of EGF-like activity by lung cancer cells raises the possibility of an autocrine loop, as epidermal growth factor is a cytokine that stimulates the growth of both normal and malignant cells. EGF-R is overexpressed in up to 80% of NSCLC cases, but its widespread distribution within normal long tissue may limit its prognostic value (MOORE and LEE 1996). Two studies have evaluated prognostic impact of EGF-R (PASTORINO et al. 1997; GIATROMANOLAKI et al. 1996). Neither a study including 515 cases of resected stage I NSCLC patients by PASTORINO et al. (1997) nor a study of 107 resected stage I patients by GIATROMANOLAKI et al. (1996) revealed any prognostic information for EGF-R in multivariate analysis.

Cyfra 21-1. Cytokeratines are epithelial markers whose expression is not lost during malignant transformation. Cyfra 21-1 is a cytokeratine-19 fragment, which is soluble in serum and may serve as a circulating tumour marker. WEISKOPF et al. (1995) performed an immunoradiometric assay of serum Cyfra 21-1 in 116 patients with NSCLC and in 71 patients with benign lung diseases. Cyfra 21-1 levels were significantly higher in advanced NSCLC than in early stage disease and were higher in NSCLC patients than in patients with benign diseases. In a multivariate analysis of survival, Cyfra 21-1 was an independent prognostic factor along with performance status and disease stage in NSCLC (WEISKOPF et al. 1995). The epithelial marker was highest in patients with squamous cell subtype. Based on this study, Cyfra 21-1 seems to be a marker of NSCLC, especially of the squamous-cell subtype. It may also reflect the extent of disease and yield independent prognostic information, which may be useful for stratifying patient populations with NSCLC if the current results can be confirmed in subsequent studies.

1.2.3.3 Tumour Cell Proteases

Plasminogen Activator System. The plasminogen activator system is a proteolytic enzyme system known to be involved in cancer invasion and metastases. Urokinase plasminogen activator (uPA), plasminogen activator inhibitor 1 (PAI-1) and the urokinase plasminogen activator receptor (uPAR) have all been examined for prognostic information in NSCLC (PAPPOT et al. 1996; PEDERSEN et al. 1994a,b). PAI-1 was an independent prognostic marker in pulmonary adenocarcinoma (PEDERSEN et al. 1994b) while uPAR was an independent prognostic marker in squamous cell carcinoma

(Pedersen et al. 1994a). The two studies did not include all the histological subtypes of NSCLC, and thus it is unclear whether PAI-1 and uPAR can be used as prognostic markers of NSCLC in general. It has been hypothesized that the variation in prognostic impact of uPAR and PAI1 between pulmonary adenocarcinoma and squamous cell carcinoma could reflect differences in tumour and stroma cell interactions with regard to plasminogen activating system.

The same group of authors have also examined uPA, PAI-1 and uPAR in a group of 228 NSCLC patients of all major histological subtypes (squamous cell carcinoma 84 patients, pulmonary adenocarcinoma 106 patients, and large cell carcinoma 38 patients) (Pappot et al. 1996). Multivariate analysis did not reveal any prognostic impact of uPA and uPAR, while PAI-1 was confined to independent information on survival (Papport et al. 1996).

Polymorphonuclear Leucocyte Elastase (PMN-E). Elastase is the only protease that can degrade insoluble elastin, which is a structural component of such elastic tissues as blood vessels, skin, breast and lung. Polymorphonuclear leucocyte elastase (PMN-E) is a neutral protease found in granulates of human polymorphonuclear leucocytes. The impact of local production of PMN-E, tumour progression and prognosis was analysed by Yamashita et al. (1996). The authors determined the production of immunoreative (ir)-PMN-E in tissue extracts from NSCLC tumours and elucidated the relationship between the tissue concentration and prognosis. In 40 specimens of NSCLC, the ir-PMN-E concentration was significantly higher in stage IIIB versus stages I, II and IIIA (Yamashita et al. 1996). Analyses of prognostic factors in a group of 101 patients with NSCLC demonstrated that those with a high ir-PMN-E had significantly shorter overall survival versus those with a low ir-PMN-E, a finding which was also significant in multivariate analysis. The results suggest that the local production of PMN-E may be involved in tumour invasion associated with the poor prognosis in patients with NSLCC.

1.2.3.4 Tumour Associated Antigenes

Blood-Group Carbohydrate Antigenes. Oncofetal antigenes are alterations of the normal classic blood group antigenes and are frequently expressed by tumour cells. The tumours often lose a major blood group A and B determinant, whereas precursor antigene H and H-related antigenes often increase reciprocally. The presence of blood group antigenes A, B and H was assessed immunohistochemically in tumour samples from 164 resected NSCLC patients by Lee et al. (1991). Survival of 28 patients with blood A or AB, who had primary tumours negative for blood group antigene A, was significantly shorter than that of 45 patients with antigene A-positive tumours ($P < 0.001$) and of the 93 patients with blood group B or 0 ($P = 0.002$). Expression of blood group antigene B or H in tumours cells did not correlate with survival. A multivariate analysis showed that the expression of blood group antigene A in tumour cells added significantly to the prediction of overall survival provided by other known prognostic factors among patients with blood type A or AB ($P = 0.004$). Thus, the expression of blood group antigene A in tumour cells sems to be an important favourable prognostic factor in NSCLC.

Miyake et al. (1992) evaluated the binding of the monoclonal antibody MIA-15-5, which defines H, Ley and Leb antigenes in a study of 149 lung cancer patients, 141 of whom had NSCLC. Survival was significantly worse for MIA-15-5 positive patients compared with MIA-15-5 negative patients and the difference was most pronounced in squamous cell carcinoma. Multivariate analysis indicated that among the variables tested MIA-15-5 positivity had the best correlation with 5-year mortality, followed by lymph node status (N-stage) and tumour size (T-stage).

CA 242. CA 242 is a tumour carbohydrate antigen which is present in serum. The prognostic impact has been evaluated in 102 NSCLC patients (Pujol et al. 1993). Patients with unresectable disease and elevated CA 242 had significantly (univariate testing) shorter survival than those with CA 242 <20 U/ml, but CA 242 was without prognostic information in patients with resectable disease. CA 242 was significantly related to the stage of disease, but was without prognostic impact in a multivariate analysis (Pujol et al. 1993).

Antigene 43-9F. Expression of antigene 43-9F, which is a tumour associated carbohydrate epitope, can be identified by a 43-9F monoclonal antibody. Battifora et al. evaluated 231 resected lung cancer patients of all cell types and observed a significant impact of antigene 43-9F on prognosis for patients with squamous cell carcinoma (Battifora et al.

1992). In multivariate analysis, 43-9 F staining was a significant independent predictor of survival.

1.2.3.5 Tumour Cell Proliferation

The proliferative fraction, as shown by analyses of DNA patterns in NSCLC, suggests that patients whose tumours have either a low proportion of cells in G-0 or G-1 phase or a high proliferative fraction have shorter survival, as discussed previously. Besides DNA patterns, other markers of proliferative activity have been examined as discussed below.

Ki-67 Proliferation Associated Nuclear Antigene. The proliferation associated Ki-67 nuclear antigene is a marker of the proliferative activity of NSCLC. Pence et al. (1992) investigated the utility of tumour proliferation index as a prognostic marker in 61 patients with NSCLC by measuring immunostaining for Ki-67 and DNA-ploidy. A significant survival advantage was observed for six patients with low proliferative activity and a multivariate analysis selected the proliferative activity as a significant survival predictor. In contrast, two subsequent studies by Giatromanolaki et al. (1996) and Harpole et al. (1996) did not observe prognostic independent information affiliated with the Ki-67 in multivariate analysis.

1.2.3.6 Other Biological Parameters

Monomeric Laminin Receptor (67 LR). The monomeric laminin receptor (67 LR) is associated with invasiveness and metastatization. Assessment of immunostaining for 67 LR was based on cellular membrane labelling in a study by Pastorino et al. (1997). The monomeric laminin receptor 67 LR in this study included 515 cases of pathologic stage I NSCLC without prognostic influence in multivariate analysis.

Motility-Related Protein 1 (MRP-1). Motility-related protein 1 (MRP-1)/CD-9 is a transmembrane glucoprotein closely associated with suppression cell motility and reduced metastatic potential of some tumour cells. NSCLC patients with low expression of MRP-1/CD-9, especially the adenocarcinoma type, have revealed a short overall survival. Higashiyama et al. (1997) investigated the expression by immunohistochemically staining in 132 patients with pulmonary adenocarcinoma undergoing potentially curative surgery. Of these patients, 44 (33%) showed reduced expression of MRP-1/CD-9 and an inverse association was observed between its expression and factors associated with tumour progression, such as nodal involvement ($P = 0.029$) or stage ($P = 0.028$). Patients with reduced expression of MRP-1/CD-9 showed significantly worse prognosis and in multivariate analysis immunohistochemical MRP-1/CD-9 expression level was an independent prognostic factor for disease free survival ($P = 0.021$), but not for overall survival (Higashiyama et al. 1997b).

1.3 Conclusions on Non-Small Cell Lung Cancer

Definite prognostic factors in complete resected NSCLC are performance status, stage, lymph node status (N), and perioperative blood transfusion, even though the latter variable may rather serve as an indicator of other yet undetermined variables of poor prognosis than being of influence by itself. Among non-resectable patients treated with chemotherapy with or without radiotherapy, definite prognostic variables predicting survival include performance status, gender, stage, division into limited and extensive disease, and pretreatment plasma-albumin level. For patients treated with radiotherapy alone, definite prognostic factors include performance status, age, gender, and weight loss.

Even with the use of the classical clinical variables mentioned above, a large variation in prognosis is observed. It is likely that this variation is due to the different biological properties of the tumour cells and accordingly, a large number of variables describing biological features of tumours have been evaluated in NSCLC patients. Most of these variables have been evaluated in relatively few trials and their current role as predictors of prognosis are as yet unclear. At present, changes in treatment policies or staging recommendations are not justified based on the studies reviewed. Future studies are warranted to document further the value of these variables to more accurately predict the prognosis of patients with NSCLC and to select the appropriate treatment option. Doing so will enable oncologists to make treatment decisions on a firmer basis than is currently possible, and more confirmatory investigations and prospective clinical trials are needed to verify the validity and reliability of the biological markers.

1.4 Prognostic Factors in Small Cell Lung Cancer

Every fifth to fourth lung cancer patient has small cell carcinoma (SCLC). This cell type differs biologically from the non-small cell types in several aspects. SCLC disseminates early and surgery is restricted to less than 5% of the patients. The TNM system (MOUNTAIN 1988) is not useful because more than 90% of the patients have stage III or IV disease. Instead, SCLC is staged as extensive or limited depending on whether or not the tumor has spread beyond one lung, excluding pleura but including regional mediastinal and supraclavicular lymph nodes. About 55%–60% of newly diagnosed patients have extensive stage disease. The principal treatment modality is chemotherapy, but in spite of intensive clinical research on treatment of this disease during the last $2^1/_2$ decades the prognosis remains sinister. Current chemotherapy plus chest irradiation in limited stage disease results in response rates of over 90% but 80% of the patients will nevertheless die from recurrent disease within the first 2 years from diagnosis and 5-year survival is a rare event seen in less than 5% of patients. Stage of disease is the principal pretreatment predictor of long-term survival. Thus, the probability of 5-year survival is three to four times higher in patients with limited disease than extensive stage disease (LASSEN et al. 1995; FUKUOKA et al. 1990). Other pretreatment clinical features and biochemical tests carry additional prognostic information, and algorithms based on such variables have proved useful to characterize survival estimates the first 2 years after initiation of treatment, which is the time interval where differences among treatment results are most apparent. Stratification based on performance status (PS) and serum lactate dehydrogenase (LDH) is widely used to reduce or to adjust for confounding evaluation of the treatment effect but international guidelines or a stratification system have not yet been established.

1.4.1 Importance of Prognostic Factors in Small Cell Lung Cancer

The aims of improving treatment results in small cell lung cancer has followed various strategies during the last 25 years such as alternation between non-cross resistant regimens, dose intensification, and various regimes of chest and brain irradiation. Many trials have evaluated efficacy of new drugs alone and in combination regimens. Pretreatment prognostic factors have been important for definition of inclusion criteria and for analysis of results.

In phase II trials prognostic factors support a standardized selection of patients. It could be preferable to exclude patients with high risk of early death, and to define a target population in the condition to tolerate intensive, potentially curative therapy, with good or with only modest chances for long term survival. Similarly, prognostic factors may be useful to characterize patients for whom a palliative regime would be most feasible.

The purpose of randomization in phase III trials is to obtain accidental and thus similar distributions of unknown prognostic patient characteristics in each treatment group. This intention is easily fulfilled if the trial includes 250–300 patients in each arm. Figures of this magnitude are normal in current trials, required to reduce the risk of type II error when differences in results between treatment arms are so modest as in small cell lung cancer. Previously, when trials typically included 100–150 patients in each arm it was regarded mandatory to stratify for important prognostic factors prior to randomization, often resulting in a complex system of closed envelopes when this technique was used (STAQUET and DALESIO 1984). With the current availability of computers and possibility for on-line randomization via telephone lines the envelope method has been replaced by the minimization method at many centres (TAVES 1974). Three or four important prognostic factors (or potentially influential factors such as treatment centre) are selected and allocation to one or the other treatment is performed to minimize imbalances (Table 1.4).

1.4.2 Clinical Prognostic Factors

The first recognized prognostic factors in small cell lung cancer were stage of disease and performance status. The impact of stage can be differentiated into influence of specific sites such as liver and bone marrow, and it can be semiquantitated according to number of sites (liver – bone marrow + distant lymph nodes, etc.) (IHDE et al. 1981), but none of these policies has been adopted in trials or in clinical routine. There may be several reasons why: the option of staging procedures varies from centre to centre, and influence of individual sites may depend on diagnostic procedure and therefore change over

Table 1.4. Allocation to treatment arm A or B by minimization procedure

Prognostic factor score	PS		P-sodium			NSE				Sum
	0	1	0	1		0	1	2	3	
Arm A	12	3	9	6		5	2	5	3	
Arm B	11	4	7	8		2	4	8	1	
New pt.		1		1	1					
Status if allocated to arm A	12	4	9	7		5	2	6	3	
Absolute difference (A–B)		0		1		2				3
Status if allocated to arm B	11	5	7	9		2	4	9	1	
Absolute difference (A–B)		2		3		4				9

Conclusion: The new patient no. 16 should be allocated to arm A.

time. The sum of metastatic sites depends on number and sensitivity of staging procedures. Furthermore, it seems dubious to equate the sum of for example pleural + cervical lymph node metastases with the sum of brain + liver metastases. The prognostic influence of performance status is independent of that of stage and of biochemical tests in multivariate analyses (Souhami et al. 1985; Østerlind and Andersen 1986). The PS characteristics may seem rough and prone to biased subjective assessments and this weakness may explain large variations from centre to centre. In two studies on aggregated data materials (Rawson and Peto 1990; Jørgensen et al. 1996), the proportions of patients in good PS varied between 7%–74% and 40%–87%, respectively. Within a joint group, however, variation can be much less. As an example the distribution on PS remained constant with time comparing data on 874 patients included in Copenhagen Lung Cancer Group protocols from 1973 to 1981 with data from 728 patients included in trials during 1981–1987: 18%, 46%, 19%, 12% and 5% vs 19%, 43%, 21%, 11%, 6%, respectively, scored to have PS 0, 1, 2, 3, or 4 according to the WHO scale (Who 1979). Death hazards related to PS changed, however, as reflected by a plot of the logarithm to median survival (in days) vs PS (Fig. 1.1). The original linear relationship was broken in the last period, where inclusion of *cis*-platin and etoposide resulted in more intensive regimens (Lassen et al. 1996).

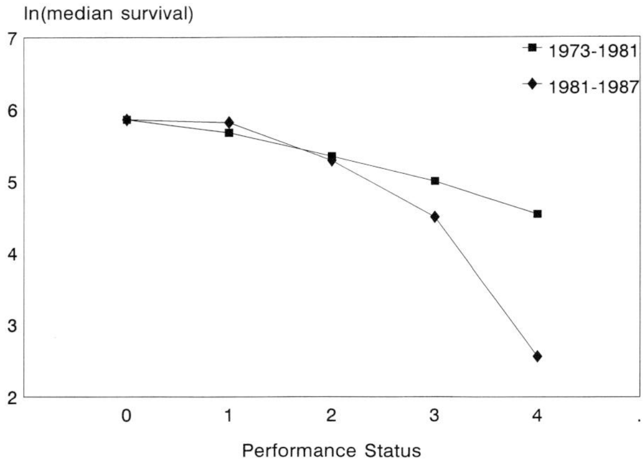

Fig. 1.1. Median survival values (logarithmically transformed) related to pretreatment performance status in 874 patients included in treatment trials 1973 to 1981 and in 728 patients included in trials 1981 to 1987. The linearity observed in the early era reflects a simple proportionality between PS and death hazard. In the recent era the prognostic impact of PS >2 was worse than expected

The role of biochemical tests, routinely obtained at diagnosing and pretreatment staging, has been evaluated in a number of multivariable analyses (Table 1.5) (Souhami et al. 1985; Østerlind and Andersen 1986; Cerny et al. 1987; Vincent et al. 1987; Spiegelman et al. 1989; Dearing et al. 1990; Albain et al. 1990; Allan et al. 1990; Sagman et al. 1991b). Increased values of serum LDH and serum alkaline phosphatase are associated with an inferior prognosis although only one of the two remains when both are included in multivariable analyses. Serum LDH is increased in 55%–60% of newly diagnosed patients compared to only 40% having abnormal values of serum alkaline phosphatase. Values of alkaline phosphatase and LDH are correlated and LDH is usually the most influential when both are included in a Cox analysis. Finally, LDH primarily seems to be a tumour marker (Sagman et al. 1991a) while increased serum alkaline phosphatase more reflects bone and liver metastases. Other laboratory values with prognostic influence include hyponatremia, anemia, hypoalbuminemia, hypouricemia, and low serum bicarbonate (Table 1.5). Hyponatremia is often caused by ectopic inappropriate secretion of antidiuretic hormone (SIADH) (List et al. 1986) and although SIADH is not a significant prognostic factor in univariate analysis the adverse influence of hyponatremia has been proven in multivariate analysis (Østerlind and Andersen 1986;

Table 1.5. Clinical prognostic factors: results from multivariate analyses 1985–1991

Factor	Author No of pts.	So 371	O 874	C 407	V 333	Sp 1521	D 411	Alb 2580	All 411	Sa 614
Performance status		s	s	s	s	s	s	s	s	s
Extensive stage		s	s	s	s	s	s	s	s	s
LDH or alkaline phosphatase		s	s	s	ns	?	s	s	s	s
Hyponatraemia		s	s	s	ns	?	ns	?	ns	ns
Male gender		ns	s	ns	ns	s	s	s	ns	ns

s, significant influence; ns, no significant influence; ?, not investigated. So, Souhami et al. 1985; O, Østerlind et al. 1986; C, Cerny et al. 1987; V, Vincent et al. 1987; Sp, Spiegelman et al. 1989; D, Dearing et al. 1990; Alb, Albain et al. 1990; All, Allan et al. 1990; Sa, Sagman et al. 1991a.

Table 1.6. Prognostic factors of early (0–6 months) and late (6–24 months) survival after initiation of chemotherapy (From Rawson and Peto 1990)

Period variable	0–6 months 1960 pts.	6–24 months 1310 pts.
Performance status	s	s
Extensive stage	s	s
Alkaline phosphatase	s	s/nm
Hyponatraemia	s/nm	s

All four variables had a statistically significant influence on survival in both periods.
s, significant (Cox analysis); nm, not mandatory for an optimal separation of patients into three equally sized prognostic strata.

Rawson and Peto 1990). In a large, cumulative series (Rawson and Peto 1990), hyponatremia proved a steady influence with little change in risk ratio from the initial 6 months to the subsequent 6–24 months after initiation of chemotherapy compared to influence of PS, stage and alkaline phosphates, which decreased relatively more with time (Table 1.6). Pretreatment hyponatremia also has negative influence on the duration of complete remission (Østerlind et al. 1987), but the attribute has no significant influence on chances of long term survival in benchmark analyses (Lassen et al. 1995).

Based on a combination of performance status and two or more laboratory tests it is possible to establish algorithms for prognostic stratification and it was once suggested that stratification by laboratory parameters could replace conventional staging (Souhami et al. 1985). A policy without staging would be cheaper, faster and less inconvenient for the patient, but more than 10 years after the proposal staging is still mandatory in trials on SCLC. The reason is that treatment in limited disease includes chest irradiation at most centres, and irradiation of primary tumour has never proved advantageous in patients with extensive stage disease.

The dual role of stage as an important prognostic factor and as criterion for a treatment policy with or without radiotherapy are intriguing conclusions in many prognostic factor studies. The enigma could be handled by making separate statistical analyses for each stage or by stratification for stage in the Cox model (Østerlind and Andersen 1986). In another statistical method: the recursive partitioning and amalgamation method (RECPAM) (Ciampi et al. 1988), stage is often responsible for the first partition or split because it is one of the most influential factors. The subsequent partitions then reflect the hierarchy of prognostic factors in limited and extensive stage, respectively (Albain et al. 1990; Sagman et al. 1991b). At amalgamation, however, patients from both stages may be mixed again. In a Canadian study (Sagman et al. 1991b), the two intermediate of four prognostic groups thus included patients from both stages. A similar mixture was seen in our own series when we stratified patients according to a simple algorithm in which performance status >1, abnormal LDH and extensive disease each counted for one point of a prognostic index. This simple algorithm resulted in an even distribution of patients in different prognostic strata and in a good separation of survival curves (Fig. 1.2) but stratum II included 33% extensive stage patients and stratum III 16% limited stage patients.

Another problem related to stage as prognostic factor is stage migration, caused by a downgrading of patients from limited to extensive stage disease after introduction of new, more sensitive imaging techniques (Feinstein et al. 1985). The result is apparently improved survival figures in both disease stages. Influence from stage migration must be considered when results from different centres are compared, in reviews of historical data and in meta-

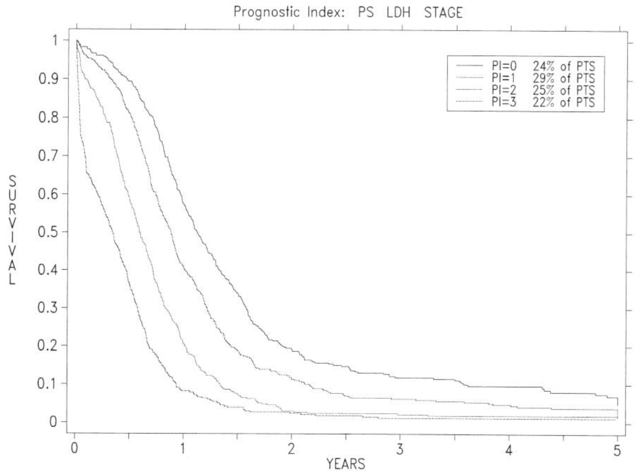

Fig. 1.2. Survival curves for 1494 patients with SCLC stratified after a prognostic index, PI = P + L + S, where P = 0 if PS < 2, P + 1 if PS ≥ 2, L = 0 if serum LDH is normal, L = 1 if LDH is increased, and S = 0 if limited stage, S = 1 if extensive stage. PI thus takes values from 0 to 3

analyses, while the phenomenon only plays a minor role in trials, where staging procedures are kept unchanged. In our own series of patients included in treatment trials from 1973 to 1981 and 1981 to 1987, respectively, the proportion of limited disease patients decreased from 51% to 46%, while the median survival increased from 324 days to 395 days. Median survival in extensive stage disease remained unchanged, maybe because poor risk patients in the extensive stage category did not tolerate the new treatment regimes so well (Fig. 1.1).

Early or Toxic Death. Some prognostic factors may be predictors of increased risk of early or toxic death, which may help to exclude susceptible patients from intensive treatment protocols. Performance status is the strongest predictive factor, followed by increased alkaline phosphatase and clinical hepatomegaly (Radford et al. 1993; Morittu et al. 1989). Age less than 50 years significantly reduces the risk of early death (Morittu et al. 1989).

Long-Term Survival. Factors related to long-term survival can be investigated in various ways. Rawson and Peto (1990) divided the time after initiation of therapy into periods: 0–6 months, 6–24 months, and >24 months. Stage of disease, performance status, alkaline phosphatase and hyponatraemia all had a significant influence on survival but the influence decreased with time and none of the variables had a significant impact in the late period >24 months. Stage of disease was the principal prognostic factor beyond 6 months. Another strategy focuses on survival at certain benchmarks such as 18 months (Østerlind et al. 1986) or 5 years (Lassen et al. 1995; Jacoulet et al. 1997). With only 8% and 3.5% of the patients alive at the two bench marks, respectively, the "signal" is weak and regression analysis will therefore only point out one or two significant predictive factors. Stage of disease is clearly the most important factor. High pretreatment serum LDH and bone marrow metastases are other negative features and males have in some series inferior chances compared to those of females (Johnson et al. 1988).

1.4.3 Tumour Markers, Growth Factors and Other Cancer Related Serum Compounds

The diagnosis of small cell lung cancer is primarily based on small bronchoscopic biopsies. These specimens are often not large enough and not sufficiently representative for the entire tumour to enable meaningful investigations of tumour cell characteristics including genetic markers such as the *myc* family oncogene, which is amplified in about 10% of untreated SCLC tumors (Johnson et al. 1987). Expression of the epithelial antigen MBr1 was a negative prognostic marker in a series of 161 patients investigated by Martignone et al. (1993), but the clinical importance is uncertain.

Many serum markers and other compounds with a direct or only indirect relationship to the cancer have been investigated during the last decade (Table 1.7) (Akoun et al. 1985; Jaques et al. 1988; Jørgensen et al. 1988; Gronowitz et al. 1990; Harding et al. 1990; van der Gaast et al. 1991; Johnson et al. 1993; Szturmowicz et al. 1993; Drivsholm et al. 1994; Vangsted et al. 1994a,b; Pujol et al. 1996; Rosenfeld et al. 1997). The prognostic influence of many of these compounds has been investigated in univariate analyses and they may not have a significant influence in multivariable analysis. Thus, serum values of NSE, TK, TPA, CK-BB and LDH are all correlated to stage of disease and pairwise correlated to each other (Gronowitz et al. 1990; Johnson et al. 1993). As a consequense of these correlations only TPA – plus age, performance status and gender sex – remained as a significant prognostic factor in a Cox analysis including TK, NSE, TPA, CEA, and LDH (Gronowitz et al. 1990). Similarly, only NSE, PS and plasma albumin were left in the final Cox model (Johnson et al. 1993) while chromogranin A, LDH and hyponatraemia were excluded. The relationship be-

Table 1.7. Tumour markers with influence on survival in small cell lung cancer

Markers	Significant impact references	No significant impact
Neuron specific enolase (NSE)	Ak Ja_1 Jø Ha Jo Sz Dr	Gr Ga
Creatinine kinase BB (CK-BB)	Ja_1	
Thymidine kinase (TK)	Ga	Ja_1
Tissue polypeptide antigen (TPA)	Gr Pu	Ga
Chromogranin A (CgA)	Dr	Jo
Pro-gastrin-releasing-peptide (proGRP)	Dr	
Carcinoembryonic antigen (CEA)	Ja_1	Jø Gr Jo
Neural cell adhesion molecule (NCAM)	Ja_2	Va
Ganglioside fucosyl-GM_1 ($FucGM_1$)		Va
Cytokeratin fragment (CYFRA 21-1)	Pu	
Serum anti-p53 antibodies		Ro

Ak, Akoun et al. 1985: 43 pts.; Ja_1, Jaques et al. 1988: 195 pts.; Ja_2, Jaques 1993: 221 pts.; Jø, Jørgensen et al. 1988: 85 pts.; Gr, Gronowitz et al. 1990: 125 pts.; Ha, Harding et al. 1990: 37 pts.; Ga, van der Gaast et al. 1991: 69 pts.; Jo, Johnson et al. 1993: 159 pts.; Sz, Szturmowicz et al. 1993: 92 pts.; Dr, Drivsholm et al. 1994: 132 pts.; Va, Vangsted et al. 1994a,b: 96 pts.; 112 pts.; Pu, Pujol et al. 1996: 91 pts.; Ro, Rosenfeld et al. 1997: 170 pts.

Table 1.8 Distribution and survival characteristics of 500 patients with SCLC[a] categorized according to prognostic indices based on stage (S), performance status (P) and NSE or LDH

Prognostic index	N	Pct.	Median survival (days)	Early death (< day 30)	2 year survival
Score PI_{NSE}					
0	44	9%	468	0%	19%
1–2	168	34%	366	0%	16%
3–6	221	44%	252	11%	5%
7	67	13%	126	21%	2%
Score PI_{LDH}					
0	113	23%	428	0%	16%
1	151	30%	333	4%	12%
2	128	25%	258	7%	7%
3	108	22%	145	21%	1%

Algorithms: $PI_{NSE} = S + 2 \cdot P + NSE$; $PI_{LDH} = S + P + LDH$; Scoring: S = 0 (stage: limited), S = 1 (stage: extensive); P = 0 (PS < 2), P + 1 (PS ≥ 2); NSE = 0 (≤12.5 µg/l); NSE = 1 (12.5–25 µg/l); NSE = 2 (25–50 µg/l NSE = 3 (50–75 µg/l); NSE = 4 (>75 µg/l); LDH = 0 (normal); LDH = 1 (increased).
[a] Data from cumulative series (Jørgensen et al. 1996).

tween NSE and LDH has been investigated in a series from one institution (Jørgensen et al. 1988) and in a large multi-institutional series including 560 patients (Jøgensen et al. 1996). NSE was increased (>12.5 µg/l) in 81% of the patients compared to 54% for LDH. LDH could be excluded, resulting in a model of NSE, PS and stage of disease. Drivsholm et al. (1994) investigated NSE and CgA plus the growth factor pro-GRP and found significant prognostic impact of all three in a Cox analysis while LDH, alkaline phosphatase and plasma sodium were excluded. These studies prove that NSE is a strong prognostic factor and suggest that prognostic investigations of new tests should include NSE plus LDH and other important clinical factors.

Of these tumor markers and growth factors, serum NSE is the only well documented marker, which has been the way through early exploratory studies followed by larger studies fulfilling most of the guidelines Simon and Altman recently (1994) set up for phase III prognostic factor studies. NSE assays have been commercially available for nearly a decade and NSE is measured at staging in many centres but NSE has, nevertheless, not yet found a definitive place in pretreatment staging of SCLC. NSE cannot be used as a surrogate for staging (Quoix et al. 1993). Prognostic stratification based on NSE, stage and performance status may not have important clinical advantages compared to an algorithm based on LDH plus stage and PS although the extremes, the subgroups of long-term survival and early death, respectively, may be better separated (Table 1.8). Realizing that treatment trials in SCLC will continue to be carried out separately for limited and extensive stage disease, it might be worthwhile to clarify the role of NSE and other factors in prognostic systems for each stage.

Increasing research in the metastatic process has put focus on compounds involved in cell adhesion, proteolysis and vascularization. Again research in SCLC is hampered by the lack of surgical specimens. Plasma levels of plasmin-α_2-plasmin inhibitor (TAGUCHI et al. 1996) and of plasma D-dimer (TAGUCHI et al. 1997) – attributes of activated fibrinolysis – have a negative influence on prognosis, independent of stage of disease and performance status. Interactions between tumour and the immune system in the patient may have a relationship to the prognosis. Thus, increased values of soluble interleukin-2 receptors are found in serum from patients with SCLC (SARANDAKOU et al. 1993). The values are correlated to NSE measured in the same sample. Interleukin-2 is secreted by white blood cells. The secretion is decreased in patients with SCLC, possibly mediated by TGFβ1 secreted by the tumour cells, and low IL-2 activity is associated with an inferior prognosis (FISCHER et al. 1997). The test requires incubation of living blood cells for 48 h, which is less appropriate for routine use.

1.4.4 Prognostic Factor Studies

From a clinical point of view the majority of these new compounds should not be regarded as new prognostic factors. These investigations should rather be regarded as human model testing of hypotheses from the laboratory, where these compounds or cellular features are intensively investigated on cell lines and on heterotransplanted tumours. Unfortunately, the clinical investigations are often suboptimal due to lack of data on principal prognostic factors such as stage, performance status, LDH and plasma sodium. Many new factors will not have a statistically significant influence on survival in a multivariable analysis including these basic variables, in which case it may be tempting to omit the Cox analysis. Other weaknesses are lack of a clear idea or hypothesis about why the new factor should have an impact on survival, lack of statistical dimensioning and of selection criteria for inclusion of patients. Laboratories build up banks of tissue specimens and plasma samples, forgetting the importance of good cooperation with the clinicians who generate the clinical data, which should be sampled as systematic and standardized as biological specimens.

The plethora of prognostic factor studies and the lack of standards have prompted the American Joint Committee on Cancer to propose criteria for evaluating putative prognostic factors (BURKE and HENSON 1993). Thus, a prognostic factor should be significant, independent and clinically important. In general, criteria for a proposed prognostic system should include the TNM criteria, i.e., limited vs extensive stage in the case of SCLC. A further 12 criteria are listed of which the first is that the test should be easy for the physician to use. Without effective therapy, prognostic information is of little value, the committee has noted. In the treatment of small cell lung cancer no new prognostic factors are necessary until significant progress in therapy is a reality.

References

Akoun GM, Scarna HM, Milleron BJ, Bénichou MP, Herman DP (1985) Serum neuron-specific enolase. A marker for disease extent and response to therapy for small-cell lung cancer. Chest 87:39–43

Alama A, Constantini M, Repetto L et al (1990) Thymidine labelling index as prognostic factor in resected non-small cell lung cancer. Eur J Cancer 26:622–625

Albain KS, Crowley JJ, LeBlanc M, Livingston RB (1990) Determinants of improved outcome in small-cell lung cancer: an analysis of the 2580-patient Southwest Oncology Group data base. J Clin Oncol 8:1563–1574

Albain KS, Crowley JJ, LeBlanne M, Livingston RB (1991) Survival determinants in extensive-stage non-small-cell lung cancer: the Southwest Oncology Group experience. J Clin Oncol 9:1618–1626

Allan SG, Stewart ME, Love S, Cornbleet MA, Smyth JF, Leonard CF (1990) Prognosis at presentation of small cell carcinoma of the lung. Eur J Cancer 26:703–705

Apolinario RM, van der Valk P, de Jong JS (1997) Prognostic value of the expression of p53, *bcl*-2 and *bax* oncoproteins, neovascularization in patients with radically resected non-small-cell lung cancer. J Clin Oncol 15:2456–2466

Battifora H, Sorensen HR, Mehta P et al (1992) Tumor-associated antigen 43-9F is of prognostic value in squamous cell carcinoma of the lung. Cancer 70:1867–1872

Berendsen HH, de Leij L, Poppema S et al (1989) Clinical characterization of non-small-cell lung cancer tumors showing neuroendocrine differentiation features. J Clin Oncol 7:1614–1620

Bonomi P, Gale M, Rowland K et al (1991) Pre-treatment prognostic factors in stage II non-small cell lung cancer patients receiving combined modality treatment. Int J Radiat Oncol Biol Phys 20:247–252

Buccheri G, Ferrigno D, Vola F (1993) Carcinomembryonic antigen (CEA) tissue polypeptide antigen (TPA) and other prognostic indicators in squamoid cell lung cancer. Lung Cancer 10:21–33

Buhr J, Berghaeuser KH, Gonner S et al (1997) The prognostic significance of tumor cell detection in intraoperative pleural lavage and lung tissue cultures for patients with lung cancer. J Thorac Cardiovasc Surg 113:683–690

Burke HB, Henson DE (1993) Criteria for prognostic factors and for an enhanced prognostic system. Cancer 72: 3131–3135
Cangemi V, Volpino P, D'Andrea N et al (1996) Lung cancer surgery in elderly patients. Tumori 82:237–241
Carles J, Ariza A, Rosell R et al (1996) Prognostic implications of P-glycoprotein, epidermal growth factor receptor and transforming growth factor alpha: immunohistochemical expression in non-small cell lung cancer. Oncol Rep 3: 787–791
Carney DN (1991) Lung cancer biology. Curr Opin Oncol 1991 3:288–296
Cerny T, Blair V, Anderson H, Bramwell V, Thatcher N (1987) Pretreatment prognostic factors and scoring system in 407 small-cell lung cancer patients. Int J Cancer 39:146–149
Chastang C, Lebeau B, Charpak Y, Decroix G (1985) Prognostic factors from a randomized clinical trial in resected lung cancer. Stat Med 4:279–285
Chiba I, Takahashi T, Nau MM et al (1990) Mutations in the p53 gene are frequent in primary, resected non-small cell lung cancer. Oncogenes 5:1603–1610
Ciampi A, Lawless JF, McKinney SM, Singhal K (1988) Regression and recursive partition strategies in the analysis of medical survival data. J Clin Epidemiol 41:737–748
Cox DR (1972) Regression models and life-tables. JR Stat Soc 34:187–220
Dalquen P, Sauter G, Torhorst J et al (1996) Nuclear p53 overexpression is an independent prognostic parameter in node-negative non-small cell lung carcinoma. J Pathol 178:53–58
Dearing MP, Steinberg SM, Phelps R, Anderson MJ, Mulshine JL, Ihde DC (1990) Outcome of patients with small-cell lung cancer: effect of changes in staging procedures and imaging technology on prognostic factors over 14 years. J Clin Oncol 6:1042–1049
Delaurier J, Brisson J, Cartier R et al (1989) Carcinoma of the lung. Evaluation of satellite nodules as a factor influencing prognosis after resection. J Thorac Cardiovasc Surg 97:504–512
Diez M, Torres A, Ortega L et al (1993) Value of serum neuron-specific enolase in non-small cell lung cancer. Oncology 50:127–131
Dosaka-Akita H, Hu SX, Fujino M et al (1997) Altered retinoblastoma protein expression in non-small cell lung cancer: its synergistic effects with altered ras and p53 protein status on prognosis. Cancer 79:1329–1337
Drivsholm L, Østerlind K, Holst J (1994) Neuron specific enolase (NSE), pro-gastrin-releasing peptide (proGRP) and chromogranin A (chromA) are significant prognostic factors in small cell lung cancer (SCLC). Lung Cancer 11:77
Ebina M, Steinberg S, Mulshine J, Linnoila I (1994) Relationship of p53 overexpression and upregulation of proliferating cell nuclear antigen with the clinical course of non-small cell lung cancer. Cancer Res 54:2496–2503
Einhorn LE, Loehrer PJ, Williams SD et al (1986) Random prospective study of vindesine versus vendesine plus high-dose cisplatin versus vendesine plus cisplatin plus mitomycin C in advanced non-small-cell lung cancer. J Clin Oncol 4:1037–1043
Espinosa E, Feliu J, Zamora P et al (1995) Serum albumin and other prognostic factors related to response and survival in patients with advanced non-small cell lung cancer. Lung Cancer 12:67–76
Esposito V, Baldi A, De Luca et al (1997) Prognostic value of p53 in non-small cell lung cancer: relationships with proliferating cell nuclear antigen and cigarette smoking. Hum Pathol 28:233–237
Evans WK, Nixon DW, Daly JM et al (1987) A randomized study of oral nutritional support versus ad lib nutritional intake during chemotherapy for advanced colorectal and non-small cell lung cancer. J Clin Oncol 5:113–124
Feinstein AR, Sosin DM, Wells CK (1985) The Will Rogers phenomenon. Stage migration and new diagnostic techniques as a source of misleading statistics for survival in cancer. N Engl J Med 312:1604–1608
Feld R, Abratt R, Graziano S et al (1997) Pretreatment minimal staging and prognostic factors for non-small cell lung cancer. Lung Cancer 17:3–10
Finkelstein DM, Ettinger DS, Ruckdeschel JC (1986) Long-term survivors in metastatic non-small cell lung cancer: an Eastern Cooperative Oncology Group study. J Clin Oncol 4:702–709
Fischer JR, Schindel M, Bülzebruck H, Lahm H, Krammer PH, Drings P (1997) Decrease of interleukin-2 secretion is a new independent prognostic factor associated with poor survival in patients with small-cell lung cancer. Ann Oncol 8:57–461
Fontanini G, Macchiarini P, Pepe S et al (1992) The expression of profilerating cell nuclear antigen in paraffin sections of peripheral, node-negative non-small cell lung cancer. Cancer 70:1520–1527
Fujino M, Dosaka-Akita H, Harada M et al (1995) Prognostic significance of p53 and ras p21 expression in non-small cell lung cancer. Cancer 76:2457–2463
Fukuoka M, Masuda N, Matsui K, Makise Y, Takada M, Negoro S, Sakai N, Kusuncki Y, Kudoh S, Ryu S, Takifuji N (1990) Combination chemotherapy with or without radiation therapy in small cell lung cancer. An analysis of a 5-year follow-up. Cancer 65:1678–1684
Gail MH, Eagan RT, Feld R et al (1984) Prognostic factors in patients with resected stage I non-small cell lung cancer. A report from the Lung Cancer Study Group. Cancer 54:1803–1813
Gasinska A, Kolodziejski L, Biesaga B (1997) Tumour cell kinetics as prognostic factor in surgically-treated-non-small cell lung cancer. Lung Cancer 18:159–170
Giatromanolaki A, Konkourakist M, O'Byrnet K et al (1996) Prognostic value of angiogenesis in operable non-small cell lung cancer. J Pathol 179:80–88
Goto I, Yoneda S, Yamamoto M, Kawajiri K (1996) Prognostic significance of germ line polymorphisms of the CYP1A1 and glutathione S-transferase genes in patients with non-small cell lung cancer. Cancer Res 56:3725–3730
Graham MV, Geitz LM, Bychardt R et al (1992) Comparison of prognostic factors and survival among black patients and white patients treated with irradiation for non-small-cell lung cancer. J Natl Cancer Inst 84:1731–1735
Graziano S (1997) Non-small cell lung cancer: clinical value of new biological predictors. Lung Cancer 17:37–58
Graziano SL, Mazid R, Newman N et al (1989) The use of neuroendocrine immunoperoxidase markers to predict chemotherapy response in patients with non-small-cell lung cancer. J Clin Oncol 7:1398–1406
Gronowitz JS, Bergström R, Nôu E, Påhlman S, Brodin O, Nilsson S, Källander, CFR (1990) Clinical and serologic markers of stage and prognosis in small cell lung cancer. A multivariate analysis. Cancer 66:722–732
Hannisdal E, Engan T (1991) Blood analyses and survival in symptom- and survey-detected lung cancer patients. J Intern Med 229:337–341
Harada M, Dosaka-Akita H, Miyamoto H, Kuzumaki N, Kawakami Y (1992) Prognostic significance of the expression of ras oncogene product in non-small cell lung cancer. Cancer 69:72–77

Harding M, McAllister J, Hulks G, Vernon D, Monie R, Paul J, Kaye SB (1990) Neurone specific enolase (NSE) in small cell lung cancer: a tumour marker of prognostic significance? Br J Cancer 61:605–607

Harpole DH Jr, Herndon JE, Young WG Jr et al (1995) Stage I non-small cell lung cancer: a multivariate analysis of treatment methods and patterns of recurrence. Cancer 76: 787–796

Harpole DH Jr, Richards WG, Herndon JE II, Sugarbaker DJ (1996) Angionesis and molecular biologic substaging in patients with stage I non-small cell lung cancer. Ann Thoracic Surg 61:1470–1476

Hespanhol V, Queiroga H, Magalhaes A et al (1995) Survival predictors in advanced non-small cell lung cancer. Lung Cancer 13:253–267

Higashiyama M, Doi O, Kodama K et al (1997a) Bcl-2 oncoprotein in surgically resected non-small cell lung cancer: possibly favorable prognostic factor in association with low incidence of distant metastasis. J Surg Oncol 64:48–54

Higashiyama M, Doi O, Kodama K et al (1997b) Immunohistochemically detected expression of motility-related protein-1 (MRP-1/CD9) in lung adenocarcinoma and its relation to prognosis. Int J Cancer 74:205–211

Hilsenbeck SG, Raub WA Jr, Sridhar KS (1993) Prognostic factors in lung cancer based on multivariate analysis. Am J Clin Oncol 16:301–309

Horio Y, Takahashi T, Kuroishi T et al (1993) Prognostic significance of p53 mutations and 3p deletions in primary resected non-small cell lung cancer. Cancer Res 53:1–4

Ihde DC, Makuch RW, Carney DN, Bunn PA, Cohen MH, Matthews MJ, Minna JD (1981) Prognostic implications of stage of disease and sites of metastases in patients with small cell carcinoma of the lung treated with intensive combination chemotherapy. Am Rev Respir Dis 123: 500–507

Ischinose Y, Hara N, Ohta M et al (1993) Is T factor of the TNM staging system a predominant prognostic factor in pathologic stage I non-small-cell lung cancer? J Thorac Cardiovasc Surg 106:90–94

Ischinose Y, Yano T, Asoh H et al (1995) Prognostic factors obtained by pathologic examination in completely resected non-small-cell lung cancer. J Thorac Cardiovasc Surg 110:601–605

Isobe H, Miyamoto H, Shimizi T et al (1990) Prognostic and therapeutic significance of the flow cytometric nuclear DNA content in non-small cell lung cancer. Cancer 65:1391–1395

Jacoulet P, Depierre A, Moro D, Rivière A, Milleron B, Quoix E, Ranfaing E, Anthoine D, Lafitte JJ, Lebeau B, Kleisbauer JP, Massin F, Fournel P, Zaegel M, Leclerc JP, Garnier G, Brambilla E, Capron F (1997) Long-term survivors of small-cell lung cancer (SCLC): a French multicenter study. Ann Oncol 8:1009–1014

Jaques GJ, Bepler G, Holle R, Wolf M (1988) Prognostic value of pretreatment carcinoembryonic antigen, neuron-s pecific enolase, and creatine kinase-BB levels in sera of patients with small cell lung cancer. Cancer 62:125–134

Jaques GJ, Auerbach B, Pritsch M, Wolf M, Madrey N, Havemann K (1993) Evaluation of Serum neural cell adhesion molecule as a new tumor marker in small cell lung cancer. Cancer 72:418–425

Jeremic B, Shibamoto Y (1996) Effect of interfraction interval in hyperfractionated radiotherapy with or without concurrent chemotherapy for stage III non-small cell lung cancer. Int J Radiat Oncol Biol Phys 34:303–308

Johnson B, Steinberg SM, Phelps R, Edison M, Veach SR, Ihde D (1988) Female patients with small cell lung cancer live longer than male patients. Am J Med 85:194–196

Johnson BE, Ihde DC, Makuch RW (1987) myc family oncogene amplification in tumor cell lines established from small cell lung cancer patients and its relationship to clinical status and course. J Clin Invest 79:1629–1634

Johnson PWM, Joel SP, Love S, Butcher M, Pandian MR, Squires L, Wrigley PFM, Slevin ML (1993) Tumour markers for prediction of survival and monitoring of remission in small cell lung cancer. Br J Cancer 67:760–766

Jørgensen LGM, Østerlind K, Hansen HH, Cooper EH (1988) The prognostic influence of serum neuron specific enolase in small cell lung cancer. Br J Cancer 58:805–807

Jørgensen LGM, Østerlind K, Genollá J, Gomm SA, Hernández JR, Johnson PWM, Løber J, Splinter TAW, Szturmowicz M (1996) Serum neuron-specific nolase (S-NSE) and the prognosis in small-cell lung cancer (SCLC): a combined multivariable analysis on data from nine centres. Br J Cancer 74:463–467

Kanters S, Lammers J-W, Voest E (1995) Molecular and biological factors in the prognosis of non-small cell lung cancer. Eur Respir J 8:1389–1397

Kawahara M, Furuse K, Kodama N et al (1991) A randomized study of cisplatin versus cisplatin plus vindesine for non-small cell lung carcinoma. Cancer 68:714–719

Kawashimi K, Nomura S, Hirai H et al (1992) Correlation of L-myc RFLP with metastasis, prognosis, and multiple cancer in lung cancer patients. Int J Cancer 50:557–561

Kern JA, Schwartz DA, Nordberg JE et al (1990) p185neu expression in human lung adenocarcinoma predicts shortened survival. Cancer Res 50:5184–5191

Kessler R, Gasser B, Massard G et al (1996) Blood vessel invasion is a major prognostic factor in resected non-small cell lung cancer. Ann Thorac Surg 62:1489–1493

Kim YC, Park KO, Kim HJ et al (1996) DNA ploidy and proliferative activity in bcl-2 expressed non-small cell lung cancer. Kor J Int Med 11:101–107

Kishimoto Y, Murakami Y, Shiraishi M, Hayakhi K, Sekia T (1992) Aberrations of the p53 tumor suppressor gene in human non-small cell carcinomas of the lung. Cancer Res 52:4799–4804

Kojima A, Shinkaii T, Eguchi K et al (1991) Analysis of three-year survivors among patients with advanced inoperable non-small cell lung cancer. Jpn Clin Oncol 21:276–281

Kolodziejski L, Niezabitowski A, Gasinska A (1997) Clinical and flow cytometric prognostic factors in surgically treated squamous cell lung cancer. Lung Cancer 16:173–182

Koukourakis MI, Giatromanolaki A, O'Byrne KJ et al (1997) Platelet-derived endothelial cell growth factor expression correlates with tumour angiogenesis and prognosis in non-small-cell lung cancer. Br J Cancer 75:477–481

Lassen U, Østerlind K, Hansen M, Dombernowsky P, Bergman B, Hansen HH (1995) Long-term survival in small-cell lung cancer: posttreatment characteristics in patients surviving 5 to 18+ years – an analysis of 1714 consecutive patients. J Clin Oncol 13:1215–1220

Lassen U, Kristjansen PEG, Østerlind K, Bergman B, Sigsgaard TC, Hirsch FR, Hansen M, Dombernowsky P, Hansen HH (1996) Superiority of cisplatin or carboplatin in combination with teniposide and vincristine in the induction chemotherapy of small-cell lung cancer. A randomized trial with 5 years follow up. Ann Oncol 7: 365–371

Lee JB, Ro JY, Sahin AA et al (1991) Expression of blood-group antigen. A – a favorable prognostic factor in non-small-cell lung cancer. N Engl J Med 324:1084–1090

Lee JS, Yoon A, Kalapurkal SK et al (1995) Expression of p53 oncoprotein in non-small-cell lung cancer: a favorable prognostic factor. J Clin Oncol 13:1893–1903

Liewald F, Hatz R, Storck M et al (1992) Prognostic value of deoxyribonucleic acid aneuploidy in primary non-small-cell lung carcinomas and their metastases. J Thorac Cardiovasc Surg 104:1476–1482

Linnoila I (1990) Pathology of non-small cell lung cancer. New diagnostic appoaches. Hematol Oncol North Am 4: 1027–1051

Linnoila RI, Jensen S, Steinberg S et al (1989) Neuroendocrine differentiation in non-small cell lung cancer correlates with favorable response to chemotherapy (abstract). Proc Am Soc Clin Oncol 8:248

Lipford HH, Sears DL, Eggleston JC, More CW, Littlemore KD, Baker RR (1984) Prognostic factors in surgically resected limited-stage, non-small cell carcinoma of the lung. Am J Surg Pathol 8:357–365

List AF, Hainsworth JD, Davis BW, Hande KR, Greco FA, Johnson DH (1986) The syndrome of inappropriate secretion of antidiuretic hormone (SIADH) in small-cell lung cancer. J Clin Oncol 4:1191–1198

Little AG, WU H-S, Ferguson MK et al (1990) Perioperative blood transfusion adversely affects prognosis of patients with stage I non-small-cell lung cancer. Am J Surg 160: 630–632

Macchiarini P, Fontanini G, Hardin JM, Pingitore R, Angeletti CA (1992) Most peripheral, node-negative, non-small-cell lung cancers have low proliferative rates and no intratumoral and peritumoral blood and lymphatic vessel invasion. J Thorac Cardiovasc Surg 104:892–899

Martignone S, Menard S, Bedini A, Paccagnella A, Fasolato S, Veggian R, Colnaghi MI (1993) Study of the expression and function of the tumour-associated antigen CaMBr1 in small cell lung carcinomas. Eur J Cancer 29A:2020–2025

Matsumoto H, Muramatsu T, Shimazu H (1992) Carbohydrate profiles shown by a lectin and a monoclonal antibody correlate with metastatic potential and prognosis of human lung carcinomas. Cancer 6:2084–2090

McLaren R, Kuzu I, Dunnill M, Harris A, Lane D, Catter KC (1992) The relationship of p53 immunostaining to survival in carcinoma of the lung. Br J Cancer 66:735–738

Miller TP, Chen TT, Coltman CA et al (1986) Effect of alternating combination chemotherapy on survival of ambulatory patients with metastatic large-cell and adenocarcinoma of the lung. A Southwest Oncology Group study J Clin Oncol 4:502–508

Mitsudomi T, Steinberg SM, Oie HK et al (1991) ras Gene mutations in non-small cell lung cancers are associated with shortened survival irrespective of treatment intent. Cancer Res 51:4999–5002

Mitsudomi T, Steinberg SM, Nau MM et al (1992) p53 Gene mutations in non-small cell lung cancer cell lines and their correlation with the presence of ras mutations and clinical features. Oncogene 7:171–180

Mitsudomi T, Oyama T, Kusano T, Osaki T, Nakanishi R, Shirakusa T (1993) Mutations of the p53 gene as a predictor of poor prognosis in patients with non-small-cell lung cancer. J Natl Cancer Inst 85:2018–2023

Miyake M, Taki T, Hitomi S, Hakomori S-I (1992) Correlation of expression of H/Ley/Leb antigenes with survival in patients with carcinoma of the lung. N Engl J Med 1992 327:14–18

Miyamoto H, Karado M, Isobe H et al (1991) Prognostic value of nuclear DNA content and expression of the ras oncogene product in lung cancer. Cancer Res 51: 6346–6350

Møller-Pedersen L, Milman N (1996) Prognostic significance of thrombocytosis in patients with primary lung cancer. Eur Respir J 9:1826–1830

Moore DF, Lee JS (1996) Staging and prognostic factors: non-small cell lung cancer. In: Pass H II, Mitchell JB, Johnson DH, Turrisi AT (eds) Lung cancer: principles and practice. Lippincott-Raven, Philadelphia

Morittu L, Earl HM, Souhami RL, Ash CM, Tobias JS, Geddes DM, Harper PG, Spiro SG (1989) Patients at risk of chemotherapy-associated toxicity in small cell lung cancer. Br J Cancer 59:801–804

Mørkve O, Halvorsen OJ, Skjaerven R, Stangeland L, Culsvik A, Lacrum OD (1993) Prognostic significance of p53 protein expression and DNA ploidy in surgically treated non-small cell lung carcinomas. Anticancer Res 12: 571–578

Mountain CF (1986) A new international staging system for lung cancer. Chest 89:225–233

Mountain CF (1988) Prognostic implications of the international staging system for lung cancer. Semin Oncol 15: 236–245

Mountain C (1995) New prognostic factors in lung cancer. Biologic prophets of cancer cell aggression. Chest 108: 246–54

Muers MF, Sherlin P, Brown J (1996) Prognosis in lung cancer: physicians' opinions compared with outcome and a predictive model. Thorax 51:894–902

Nishio M, Koshikawa T, Kuoishi T et al (1996) Prognostic significance of abnormal p53 accumulation in primary, resected non-small-cell lung cancers. J Clin Oncol 14: 497–502

O'Connell JP, Kris MG, Ralla RJ et al (1986) Frequency and prognostic importance of pretreatment clinical characteristics in patients with advanced non-small cell lung cancer treated with combination chemotherapy. J Clin Oncol 4:1604–1614

Ogawa J, Tsurumi T, Inoue H, Shohtsu A (1992) Relationship between tumor DNA ploidy and regional lymph node changes in lung cancer. Cancer 69:1688–1695

Ogawa JI, Inoue H, Koide S (1997) Glucose-transporter-type-I-gene amplification correlates with sialyl-Lewis-X synthesis and proliferation in lung cancer. Int. J Cancer 74:189–192

Østerlind K, Andersen PK (1986) Prognostic factors in small cell lung cancer: multivariate model based on 778 patients treated with chemotherapy with or without irradiation. Cancer Res 46:4189–4194

Østerlind K, Hansen HH, Hansen M, Dombernowsky P, Andersen PK (1986) Long-term disease-free survival in small-cell carcinoma of the lung: a study of clinical determinants. J Clin Oncol 4:1307–1313

Østerlind K, Hansen HH, Dombernowsky P, Hansen M, Andersen PK (1987) Determinants of complete remission induction and maintenance in chemotherapy with or without irradiation of small cell lung cancer. Cancer Res 47:2733–2736

Pappot H, Brünner N (1995) The plasminogen activation system and its role in lung cancer. Lung Cancer 12:1–12

Pappot H, Francis D, Brünner N et al (1996) p53 Protein in non-small cell lung cancer as quantitated by enzyme-linked immunosorbent assay: relation to prognosis. Clin Cancer Res 2:155–160

Pastorino U, Andreola S, Tagliabue E et al (1997) Immunocytochemical markers in stage I lung cancer: relevance to prognosis. J Clin Oncol 15:2858–2865

Pedersen H, Brünner N, Grøndahl-Hansen J, Francis D, Østerlind K, Rønne E, Hansen HH, Danø K (1994a) Prognostic impact of urokinase, urokinase receptor, and type 1 plasminogen activator inhibitor in squamous and large cell lung cancer tissue. Cancer Res 54:4671–4675

Pedersen H, Francis D, Grøndahl-Hansen J, Østerlind K, Hansen HH, Danø K, Brünner N (1994b) Urokinase and plasminogen activator inhibitor type 1 in pulmonary adenocarcinoma. Cancer Res 54:120–123

Pena CM, Rice TW, Ahmad M, Medendorp S (1992) Significance of perioperative blood transfusions in patients undergoing resection of stage I and II non-small cell lung cancers. Chest 102:84–88

Pence JC, Kerns BM, Kerns MT et al (1992) Prognostic significance of the proliferation index in surgically resected non-small cell lung cancer. Arch Surg 128: 1382–1390

Pujol JL, Cooper EH, Lehmann M et al (1993) Clinical evaluation of serum tumour marker CA 242 in non-small cell lung cancer. Br J Cancer 67:1423–1429

Pujol J-L, Grenier J, Parrat E, Lehmann M, Lafontaine T, Quantin X, Michel F-B (1996) Cytokeratins as serum markers in lung cancer: a comparison of CYFRA 21-1 and TPS. Am J Respir Crit Care Med 154:725–733

Quinlan DC, Davidson AG, Summers CL. Wender HE, Doshi HM (1992) Accumulation of p53 protein correlation with a poor prognosis in human lung cancer. Cancer Res 52:4828–4831

Quoix E, Charloux A, Popin E, Pauli G (1993) Inability to predict disease extent in small cell lung cancer based on initial level of serum neuron-specific enolase. Eur J Cancer 16:2248–2250

Radford JA, Ryder WDJ, Dodwell D, Anderson H, Thatcher N (1993) Predicting septic complications of chemotherapy: an analysis of 382 patients treated for small cell lung cancer without dose reduction after major sepsis. Eur J Cancer 29A:81–86

Rapp E, Pater JL, William A et al (1988) Chemotherapy can prolong survival in patients with advanced non-small-cell lung cancer: report of a Canadian multicenter randomized trial. J Clin Oncol 6:633–641

Rawson NSB, Peto J (1990) An overview of prognostic factors in small cell lung cancer. A report from the subcommittee for the management of lung cancer of the United Kingdom coordinating committee on cancer research. Br J Cancer 61:597–604

Rodenhuis S, Slebos RJC (1992) Clinical significance of ras oncogene activation in human lung cancer. Cancer Res 52[Suppl 6]:26658–26698

Rosenfeld MR, Malats N, Schramm L, Graus F, Cardenal F, Vinolas N, Rosell R, Tora M, Real FX, Posner JB, Dalmau J (1997) Serum anti-p53 antibodies and prognosis of patients with small-cell lung cancer. JNCI 89: 381–385

Sagman U, Feld R, Evans WK, Warr D, Shepherd FA, Payne D, Pringle J, Yeoh J, DeBoer G, Malkin A, Ginsberg R (1991a) The prognostic significance of pretreatment serum lactate dehydrogenase in patients with small-cell lung cancer. J Clin Oncol 9:954–961

Sagman U, Maki E, Evans WK, Warr D, Shepherd FA, Sculier JP, Haddad R, Payne D, Pringle F, Yeoh JL, Ciampi A, DeBoer G, McKinney S, Ginsberg R, Feld R (1991b) Small-cell carcinoma of the lung: derivation of a prognostic staging system. J Clin Oncol 9:1639–1649

Sarandakou A, Poulakis N, Rizos D, Trakakis E, Phocas I (1993) Anticancer Res 13:173–176

Sceagliotti GV, Micela M, Gubetta L et al (1993) Prognostic significance of Ki67 labelling in resected non small cell lung cancer. Eur J Cancer 29A:363–365

Scott C, Sause WT, Byhardt R et al (1997) Recursive partitioning analysis of 1592 patients on four radiation therapy oncology group studies in inoperable non-small cell lung cancer. Lung Cancer 17:59–74

Sculier JP, Paesmans M, Libert P et al (1994) Long-term survival after chemotherapy containing platinum derivatives in patients with advanced unresectable non-small cell lung cancer. Eur J Cancer 30A:1342–1347

Shinkai T, Eguchi K, Sasaki Y et al (1992) A prognostic-factor risk index in advanced non-small-cell lung cancer treated with cisplatin-containing combination chemotherapy. Cancer Chemother Pharmacol 30:1–6

Simon R, Altman DG (1994) Statistical aspects of prognostic factor studies in oncology. Br J Cancer 69:979–985

Skov, BG, Sørensen JB, Hirsch FR, Larsson LI, Hansen HH (1991) Prognostic impact of histologic demonstration of chromogranin A and neuron-specific enolase in pulmonary adenocarcinoma. Ann Oncol 2:355–360

Slebos RJC, Kibbaellar RE, Dalesio O et al (1990) K-ras oncogene activation as a prognostic marker in adeno-carcinoma of the lung. N Engl J Med 32:561–565

Sørensen JB (1994) Prognostic factors in non-small cell lung cancer. Radiol Oncol 28:301–308

Sørensen JB, Badsberg JH (1990) Prognostic factors in resected stage I and II adenocarcinomas of the lung. A multivariate regression analysis of 137 consecutive patients. J Thorac Cardiovasc Surg 99:218–226

Sørensen JB, Badsberg JH, Olsen J (1989) Prognostic factors in iniperable adenocarcinoma of the lung: a multivariate regression analysis of 259 patients. Cancer Res 49: 5748–5754

Souhami RL, Bradbury I, Geddes DM, Spiro SG, Harper PG, Tobias JS (1985) Prognostic significance of laboratory parameters measured at diagnosis in small cell carcinoma of the lung. Cancer Res 45:2878–2882

Spiegelman D, Maurer LH, Ware JH, Perry MC, Chahinian AP (1989) Prognostic factors in small-cell carcinoma of the lung: an analysis of 1521 patients. J Clin Oncol 7: 344–354

Staquet M, Dalesio O (1984) Cancer clinical trials. In: Buyse ME, Staquet MJ, Sylvester RJ (eds) Methods and practice. Oxford University Press, Oxford, pp 261–275

Stevenson II, Gazdar AF, Phelps R et al (1990) Tumor cell lines established in vitro: an independent prognostic factor for survival in non-small-cell lung cancer. Ann Intern Med 113:764–770

Stipa S, Danesi DT, Modini C et al (1993) The importance of heterogeneity and of multiple site sampling in the prospective determination of deoxyribonucleic acid flow cytometry. Surg Gynecol Obst 176:427–434

Sugio K, Ishida T, Yokoyama H, Inoue T, Sugimachi K, Sasazuki T (1992) ras Gene mutation as a prognostic marker in adenocarcinoma of the human lung without lymph node metastases. Cancer Res 52:2903–2906

Sukurai M, Shinkai T, Eguchi K et al (1987) Prognostic factors in non-small cell lung cancer: multiregression analysis in the National Cancer Center Hospital (Japan). J Cancer Res Clin Oncol 115:563–566

Szabo E, Mulshine J (1993) Epidemiology, prognostic factors and prevention of lung cancer. Curr Opin Oncol 5:302–309

Szturmowicz M, Roginska E, Roszkowski K, Kwiek S, filipecki S, Rowinska-Zakrzewska E (1993) Prognostic value of neuron-specific enolase in small cell lung cancer patients. Lung Cancer 8:259–264

Taguchi O, Gabazza EC, Yoshida M, Yamakami T, Kobayashi H, Shima T (1996) High plasma level of plasmin-α_2-

plasmin inhibitor complex is predictor of poor prognosis in patients with lung cancer. Clin Chim Acta 244:69–81

Taguchi O, Gabazza EC, Yasui H, Kobayashi T, Yoshida M, Kobayashi H (1997) Prognostic significance of plasma D-dimer levels in patients with lung cancer. Thorax 52:563–565

Takigawa N, Segawa Y, Okahara M et al (1996) Prognostic factors for patients with advanced non-small cell lung cancer: univariate and multivariate analyses including recursive partitioning and amalgamation. Lung Cancer 15:67–77

Tartter PI, Burrows L, Kirschner P (1984) Perioperative blood transfusion adversely affects prognosis after resection of stage I (subset NO) non-oat cell lung cancer. J Thorac Cardiovasc Surg 88:659–662

Tateishi M, Ishidu T, Mitsudomi T, Kanedo S, Sugimachi K (1991) Prognostic value of c-erb B-2 protein expression in human lung adenocarcinoma and squamous cell carcinoma. Eur J Cancer 27:1372–1375

Taves DR (1974) Minimization: a new method of assigning patients to treatment and control groups. Clin Pharm Ther 15:443–453

Thiberville L, Bourguignon J, Metayer J et al (1995) Frequency and prognostic evaluation of 3p21–22 allelic losses in non-small lung cancer. Int J Cancer 64:371–377

van Bodegom PC, Baak JPA, Stroet-van Galen C et al (1989) The percentage of aneuploid cells is significantly correlated with survival in accurately staged patients with stage I resected squamous cell lung cancer and long-term follow up. Cancer 63:143–147

van der Gaast A, van Putten WLJ, Oosterom R, Cozijnsen M, Hoekstra R, Splinter TAW (1991) Prognostic value of serum thymidine kinase, tissue polypeptide antigen and neuron specific enolase in patients with small cell lung cancer. Br J Cancer 64:369–372

Vangsted A, Drivsholm L, Andersen E, Bock E (1994a) New serum markers for small-cell lung cancer. II. The neural cell adhesion molecule, NCAM. Cancer Detect Prev 18:221–229

Vangsted A, Drivsholm L, Andersen E, Pallesen T, Zeuthen J, Wallin H (1994b) New serum markers for small-cell lung cancer. I. The ganglioside Fucosyl-GM1. Cancer Detect Prev 18:221–229

Veale D, Kerr N, Gibson GJ, Harris AL (1989) Characterisation of epidermal growth factor receptor in primary human non-small cell lung cancer. Cancer Res 49:1313–1317

Veale D, Kerr N, Gibson GJ, Kelly PJ, Harris AL (1993) The relationship of quantitative epidermal growth factor receptor expression in non-small cell lung cancer to long term survival. Br J Cancer 68:162–165

Vincent MD, Ashley SE, Smith IE (1987) Prognostic factors in small cell lung cancer: a simple prognostic index is better than conventional staging. Eur J Cancer Clin Oncol 23:1589–1599

Visakorpi T, Holli K, Hakama M (1995) High cell proliferation activity determined by DNA flow cytometry and prognosis in epidermoid lung carcinoma. Acta Oncol 34:605–609

Volm M, Mattern J, Müller T, Drings P (1988) flow cytometry of epidermoid lung carcinomas: relationship of ploidy and cell cycle phases to survival. A five-year follow up study. Anticancer Res 8:105–112

Weiskopf B, Demangeat C, Purohit A et al (1995) Cyfra 21-1 as biologic marker of non-small cell lung cancer: evaluation of sensitivity, specificity, and prognostic role. Chest 108:163–169

WHO Handbook for Reporting Results of Cancer Treatment (1979) WHO, Geneva

Xu H-J, Hu S-X, Cagle PT et al (1991) Absence of RB protein expression in primary non-small cell lung carcinomas. Cancer Res 51:2735

Yamashita JI, Tashiro K, Yoneda S et al (1996) Local increase in polymorphonuclear leukocyte elastase is associated with tumor invasiveness in non-small cell lung cancer. Chest 109:1328–1334

Zimmermann PV, Hawson GAT, Bint MH, Parsons PG (1987) Ploidy as a prognostic determinant in surgically treated lung cancer. Lancet 230:530–533

2 Radiological Evaluation of Intrathoracic Extension and Resectability of Non-Small Cell Lung Cancer

J.A. Hanson and P. Armstrong

CONTENTS

Chest imaging makes an important contribution to the pre-operative assessment of patients with lung cancer. Whilst there are accepted standard approaches for most operable patients, based on the International Staging System, there is variation in surgical strategy for those with more extensive tumours at the limits of resectability. The International Staging System, and the operative management of non-small cell lung cancer, will, therefore, be briefly discussed, before the radiological evaluation of intrathoracic non-small cell cancer is considered.

2.1 International Staging System

The newly revised International Staging System for non-small cell lung cancer stratifies disease extent in terms of prognosis (Mountain 1997). It is based on the TNM grading of the primary tumour, regional nodes and distant metastases (Tables 2.1, 2.2).

Stage I tumours are confined to the lung, without extension to the parietal pleura; when in major bronchi the tumour is more than 2 cm beyond the tracheal carina. Stage I tumours have no nodal or distant spread. This stage is divided into A and B according to whether the tumour is T1 or T2.

Stage IIA tumours are the same as stage IA, but with ipsilateral hilar nodal metastasis.

Stage IIB tumours can be either the same as stage IB, but with ipsilateral hilar nodal metastasis, *or* are tumours without nodal or distant spread but which have invaded the adjacent chest wall, mediastinum or diaphragm and are potentially surgically resectable (Scott et al. 1988; Martini et al. 1994). Included are tumours which extend along the main bronchi to within 2 cm of the carina but do not involve it, which may be resected with bronchoplastic techniques (Belli et al. 1985).

Stage IIIA comprises (a) T3 tumours in which the only spread is to hilar nodes or (b) T1-T3 tumours without distant metastases which have spread to ipsilateral mediastinal and/or subcarinal nodes (N2). These patients may benefit from mediastinal lymphadenectomy (Goldstraw et al. 1994; Mountain 1994).

Stage IIIB tumours involve critical mediastinal structures such as the great vessels, oesophagus, and trachea (T4), or have spread to contralateral mediastinal nodes (N3). These patients are not considered to be conventional surgical candidates (Naruke et al. 1988a; Mountain 1997). However, a few surgeons have recently proposed extending the surgical option to the occasional highly selected patient with stage IIIB disease. Further work is required, and definitive results may take years to evaluate.

Stage IV: Patients with distant metastatic disease (M1).

These stages have been devised to produce groups which reflect the management options and survival figures with appropriate treatment (Tables 2.3, 2.4).

J.A. Hanson, Department of Diagnostic Imaging, St. Bartholomew's Hospital, West Smithfield, London EC1A 7BE, UK
P. Armstrong, Department of Academic Radiology, St. Bartholomew's Hospital, West Smithfield, London EC1A 7BE, UK

Table 2.1. TNM classification of tumour extent (From MOUNTAIN 1997)

Primary tumour (T)

Tx	Primary tumour cannot be assessed, or tumour proven by the presence of malignant cells in sputum or bronchial washings but not visualised by imaging or bronchoscopy.
T0	No evidence of primary tumour.
Tis	Carcinoma in situ
T1	Tumour ≤3 cm in greatest dimension, surrounded by lung or visceral pleura, without bronchoscopic evidence of invasion more proximal than the lobar bronchus[a] (i.e. not in the main bronchus).
T2	Tumour with any of the following features of size or extent: >3 cm in greatest dimension; involves main bronchus, ≥2 cm distal to the carina; invades the visceral pleura; associated with atelectasis or obstructive pneumonitis that extends to the hilar region but does not involve the entire lung.
T3	Tumour of any size that directly invades any of the following: chest wall (including superior sulcus tumours), diaphragm, mediastinal pleura, parietal pericardium; or tumour in the main bronchus <2 cm distal to the carina, but without involvement of the carina; or associated atelectasis or obstructive pneumonitis of the entire lung.
T4	Tumour of any size that invades any of the following: mediastinum, heart, great vessels, trachea, oesophagus, vertebral body, carina; or tumour with a malignant pleural or pericardial effusion[b], or with satellite tumour nodule(s) within the ipsilateral primary-tumour lobe of the lung.

Regional lymph nodes (N)

Nx	Regional lymph nodes cannot be assessed.
N0	No regional lymph node metastasis.
N1	Metastasis to ipsilateral peribronchial and/or ipsilateral hilar lymph nodes, and intrapulmonary nodes involved by direct extension of the primary tumour.
N2	Metastasis to ipsilateral mediastinal and/or subcarinal lymph node(s).
N3	Metastasis to contralateral mediastinal, contralateral hilar, ipsilateral or contralateral scalene, or supraclavicular lymph node(s).

Distant metastasis (M)

Mx	Presence of distant metastasis cannot be assessed.
M0	No distant metastasis.
M1	Distant metastasis present[c]

[a] The uncommon superficial tumour of any size with its invasive component limited to the bronchial wall, which may extend proximal to the main bronchus, is also classified T1.

[b] Most pleural effusions associated with lung cancer are due to tumour. However, there are a few patients in whom multiple cytopathologic examinations of pleural fluid show no tumour. In these cases, the fluid is nonbloody and is not an exudate. When these elements and clinical judgement dictate that the effusion is not related to the tumour, the effusion should be excluded as a staging element and the patient's disease should be staged T1, T2, or T3. Pericardial effusion is classified according to the same rules.

[c] Separate metastatic tumour nodule(s) in the ipsilateral nonprimary-tumour lobe(s) of the lung also are classified M1.

Table 2.2. Stage grouping by TNM subsets (From MOUNTAIN 1997)

Stage	Definition	Stage	Definition
IA	T1N0M0	IIIB	T4N0M0
IB	T2N0M0		T4N1M0
			T4N2M0
IIA	T1N1M0		T1N3M0
IIB	T2N1M0		T2N3M0
	T3N0M0		T3N3M0
			T4N3M0
IIIA	T3N1M0		
	T1N2M0	IV	Any T, any N, M1
	T2N2M0		
	T3N2M0		

Staging is not relevant for occult carcinoma, designated TxN0M0.

Table 2.3. Five-year survival figures (%) according to stage (From MOUNTAIN 1997)

Stage	Clinical staging	Pathological staging
IA	61	67
IB	38	57
IIA	34	55
IIB	22–24	38–39
IIIA	9–13	23–25
IIIB	1–8	
IV	1	

Table 2.4. Summary of staging of non-small cell lung cancer

Stage I
No nodal metastases and totally removable by lobectomy or pneumonectomy. Divided into A or B based on tumour size/involvement of major bronchi
Stage II
Adds hilar node involvement (IIA) *or* resectable chest wall/resectable mediastinal involvement (IIB)
Stage IIIA
Extensive but resectable disease (T3N1, T1N2, T2N2, T3N2)
Stage IIIB
Irresectable disease by conventional criteria but still confined to chest, so eligible for radical radiotherapy
Stage IV
Distant metastases

2.2 Surgical Management of Non-Small Cell Lung Cancer

Surgery remains the most effective treatment for non-small cell lung cancer (Bains 1991). Appropriate selection of patients is critical, and the possibility of cure depends on the complete removal of all apparent disease. Surgery should be avoided when it can be confidently predicted that the tumour is too extensive to permit complete macroscopic clearance. Surgery is also inappropriate in patients with physiological contraindications, although decisions regarding operability (Friedman 1988) vary between clinicians. In addition to the stage, assessment of prognosis should take into account the histological type and grade of tumour, individual patient factors and local institutional experience.

Stage I tumours can be completely removed, lobectomy being the procedure of choice (Bains 1991). Small peripheral tumours may be technically suitable for wedge resection or segmentectomy in patients with poor cardiorespiratory reserve. Pneumonectomy becomes necessary if the tumour crosses a fissure or extends to the main bronchus. The resection is accompanied by mediastinal node dissection, varying in degree from sampling of suspect nodes to more meticulous mediastinal lymphadenectomy. The latter approach is preferred as it permits more accurate staging (Bollen et al. 1993; Izbicki et al. 1995). Five-year survival figures of 55%–75% are reported (Naruke et al. 1988a; Mountain 1997) (Table 2.3).

Stage II tumours are also treated by resection. The presence of ipsilateral hilar node metastases does not preclude pneumonectomy, but the 5-year survival is significantly reduced to 35%–55% (Naruke et al. 1988a; Mountain 1997) (Table 2.3). There may be roles for post-operative radiotherapy to improve control of local recurrence and combination chemotherapy to achieve survival benefit.

The presence of positive mediastinal (N2) nodes converts the disease to stage IIIA. It is accepted that a subgroup of patients with IIIA disease benefit from surgery (Table 2.3), although the appropriate selection of cases is debated. There is considerable variation of prognosis within the N2 group depending on site and number of involved nodes, extranodal spread, the size and histology of the primary tumour.

Surgery is inappropriate in N2 disease presenting with dysphagia or dysphonia, as this implies extranodal spread, but the surgical management of lesser degrees of N2 disease is controversial. Conflicting published results are partly due to differences in selection criteria and data analysis. Prognosis correlates with the method by which N2 disease is established. Positive nodal disease discovered preoperatively by mediastinal biopsy or CT, with otherwise favourable surgical features, is associated with a worse outcome than when nodal involvement is established only after mediastinal dissection (Pearson et al. 1982; Cybulsky et al. 1992). In a study based on mediastinoscopy, Pearson et al. showed a 5-year survival of 9% vs 24% respectively for these two groups (Pearson et al. 1982). Two recent series have confirmed that a reasonable survival dividend can be achieved in certain patient subsets, provided that complete removal of tumour is possible. In the large series reported by Mountain, 307 patients finally staged as N2 showed a 5-year survival of 31% (Mountain 1994). Improved outcome correlated with small primary tumour (less than 3 cm, T1), and was inversely correlated with the number and extent of positive mediastinal nodes. Similarly, Goldstraw et al. found that improved survival was associated with single as opposed to multiple level mediastinal nodal involvement (Goldstraw et al. 1994). In addition, this study noted more favourable outcome with squamous carcinoma when compared with other cell types, although there are conflicting reports in the literature regarding the influence of histological type on the prognosis of patients with N2 disease (Martini et al. 1983; Naruke et al. 1988b).

The use of neoadjuvant chemoradiotherapy in N2 disease is an area of promising research (Rusch et al. 1993a). The intention is to render bulky nodal disease technically resectable, and to improve prognosis. The appropriate indications remain to be defined. Refinements to radiological staging may be necessary to reflect changes in node appearance.

Involvement of contralateral mediastinal nodes, or supraclavicular nodes on either side (N3), is a manifestation of distant spread and these patients are inoperable. They are included in the regional nodal staging because of their suitability for radical radiotherapy.

In terms of mediastinal invasion, the distinction between T3 and T4 disease is critical, because for most surgeons it reflects the dividing line between surgical and non-surgical management. The results of operation for T3 tumours affecting the mediastinum are poor (BURT et al. 1987; MARTINI et al. 1994), even when complete clearance is possible (5%–10% 5-year survival). This may be improved with adjuvant brachytherapy by implanting isotope sources perioperatively (BURT et al. 1987). Subsets of patients have been identified with a better prognosis: there are reports of 5-year survival of 30% if patients with coexistent N2 disease are excluded (MARTINI et al. 1994).

Some salvage can be achieved in highly selected patients with T4 disease, provided complete resection can be achieved. Limited aortic arch, superior vena cava or left atrial invasion can be resected, and repaired or bypassed with prosthetic grafts, with occasional 5-year survival (DARTEVELLE et al. 1987; NAKAHARA et al. 1989; TSCHIUYA et al. 1994). Recently the successful resection of tumours invading thoracic vertebrae has been reported in highly selected cases (GRUNENWALD et al. 1996). A course of neoadjuvant chemotherapy is given initially to "sterilise" the tumour. If repeat assessment is favourable, vertebrectomy and bone grafting procedures are performed. Further work is needed to determine long-term outcome. Usually, however, such radical surgery is not justified.

Localised invasion of the chest wall (T3) is not a contraindication to surgery (PIEHLER et al. 1982; MCCAUGHAN et al. 1985; ALLEN et al. 1991). Resection can be performed by extrapleural mobilisation if the tumour appears limited to the parietal pleura, or en bloc resection of tumour and skeletal structures with reconstruction of the chest wall defect (MCCAUGHAN 1994). Although the spread of tumour beyond the parietal pleura into the chest wall is an adverse feature, the main determinant of outcome is the coexistence of mediastinal nodal disease, rather than the presence or depth of chest wall invasion. Five-year survival figures of 25%–40% can be achieved in patients with normal regional lymph nodes (PIEHLER et al. 1982; MCCAUGHAN et al. 1985; ALLEN et al. 1991). The recently revised International Staging System now classifies T3 N0 M0 tumours as Stage IIB disease to reflect this relatively favourable outlook.

In contrast, diffuse pleural involvement by malignant effusion or nodular seeding indicates tumour dissemination and inoperable T4 disease.

Superior sulcus tumours (the so-called Pancoast's tumour) invade the adjacent chest wall and root of neck, and can involve neural structures. Multidisciplinary treatment may be effective, using preoperative radiotherapy, followed by en bloc chest wall resection, with laminectomy or vertebrectomy as necessary, and brachytherapy. Such an approach can result in survival figures little worse than for other sites of chest wall invasion (PAULSON 1979; MILLER et al. 1979).

Because there are so-many factors affecting the surgical resectability of non-small cell lung cancer, the value of imaging is best judged by measuring the accuracy with which radiology can determine the final surgicopathological tumour stage of the International Staging System. The overall aim is to permit all suitable patients to undergo thoracotomy with the hope of cure, whilst preventing unnecessary debilitating surgery in those who will not benefit.

2.3 Staging Regional Nodal Disease

The position of hilar and mediastinal nodes should be described according to the recently unified American Thoracic Society (ATS) and American Joint Committee on Cancer (AJCC) classification (MOUNTAIN and DRESLER 1997). This system uses fixed anatomical landmarks to localise individual nodal stations. The upper and lower paratracheal stations are designated 2R/2L and 4R/4L respectively. Aortopulmonary nodes (station 5) lie lateral to the aortic arch and ligamentum arteriosum. Station 6 nodes lie anterior to the aortic arch and great vessels. No right/left distinction exists for subcarinal nodes, at station 7, and therefore these always represent N2 disease. The paraoesophageal nodes (station 8) lie at least 3 cm below the tracheal carina and should include nodes within the inferior pulmonary ligament as these cannot be distinguished radiologically (FRIEDMAN 1988). The significance of diaphragmatic nodes has been recognised and they are included with mediastinal N2 nodes.

By definition, hilar nodes are intrapulmonary and lie outside the mediastinal pleura. At surgery this position varies with the force of retraction of the lung, and there may be some difficulty in distinguishing N1 from N2 nodes. The intrapulmonary nodes (11R/11L) are designated N1 and can be further classified into lobar and interlobar positions. The differentiation of the 10R/10L tracheobronchial nodes causes a problem, and Friedman suggests that ipsilateral 10R nodes be designated N1, wheras 10L nodes be classified as mediastinal because of the relative ease of surgical exposure (FRIEDMAN 1988). The presence of supraclavicular nodes (1R/1L) reflects distant spread of disease, and involvement of these nodes is classified N3.

Spread of tumour to hilar or mediastinal lymph nodes is a common finding in patients presenting with lung cancer. Non-sequential spread to mediastinal nodes, bypassing hilar nodes, may occur in up to one-third of cases (LIBSHITZ et al. 1986; TATEISHI et al. 1994). The radiological detection of lymph node metastases is generally based on the demonstration of nodal enlargement, an approach which is fundamentally flawed. Microscopic involvement may not cause enlargement, and conversely nodal enlargement can be due to benign diseases. The presence of microscopically involved normal sized nodes has been increasingly recognised by studies employing complete mediastinal lymphadenectomy as a reference standard. In 1985, MCKENNA et al. noted that 40% of patients with mediastinal metastases had normal sized nodes at CT (MCKENNA et al. 1985). Other authors have confirmed the high frequency of metastases to normal sized nodes, although the figures vary between patient populations (GROSS et al. 1986; KERR et al. 1992; DALY et al. 1993). In a rigorous study by MCLOUD et al., 13% of nodes <1 cm diameter contained tumour (MCLOUD et al. 1992). However, these comprised a sufficiently large proportion of the total number of nodes dissected that almost half of the nodal deposits were found in normal sized nodes. Furthermore, a recent Japanese study has reported similar size distributions for both benign and malignant lymph nodes (ARITA et al. 1996).

Nodal enlargement may be a benign process due to reactive change initiated by the tumour or distal infection, or coincidental occupational or granulomatous lung disorders (LIBSHITZ and MCKENNA 1984). These latter factors are subject to considerable geographic variation. MCLOUD's study found that 37% of substantially enlarged nodes 2–4 cm in diameter were tumour free (MCLOUD et al. 1992). The high prevalence of histoplasmosis in certain parts of the United States exacerbates this problem.

The choice of the upper limit for normal nodal size is complex. Published limits vary according to the position within the mediastinum, from 11 mm in the paratracheal regions to 3 mm in the hila (SCHNYDER and GAMSU 1981; G.M. GLAZER et al. 1985; KIYONO et al. 1985; INGRAM et al. 1989; REMY-JARDIN et al. 1995). The maximum diameter of any node varies with its orientation in the cross-sectional imaging plane. Short axis diameter measurements are therefore widely used to avoid this variation (G.M. GLAZER et al. 1985). A common policy is to use the convenient and reasonably accurate figure of 10 mm as the upper limit for normal. This gives a relatively high sensitivity for metastatic disease, but requires the routine use of biopsy to maintain specificity (Fig. 2.1).

CT is the standard imaging modality for diagnosing nodal enlargement (Fig. 2.2), and many studies have been performed to measure its accuracy (BARON et al. 1982; OSBORNE et al. 1982; DALY et al. 1987; PATTERSON et al. 1987; IKEZOE et al. 1990; DILLEMANS et al. 1994). Early work suggested that CT would be sufficiently accurate to allow decisions regarding thoracotomy without the need for an invasive surgical staging procedure such as mediastinoscopy. However, more recent studies

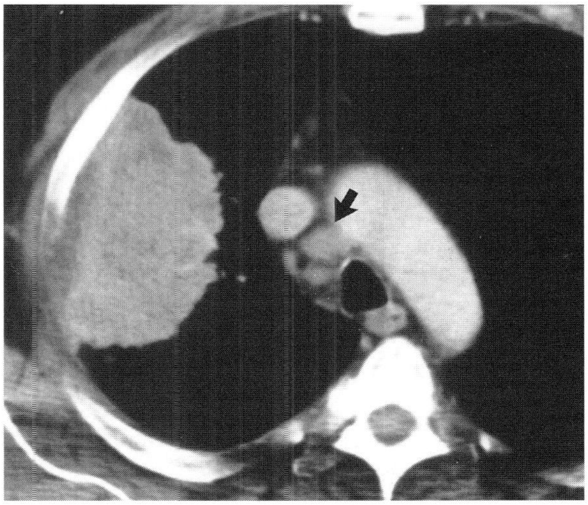

Fig. 2.1. False positive mediastinal lymphadenopathy, and indeterminate chest wall invasion, shown by CT. The enlarged paratracheal node (→) measures 1.5 cm in short-axis diameter. There is extensive contact between the primary tumour and chest wall with no visible extrapleural fat plane. The patient initially underwent mediastinoscopy and sampling of the enlarged paratracheal node, which revealed no evidence of malignancy. At surgery the lymph node was removed and shown to be clear of metastasis. The primary tumour could be dissected off the chest wall, with histopathological extension only to the parietal pleura

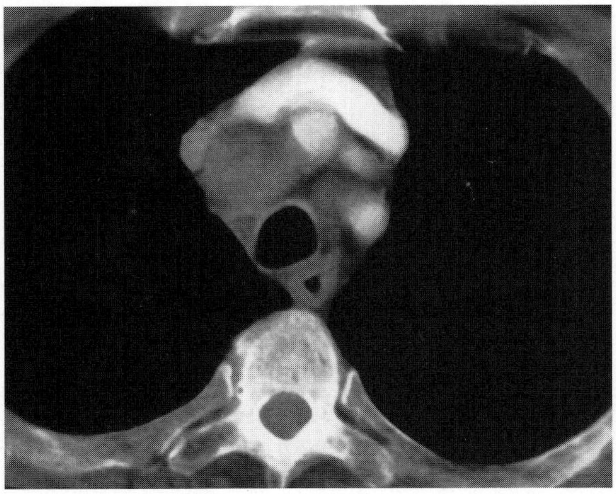

Fig. 2.2. Mediastinal lymphadenopathy shown by CT. Enlarged right paratracheal lymph node in a patient with a left upper lobe squamous cell carcinoma. This node was proven to contain metastatic tumour (N3) by transthoracic CT guided needle biopsy

using rigorous surgical/pathological correlation and more complete lymph node dissection have given less favourable results with sensitivities and specificities of the order of 60%–70% using a short axis diameter of 10 mm as the upper limit of normal (LIBSHITZ and MCKENNA 1984; MCLOUD et al. 1992; STAPLES et al. 1988; WEBB et al. 1991). It has been shown that formal mediastinal lymphadenectomy can detect up to twice the number of positive node stations found by more limited sampling (IZBICKI et al. 1995).

Some of the apparent variation in published results is accounted for by the discrepancy between patient-based analyses and individual nodal station analysis. If the enlarged node identified at CT does not correspond to the positive node confirmed pathologically, the CT is classified as false positive even though the correct N stage has been predicted (STAPLES et al. 1988). The considerable interobserver variation in the interpretation of mediastinal CT, even between experienced chest radiologists, has been recently highlighted. The kappa statistic is used to assess the degree of agreement between observers that is not chance-related, with values >0.6 indicating reasonable agreement. A range of kappa values have been reported for mediastinal node staging in non-small cell lung cancer, between 0.24 and 0.46 for all mediastinal nodes taken together, and generally higher values of 0.58–0.68 for individual nodal station analysis (WEBB et al. 1993; BOLLEN et al. 1994; GUYATT et al. 1995). The left superior mediastinal nodes are subject to the most marked interobserver error.

Analysis of the distribution of enlarged lymph nodes has been proposed to improve specificity. A European study from BUY et al. showed that if a node within the draining territory of the tumour was both enlarged (>10 mm short axis diameter) and at least 5 mm larger than other nodes, then the positive predictive value approached 95% (BUY et al. 1988).

Peripheral T1 tumours have a lower incidence of mediastinal nodal metastases than T2 and T3 tumours, and some authors have suggested that CT is not cost-effective in these cases, particularly for tumours <2 cm diameter, because of the relatively high false positive rates and low yield (PEARLBERG et al. 1985; DALY et al. 1987). However, other authors argue in favour of staging CT, as more recent studies suggest a higher incidence of N2 disease in T1N0M0 lesions than previously recognised, and the detection of additional important information (DUNCAN et al. 1993; SEELY et al. 1993).

Mediastinal node enlargement can also be imaged with MRI using the same anatomical criteria as for CT (MARTINI et al. 1985; WEBB et al. 1985; HEELAN et al. 1985; MUSSET et al. 1986; POON et al. 1987; STIGLBAUER et al. 1991). Various scanning techniques have been proposed. We have obtained the best spatial and contrast resolution using multiplanar spin echo T1-weighted sequences with ECG gating. Advantages of MRI over CT are limited; the most significant is the capability to image in any plane (BATRA et al. 1988). There are circumstances in which coronal or sagittal imaging is helpful to more clearly visualise lymphadenopathy in the aortopulmonary (station 5) and subcarinal (station 7) regions. CT is compromised by partial volume averaging in these areas. Oblique sagittal scans aligned along the left pulmonary artery may be useful. A second advantage of MRI is the ease with which small hilar lymph nodes can be detected without the need for intravenous contrast medium (MUSSET et al. 1986; WEBB et al. 1984). This is due to the striking contrast between fast flowing blood in the hilar vessels producing signal voids. However, the improved detection of hilar lymphadenopathy has low clinical impact owing to the limited relevance of N1 disease in surgical planning.

The increased contrast resolution of MRI has not proved useful. There is little difference in signal characteristics between benign and malignant nodes (WEBB et al. 1985; MUSSET et al. 1986; G.M. GLAZER et al. 1988). One small study using gadolinium-enhanced breath-held gradient echo sequences has suggested that nodal metastases from squamous cell carcinoma can be distinguished from anthracotic nodes on the basis of dynamic enhancement patterns, but further work is needed (LAISSY et al. 1994). Indeed, MRI has several disadvantages. Cardiac and respiratory motion artefact can result in blurring of a cluster of small nodes to resemble pathological enlargement (Fig. 2.3) (WEBB et al. 1984; MUSSET et al. 1986). The presence of calcification within an enlarged node is an important sign favouring a benign process, but this is difficult to appreciate on MRI (LEVITT et al. 1985).

Several studies have compared the accuracies of CT and MRI for nodal staging, and have generally shown little difference (GEORGIAN et al. 1990; MAYR et al. 1992). Both techniques are subject to considerable interobserver variation (WEBB et al. 1993). The most comprehensive comparison is the multi-centre Radiologic Diagnostic Oncology Group (RDOG) study which constructed receiver operating characteristic curves for both modalities, and reported sensitivities of 52% and 48%, and specificities of 69% and 64% for CT and MRI respectively (WEBB et al. 1991).

It is now established that the positive predictive value of CT for the presence of enlarged mediastinal nodes is too low to deny a patient surgery. Positive findings should be confirmed histologically, the prime role of CT or MRI being to target the biopsy procedure. A variety of methods have been used to sample mediastinal nodes, including a transbronchial approach. Mediastinoscopy or anterior mediastinotomy are performed by the surgeon (GINSBERG 1994), but lower mediastinal stations are inaccessible. Video assisted thoracoscopy allows mediastinal staging by direct visualisation and biopsy, and is well tolerated (LANDRENEAU et al. 1993; RENDIAN et al. 1994; ROVIARO et al. 1995). CT guided transthoracic biopsy is a further contribution of radiology to the staging process (PROTOPAPAS and WESTCOTT 1996). It is a reliable, minimally invasive procedure allowing most enlarged nodes to be reached (Fig. 2.2).

The most important recent advance in lung cancer imaging has been the development of positron emission tomography (PET) using the tracer fluorine-18 fluorodeoxyglucose (FDG). This technique produces cross-sectional thoracic images of metabolic activity for glucose, with neoplastic tissues having high metabolic rates. Metastatic nodes can be identified by virtue of abnormal function, an additional diagnostic parameter. Several centres have published results comparing CT and FDG PET for the staging of mediastinal nodal disease in non-small cell lung cancer (SCOTT et al. 1994; WAHL et al. 1994; STEINERT et al. 1997; GUHLMANN et al. 1997). These papers consistently show that FDG PET is superior, with sensitivities/specificities of the order of 80%–90%. WAHL et al. found that FDG PET data combined with the anatomic information from

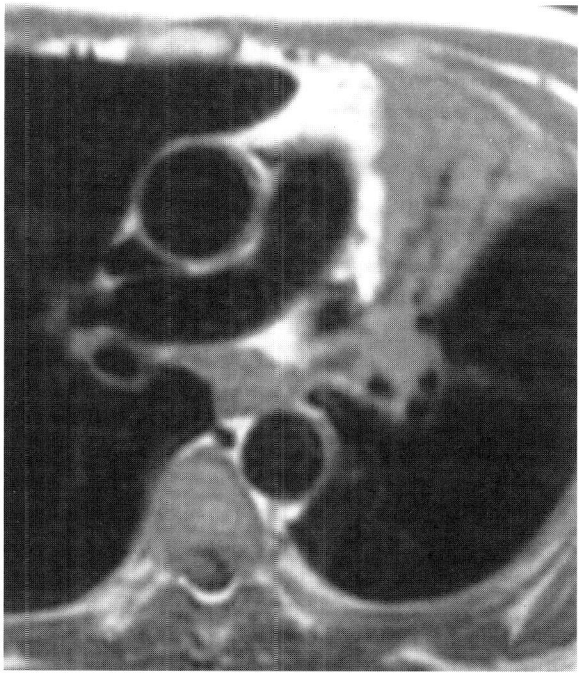
a

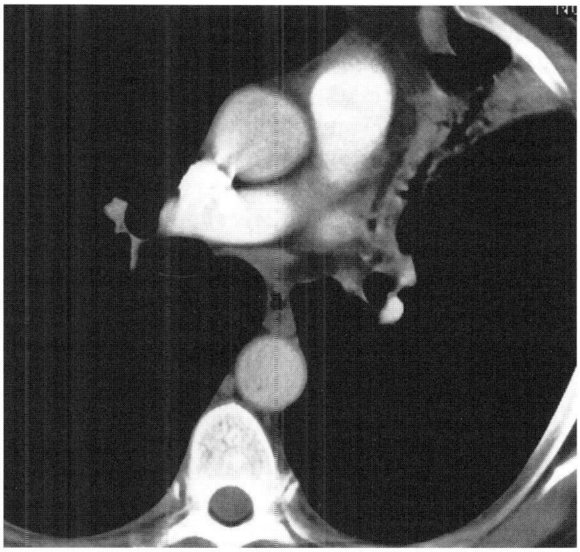
b

Fig. 2.3. **a** Subcarinal node enlargement: false positive MRI. Axial T1-weighted scan shows apparent subcarinal node enlargement in a patient with a left upper lobe cancer, due to blurring of the oesophagus and subcarinal tissues. **b** Enhanced CT scan in the same patient shows normal subcarinal anatomy. At thoracotomy the largest subcarinal node measured ≤10 mm and was clear of tumour. (From HANSON and ARMSTRONG 1997)

CT can predict resectability of T3 tumours with reasonable accuracy. In an influential study, GLAZER et al. identified three features of the tumour which predicted surgically resectable tumour: (a) less than 3 cm of mediastinal contact, (b) maintained fat plane of separation from the mediastinum, and (c) less than 90° angle of circumferential aortic contact (H.S. GLAZER et al. 1989). The presence of at least one of these signs was associated with successful resection in 36/37 cases. Unfortunately, predicting irresectability is more difficult (Fig. 2.7) (MCLOUD 1989), and in GLAZER's series, almost half the operable cancers showed more than 3 cm of mediastinal contact. Loss of fat plane is of limited significance, as this may be produced by reactive inflammatory change, fibrosis or motion artefact. Other studies have evaluated similar criteria and have confirmed the disappointing results (MARTINI et al. 1985; MUSSET et al. 1986; SCOTT et al. 1988). WHITE et al. reported the sensitivity of CT for inoperable mediastinal invasion to be only 27% (WHITE et al. 1994). Another study found that even anatomical distortion of mediastinal structures did not indicate invasion of those structures approximately half the time (HERMAN et al. 1994).

Attempts have been made to improve the detection of fixation of tumour. Dynamic studies using electron beam CT with respiratory and cardiac gating can reveal movement between the mass and mediastinal structures, implying lack of invasion (MURATA et al. 1994). Similarly, CT performed following the induction of a pneumothorax can show mobile, and therefore resectable, tumour (YOKOI et al. 1991). These small series describe useful methods for excluding mediastinal invasion, but do not address the problem of diagnosis of inoperable T4 disease, as benign adhesions may also result in tumour fixation. The inconvenience of performing the examination precludes widespread use.

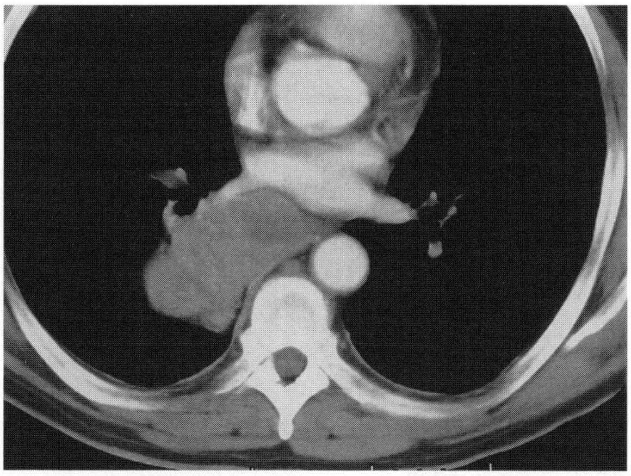

Fig. 2.7. False positive mediastinal invasion at CT. Right lower lobe tumour showing extensive contact with the oesophagus and indentation of the left atrium. However, at surgery the tumour was easily dissected off the mediastinal pleura and resected by right lower lobectomy. Histology showed that the tumour had only invaded as far as the visceral pleura. (From HANSON and ARMSTRONG 1997)

Spiral CT is now widely available, and has theoretical advantages, including more optimal contrast opacification of vascular structures, and reduced respiratory motion artefact. The reduction of partial volume averaging by overlapping slice reconstruction, and high quality multiplanar reformations, should improve assessment of regions such as the tracheal carina and aortopulmonary window. Visualisation of the bronchial tree using multiplanar and 3D techniques and virtual bronchoscopy are now established practices (REMY-JARDIN and REMY 1996). Formal studies of the utility of these new techniques in staging non-small cell lung cancer are awaited.

MRI in the axial plane displays the same anatomy as CT, and can also be used to stage mediastinal spread. In certain specific situations MRI may be used to advantage (LEVITT et al. 1985; MARTINI et al. 1985; MUSSET et al. 1986; LAURENT et al. 1988; WEBB et al. 1991). The routine use of ECG triggering to limit cardiac motion artefact compensates for the slightly reduced spatial resolution, and results in images which may be subjectively superior to CT, particularly in regions adjacent to cardiovascular structures. There is no need for intravenous contrast for vascular opacification (MAYR et al. 1992), and endoluminal tumour spread along venous pathways and within the atria can be elegantly shown. Pericardial transgression can be discerned. A further advantage of MRI is the availability of multiplanar imaging (Fig. 2.8), optimised for the subcarinal, aortic arch and aortopulmonary regions. However, MRI has the same limitations as CT in regard to the diagnosis of inoperable tumour invasion, since signal changes within the mediastinal fat are produced by both inflammatory and neoplastic processes (MUSSET et al. 1986; STIGLBAUER et al. 1991; MAYR et al. 1992).

A number of studies have compared MRI and CT for diagnosing mediastinal invasion, and show no difference in overall accuracy (MARTINI et al. 1985; MUSSET et al. 1986; LAURENT et al. 1988; KAMEDA et al. 1988). In the Radiologic Diagnostic Oncologic Group (RDOG) study, there was a non-significant advantage for MRI in a small number of patients (WEBB et al. 1991). However, the imaging modality of choice remains CT, because of practical and economic factors in its favour, and the likely, but as yet unproven, benefits of state-of-the-art spiral CT techniques.

It is worth noting that some authors have highlighted the value of endoscopic ultrasonography for evaluating the primary tumour within the mediastinum, in addition to its role in nodal staging (TATSUMURA 1995). This technique permits real-time visualisation of the tumour relationship with moving cardiovascular structures, and may be the imaging method of choice in occasional circumstances. Also, it may be used peroperatively.

Unfortunately, there are limitations with all radiological studies of mediastinal invasion and, therefore, a number of patients continue to undergo inappropriate thoracotomy because it is not possible to establish preoperatively that their disease is beyond surgical cure.

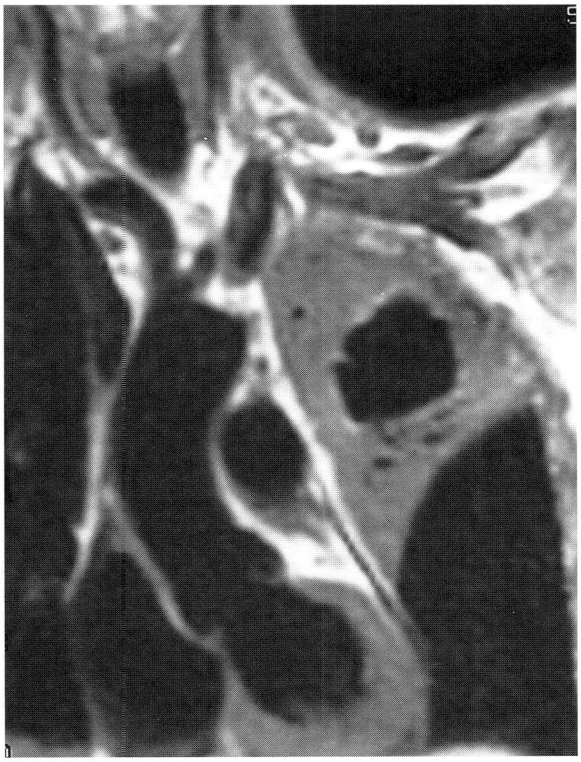

Fig. 2.8. Assessment of mediastinal invasion by MRI. Coronal T1-weighted image showing left upper lobe abscess distal to an obstructing squamous cell carcinoma. A clear line of mediastinal fat separates the tumour and collapsed lobe from the pericardium and great vessels. The carcinoma was resected by left upper lobectomy. Histology showed that the lobe was diffusely infiltrated by tumour to within 1 mm of the visceral pleural surface pleura. (From HANSON and ARMSTRONG 1997)

2.4.2 Chest Wall Invasion

Even though localised invasion of the ribs and intercostal muscles by a peripheral tumour is not a contraindication to surgery (PAULSON 1979; MCCAUGHAN et al. 1985; ALLEN et al. 1991), preoperative diagnosis is desirable as the balance of operability is altered and modified surgical techniques are required.

Advanced rib destruction may be evident on the plain chest radiograph, but even moderate degrees of chest wall invasion can be overlooked. Technetium-99m diphosphonate radionuclide scans are a very sensitive modality for bone involvement, and in the appropriate setting and location positive findings are fairly specific. Cortical bone erosion can be demonstrated with CT, and can localise the destructive process to rib (T3) or vertebral body (T4).

Although extensive tumour spread within the chest wall soft tissues is well seen at CT (Fig. 2.9), or MRI, the accuracy for detecting borderline invasion of the parietal pleura is less good, and subject to the same limitations as the assessment of mediastinal invasion (H.S. GLAZER et al. 1985; PENNES et al. 1985; PEARLBERG et al. 1987; SCOTT et al. 1988). The CT signs of parietal pleural transgression by tumour include obtuse angle of contact, obliteration of the extrapleural fat plane, pleural thickening, and the presence of extrapleural soft tissue. These signs, particularly in combination, are sensitive but nonspecific for parietal pleural invasion (H.S. GLAZER

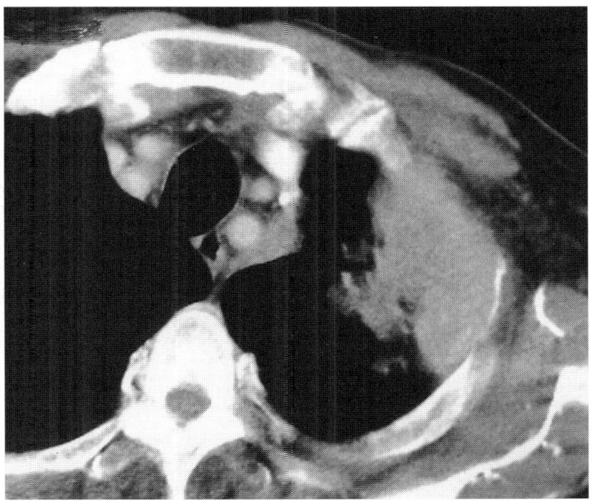

Fig. 2.9. Definite chest wall invasion by tumour. CT scan showing left upper lobe tumour invading the chest wall, showing rib destruction and extension of soft tissue beyond the line of the ribs

et al. 1985). Inflammatory change and fibrosis excited by the cancer can be indistinguishable from chest wall invasion by tumour. Local chest wall pain may be a more specific finding. Conversely, lack of chest wall extension is reliably predicted by the presence of acute angle and less than 3 cm of tumour contact. Preservation of the extrapleural fat line suggests that the tumour has not extended beyond the visceral pleura.

Dynamic CT methods, as previously discussed, may also help with the assessment of tumours contiguous with the chest wall, by studying relative movement of the tumour and pleural surface. Lack of fixation with respiration can be detected with conventional or electron beam cine CT (Murata et al. 1994; Shirakawa et al. 1994). Similarly, tumours which move away from the chest wall following induction of a diagnostic pneumothorax are staged T2 (Yokoi et al. 1991). A recent study utilised spiral CT to generate 3D surface-shaded reformations (Kuriyama et al. 1994). The authors were able to distinguish visceral from parietal pleural invasion with 80% accuracy by analysing pleural configuration. The rationale for this approach was based on the hypothesis that neoplastic disruption of the visceral pleural elastic lamina would result in loss of mechanical stability and therefore inward puckering of thickened pleura towards the tumour. The presence of thin membranous tags between the tumour and the pleural surface, in the absence of pleural puckering, did not constitute pleural invasion. However, larger studies are required to establish the value of these methods of imaging the physical attachment of tumour to the chest wall, as inflammatory adhesions may mimic many of the findings.

Tumours at the lung apex and base are difficult to evaluate by CT (Pennes et al. 1985). Multiplanar reformations generated with spiral data acquisition may be of use at the lung base to show the relationship to the diaphragm (Brink et al. 1994). However, the longitudinal spatial resolution of even these image reformations will remain compromised by partial volume averaging at the lung apex.

Pleural disease is often observed at CT. This usually takes the form of pleural fluid, which may not be apparent on the plain chest radiograph. It generally indicates tumour dissemination. Even in the rare case where repeated cytological examinations of the fluid are negative, the outlook is poor (Decker et al. 1978). Tiny pleural nodules and thickening of the interlobar fissures may be easily overlooked, but the presence of these signs has profound significance as they may indicate T4 disease (Murayama et al. 1996).

MRI may also be used to stage chest wall extension, although initial enthusiasm has been tempered (Musset et al. 1986; Haggar et al. 1987; Mayr et al. 1992). The key observation of the thin line of extrapleural fat is perhaps more conspicuous as a bright white line on T1-weighted MRI than as a black line at CT. In a recent study, the presence of lower signal material extending within this high intensity layer was 85% sensitive for chest wall invasion (Padovani et al. 1993). However, there is overlap between signal changes from neoplastic and benign inflammatory tissues, and when prospectively compared in the RDOG study, MRI and CT had similarly disappointing accuracies (Webb et al. 1991).

It is the familiar multiplanar capability of MRI which has most to offer, particularly for cancers at the lung apex and close to the diaphragm. When aggressive multimodality treatment of superior sulcus tumours is contemplated, MRI is the imaging technique of choice (Heelan et al. 1989; Takasugi et al. 1989; McLoud et al. 1989). Extrapleural extension of tumour can be traced into the root of the neck (Fig. 2.10). Neural and vascular structures are elegantly shown. STIR sequences, surface coils and thin sections may be a helpful choice (Castagno

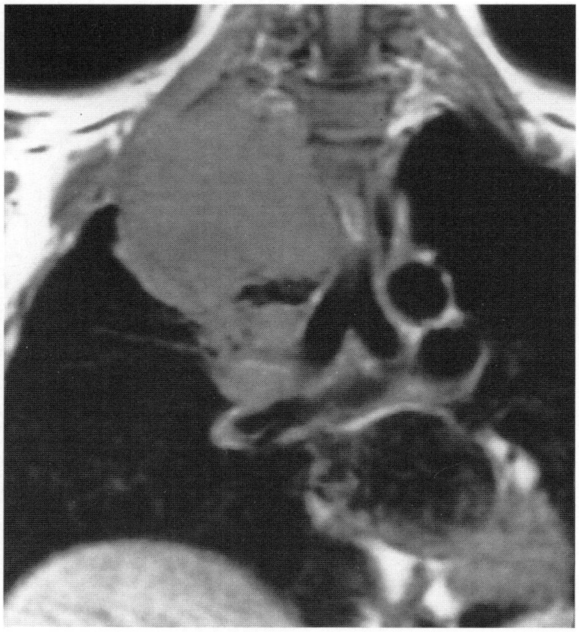

Fig. 2.10. MRI demonstration of superior sulcus tumour. Coronal T1-weighted scan shows right upper lobe adenocarcinoma extending across the extrapleural fat into the root of the neck and involving the brachial plexus

and Shuman 1987; Rapoport et al. 1988; Heelan et al. 1989; McLoud et al. 1989).

There are reports from Japan regarding the ultrasonographic assessment of chest wall invasion. Using high frequency probes, the pleural surface appears as a brightly echogenic interface. Disruption of this line suggests parietal pleural invasion. Fixation of the tumour during respiration can be observed. One report found that ultrasound was superior to CT for the diagnosis of chest wall invasion, with more than 95% sensitivity and specificity (Suzuki et al. 1993). However, these results were not confirmed by another study, which suggested that ultrasound guided biopsy was required for more reliable results (Nakano et al. 1994).

Accurate preoperative assessment of the extent of chest wall disease is helpful to the surgeon, but does not have the same critical implications for management as does the determination of inoperable T4 mediastinal invasion. This is because of the flexibility of surgical procedures. The important message is that radiology may overestimate chest wall invasion, but should not label the patient as inoperable. In the case of superior sulcus tumours, however, the clear demonstration of tumour extension into the root of the neck by MRI will influence management.

2.5 Summary: Staging Intrathoracic Non-Small Cell Lung Cancer

Thoracic CT is widely used in the pre-operative regional staging of non-small cell lung cancer. While the overall value is believed to be considerable, the limitations of CT should be clearly appreciated (Armstrong et al. 1995; Hanson and Armstrong 1997). At best, both the sensitivity and specificity for mediastinal nodal disease are of the order of 65%, and therefore biopsy confirmation should be obtained before denying a patient surgery on the basis of CT alone. Similarly, CT is poor at identifying irresectable tumours contiguous with the mediastinum or chest wall (sensitivity 25%–40%), although it has good accuracy in predicting resectability.

As yet MRI offers few established advantages over CT, but can be used effectively as a problem solving technique in specific situations. Other modalities such as ultrasound, endosonography and radionuclide imaging may find a role in resolving indeterminate CT and plain film findings.

References

Allen MS, Mathisen DJ, Grillo HC, Wain JC, Moncure AC, Hilgenberg AD (1991) Bronchogenic carcinoma with chest wall invasion. Ann Thorac Surg 51:948–951

Arita T, Matsumoto T, Kuramitsu T, Kawamura M, Matsunaga N, Sugi K, Esato K (1996) Is it possible to differentiate malignant mediastinal nodes from benign nodes by size? Reevaluation by CT, transoesophageal echocardiography and nodal specimen. Chest 110:1004–1008

Armstrong P, Wilson AG, Dee P, Hansell DM (1995) Imaging of diseases of the chest. Mosby, St Louis

Bains MS (1991) Surgical treatment of lung cancer. Chest 100:826–837

Baron RL, Levitt RG, Sagel SS, White MJ, Roper CL, Marbarger JP (1982) Computed tomography in the preoperative evaluation of bronchogenic carcinoma. Radiology 145:727–732

Batra P, Brown K, Steckel RJ, Collins JD, Ovenfors CO, Aberle D (1988) MR imaging of the thorax: a comparison of axial, coronal and sagittal imaging planes. J Comput Assist Tomogr 12:75–81

Belli L, Meroni A, Roncinara G, Beati CA (1985) Bronchoplastic procedures and pulmonary artery reconstruction in the treatment of bronchogenic cancer. J Thorac Cardiovasc Surg 90:167–171

Bollen ECM, van Duin CJ, Theunissen PH, van't Hof-Grootenboer AE, Blijham GH (1993) Mediastinal lymph node dissection in resected lung cancer: morbidity and accuracy of staging. Ann Thorac Surg 55:961–966

Bollen ECM, Goei R, van't Hof-Grootenboer AE, Versteege CWM, Engelshove HA, Lamers RJS (1994) Interobserver variability and accuracy of computed tomographic assessment of nodal status in lung cancer. Ann Thorac Surg 58:158–162

Bourgouin PM, McLoud TC, Fitzgibbon JF et al (1991) Differentiation of bronchogenic carcinoma from post-obstructive pneumonitis by magnetic resonance imaging: histopathologic correlation. J Thorac Imaging 6:22–27

Breitz HB, Sullivan K, Nelp WB (1993) Imaging lung cancer with radiolabeled antibodies. Semin Nucl Med 23:127–132

Brink J, Heiken JP, Semenkowich J, Teefey SA, McClennan BL, Sagel SS (1994) Abnormalities of the diaphragm and adjacent structures: findings on multiplanar spiral CT scans. AJR 163:307–310

Brown JS, Rudd R (1995) New staging investigations for lung cancer: what will they have to offer to be clinically useful? Eur J Nucl Med 22:497–498

Burt ME, Pomerantz AH, Bains MS, McCormack PM, Kaiser LR, Hilaris BS, Martini N (1987) Results of surgical treatment of stage III lung cancer invading the mediastinum. Surg Clin North Am 67:987–1000

Buy JN, Ghossain MA, Poirson F (1988) Computed tomography of mediastinal lymph nodes in non-small cell lung cancer: a new approach based on the lymphatic pathway of tumour spread. J Comput Assist Tomogr 12:545–552

Castagno AA, Shuman WP (1987) MR imaging in clinically suspected brachial plexus tumor. AJR 149:1219–1222

Chiti A, Maffioli LS, Infante M et al (1996) Assessment of mediastinal involvement in lung cancer with technetium-99m sestamibi SPECT. J Nucl Med 37:938–942

Cybulsky IJ, Lanza LA, Ryan B, Putnam JB, McMurtrey MM, Roth JA (1992) Prognostic significance of computed tomography in resected N2 lung cancer. Ann Thorac Surg 54:533–537

Daly BDT Jr, Faling LJ, Gunars Bite et al (1987) Mediastinal lymph node evaluation by computed tomography in lung cancer: an analysis of 345 patients grouped by TNM staging, tumour size, and tumour location. J Thorac Cardiovasc Surg 94:664–672

Daly BDT, Mueller JD, Faling LJ, Diehl JT, Bankoff MS, Karp DD, Rand WM (1993) N2 lung cancer: outcome in patients with false-negative computed tomographic scans of the chest. J Thorac Cardiovasc Surg 105:904–911

Dartevelle P, Chapelier A, Navajas M et al (1987) Replacement of the superior vena cava with polytetrafluoroethylene grafts combined with resection of mediastinal-pulmonary malignant tumors. J Thorac Cardiovasc Surg 94:361–366

Decker DA, Dines DE, Payne WS, Bernatz PE, Pairolero PC (1978) The significance of a cytologically negative pleural effusion in bronchogenic carcinoma. Chest 74:640–642

Dillemans B, Deneffe G, Verschakelen J, Decramer M (1994) Value of computed tomography and mediastinoscopy in preoperative evaluation of mediastinal nodes in non-small cell lung cancer. A study of 569 patients. Eur J Cardiothorac Surg 8:37–42

Duncan KA, Gomersall LN, Weir J (1993) Computed tomography of the chest in T1N0M0 non-small cell bronchial carcinoma. Br J Radiol 66:20–22

Friedman PJ (1988) Lung cancer: update on staging classifications. AJR 150:261–264

Gambhir SS, Hoh CK, Phelps ME, Madar I, Maddahi J (1996) Decision tree sensitivity analysis for cost-effectiveness of FDG-PET in the staging of non-small cell lung cancer. J Nucl Med 37:1428–1436

Georgian D, Rice TW, Mehta AC, Wiedemann HP, Stoller JK, O'Donovan PB (1990) Intrathoracic lymph node evaluation by CT and MRI with histopathologic correlation in non-small cell bronchogenic carcinoma. Clin Imaging 14:35–40

Ginsberg RJ (1994) Role of preoperative surgical staging in left upper lobe tumours. Ann Thorac Surg 57:526–527

Glazer GM, Gross BH, Quint LE, Francis IR, Bookstein FL, Orringer MB (1985) Normal mediastinal lymph nodes: number and size according to American Thoracic Society mapping. AJR 144:261–265

Glazer GM, Orringer MB, Chenevert TL et al (1988) Mediastinal lymph nodes: relaxation time/pathologic correlation and implications of lung cancer staging with MR imaging. Radiology 168:429–431

Glazer HS, Duncan-Meyer J, Aronberg DJ, Moran JF, Levitt RG, Sagel SS (1985) Pleural and chest wall invasion in bronchogenic carcinoma: CT evaluation. Radiology 157:191–194

Glazer HS, Kaiser LR, Anderson DJ, Molina PL, Emami B, Roper CL, Sagel SS (1989) Indeterminate mediastinal invasion in bronchogenic carcinoma: CT evaluation. Radiology 173:37–42

Goldstraw P, Mannam GC, Kaplan DK, Michail P (1994) Surgical management of non-small cell lung cancer with ipsilateral mediastinal node metastasis (N2 disease). J Thorac Cardiovasc Surg 107:19–27

Gross BH, Glazer GM, Orringer MB, Spizamy DL, Flint A (1986) Bronchogenic carcinoma metastatic to normal-sized lymph nodes: frequency and significance. Radiology 166:71–74

Grunenwald D, Mazel C, Girard P, Berthiot G, Dromer C, Baldeyrou P (1996) Total vertebrectomy for en bloc resection of lung cancer invading the spine. Ann Thorac Surg 61:723–725

Guhlmann A, Storck M, Kotzerke J, Moog F, Sunder-Plassman L, Reske SN (1997) Lymph node staging in non-small cell lung cancer: evaluation by [^{18}F]FDG positron emission tomography (PET). Thorax 52:438–441

Guyatt GH, Lefcoe M, Walter S et al (1995) Interobserver variation in the computed tomographic evaluation of mediastinal lymph node size in patients with potentially resectable lung cancer. Chest 107:116–119

Haggar AM, Pearlberg JL, Froelich JW et al (1987) Chest wall invasion by carcinoma of the lung: detection by MR imaging. AJR 148:1075–1078

Hanson JA, Armstrong P (1997) Staging intrathoracic non-small cell lung cancer. Eur Radiol 7:161–172

Harker CP, Stern EJ, Frank MS (1994) Hemidiaphragm paralysis: CT diagnosis. J Thorac Imaging 9:166–168

Hawes RH, Gress F, Kesler KA, Cummings OW, Conces DJ Jr (1994) Endoscopic ultrasound versus computed tomography in the evaluation of the mediastinum in patients with non-small cell lung cancer. Endoscopy 26:784–787

Heelan RT, Martini N, Westcott JW et al (1985) Carcinomatous involvement of the hilum and mediastinum: computed tomographic and magnetic resonance evaluation. Radiology 156:111–115

Heelan RT, Demas BE, Caravelli JF et al (1989) Superior sulcus tumors: CT and MR imaging. Radiology 170:637–641

Herman SJ, Winton Tl, Weisbrod GL, Towers MJ, Mentzer SJ (1994) Mediastinal invasion by bronchogenic carcinoma: CT signs. Radiology 190:841–846

Houston JG, Fleet M, McMillan N, Cowan MD (1995) Ultrasonic assessment of hemidiaphragmatic movement: an indirect method of evaluating mediastinal invasion in non-small cell lung cancer. Br J Radiol 68:695–699

Ikezoe J, Kadowaki K, Morimoto S (1990) Mediastinal lymph node metastases from non-small cell bronchogenic carcinoma: reevaluation with CT. J Comput Assist Tomogr 14:340–344

Ingram CE, Belli AM, Lewars MD, Reznek RH, Husband JE (1989) Normal lymph node size in the mediastinum: a retrospective study in two patient groups. Clin Radiol 40:35–39

Izbicki JR, Passlick B, Karg O, Bloechle C, Pantel K, Knoefel WT, Thetter O (1995) Impact of radical systematic mediastinal lymphadenectomy on tumor staging in lung cancer. Ann Thorac Surg 59:209–214

Kameda K, Adachi S, Kono M (1988) Detection of T-factor in lung cancer using magnetic resonance imaging and computed tomography. J Thorac Imaging 3:73–80

Kerr KM, Lamb D, Wathen CG, Walker WS, Douglas NJ (1992) Pathological assessment of mediastinal lymph nodes in lung cancer: implications for noninvasive staging. Thorax 47:337–341

Kiyono K, Sone S, Sakai F et al (1985) The number and size of normal mediastinal lymph nodes: a postmortem study. AJR 150:771–776

Kondo D, Imaizumi M, Abe T, Naruke T, Suemasu K (1990) Endoscopic ultrasound examination for mediastinal lymph node metastases of lung cancer. Chest 98:586–593

Kramer EL, Noz ME, Liebes L, Murthy S, Tiu S, Goldenberg DM (1994) Radioimmunodetection of non-small cell lung cancer using technetium-99m-anticarcinoembryonic antigen IMMU-4 Fab' fragment: preliminary results. Cancer 73:890–895

Kuriyama K, Tateishi R, Kumatani T et al (1994) Pleural invasion by peripheral bronchogenic carcinoma: assessment with three-dimensional helical CT. Radiology 191:365–369

Laissy J-P, Gay-Depassier P, Soyer P et al (1994) Enlarged mediastinal lymph nodes in bronchogenic carcinoma: assessment with dynamic contrast-enhanced MR imaging. Radiology 191:263–267

Landreneau RJ, Hazelrigg SR, Mack et al (1993) Thoracoscopic mediastinal lymph node sampling: useful for mediastinal lymph node stations inaccessible by cervical mediastinoscopy. J Thorac Cardiovasc Surg 106:554–558

Laurent F, Drouillard J, Dorcier F (1988) Bronchogenic carcinoma staging: CT vs MR imaging – assessment with surgery. Eur J Cardiothorac Surg 2:31–36

Levitt RG, Glazer HS, Roper CL, Lee JK, Murphy WA (1985) Magnetic resonance imaging of mediastinal and hilar masses: comparison with CT. AJR 145:9–14

Lewis JW Jr, Pearlberg JL, Beute GH, Alpern M, Kvale PA, Gross BH, Magilligan DJ Jr (1990) Can computed tomography of the chest stage lung cancer? Yes and no. Ann Thorac Surg 49:591–596

Libshitz HI, McKenna RJ Jr (1984) Mediastinal lymph node size in lung cancer. AJR 143:715–718

Libshitz HI, McKenna RJ Jr, Mountain CF (1986) Patterns of mediastinal metastases in bronchogenic carcinoma. Chest 90:229–232

Martini N, Flehinger BJ, Zaman MB (1983) Results of resection in non-oat cell carcinoma of the lung with mediastinal lymph node metastases. Ann Surg 198:386–397

Martini N, Heelan R, Westcott J et al (1985) Comparative merits of conventional computed tomographic and magnetic resonance imaging in assessing mediastinal involvement in surgically confirmed lung carcinoma. J Thorac Cardiovasc Surg 90:639–648

Martini N, Yellin A, Ginsberg RJ, Bains MS, Burt ME, McCormack PM, Rusch VW (1994) Management of non-small cell lung cancer with direct mediastinal involvement. Ann Thorac Surg 58:1447–1451

Mayr B, Lenhard M, Fink U, Heywang-Kobrunner SH, Sunder-Plassman L, Permanetter W (1992) Preoperative evaluation of bronchogenic carcinoma: value of MR in T- and N-staging. Eur J Radiol 14:245–251

McCaughan BC (1994) Primary lung cancer invading the chest wall. Chest Surg Clin North Am 4:17–28

McCaughan BC, Martini N, Bains MS, McCormack PM (1985) Chest wall invasion of carcinoma of the lung: therapeutic and prognostic implications. J Thorac Cardiovasc Surg 89:836–841

McKenna RJ, Libshitz HI, Mountain CF, McMurtrey MM (1985) Roentgenographic evaluation of mediastinal nodes for preoperative assessment in lung cancer. Chest 88:206–210

McLoud TC (1989) CT of bronchogenic carcinoma: indeterminate mediastinal invasion. Radiology 173:15–16

McLoud TC, Filion RB, Edelman RR, Shepard JA (1989) MR imaging of superior sulcus carcinoma. J Comput Assist Tomogr 13:233–239

McLoud TC, Bourgouin PM, Greenberg RW et al (1992) Bronchogenic carcinoma: analysis of staging in the mediastinum with CT by correlative lymph node mapping and sampling. Radiology 182:319–323

Miller JI, Mansour KA, Hatcher CR (1979) Carcinoma of the superior pulmonary sulcus. Ann Thorac Surg 28:44–47

Mountain CF (1994) Surgery for stage IIIa-N2 non-small cell lung cancer. Cancer 73:2589–2598

Mountain CF (1997) Revisions in the International System for Staging Lung Cancer. Chest 111:1710–1717

Mountain CF, Dresler CM (1997) Regional lymph node classification for lung cancer staging. Chest 111:1718–1723

Murata K, Takahashi M, Mori M et al (1994) Chest wall and mediastinal invasion by lung cancer: evaluation by multisection expiratory dynamic CT. Radiology 191:251–255

Murayama S, Murakami J, Yoshimitsu K, Torii Y, Ishida T, Masuda K (1996) CT diagnosis of pleural dissemination without pleural effusion in primary lung cancer. Radiat Med 14:117–119

Musset D, Grenier P, Carette MF et al (1986) Primary lung cancer staging: prospective comparative study of MR imaging with CT. Radiology 160:607–611

Nakahara K, Ohno K, Mastumura K et al (1989) Extended operation for lung cancer invading the aortic arch and superior vena cava. J Thorac Cardiovasc Surg 97:428–433

Nakano N, Yasumitsu T, Kotake Y, Morino H, Ikezoe J (1994) Preoperative histologic diagnosis of chest wall invasion by lung cancer using ultrasonically guided biopsy. J Thorac Cardiovasc Surg 107:891–895

Naruke T, Goya T, Tsuchiya R, Suemasu K (1988a) Prognosis and survival in resected lung carcinoma based on the new international staging system. J Thorac Cardiovasc Surg 96:440–447

Naruke T, Goya T, Tsuchiya R, Suemasu K (1988b). The importance of surgery to non-small cell carcinoma of lung with mediastinal lymph node metastasis. Ann Thorac Surg 46:603–610

Onitsuka H, Tsukuda M, Araki A, Murakami J, Torii Y, Masuda K (1991) Differentiation of central lung tumor from postobstructive lobar collapse by rapid sequence computed tomography. J Thorac Imaging 6:28–31

Osborne DR, Korobkin M, Ravin CE et al (1982) Comparison of plain radiography, conventional tomography and computed tomography in detecting intrathoracic metastases from lung carcinoma. Radiology 142:157–161

Padovani B, Mouroux J, Seksik L et al (1993) Chest wall invasion by bronchogenic carcinoma: evaluation with MR imaging. Radiology 187:33–38

Patterson GA, Ginsberg RJ, Poon et al (1987) A prospective evaluation of magnetic resonance imaging, computed tomography, and mediastinoscopy in the preoperative assessment of mediastinal node status in bronchogenic carcinoma. J Thorac Cardiovasc Surg 94:679–684

Paulson DL (1979) Carcinoma in the superior pulmonary sulcus. Ann Thorac Surg 28:3–4

Pearlberg JL, Sandler MA, Beute GH, Madrazo BL (1985) T1N0M0 bronchogenic carcinoma: assessment by CT. Radiology 157:187–190

Pearlberg JL, Sandler MA, Beute GH, Lewis JR Jr, Madrazo BL (1987) Limitations of CT in evaluation of neoplasms involving chest wall. J Comput Assist Tomogr 11:290–293

Pearson FG, DeLarue NC, Ilves R, Todd TRJ, Cooper JD (1982) Significance of positive superior mediastinal nodes identified at mediastinoscopy in patients with resectable cancer of the lung. J Thorac Cardiovasc Surg 83:1–11

Pennes DR, Glazer GM, Wimbish KJ, Gross BH, Long RW, Orringer MB (1985) Chest wall invasion by lung cancer: limitations of CT evaluation. AJR 144:507–511

Piehler JM, Pairolero PC, Weiland LH, Offord KP, Payne WS, Bernatz PE (1982) Bronchogenic carcinoma with chest wall invasion: factors influencing survival following enbloc resection. Ann Thorac Surg 34:684–691

Poon PY, Bronskill MJ, Henkelman RM et al (1987) Mediastinal lymph node metastases from bronchogenic carcinoma: detection with MR imaging and CT. Radiology 162:651–656

Potepan P, Meroni E, Spagnoli I et al (1996) Non-small-cell lung cancer: detection of mediastinal lymph node metastases by endoscopic ultrasound and CT. Eur Radiol 6:19–24

Protopapas Z, Weskott JL (1996) Transthoracic needle biopsy of mediastinal lymph nodes for staging lung and other cancers. Radiology 199:489–496

Quint LE, Glazer GM, Orringer MB (1987) Central lung masses: prediction with CT of need for pneumonectomy versus lobectomy. Radiology 165:735–738

Rapoport S, Blair DN, McCarthy SM, Desser TS, Hammers LW, Sostman HD (1988) Brachial plexus: correlation of MR imaging with CT and pathologic findings. Radiology 167:161–165

Remy-Jardin M, Remy J (1996) Spiral CT of the chest. Springer, Berlin Heidelberg New York

Remy-Jardin M, Duyck P, Remy J et al (1995) Hilar lymph nodes: identification with spiral CT and histologic correlation. Radiology 196:387–394

Rendina EA, Venuta F, De Giacomo T et al (1994) Comparative merits of thoracoscopy, mediastinoscopy, and mediastinotomy for mediastinal biopsy. Ann Thorac Surg 57:992–995

Roviaro G, Varoli F, Rebuffat C et al (1995) Videothoracoscopic staging and treatment of lung cancer. Ann Thorac Surg 59:971–974

Rusch VW, Albain KS, Crowley JJ et al (1993a) Surgical resection of stage IIIA and stage IIIB non-small cell lung cancer after concurrent induction chemoradiotherapy. A Southwest Oncology Group trial. J Thorac Cardiovasc Surg 105:97–104

Rusch V, Macapinlac H, Heelan R et al (1993b) NR-LU-10 monoclonal antibody scanning: a helpful new adjunct to computed tomography in evaluating non-small cell lung cancer. J Thorac Cardiovasc Surg 106:200–204

Schnyder PA, Gamsu G (1981) CT of the pretracheal retrocaval space. AJR 136:303–308

Scott IR, Muller NL, Miller RR, Evans KG, Nelems B (1988) Resectable stage III lung cancer: CT, surgical and pathologic correlation. Radiology 166:75–79

Scott WJ, Schwabe JL, Gupta NC, Dewan NC, Reeb SD, Sugimoto JT, and members of the PET-Lung Tumour Study Group (1994) Positron emission tomography of lung tumors and mediastinal lymph nodes using [F-18] fluorodeoxyglucose. Ann Thorac Surg 58:698–703

Seely JM, Mayo JR, Miller RR, Muller NL (1993) T1 lung cancer: prevalence of mediastinal nodal metastases and diagnostic accuracy of CT. Radiology 186:129–132

Shirakawa T, Fukuda K, Miyamoto Y, Tanabe H, Tada S (1994) Parietal pleural invasion of lung masses: evaluation with CT performed during deep inspiration and expiration. Radiology 192:809–811

Staples CA, Muller NL, Miller RR, Evans KG, Nelems RG (1988) Mediastinal nodes in bronchogenic carcinoma: comparison between CT and mediastinoscopy. Radiology 167:367–372

Steinert HC, Hauser M, Allemann F, Engel H, Bethold T, von Schulthess GK, Weder W (1997) Non-small cell lung cancer: nodal staging with FDG PET versus CT with correlative lymph node mapping and sampling. Radiology 202:441–446

Stiglbauer R, Schurawitzki H, Klepetko W, Kramer J, Schratter M, Tscholakoff D, Eckersberger F (1991) Contrast-enhanced MRI for the staging of bronchogenic carcinoma: comparison with CT and histopathologic staging – preliminary results. Clin Radiol 44:293–298

Suzuki N, Saitoh T, Kitamura S (1993) Tumor invasion of the chest wall in lung cancer: diagnosis with US. Radiology 187:39–42

Takasugi JE, Rapoport S, Shaw C (1989) Superior sulcus tumours: the role of imaging. J Thorac Imaging 4:41–48

Tateishi M, Fukuyama Y, Hamatake M, Kohdono S, Ishida T, Sugimachi K (1994) Skip mediastinal lymph node metastasis in non-small cell lung cancer. J Surg Oncol 57:139–142

Tatsumura T (1995) Preoperative and intraoperative ultrasonographic examination as an aid in lung cancer operations. J Thorac Cardiovasc Surg 110:606–612

Tobler J, Levitt RG, Glazer HS, Moran J, Crouch E, Evens RG (1987) Differentiation of proximal bronchogenic carcinoma from postobstructive lobar collapse by magnetic resonance imaging. Invest Radiol 22:538–543

Tschiuya R, Asamura H, Kondo H, Goya T, Naruke T (1994) Extended resection of the left atrium, great vessels, or both for lung cancer. Ann Thorac Surg 57:960–965

Wahl RL, Quint LE, Greenough RL, Meyer CR, White RI, Orringer MB (1994) Staging of mediastinal non-small cell lung cancer with FDG PET, CT and fusion images: preliminary prospective evaluation. Radiology 191:371–377

Webb WR, Gamsu G, Stark DD, Moon KL Jr, Moore EH (1984) Magnetic resonance imaging of the normal and abnormal pulmonary hila. Radiology 178:705–713

Webb WR, Jensen BG, Sollitto R, Geer G de, McCowin M, Gamsu G, Moore E (1985) Bronchogenic carcinoma: staging with MR compared with CT and surgery. Radiology 156:117–124

Webb WR, Gatsonis C, Zerhouni EA, Heelan RT, Glazer GM, Francis IR, McNeil BJ (1991) CT and MR imaging in staging non-small cell bronchogenic carcinoma: report of the Radiologic Diagnostic Oncologic Group. Radiology 178:705–713

Webb WR, Sarin M, Zerhouni EA, Heelan RT, Glazer GM, Gatsonis C (1993) Interobserver variability in CT and MR staging of lung cancer. J CAT 17:841–846

White PG, Adams H, Crane MD, Butchart EG (1994) Preoperative staging of carcinoma of the bronchus: can computed tomographic scanning reliably identify stage III tumours? Thorax 49:951–957

Wiersema MJ, Kochman ML, Cramer HM, Wiersema LM (1994) Preoperative staging of non-small cell lung cancer: transoesophageal US-guided fine-needle aspiration biopsy of mediastinal lymph nodes. Radiology 190:239–242

Yokoi K, Mori K, Miyazawa N, Saito Y, Okuyama A, Sasagawa M (1991) Tumor invasion of the chest wall and mediastinum in lung cancer: evaluation with pneumothorax CT. Radiology 181:147–152

Yokoi K, Okuyama A, Mori K, Tominaga K, Miyazawa N, Takizawa I, Sasagawa M (1994) Mediastinal lymph node metastasis from lung cancer: evaluation with Tl-201 SPECT – comparison with CT. Radiology 192:813–817

3 Positron Emission Tomography: A New Tool in Diagnosing, Staging, and Treatment Monitoring of Lung Cancer

C. SCHIEPERS

CONTENTS

3.1 Introduction

Lung cancer is presently the most common cancer in the United States and its incidence around the world is increasing. Early detection and subsequent treatment have led to an improved survival in certain types of cancer, but major problems remain both in detection and staging of disease. The type most frequently seen is non-small cell cancer (NSCLC). Anatomic imaging modalities such as computed tomography (CT) and magnetic resonance imaging (MRI) have superb resolution, but cannot always reliably differentiate a benign from a malignant lesion. Certain parameters such as lesion size and absence of calcification may indicate a higher likelihood of being malignant, but definite diagnosis still relies on invasive procedures such as bronchoscopy and percutaneous or open biopsy to provide tissue specimens for histopathology.

As has been pointed out by various authors, the sensitivity and specificity of staging with CT and MRI is rather low (WEBB et al. 1991; DALES et al. 1990; MCLOUD et al. 1992; DILLEMANS et al. 1994). In the prospective NIH sponsored trial of the RDOC (Radiological Diagnostic Oncology Group) in staging NSCLC, CT had a sensitivity of 52% and MRI 48%, and a somewhat higher specificity for both modalities with 69% for CT and 64% for MRI (WEBB et al. 1991). This is not too surprising given the size criteria that are used in differentiating benign from malignant tissue.

Positron emission tomography (PET) is also a tomographic method, based on imaging of biochemical processes in vivo, such as glucose or oxygen metabolism or synthesis of proteins and nucleic acids. The application of PET as a clinical tool has expanded in recent years, and presently this sophisticated technique is available in most of the major university hospitals. Currently, there is an enormous growth of PET centers in Europe. PET is unique since it creates functional images by exploiting fundamental biochemical properties of tissues, and thus reveals differences between benign and malignant disease. At the cellular level, Warburg observed in 1930 that increased glucose consumption was a marker of the malignant state and "aerobic glycolysis" was accelerated with increasing grades of tumor (WARBURG 1930, 1956). More recently, elevated numbers of glucose transporters have been identified in neoplastic tissue, responsible for the increased uptake and metabolism. This is both at the level of glucose membrane transporters and key enzymes of the glycolytic pathway. Most of the experience in PET oncology has been using a tracer which is a glucose analogue: FDG (^{18}F-fluoro-deoxy-glucose). The images are of high quality and are easy to interpret. Tumor tissue perfusion has also been investigated and studies have been performed with flow tracers such as ^{15}O-water and ^{13}N-ammonia. In general, flow varies greatly between tumor types and is not clearly associated with disease prognosis. The oxygen metabolism experience is limited because of the requirement of an on-site cyclotron and time consuming data acquisition and processing. Studies with amino acids such as methionine, tyrosine, and leucine have been done with success, but the signal is

C. SCHIEPERS, UCLA School of Medicine, Nuclear Medicine, CHS-AR144, 10833 Le Conte Avenue, Los Angeles, CA 90095-6942, USA

weaker than with FDG. Thymidine, presumably, is the best marker for tumor proliferation, but studies so far are limited and the signal is even weaker than that obtained with amino acids (Hawkins et al. 1992). In this overview we will mainly deal with FDG as the tumor tracer of choice for PET in oncology.

Recently, several reviews have been published on the applicability of nuclear medicine techniques in lung cancer (Abdel-Dayem et al. 1994), or the emerging role of PET in oncology (Rigo et al. 1996; Hoh et al. 1997).

3.2 Imaging Method

The typical PET oncology protocol is usually performed with a dedicated PET system, which includes a positron camera, a fast computer, and sophisticated hardware and software to reconstruct and display the images.

The patient preparation consists of a prolonged fast (>6 h), preferably overnight, to decrease glucose consumption of the normal tissues. A dose of 350–500 MBq (10–15 mCi) FDG is administered, and after an uptake period the images are acquired. An interval of 60–90 min after tracer administration is usually sufficient to achieve increased uptake in abnormal tissues relative to normal lung activity. Images that are generated are discussed in the following paragraphs.

3.2.1 Static Tomographic Imaging

Transverse slices of selected body areas are reconstructed, from which coronal and sagittal planes can be extracted and displayed as volumetric datasets (Hawkins et al. 1992). The axial size of the images is determined by the scanner, and is 10–25 cm in current systems. PET images can be acquired:

3.2.1.1 With Attenuation Correction

The images can be corrected for the loss of photons traveling through the tissues. This is done by acquisition of a separate transmission scan which has to be performed before tracer administration in older PET systems. In the newer generation PET scanners this can be done after tracer injection, thereby allowing the tracer uptake period to be done outside the scanner, which will enhance patient throughput. This acquisition mode also permits true quantitation of metabolic activity in units of micromoles per minute per gram.

3.2.1.2 Without Attenuation Correction

These images only permit visual interpretation; quantitative analysis is not possible.

3.2.2 Whole Body Imaging

This imaging mode was introduced in the late 1980s by UCLA School of Medicine, and subsequently became the standard for PET imaging in oncology (Hawkins et al. 1992; Hoh et al. 1993). The main advantage is the large size of covered area, i.e., 80–150 cm, which greatly facilitates interpretation by supplying body landmarks.

1. Planar projections are created, in which the total activity distribution is viewed from different angles around the patient. A rotating cine display is subsequently used to inspect the data and to focus on specific zones.
2. Tomographic slices (transverse, coronal and sagittal) are reconstructed for volumetric review of the whole body. This is the favorite mode for diagnosing and staging of disease outside the limited primary field of view, i.e., thorax. In general, these images are not corrected for attenuation, since that would increase acquisition times prohibitively. However, new techniques and algorithms are being investigated to overcome this problem.

The spatial resolution of a modern CT or MRI system is much better than that of a PET system. However, this is not the only determining factor in detecting abnormalities. The ratio between metabolic activity of the lesion and its surroundings (tissue-to-background ratio) or the "contrast" resolution helps determine the presence of disease. Thus, very active metabolic lesions of 5 mm have been detected with FDG-PET. As a rule of thumb, the attenuation corrected PET can detect lesions of about 1 cm and with the nonattenuation corrected whole-body PET technique the lower limit is around 1.5 cm.

3.3 Image Interpretation

Besides visual interpretation of the images, in which abnormally increased uptake is localized, various quantitative methods have been developed. PET with FDG is a true quantitative technique that provides estimates of the glucose metabolism in micromoles per minute per gram of selected lesions, but this requires arterial blood sampling and dynamic imaging over the entire tracer uptake period (Nolop et al. 1987; Minn et al. 1995). Thus, the procedure is complicated and performed mainly for research purposes. In clinical practice, a simpler quantitative approach is used such as the SUV (standardized uptake value), which is the ratio of the tracer concentration in the lesion relative to the expected tracer distribution if the injected dose were distributed uniformly throughout the body. For a lung lesion, an SUV of 2.5 or more indicates a 96% probability for neoplasm, whereas a value of 2.0 or less is predictive of a benign lesion or normal tissue (Zasadny et al. 1996; Miyauchi and Wahl 1996; Knopp et al. 1990).

In Fig. 3.1 a typical patient is presented in which the work-up diagnosed stage III disease. The PET was ordered and confirmed stage IIIA disease and ruled out distant metastases (stage IV), for which surgery is not an option.

False positive results have been reported, mainly inflammatory in nature. In the thorax these include: tuberculosis, fungal infections, sarcoidosis, nonspecific granulomas, suture granulomas, benign fibrous

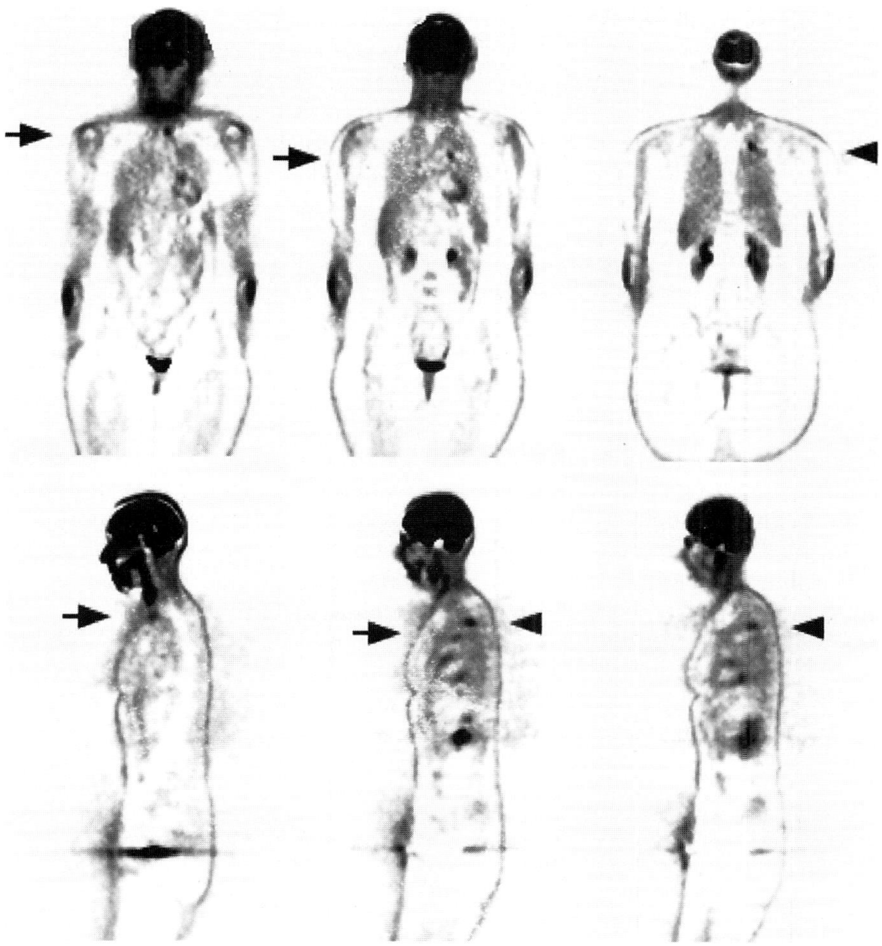

Fig. 3.1. Coronal (*top row*) and sagittal images obtained with FDG PET of a 39-year-old white woman. She presented with bilateral joint swelling of both lower extremities. A routine chest radiograph revealed a left upper lobe mass, not seen on prior chest films. CT showed lymph adenopathy and was considered stage III. PET revealed the primary lesion (*arrowhead*) and two affected lymph nodes (*arrows on the left side of the image*, indicating level). There was no contralateral or distal disease, rendering this stage IIIA. Subsequent surgery confirmed the absence of contra-lateral lymph node involvement

mesotheliomas, acute postoperative and radiation changes.

3.4 Clinical Applications

In reviewing the literature, studies were selected that met the criteria of being published in peer reviewed journals. Abstracts were, therefore, not considered. The papers have been subdivided into initial attempts and feasibility studies of PET in lung cancer. Subsequently, two well established indications, reimbursed by most insurance companies, will be discussed. Finally, the diagnosis of recurrent disease and monitoring of therapy are dealt with.

A first problem encountered in this review process was the publication of the same group of data (or subsets) by different authors from the same institution. This was especially the case in the characterization of lung nodules. The most active in this respect were the Duke and Creighton University groups. Moreover, these data were also included in the multicenter trial. Fortunately, in the staging of lung cancer, a greater variety of institutions from different countries reported results, with well defined study groups, a prospective approach and mainly NSCLC. The number of studies that have evaluated therapy response is still limited.

3.4.1 Initial Studies

The first imaging attempts revealed increased FDG uptake in lung tumors and shed light on the utility of the technique. In 1987 the Hammersmith group showed in vivo the applicability of PET in pulmonary neoplasms (Nolop et al. 1987). The average tumor uptake was sevenfold increased over normal lung tissue.

In 1990, Knopp and colleagues from Heidelberg reported a study on 80 patients at the annual meeting of the Radiological Society in Chicago. This was an early prospective study which showed very high sensitivity and specificity in detecting bronchogenic carcinoma. High FDG uptake in adenopathy revealed tumor involvement at histology in all cases. PET provided additional information to CT and MR, and tumor stage was changed in 20% of patients. Unfortunately, this study was never published in an international journal.

Kubota and colleagues (1988, 1990, 1992, 1993) have studied lung cancer with two different tracers: FDG to evaluate the glucose metabolism and methionine for the protein synthesis. They have reported their results and favor methionine as the tracer of choice. However, the short half-life of C-11 (20 min) makes an on-site cyclotron necessary for the production of the radiopharmaceutical, limiting its use to those centers.

The first study using the whole body technique in lung cancer was published by Rege et al. from UCLA (Rege et al. 1993). In 4/16 patients extrathoracic metastases were detected. Several other centers attempted to characterize chest masses with FDG. In these studies a semiquantitative criterion of SUV >2.5 was used to diagnose malignancy (Lewis et al. 1994; Hubner et al. 1995; Sazon et al. 1996; Slosman et al. 1993). Table 3.1 gives an overview of early PET imaging studies and their indication.

3.4.2 Solitary Pulmonary Nodules

The first well-established application of PET in lung cancer was the characterization of solitary pulmonary nodules (size <4 cm) and/or chest masses. CT cannot reliably distinguish benign from malignant nodules (Keogan et al. 1993). The utility of FDG-PET in indeterminate lung nodules has been extensively evaluated and yields sensitivities over 90% as reported by various institutions (Dewan et al. 1993, 1995; Scott et al. 1994; Patz et al. 1993; Gupta et al.

Table 3.1. Early reports on PET with FDG in the detection, assessment of extent and work-up of lung cancer

Author	Year	Tumor type	Patients	True positive	PET technique	Objective
Nolop et al.	1987	Mixed	12	12/12	Cross sectional	Tumor glucose consumption
Abe et al.	1990	Mixed	5	5/5	Cross sectional	Therapy response
Kubota et al.	1990	Mixed	22	10/12	Cross sectional	Characterization masses
Rege et al.	1993	Mixed	16	14/16	Whole body	Lesion detection
Lewis et al.	1994	NSCLC	34	34/34	Whole body	Surgical management
Slosman et al.	1993	Mixed	31	29/31	Cross sectional	Pre-op. evaluation

Table 3.2. Overview of sensitivity (*Sens*), specificity (*Spec*), positive and negative predictive value (*PPV, NPV*) PET in the differentiation of solitary pulmonary nodules between benign and malignant, and study design

Author	Year	Patients	Study	Comparison	Sens	Spec	PPV	NPV
Dewan et al.	1993	30	Prospective	CT+biopsy	95	80	90	89
Scott et al.	1994	62	Retrospective	CT+biopsy	94	80	94	80
Dewan et al.	1995	33	Retrospective	TTNA[a]	100	78	93	100
Patz et al.	1993	51	Prospective	CT+biopsy	89	100		
Duhaylongsod et al.	1995b	100	Retrospective	CT+biopsy	97	82		
ICP	1993	237	Retrospective	CT+biopsy	96	90		
Lowe et al.	1997	197	Retrospective	CT+biopsy	96	77	86	92

[a] Trans thoracic needle aspiration.

1992; Duhaylongsod et al. 1995; Lowe et al. 1994, 1997; see Table 3.2). In general, false positive PET lesions can easily be assessed by conventional radiography. Thus, the FDG-PET scan was best suited after conventional imaging to discriminate a suspicious nodule of being benign or malignant.

The researchers from Duke University published several papers on the classification of pulmonary nodules, initiated the first multicenter trial, and proposed an algorithm for screening which is cost effective (Patz et al. 1993; Gupta et al. 1992; Duhaylongsod et al. 1995a; Lowe et al. 1994). Authors from different institutions have corroborated these findings (Hubner et al. 1995; Sazon et al. 1996; Slosman et al. 1993) and the Institute of Clinical PET (ICP) presented the data of ten participating centers in 1994. The pulmonary task force of the ICP has developed algorithms for solitary pulmonary nodules based on this multicenter study. This investigation has convincingly demonstrated that a reduction in costs can be obtained if PET were included after the conventional work-up and before performing a CT of the chest.

The latest report from Lowe et al. (1997) on 197 patients in the Duke University series revealed a lower specificity, which the authors attributed to a "verification bias," i.e., the referring physicians no longer chose biopsy to verify "negative" PET studies.

Dewan et al. (1995) have shown PET with FDG to be highly accurate and as efficacious as transthoracic needle aspiration without the morbidity of the latter. PET is an attractive alternate non-invasive procedure in the management of suspicious pulmonary nodules.

3.4.3 Mediastinal Staging

The second major field of application in lung cancer concerns the presurgical staging of nodes in the mediastinum. The relevance of the mediastinum is related to the close correspondence between disease involvement and prognosis. Also, distant metastases can be evaluated with PET, e.g., the presence of contralateral metastases excludes surgery as a therapeutic option (see Fig. 3.1).

Dales et al. (1990) in their meta-analysis study of 1990 have argued that non-invasive detection of lymph node metastasis must await an approach fundamentally different from the node size determination. In the prospective NIH sponsored trial of the RDOC (Webb et al. 1991), both CT and MR imaging had a sensitivity around 50% and a somewhat higher specificity around 65%. These results are not unexpected since node size is the criterion for diagnosing cancer. On the other hand, in about one-third of nodes with sizes between 2 and 4 cm no tumor cells were detected with histopathology. Similar reports on the relative insensitivity of CT have come from Harvard (McLoud et al. 1992) and Belgium (Dillemans et al. 1994).

Wahl and associates (1994) have established that metabolic imaging with FDG PET is considerably more accurate than CT in staging mediastinal involvement with non-small cell cancer. They emphasized that these findings are not totally unexpected given the tumor localizing properties of FDG. Minn et al. (1995), also at the University of Michigan, studied the reproducibility of quantitative indices in lung cancer and obtained variations of 5%–6%. Subsequent studies (Chin et al. 1995; Valk et al. 1995) underscore the excellent results in assessing disease involvement of the mediastinum.

The whole-body PET technique is not only able to evaluate the primary lesion and mediastinum, but is especially suited for detection of occult metastases and/or disease involvement of lymphadenopathy. Various studies are available in the literature revealing for PET a sensitivity of about 85% and a specificity of 90%, which compares favorably to 60% and 80%, respectively, for CT in the same groups of

Table 3.3. Results on sensitivity (*Sens*) and specificity (*Spec*) of CT and PET with FDG in lymph node assessment staging of the mediastinum

Author	Year	Patients	Histology	CT		PET	
				Sens	Spec	Sens	Spec
WAHL et al.	1994	23	NSCLC	64	44	82	81
CHIN et al.	1995	30	NSCLC	56	86	78	81
VALK et al.	1995	76	NSCLC	63	73	83	94
SASAKI et al.	1996	29	NSCLC	65	87	76	98
BURY et al.	1996	50	NSCLC	72	81	90	86
GUHLMANN et al.	1997	46	NSCLC	50	75	80	100
STEINERT et al.	1997	47	NSCLC	57	94	89	99

patients (Table 3.3). To date, the largest series is from VALK et al. (1995).

The findings of the aforementioned institutions have now been corroborated in Japan by SASAKI et al. (1996), in Belgium by BURY et al. (1996), in Germany by GUHLMANN et al. (1997), and in Switzerland by STEINERT et al. (1997). Table 3.3 gives an overview of lymph node staging of lung cancer reported in peer reviewed journals.

GAMBHIR et al. (1996) have performed a study on cost-effectiveness of FDG-PET in NSCLC staging and management. By using rigorous decision tree analysis, they were able to show that CT plus PET was the most economical way to work up primary lung cancer, with a marginal increase in patient life expectancy when compared with staging by CT alone.

Based on the evidence above, it is warranted to conclude that PET has a place in pre-operative staging of NSCLC.

3.4.4 Diagnosis of Recurrence

A third application for PET in lung cancer is the detection of recurrence, in other words re-staging of the patient during the routine work-up. The major contribution is the evaluation for distant metastases, detection of occult disease, and staging of the mediastinum. Thus, the certainty for selecting surgical candidates may be enhanced. This may be considered as a special case of staging as discussed under 3.4.3. Studies that specifically addressed recurrence are those of PATZ et al. (1994), FRANK et al. (1995), INOUE et al. (1995), and KUBOTA et al. (1992).

3.4.5 Therapy Monitoring

The fourth area where PET is a valuable adjunct is assessment of response to treatment (ABE et al. 1990; HEBERT et al. 1996; HAMBERG et al. 1994; DUHAYLONGSOD et al. 1995b). Usually, metabolic indices change earlier than tumor size as detected with morphological imaging modalities such as CT and MRI. However, inflammatory changes may cause false positive responses and need to be excluded. The effect of chemotherapy alone was studied by ABE et al. (1990), and of radiation therapy by HEBERT et al. (1996). Results on combination therapy were reported by HAMBERG et al. (1994) and KUBOTA et al. (1993).

In general, the changes due to radiation therapy last longer than those of chemotherapy. Therefore, repeat PET studies should be interspaced 4–8 weeks after chemo- and 2–3 months after radiotherapy. Further research is needed to clarify this.

3.4.6 Future Outlook

Different tracers can be utilized such as labeled amino acids or peptides, but at present only a few studies have been reported. An interesting tracer is FMISO, which is a hypoxia binding radiopharmaceutical, and therefore well suited to evaluate the effects of radiation therapy (RASEY et al. 1996). Also, conventional nuclear medicine tracers such as thallium-201 chloride and technetium-99m sestamibi have been used in lung cancer. Only one study has directly compared the value of sestamibi to FDG-PET in the same group of patients (WANG et al.

1997). More studies are necessary to elucidate the scope of these tracers in clinical practice.

3.5 Conclusions

Established indications for PET imaging in lung cancer are the following:

1. Diagnosis: Differentiation of solitary or indeterminate lung nodules as benign or malignant.
2. Staging: In newly diagnosed patients, especially for node involvement; to evaluate suspicious lesions seen on anatomic imaging modalities and their extent; detection of distant disease.

At this moment there are limited data available to suggest that PET is valuable for:

1. Restaging: Evaluation of recurrent tumor and involved nodes. Detection of occult metastases.
2. Therapy monitoring: Evaluation of response to surgery, radiation and/or chemotherapy. Tumor glucose metabolism changes rapidly in patients responding to treatment.

References

Abdel-Dayem HM, Scott A, Macapinlac H, Larson S (1994) Tracer imaging in lung cancer. Eur J Nucl Med 21:57–81

Abe Y, Matzuzawa T, Fujiwara T et al (1990) Clinical assessment of therapeutic effects on cancer using FDG and PET: preliminary study of lung cancer. Int J Radiat Oncol Biol Phys 19:1005–1010

Bury T, Dowlati A, Paulus P et al (1996) Staging of non-small-cell lung cancer by whole-body fluorine-18 deoxyglucose positron emission tomography. Eur J Nucl Med 23:204–206

Chin R Jr, Ward R, Keyes JW et al (1995) Mediastinal staging of non-small-cell lung cancer with positron emission tomography. Am J Respir Critic Care Med 152:2090–2096

Dales RE, Stark RM, Raman S (1990) Computed tomography to stage lung cancer: approaching a controversy using meta-analysis. Am Rev Respir Dis 141:1096–1101

Dewan NA, Gupta NC, Redepenning LS et al (1993) Diagnostic efficacy of PET-FDG in solitary pulmonary nodules. Chest 104:997–1002

Dewan NA, Reeb SD, Gupta NC, Gobar LS, Scott WJ (1995) PET-FDG imaging and trans-thoracic needle lung aspiration biopsy in evaluation of pulmonary lesions: a comparative risk-benefit analysis. Chest 108:441–446

Dillemans B, Deneffe G, Verschakelen J, Decramer M (1994) Value of computed tomography and mediastinoscopy in preoperative evaluation of mediastinal nodes in non-small cell lung cancer. Eur J Cardio Thorac Surg 8:37–42

Duhaylongsod FG, Lowe VJ, Patz EF Jr et al (1995a) Detection of primary and recurrent lung cancer by means of F-18 fluorodeoxyglucose positron emission tomography (FDG PET). J Thor Cardiovasc Surg 110:130–140

Duhaylongsod FG, Lowe VJ, Patz EF Jr et al (1995b) Lung tumor growth correlates with glucose metabolism measured by fluoride-18 FDG-PET. Ann Thorac Surg 60:1348–1352

Frank A, Lefkowitz D, Jaeger S et al (1995) Decision logic for retreatment of asymptomatic lung cancer recurrence based on positron emission tomography findings. Int J Rad Oncol Biol Phys 32:1495–1512

Gambhir SS, Hoh CK, Phelps ME, Madar I, Maddahi J (1996) Decision tree sensitivity analysis for cost-effectiveness of FDG-PET in the staging and management of non-small-cell lung carcinoma. J Nucl Med 37:1428–1436

Guhlmann A, Storck M, Kotzerke J et al (1997) Lymph node staging in non-small cell lung cancer: evaluation by [^{18}F]FDG positron emission tomography (PET). Thorax 52:438–441

Gupta NC, Frank AR, Dewan NA et al (1992) Solitary pulmonary nodules: detection of malignancy with PET with FDG. Radiology 184:441–444

Hamberg LM, Hunter GJ, Alpert NM et al (1994) The dose uptake ratio as an index of glucose metabolism: useful parameter or oversimplification? J Nucl Med 35:1308–1312

Hawkins RA, Hoh CK, Glaspy et al (1992) The role of positron emission tomography in oncology and other whole body applications. Semin Nucl Med 22:268–284

Hebert ME, Lowe VJ, Hoffman JM, Patz EF, Anscher MS (1996) Positron emission tomography in the pretreatment evaluation and follow-up of non-small cell lung cancer patients treated with radiotherapy: preliminary findings. Am J Clin Oncol 19:416–421

Hoh CK, Hawkins RA, Glaspy JA et al (1993) Cancer detection with whole-body PET using 2-[^{18}F]fluoro-2-deoxy-D-glucose. J Comp Assist Tomogr 17:582–589

Hoh CK, Schiepers C, Seltzer MA et al (1997) PET in oncology: will it replace the other modalities? Semin Nucl Med 27:94–106

Hubner KF, Buonocore E, Singh SK et al (1995) Characterization of chest masses by FDG PET. Clin Nucl Med 20:293–298

ICP (1997) ICP Solitary Pulmonary Nodule Task Force (R. Edward Coleman, Chair) Clinical application and economic implications of PET in the assessment of solitary pulmonary nodules: a retrospective study. *For reprints contact*: Institute for Clinical PET, 11781 Lee Jackson Memorial Highway, Suite 360, Fairfax, VA 22033, USA

Inoue T, Kim EE, Komaki R et al (1995) Detecting recurrent or residual lung cancer with FDG-PET. J Nucl Med 36:788–793

Keogan MT, Tung KT, Kaplan DK et al (1993) The significance of pulmonary nodules detected on CT staging for lung cancer. Clin Radiol 48:94–96

Knopp MV, Strauss LG, Haberkorn U et al (1990) PET of the thorax: assessment of its clinical application in tumor staging. Radiology 177:174

Kubota K, Matzuzawa TM, Fujiwara T et al (1988) Differential diagnosis of solitary pulmonary nodules with PET using C-11 methionine. J Comput Assist Tomogr 12:794–796

Kubota K, Matzuzawa T, Fujiwara T et al (1990) Differential diagnosis of lung tumor with positron emission tomography: a prospective study. J Nucl Med 31:1927–1933

Kubota K, Yamada S, Ishiwata K, Ito M, Ido T (1992) Positron emission tomography for treatment evaluation and recurrence detection compared with CT in long-term follow-up cases of lung cancer. Clin Nucl Med 17:877–881

Kubota K, Yamada S, Ishiwata K et al (1993) Evaluation of the treatment response of lung cancer with positron emission tomography and L-[methyl-^{11}C]methionine: a preliminary study. Eur J Nucl Med 20:495–501

Lewis P, Griffin S, Marsden P et al (1994) Whole body FDG PET in pre-operative evaluation of lung cancer. Lancet 344:1265–1266

Lowe VJ, Hoffman JM, DeLong DM et al (1994) Semiquantitative and visual analysis of FDG-PET images in pulmonary abnormalities. J Nucl Med 35:1771–1776

Lowe VJ, Duhaylongsod FG, Patz EF et al (1997) Pulmonary abnormalities and PET data analysis: a retrospective study. Radiology 202:435–439

McLoud TC, Bourgouin PM, Greenberg RW et al (1992) Bronchogenic carcinoma: analysis of staging in the mediastinum with CT by correlative lymph node mapping and sampling. Radiology 182:319–323

Minn H, Zasadny KR, Quint LE, Wahl RL (1995) Lung cancer: reproducibility of quantitative measurements for evaluating 2-[F-18]-fluoro-2-deoxy-D-glucose uptake at PET. Radiology 196:167–173

Miyauchi T, Wahl RL (1996) Regional 2-[^{18}F]fluoro-2-deoxy-D-glucose uptake varies in normal lung. Eur J Nucl Med 23:517–523

Nolop KB, Rhodes, Brudin LH et al (1987) Glucose utilization in vivo by human pulmonary neoplasms. Cancer 60:2682–2689

Patz EF, Lowe VJ, Hoffman JM et al (1993) Focal pulmonary abnormalities: evaluation with F-18 fluorodeoxyglucose PET scanning. Radiology 188:487–490

Patz EF, Lowe VJ, Hoffman JM et al (1994) Persistent or recurrent bronchogenic carcinoma: detection with PET and F-18 fluorodeoxyglucose. Radiology 191:379–382

Rasey JS, Koh WJ, Evans ML et al (1996) Quantifying regional hypoxia in human tumors with positron emission tomography of [^{18}F]fluoromisonidazole: a pre-therapy study of 37 patients. Int J Radiat Oncol Biol Phys 36:417–428

Rege SD, Hoh CK, Glaspy JA et al (1993) Imaging of pulmonary mass lesions with whole body PET and FDG. Cancer 72:82–90

Rigo P, Paulus P, Kaschten BJ et al (1996) Oncological applications of positron emission tomography with fluorine-18 fluorodeoxyglucose. Eur J Nucl Med 23:1641–1674

Sasaki M, Ichiya Y, Kuwabara Y et al (1996) The usefulness of FDG positron emission tomography for the detection of mediastinal lymph node metastases in patients with non-small cell lung cancer: a comparative study with X-ray computed tomography. Eur J Nucl Med 23:741–747

Sazon DA, Santiago SM, Soo Hoo GW et al (1996) FDG-PET in the detection and staging of lung cancer. Am J Respir Critic Care Med 153:417–421

Scott WJ, Schwabe JL, Gupta NC et al (1994) PET of lung tumors and mediastinal lymph nodes using FDG. Ann Thorac Surg 58:698–703

Slosman DO, Spiliopoulos A, Couston F et al (1993) Satellite PET and lung cancer: a prospective study in surgical patients. Nucl Med Commun 14:955–961

Steinert HC, Hauser M, Allemann F et al (1997) Non-small cell lung cancer: nodal staging with FDG PET versus CT with correlative lymph node mapping and sampling. Radiology 202:441–446

Valk PE, Pounds, TR, Hopkins DM et al (1995) Staging lung cancer by PET imaging. Ann Thor Surg 60:1573–1581

Wahl RL, Quint LE, Greenough RL et al (1994) Staging of mediastinal non-small cell lung cancer with FDG PET, CT, and fusion images: preliminary prospective evaluation. Radiology 191:371–377

Wang H, Maurea S, Mainolfi C et al (1997) Tc-99m MIBI scintigraphy in patients with lung cancer. Comparison with CT and fluorine-18 FDG PET imaging. Clin Nucl Med 22:243–249

Warburg O (1930) The metabolism of tumors. Constable, London

Warburg O (1956) On the origin of cancer cells. Science 123:309–314

Webb WR, Gatsonis C, Zeerhouni EA et al (1991) CT and MR imaging in staging non-small cell bronchogenic carcinoma: report of the Radiological Diagnostic Oncology Group. Radiology 178:705–713

Zasadny KR, Kison PV, Quint LE, Wahl RL (1996) Untreated lung cancer: quantification of systematic distortion of tumor size and shape on non-attenuation-corrected 2-[fluorine-18]fluoro-2-deoxy-D-glucose PET scans. Radiology 201:873–876

4 Exclusive Surgery for Stage III Disease: Is It Still Ethical?

P. Rocmans, M. Cappello, and P. de Francquen

CONTENTS

4.1 Rationale

Ethical: Means a proven and clear-cut positive benefit/risk ratio.

Proven: If phase II studies suggest a benefit, it should be confirmed by further phase III trials (or supported by meta-analysis).

Benefit: Mainly prolonged survival, ideally free of disease. Moreover, fewer/lesser symptoms, better quality of life. Also minimal treatment-related toxicity (pain, cardiorespiratory impairments, disability). Practically, better survival than natural history of the lung cancer (Vrdoljak et al. 1994).

Risk: Thirty-day postoperative mortality should be less than 5%. Quality of life should be preserved or improved. Failure rate has to be assessed (relapse pattern, disease-free interval, survival rate).

Ratio: The surgical decision is based on healing probability, expected treatment-related morbidity or mortality, possible alternative therapies and the natural history of the disease.

4.2 Resectability of Stage III NSCLC

Practically, surgery for stage III disease should achieve local control of the disease with limited morbidity. Resectability is still ill-defined: "capacity to achieve a complete resection of tumour and local extension with negative margins" (Rocmans et al. 1991). Criteria of resectability are surgeon-dependent: experience, aggressiveness, multidisciplinary support. Moreover, they vary in time with the changing profile of every thoracic surgeon.

The degree of local extension of any tumour is still clinically poorly assessed: the discrepancy between preoperative cTNM and pTNM after initial surgery reaches 30% in the best institutions (Bülzebruck et al. 1992). Therapeutic decisions are taken on cTNM. Survival rates after surgery are reported by pTNM classes. Unexpected peritumoral infiltration or intrathoracic dissemination discovered at thoracotomy or on the final pathology report restage the TNM upwards in 20–40% of cases. The best locoregional preoperative staging relies on clinical examination, computer tomography, magnetic resonance imaging, positron emission tomography, fiber bronchoscopy, mediastinoscopy, mediastinotomy, percutaneous fine needle aspiration cytology and thoracoscopy.

The rate of unexpected mediastinal lymph node dissemination (N2) ranges from 40% without preliminary mediastinoscopy to 16% in very selected cases (Goldstraw et al. 1994), even in small peripheral tumours (Koike et al. 1998: 21%). Unexpected positive pleural cytology is discovered at

---

P. Rocmans, MD, M. Cappello, MD, P. de Francquen, MD, Department of Thoracic Surgery, Hôpital Erasme, Université Libre de Bruxelles, 808 Route de Lennik, B-1070 Brussels, Belgium

thoracotomy in minimal pleural fluid or by lavage (Kondo et al. 1993; Buhr et al. 1997). Such unexpected minimal disseminations detected at thoracotomy are classified stage III, with better prognosis than cT3 N1 or cN2 cases. Tumour and extension are indeed resectable with margins free of disease.

Stage III lung cancer: As defined by the new 1997 TNM classification, stage III covers:

IIIA T3 N1 M0; any N2 M0
IIIB T4 or N3

Non resectable or marginally resectable tumours are selected for radiochemotherapy, eventually as a neoadjuvant procedure. Apparently resectable tumours are candidate for initial surgery. Postoperative adjuvant radiotherapy (or chemoradiotherapy) is advised in incomplete resections (marginal residues). Such adjuvant therapy is optional after apparently complete resection, knowing that distant relapses occur in 2/3 of the patients (Van Houtte et al. 1998).

4.3 Surgery for Stage III NSCLC

Practically, which stage III cases could benefit from exclusive surgery?

4.3.1 T3 N1 M0

N1 disease is poorly assessed preoperatively (CT, PET). N1 disease is mainly an indicator of potential downstream dissemination. It has not been proven to be a negative prognostic factor, and survival is not improved by postoperative adjuvant therapy (PORT Meta-analysis Trialists Group 1998). Very limited T3 disease clearly benefits from radical resection with free margins without adjuvant therapy. Such a policy is valuable for most T3 positions: less than 2 cm from carina, invasion of parietal pleura, pericardium, phrenic nerve, chest wall, diaphragm or mediastinal fat, whole lung atelectasis or obstructive pneumopathy (T3a). Controversy exists regarding superior sulcus tumours (usually marginally resectable) and central tumours invading the ipsilateral pulmonary artery, left subaortic space (excluding recurrent nerve) or right tracheobronchial area including the azygos vein.

For superior sulcus tumours, resectability requires the initial assessment of lack of prescalenic N3 dissemination and is related to the degree of local invasion. Initial aggressive surgery is the best choice if local extension is limited to the parietal pleura, the intercostal space and the inner cortex of the ribs. Resection is followed by adjuvant radiotherapy, especially in case of positive margins (Komaki et al. 1990; Dartevelle 1997; Rocmans 1998).

4.3.2 N2: Dissemination in Homolateral Mediastinal Lymph Nodes

Minimal N2 disease (intranodal, one level, normal size) is usually unexpected, detected at thoracotomy, identified by frozen section. Minimal N2 disease requires radical mediastinal dissection with free margins and downstream lymph nodes free of disease. Adjuvant radiation decreases the rate of mediastinal recurrence but has no impact on the survival rate (PORT Meta-analysis Trialists Group 1998). All other forms of N2 dissemination, preselected or not by mediastinoscopy, require very aggressive radical mediastinal dissection in selected cases: the 5-year survival rate is less than 20%, and more than two-thirds of patients develop distant metastases as first recurrence.

Clinical N2 disease or mediastinoscopy-proven multilevel N2 disease have been resected with less than 10% 5-year survival rate and increased postoperative morbidity (Vansteenkiste et al. 1998a). Many upper N2 disseminations have indeed spread to infraclinical, supraclavicular N3 metastases (Lee and Ginsberg 1996).

In conclusion, exclusive surgery is limited to unexpected minimal N2 disease and requires radical mediastinal dissection. Enlarged mediastinal peritracheal lymph node detected on the chest CT should be explored by cervical mediastinoscopy to confirm or eliminate N2–N3 disease and assess resectability. For left upper lobe tumour with enlarged lymph node(s) in the left anterior mediastinal chain, left prescalenic exploration is advocated to eliminate N3 and authorizes further left upper lobectomy with radical mediastinal dissection (Rocmans, unpublished data). Left parasternal mediastinoscopy is advisable for invasive, multilevel lymph nodes of the left anterior mediastinal chain, precluding thoracotomy if metastasis is demonstrated.

4.3.3 T4: Tumours Invading Central, Vital Structures

Very limited T4 tumours at the level of the carina (T4b), proximal pulmonary artery, superior vena cava, left atrium and recurrent nerve are often completely resectable. Exclusive surgery may ensure 20–40% 5-year survival rate if mediastinal lymph nodes are free of disease (Van Raemdonck et al. 1992). Proven aortic or oesophageal wall infiltration is in most institutions a criterion of nonresectability.

Superior sulcus tumours are mostly staged T3 but are T4 if they invade subclavian vessels, vertebral bodies, spinal cord or lower branches of the brachial plexus (C8, C7, C6). Aggressive, meticulous surgery may achieve apparently complete resection (Komaki et al. 1990; Dartevelle 1997), but is usually followed by adjuvant radiotherapy. The accepted policy in most groups for the past 30 years has been to apply preoperative radiation (30–40 Gy) in selected non-N2 (negative mediastinoscopy), non-N3 (negative prescalenic biopsies) cases followed by en bloc resection with upper lobectomy (Rocmans 1998).

Unexpected positive cytology at thoracotomy, in pleural lavage or minimal pleural fluid residue (Kondo et al. 1993; Buhr et al. 1997), is classified T4b and does not contraindicate resection. It has, however, been shown to be a negative prognostic factor, even if pleural relapses are poorly documented.

Any ipsilateral malignant nodule (satellite nodule) discovered in another lobe is classified pT4 (unless a different cell type suggests a second simultaneous tumour). Complete resection without adjuvant treatment is the common strategy easily achieved.

4.3.4 N3: Criteria of Nonresectability

Contralateral mediastinal lymph node dissemination (mediastinal N3a) – in some cases previously detected, in others found on thoracotomy – has been resected if unexpected or on purpose (Funatsu et al. 1992). Aggressive radical mediastinal dissection is feasible at thoracotomy or by further median sternotomy for left-sided tumours (Hata et al. 1990). Exceptional survivors have been observed at 2 years. Most patients received mediastinal irradiation to reduce the risk of local relapse.

Contralateral hilar lymph node dissemination (identically classified N3a) precludes surgery.

Supraclavicular, prescalenic lymph node dissemination (prescalenic N3b) may be expected in superior sulcus tumours and upper lobe tumours extending to the apex. Infraclinical dissemination is probable in the presence of upper mediastinal N2 or N3 disease (Lee and Ginsberg 1997). The prescalenic N3 classification was introduced in 1985 (previously M1) to be part of a locoregional concept, even if contralateral.

4.4 Potential Exclusive Surgery for Stage III NSCLC

4.4.1 Selection Criteria

- Only very limited stage III disease
- Only one factor for stage III disease (T3 or N2 or T4)
- Potential complete resection (free margins, no residue)
- No proven benefit from either neoadjuvant or postoperative adjuvant treatment
- cN3 carefully excluded (CT, fine needle aspiration cytology, mediastinoscopy, mediastinotomy, thoracoscopy, prescalenic exploration, PET)

4.4.2 Selected cTNM

- T3: Main stem bronchus, parietal pleura, pericardium, phrenic nerve, chest wall, diaphragm, mediastinal fat, whole lung atelectasis or obstructive pneumopathy (same policy for cT3 N1 stage IIIa as for T3 N0 stage IIb)
- T3: Limited superior sulcus tumour (non-N2, non-N3, non-T4)
- N2: Minimal N2 disease (unexpected or mediastinoscopy proven) and very limited N2 disease
- T4: Carina, proximal pulmonary artery, superior vena cava, left atrium, recurrent nerve, infraclinical pleural cytology, ipsilateral nodule in other lobe
- T4: Limited superior sulcus non-N2, non-T3

4.4.3 Absolute Exclusion Criteria

- Any N3
- Massive T3 infiltration (potential need for neoadjuvant treatment)
- T3 N2 (need for neoadjuvant and/or postoperative adjuvant therapy)
- Multilevel or bulky N2
- Any T4 infiltration into aorta or oesophagus
- Deep T4 invasion
- Clinical, cytologically positive pleural effusion (T4)

Such criteria, balanced by the individual experience of every thoracic surgeon, are part of the multidisciplinary surgical decision procedure. Several parameters reflect the staging performance of every institution or cooperative groups:

(a) The cTNM/pTNM discrepancy
(b) The rate of exploratory thoracotomies without possible resection (ideally less than 2%)
(c) The rate of incomplete resections requiring further adjuvant therapy (ideally less than 8%)
(d) The local disease-free interval and rate of local relapse as first recurrence
(e) The distant disease-free interval and rate of distant metastases as first recurrence

Such data are often absent from congress presentations and published reports.

We are aware that some thoracic surgeons base their policy mainly on exceptional long-term survivors attending the outpatient department. They sometimes cannot even report on global data including early postoperative deaths (Spodick 1975). Such lack of objectivity has been also demonstrated in some multidisciplinary teams for assessment of N2 or response to chemo(radio)therapy, leading to incorrect selection, misleading conclusions and further ill-founded strategies. Such a non-Cartesian approach is fortunately exceptional.

Within the limits stressed above, exclusive surgery is still indicated in many early stage III diseases. In large series involving advanced stage III cases, it may not appear to be a valuable option. More early stage III could be detected by routine annual screening of all smokers. Accelerated investigation procedure and early consultation of a thoracic surgeon may increase the successful surgical resection rate (Laroche et al. 1998). Staging should be based on pathological specimens whenever possible, limiting false-positive and false-negative assessments to a minimum.

4.5 Failure of Exclusive Surgery

Nonresectability of stage III tumour necessitates adjuvant therapy:

- For unresectable tumours discovered at exploratory thoracotomy, chemoradiotherapy is advised, possibly in a neoadjuvant setting.
- Incomplete resections with macroscopically or microscopically visible residual tumour may benefit from adjuvant treatment. Irradiation of mediastinum or other residual sites decreases the rate of local relapse but has not been shown to increase the survival rate (Van Houtte et al. 1998). Indeed, the concept of incomplete resection probably needs to be reassessed (Lacasse et al. 1998). As two-thirds of resected stage III tumours relapse at distant sites, adjuvant chemotherapy has been proposed, with some benefits but many failures (Lad 1994).

4.6 Unresectable or Marginally Resectable Tumours

Neoadjuvant treatment has been achieved and feasibility is confirmed. Results have been reported in 24 phase II and 3 small-size randomised trials (Vansteenkiste et al. 1998b). The survival benefit is limited to the best responders among the 60% response rate group: improved resectability, more chance of complete resection (60%), 10–15% complete pathological response.

Limiting factors are the ill-defined criteria of resectability, the discrepancy between cTNM and pTNM, the 40% nonresponse rate and the significant treatment-related toxicity, including surgical morbidity after radiation and/or chemotherapy.

Analysis of the data collected during the recent over-enthusiastic period led to wise, better selected strategies (see Chap. 5).

4.7 Do Completely Resected Stage III Tumours Need Further Postoperative Adjuvant Treatment?

The relapse pattern after such surgery is 10–40% local and 20–70% distant metastases. A two-thirds rate of distant recurrence is commonly observed. Postoperative irradiation may reduce the rate of local relapses but had no impact on 5-year survival rate in nine randomised trials for resected N1–N2 disease (Van Houtte et al. 1998; PORT Meta-analysis Trialists Group 1998); moreover, it appears detrimental in resected stage I and II (PORT Meta-analysis Trialists Group 1998). The potential role of chemotherapy, eliminating infraclinical micrometastases or delaying the emergence of distant metastasis, is supported by a few reports (NSCLC Collaborative Group 1995). Ongoing phase III trials may provide some answers (Intergroup Trial 0115, IALT, ALPI-EORTC, ANITA, Big Lung Trial).

4.8 Conclusions

1. Exclusive surgery is perfectly ethical in very limited stage III disease with expected complete resection.
2. Marginal residues imply postsurgical adjuvant treatment, selected in agreement with phase III trial data.
3. Complete resection may benefit from adjuvant therapy, still part of ongoing phase III prospective trials.
4. If nonresectable, clinically or after exploratory thoracotomy, stage III tumour may benefit from chemo- and/or radiotherapy, whether in a neoadjuvant setting or with curative intent.

The most difficult step is still to assess accurately the cTNM and to quantify the degree of local extension of the tumour, with further appreciation of resectability.

References

Buhr J, Berghäuser KH, Gonner S, Kelm C, Burkhardt EA, Padberg WM (1997) The prognostic significance of tumor cell detection in intraoperative pleural lavage and lung tissue cultures for patients with lung cancer. J Thorac Cardiovasc Surg 113:683–690

Bülzebruck H, Bopp R, Drings P, Bauer E, Krysa S, Probst G, van Kaick G, Müller KM, Vogt-Moykopf I (1992) New aspects in the staging of lung cancer. Prospective validation of the International Union Against Cancer TNM Classification. Cancer 70:1102–1110

Dartevelle PG (1997) Extended operations for the treatment of lung cancer. Ann Thorac Surg 63:12–19

Funatsu T, Matsubara Y, Hatakenaka R, Kosaba S, Yasuda Y, Ikeda S (1992) The role of mediastinoscopic biopsy in preoperative assessment of lung cancer. J Thorac Cardiovasc Surg 104:1688–1695

Goldstraw P, Mannam GC, Kaplan DK, Michail P (1994) Surgical management of non-small-cell lung cancer with ipsilateral mediastinal node metastasis (N2 disease). J Thorac Cardiovasc Surg 107:19–23

Hata E, Hayakawa K, Miyamoto H, Hayashida R (1990) Rationale for extended lymphadenectomy for lung cancer. Theor Surg 5:19–25

Koike T, Terashima M, Takizawa T, Watanabe T, Kurita Y, Yokoyama A (1998) Clinical analysis of small-sized peripheral lung cancer. J Thorac Cardiovasc Surg 115:1015–1020

Komaki R, Mountain CF, Holbert JM, Garden AS, Shallenberger R, Cox JD, Maor MH, Guinee VF, Samuels B (1990) Superior sulcus tumors: treatment selection and results for 85 patients without metastasis (M0) at presentation. Int J Radiat Oncol Biol Phys 19:31–36

Kondo H, Asamura H, Suemasu K, Goya T, Tsuchiya R, Naruke T, Yamagishi K, Uei Y (1993) Prognostic significance of pleural lavage cytology immediately after thoracotomy in patients with lung cancer. J Thorac Cardiovasc Surg 106:1092–1097

Lacasse Y, Bucher HC, Wong E, Griffith L, Walter S, Ginsberg RJ, Guyatt GH (1998) "Incomplete resection" in non-small cell lung cancer: need for a new definition. Ann Thorac Surg 65:220–226

Lad T (1994) The comparison of CAP chemotherapy and radiotherapy to radiotherapy alone for resected lung cancer with positive margin or involved highest sampled paratracheal node (stage IIIa) LCSG 791. Chest 106 [Suppl]:302S–306S

Laroche C, Wells F, Coulden R, Stewart S, Goddard M, Lowry E, Price A, Gilligan D (1998) Improving surgical resection rate in lung cancer. Thorax 53:445–449

Lee JD, Ginsberg RJ (1996) Lung cancer staging: the value of ipsilateral scalene lymph node biopsy performed at mediastinoscopy. Ann Thorac Surg 62:338–341

NSCLC Collaborative Group (1995) Chemotherapy in non-small cell lung cancer: a meta-analysis using updated data on individual patients from 52 randomised clinical trials. BMJ 311:899–909

PORT Meta-analysis Trialists Group (1998) Postoperative radiotherapy in non-small lung cancer: systematic review and meta-analysis of individual patient data from nine randomised controlled trials. Lancet 352:257–263

Rocmans P, Emami B, Cox J, Pacagnella A, Holsti L, Monteau M, Helle P, Comis R, Schaake C (1991) Quality control in NSCLC treatment: a consensus report. Lung Cancer 7:19–20

Rocmans P (1993) Les cancers de l'apex. In: Milleron B, Depierre A (eds) Cancers broncho-pulmonaires. Arnette Initiatives Santé, Vélizy-Villacoublay, France, pp 451–458

Spodick DH (1975) Numerators without denominators: there is no FDA for the surgeon. Lancet 232:35–37

Van Houtte P, Mornex F, Rocmans P (1998) Limites et perspectives de la radiothérapie postopératoire dans le cancer bronchique. Cancer/Radiother 2:252–259

Van Raemdonck DE, Schneider A, Ginsberg RJ (1992) Surgical treatment for higher stage non-small cell lung cancer. Ann Thorac Surg 54:999–1013

Vansteenkiste JF, De Leyn PR, Deneffe GJ, Lerut TE, Demedts MG (1998a) Clinical prognostic factors in surgically treated stage IIIA-N2 non-small cell lung cancer: analysis of the literature. Lung Cancer 19:3–13

Vansteenkiste J, De Leyn P, Deneffe G, Menten J, Lerut T, Demedts M, The Leuven Lung Cancer Group (1998b) Present status of induction treatment in stage IIIA-N2 non-small cell lung cancer: a review. Eur J Cardiothorac Surg 13:1–12

Vrdoljak E, Mise K, Sapunar D, Rozga A, Marusic M (1994) Survival analysis of untreated patients with non-small cell lung cancer. Chest 106:1797–1800

5 Induction Chemotherapy with or without Radiotherapy Followed by Surgery in Non-Small Cell Lung Cancer

Kathy S. Albain

CONTENTS

Kathy S. Albain, Division of Hematology/Oncology, Loyola University Medical Center, Cardinal Bernadin Cancer Center, Room 109, 2160 South First Avenue, Maywood, IL 60153, USA

5.1 Induction Therapy Before Surgery: An Ongoing Controversy

5.1.1 A Paradigm Shift

There is great debate regarding the proper application of chemotherapy with or without radiotherapy (RT) as induction therapy prior to surgical resection in stage IIB (T3N0-1) and stage III non-small cell lung cancer (NSCLC). Nearly as many reviews and position papers have been written on this subject as there are clinical trials (Strauss et al. 1992a; Rusch and Benfield 1993; Green et al. 1994; Johnson and Piantadosi 1994; Edelman et al. 1996; Albain 1997a; Perry et al. 1997). As these reviewers point out, initially the paradigm was to view the "neoadjuvant" or induction modality(ies) as the means to render unresectable disease resectable. However, with the recognition that early eradication of systemic micrometastases was critical to the success of any local approach, the paradigm shifted: the goal in current studies is to provide initial control of both bulk disease and distant micrometastases with induction therapy, and then employ surgical resection for definitive local control.

Under this new paradigm, the advantages of a successful induction program include optimal and concurrent cytoreduction of distant and local disease, improvement of odds of resectability in technically difficult cases, the possibility of sparing more normal lung tissue, and an "in vivo" test of chemosensitivity. These advantages must be weighed against concerns regarding increased morbidity and mortality from combined modality induction regimens, in particular, greater incidence of postoperative pulmonary complications and deaths; greater technical challenges at operation in the face of radiation fibrosis; and the small but real possibility of progression of disease during induction.

5.1.2 The Current Debate in Two Subsets

In the course of this paradigm shift, numerous small trials, and more recently larger phase II and phase III studies, were conducted that yielded a broad spectrum of outcomes that fueled the current controversy. As shown in Table 5.1, this debate can be separated into two major questions based upon the amount of disease burden. First, there is the group with nonbulky or minimal disease. These stage subsets include selected IIB (T3N0), IIIA(N1) and IIIA(N2), with either non-enlarged N2 nodes on computerized tomography (CT) scan, or microscopic N2 nodal involvement with a normal CT scan of the mediastinum. Initial surgical resection has long been the standard of care for this group and the bulk of mediastinal disease is critical in determining potential for cure after the surgical resection (MARTINI et al. 1983; MARTINI and FLEHINGER 1987; VANSTEENKISTE et al. 1998). Despite a complete surgical resection, however, the majority of these patients die of metastatic disease. Thus, the debate in this group is whether induction chemotherapy ± RT (chemoRT) definitively improves survival over surgery alone.

The second group for which there is controversy regarding the role of the three treatment modalities contains the stage subsets that have bulky disease on presentation (Table 5.1). These tumors include bulky N2 disease on CT scan or chest radiograph, T4 (no effusion) primaries, or N3 disease. The standard of care, as reviewed elsewhere (STRAUSS et al. 1992a; EDELMAN et al. 1996) and in this volume, is any one of several published chemoRT programs that demonstrated significant benefit over RT alone. The debate in this group is whether surgical resection after induction chemoRT improves outcome over chemoRT alone.

This controversy regarding optimal management within both types of disease burdens exists in large part because the published pilot studies, and now several small randomized trials, addressed a wide range of stage III/stage IIB(T3N0) subsets of NSCLC, not only across trials but also within each study. In many of the early studies, there was inconsistent pathologic documentation of nodal status and variable staging criteria were utilized. Thus, the interpretation of bi- and trimodality trials that include surgery requires close attention to the definition of stage subsets and method of documentation of such (radiograph only versus biopsy-proof of N2, N3 or T4 status).

Furthermore, these trials varied in the definition of "bulky" disease, such as variable CT size criteria for nodes, number of positive nodes, extranodal extension of tumor and various combinations of these criteria. The published studies utilized different criteria for resection after induction therapy (resection of stable disease or just the responding tumors) as well the definition of complete resection (most required resection of gross disease, whereas a few mandated negative margins or negative highest node). Other factors that may influence survival were variably available in these reports: the presence of single intranodal N2 disease, involvement of nodal stations N5 or N6 only, and positive N7 nodes (VANSTEENKISTE et al. 1998). It is also critical

Table 5.1. Induction therapy prior to surgery: two subsets and controversies

Disease burden	Stage subsets	Standard of care	Controversy
Nonbulky or minimal	• T3N0 or N1 • Non-enlarged N2 nodes on CT scan • Microscopic N2 only with normal CT scan	Initial surgical resection	Should preoperative chemotherapy ± RT be given routinely?
Bulky	• Significant N2 enlargement on CT scan or chest X-ray • T4 (no effusion) • N3 disease	ChemoRT	Does subsequent resection improve survival?

RT, radiotherapy; CT, computerized tomography.
Modified from ALBAIN (1997a).

that resection rates and overall survival are presented of the entire denominator, not just for those patients taken to thoracotomy. Other important data sporadically available are local and distant relapse rates, cause of death, and predictors of long term survival that optimally are addressed in multivariate models.

5.1.3
Objectives of this Review

The objectives of this chapter are to provide a perspective on these two critical questions (Table 5.1) in the context of a review of early studies, second and third generation trials and ongoing approaches. Wherever possible, the disease bulk and stage subsets contained within a given study along with the other factors outlined above will be stated. Throughout, stage classifications will be those employed at the time of the particular study, but with the current modifications of the International Staging System mentioned where appropriate (usually a change in classification of the T3N0 subset from stage IIIA to IIB) (Mountain 1988, 1997). The conclusion of the chapter will consider if data are sufficient to recommend new standards of care for these two groups, that is, whether the answer to the two questions posed in Table 5.1 should be "yes." Along the way to this conclusion, several other aspects of the debate will be addressed: Is there an optimal induction regimen? Is RT required in the induction program? Should RT be sequenced or given concurrent with chemotherapy? And, is there a defined role yet for the newer agents with or without RT prior to surgery?

5.2
The First Generation Studies

5.2.1
Induction RT Alone

The earliest induction trials used preoperative RT alone in an attempt to convert unresectable disease to resectable (Bromley and Szur 1955; Bloedorn et al. 1961; Shields et al. 1970; Warram 1975). These initial trials were conducted in the 1950s, 1960s and early 1970s, often without the benefit of modern staging technologies. The first results were provocative. Pathologic complete remissions were reported in up to 15% patients, but operative complications increased with doses of RT greater than 40 Gy. The consensus was that the resections were technically easier, although most cases were probably initially resectable in terms of bulk and extent by modern standards. However, this early enthusiasm for preoperative RT alone waned when randomized trials showed no survival benefit (Payne 1991). The most recent study was one arm of a randomized phase II trial of the Lung Cancer Study Group, LCSG 881 (Lad et al. 1991). Patients who had pathologic stage IIIA(N2) disease were given 44 Gy before surgery. There was only one pathologic complete remission and the median survival was 12 months. Thus, preoperative radiotherapy is no longer recommended as the sole induction modality.

5.2.2
Early Trials of Induction Chemotherapy with or without RT

The next group of studies, generally conducted in the 1980s, were the first to test first generation cisplatin-based chemotherapy with or without sequential RT prior to surgery (Skarin et al. 1989; Eagan et al. 1987; Bitran et al. 1986; Elias et al. 1994; Darwish et al. 1994). As shown in Table 5.2, the studies were small, accrued a wide mix of stage subsets and had broad variability in both the amount of minimal versus bulky disease and in the percentage of biopsy-proven N2 disease. Three trials employed the CAP regimen (cyclophosphamide, doxorubicin and low dose cisplatin), whereas two studies were cisplatin- and etoposide-based, as depicted in Table 5.2. Response rates from the induction therapy were 39%–82%, resection rates (percent of original number accrued) were 14%–88% and the survivals were highly variable (Table 5.3). Although the stage and bulk mix within these trials preclude conclusions regarding outcome, these were pivotal studies in that they demonstrated the general safety of surgery after induction therapy and, in certain cases, provided intriguing survival data.

Therefore, based on provocative findings and safety data from these first generation trials, impetus existed for the second generation trials. These studies were larger, many of which had more selected stage subsets and most documented disease pathologically. The next three sections review two categories of second generation studies and long-term survival from selected trials.

Table 5.2. First-generation induction trial designs

Group or study	Reference	Number of patients	Stage subsets	Biopsy-proven N2 (%)	Treatment program
Dana Farber I	SKARIN et al. 1989	41	T3 or low-bulk stage III (N2)	68	CAP × 2 → RT → surgery → RT → CAP × 3
LCSG 831	EAGAN et al. 1987	39	T3 or low-bulk stage III (N2)	51	CAP × 3 with split RT → surgery
University of Chicago	BITRAN et al. 1986	21	Bulky T3 or T4N2 or N3	100	VdEP × 2 → surgery → RT
Dana Farber II	ELIAS et al. 1994	54	T1-3N2 (mixed bulk)	94	CAP × 4 ± RT → surgery → RT
Perugia	DARWISH et al. 1994	42	T1-3N2 (clinically bulky)	0	EP × 2–3 → surgery → variable RT

LCSG, Lung Cancer Study Group; C, cyclophosphamide; A, doxorubicin; P, cisplatin; RT, radiotherapy; Vd, Vindesine; E, etoposide.

Table 5.3. Outcome of first generation induction trials

Group[a] or study	Response rate (%)	Resection rate (% original n)	Median survival (months)	Long-term survival
Dana Farber I	43	88	32	31%, 3-year
LCSG 831	51	33	11	8%, 2-year
University of Chicago	70	14	8	34%, 1-year
Dana Farber II	39	56	18	22%, 5-year
Perugia	82	72	24	24%, 3-year

[a] References for studies given in Table 5.2.

5.3 Second Generation Trials of Induction Chemotherapy

5.3.1 Description of Studies

All five second generation induction trials of preoperative chemotherapy alone required pathologic documentation of N2 disease. These studies are summarized in Table 5.4 (LAD et al. 1991; MARTINI et al. 1993; PISTERS et al. 1993; BURKES et al. 1994; ELIAS et al. 1997; SUGARBAKER et al. 1995). However, tumors with a wide range of disease bulk were accrued across the trials. Furthermore, the RT was variably given (intraoperative, postoperative, or not at all) and information regarding why RT was either given or withheld was not provided in detail for some of the studies. Thus, lack of concordance on these variables makes comparison of outcomes among the studies difficult. Four of the studies utilized preoperative vinblastine and cisplatin with or without mitomycin

Table 5.4. Second generation trials of induction chemotherapy of pathologic stage IIIA (N2) disease

Group or study	Reference	No. patients	Disease bulk	Chemotherapy	Radiotherapy
LCSG 881	LAD et al. 1991	28	Most bulky	MVP	None
Memorial	MARTINI et al. 1993 PISTERS et al. 1993	136	Most only one nodal station positive; mixed bulk	MVP	Variable, either intra- or postoperative
Toronto	BURKES et al. 1994	55	Mixed bulk	MVP	Postoperative
Dana Farber III	ELIAS et al. 1997	34	Mixed bulk	PFL (continuous infusion)	Postoperative
CALGB II	SUGARBAKER et al. 1995	74	Most bulky	VP	Postoperative

Abbreviations: as given in Table 5.2; V, vinblastine; M, mitomycin C; F, 5-fluorouracil; L, leucovoran; CALGB, Cancer and Leukemia Group B.

Table 5.5. Outcome of second generation induction chemotherapy trials

Group[a] or study	Response rate (%)	Complete resection rate (% initial n)	Operative mortality (%)	Median survival (months)
LCSG 881	46	68	17.0	12
Memorial	78	65	4.4	19
Toronto	71	51	8.0	21
Dana Farber III	65	62	0	18
CALGB II	64[b]	62	3.1	15

[a] References for studies given in Table 5.4.
[b] Includes stable disease.

C (MVP, VP) and the fifth trial tested continuous infusion cisplatin and 5-fluorouracil with leucovorin rescue.

5.3.2 Outcomes

The outcomes reported in these five studies are shown in Table 5.5. The response rates were 46%–78% and resection rates (of the entire denominator) were 51%–68%. Operative mortalities were 0%–17% and were predominantly pulmonary or cardiopulmonary events. Significant pulmonary morbidity was observed in these studies, usually in the postoperative time period. For example, 13% of patients treated with MVP in the Memorial Sloan Kettering Cancer Center study and 12% of those who received VP in the CALGB trial experienced major pulmonary events (Martini et al. 1993; Sugarbaker et al. 1995). It was difficult to give full dose RT in the "posterior" or postoperative time period. For instance, completion of the planned treatment (all RT given postoperatively) was possible for only 42% of patients in the CALGB study.

The median survivals (Table 5.5) were 12–21 months in these five studies of induction chemotherapy. Sites of first failure were included in three of these reports: local-regional disease as the only site of first relapse occurred in 26%, 24%, and 25% of patients, respectively (Martini et al. 1993; Elias et al. 1997; Sugarbaker et al. 1995). All of these local-only recurrences occurred in the subgroup with residual disease at surgery in the Memorial Sloan Kettering Cancer Center trial. The Dana Farber investigators noted that 15% of first relapses were in the brain only.

5.4 Second Generation Trials of Induction Chemoradiotherapy

5.4.1 Description of Studies

The other type of second generation study utilized concurrent chemoRT in which the RT began on day 1 of the chemotherapy, as outlined in Table 5.6 (Albain et al. 1995; Weiden et al. 1991; Faber et al.

Table 5.6. Second generation trials of induction chemoradiotherapy (standard fractionation) followed by surgery

Group or study	References	No. patients	Biopsy of mediastinal node or T4 required?	T3N0-1/ T4 or N3 (%)	IIIA (N2) (%)	Induction RT	Induction chemotherapy
SWOG 8805	Albain et al. 1995	126	Yes	0/40	60	Continuous, 45 Gy	EP
LCSG 852	Weiden et al. 1991	85	Yes	0/13	87	Continuous, 30 Gy	PF
Rush-Presbyterian	Faber et al.	85	Yes	21/6	73	Split, 40 Gy	PF/PEF
CALGB I	Strauss et al. 1992b	41	Yes	20/0	80	Continuous, 30 Gy	PVF
Tufts	Law et al. 1997	55	No	0/53	47	Continuous, 59 Gy	EP

Abbreviations: as given in Tables 5.2 and 5.4; SWOG, Southwest Oncology Group.

1989; Strauss et al. 1992b; Law et al. 1997). Although the RT was started on day 1 in each of the five studies, it varied across trials from continuous to split course and from 30 Gy to 59 Gy. All induction chemotherapy was cisplatin-based, with either etoposide, 5-fluorouracil, vinblastine or some combination of these drugs (Table 5.6).

Eligibility for these five trials was more variable than for the studies of induction chemotherapy alone, in that biopsy documentation of mediastinal nodal disease or T4 status was not always required. Furthermore, a wider range of stage subsets were included: stage IIIA(N2) accounted for 47%–87% of patients per trial. Two studies included T3N0 or T3N1 (21% and 20% in the Rush Presbyterian and CALGB studies, respectively), whereas all patients with stage IIIA disease in the SWOG 8805, LCSG 852 and Tufts trials had N2 nodal involvement. Selected stage IIIB subsets of T4 and/or N3 were allowed in all but the CALGB study and accounted for 6%–53% of patients per trial (Table 5.6). The SWOG 8805 and Tufts trials were designed only for bulky disease, whereas the others allowed a mix of minimal bulk and bulky presentations.

5.4.2 Outcomes

Outcome of the chemoRT induction trials is summarized in Table 5.7. Response or "response plus stable" rates were 56%–92% and resection rates were 52%–76% of patients accrued to each study. The operative mortalities were 4%–15% and, as was observed in the induction chemotherapy trials, these events were predominantly pulmonary-related, often very similar to the adult respiratory distress syndrome (ARDS). The Tufts trial was unique in that no postoperative ARDS events were observed, despite the high total dose of induction RT (Law et al. 1997). A rigid protocol to minimize fluids, transfusions and the FiO_2 was employed in this study. The treatment rendered after surgical resection was highly variable among these five studies. There was no further therapy in the Rush Presbyterian and LCSG 852 trials, two cycles of additional chemotherapy plus 14 Gy were given in the SWOG 8805 study (if residual disease or mediastinal node positivity) and one cycle plus 30 Gy was used in the CALGB trial (all patients). The Tufts investigators initially gave etoposide plus cisplatin postoperatively, but later in the trial allowed use of the carboplatin plus paclitaxel regimen. In general across trials, it is uncertain whether this "posterior" treatment, in particular the additional relatively small doses of RT, added to the efficacy of the program versus contributed more morbidity. However, the SWOG investigators reported no difference in the toxicity profile between the induction and postsurgical phases.

The median survivals for the two studies that excluded T3N0-1 tumors and required pathologic staging were 15 and 13 months (Albain et al. 1995; Weiden et al. 1991). Whereas, in the other three trials that included this better prognostic group and did not require biopsy proof of the T and N substages the median survivals were 22, 16 and 20 months (Faber et al. 1989; Strauss et al. 1992b; Law et al. 1997). Patterns of first recurrence were reported in the SWOG 8805 trial: 11% were locoregional only, whereas 61% were distant alone (Albain et al. 1995). There was no difference in the sites of relapse between those patients with negative mediastinal nodes at the time of operation (but originally positive) versus those who had persistent involvement of the mediastinal nodes. A significant proportion of the isolated distant first relapses (and in many cases, the only relapse or the sole cause of mortality) occurred in the brain only. The Tufts investigators

Table 5.7. Outcome of second generation induction chemoradiotherapy trials

Group or study[a]	Response rate (%)	Complete resection rate (% initial *n*)	Operative mortality (%)	Postoperative treatment	Median survival (months)
SWOG 8805	59	71	8	Chemo × 2 + RT 14 Gy if positive nodes or margins or if unresectable	15
LCSG 852	56	52	7	None	13
Rush-Presbyterian	92[b]	71	4	None	22
CALGB I	64[b]	61	15	Chemo × 1 + RT 30 Gy	16
Tufts	69[b]	76	5	PE or carboplatin + paclitaxel	20

[a] References for studies given in Table 5.6.
[b] Includes stable disease.

also reported a very high rate of isolated brain metastases, all of which occurred within the first 32 months of follow-up (LAW et al. 1997).

5.4.3 The Stage IIIB Subgroup

Fewer data are available regarding outcome of induction therapy followed by surgery in selected stage IIIB subsets. All patients enrolled in the second generation trials of induction chemotherapy had stage IIIA(N2) disease, whereas all but one of the chemoRT trials included patients with stage IIIB tumors. The LCSG 852 trial and the Rush Presbyterian study (Table 5.6) included 13% "minimal T4" and 6% "selected T4" lesions (clinically staged), respectively. Separate survival data for this subset were not provided. Two groups reported equivalence in outcome in combined modality trials (no surgery) for clinical stage IIIA and IIIB disease (BONOMI et al. 1992; CURRAN and STAFFORD 1995). It was suggested that the T4N0 subset may have a better outcome and perhaps should be removed from the IIIB category, just as the T3N0 subset was recently reassigned to the IIB subset instead of its former designation of IIIA (MOUNTAIN 1997). This question was explored in the SWOG 8805 study, since it was designed prospectively to include a sufficient sample of stage IIIB presentations.

The SWOG 8805 trial is unique among the other chemoRT trials that included stage IIIB disease in that pathologically documented T4 or N3 disease was required and outcome was analyzed separately for this subset (ALBAIN et al. 1995; RUSCH et al. 1994). The Tufts investigators also reported outcome separately for the IIIB group, but the staging requirements were radiographic rather than pathologic (LAW et al. 1997). The resection rates in these two studies for stage IIIA(N2) were 76% and 76%, respectively, and for stage IIIB, 63% and 50%. The median, 2-year and 3-year survivals were identical for the IIIA(N2) versus the IIIB group in the SWOG 8805 study, and the 3-year survivals were 73% and 32%, respectively, in the Tufts trial. Of note, in the SWOG 8805 study, the T4N0-1 subset had an outcome identical to the T1N2 substage and achieved a 2-year survival of 64%. In fact, this substage variable was the only independent predictor of favorable outcome from the time of registration to the study. Exploratory survival analyses were conducted within the N3 subset, of which 27 patients were accrued. The 2-year survival of the contralateral nodal N3 subgroup was zero, whereas it was 35% for the supraclavicular N3 subset. The resectability rate in this latter group was only 39%.

In the follow-up trial for pathologic stage IIIB disease conducted by the SWOG (SWOG 9019), identical induction chemoRT was utilized as in SWOG 8805, but no surgery was given; instead, the RT was continued without a break to 61 Gy and two additional cycles of EP were given (ALBAIN et al. 1997). The overall survival in this study was identical to that observed for the stage IIIB group in SWOG 8805, hinting that in an identically staged patient population, additional chemoRT may achieve the same benefit as surgical resection after induction chemoRT. However, in SWOG 9019, the recent study without surgery, the 2-year survival was only 33% for the T4N0-1 subset, compared to 64% in the surgical study, SWOG 8805. This historical comparison of consecutive trials in pathologically staged IIIB disease suggests that surgery might be beneficial in this select group, but a prospective randomized study is required to validate this observation (ALBAIN 1997b).

5.5 Long-Term Survival and Predictors of Outcome

5.5.1 Trials with Mature Follow-up

Long-term survival and its predictors were provided in several of the trials of induction chemotherapy and induction chemoRT that were reviewed in the preceding two sections. Selected studies with a minimum of 3 years of long-term survival data are summarized in Table 5.8 (MARTINI et al. 1993; PISTERS et al. 1993; BURKES et al. 1994; ALBAIN et al. 1995; ALBAIN 1997b; STRAUSS et al. 1992b; STRAUSS 1997; SUGARBAKER et al. 1995; FABER et al. 1989; LAW et al. 1997). Note that the SWOG 8805 trial follow-up is updated for this chapter (ALBAIN and CROWLEY 1998, personal communication), as is the Toronto study (BURKES 1996, personal communication). These studies with available long-term follow-up (Table 5.8) differed in several critical aspects: (a) disease bulk, (b) the inclusion of T3N0 or N1 subsets, (c) whether or not pathologic documentation of N2 disease was required and (d) the inclusion of IIIB subsets. These disease bulk and stage subset variations and potential inaccurate staging on clinical grounds may to a major degree explain the wide range of 3–7 year survivals shown in Table 5.8.

Table 5.8. Selected studies of induction therapy followed by surgery: long-term survival and predictors of outcome

Group or study[a]	Bulky disease only?	T3N0 or N1 included?	Biopsy proof of N2?	Selected IIIB included?	Long-term survival	Predictors of favorable outcome
Memorial	No	No	Yes	No	17%, 5-year	Pathologic CR
Toronto	No	No	Yes	No	34%, 5-year	Complete resection
SWOG 8805	Yes	No	Yes	Yes	N2: 21%, 5-year IIIB: 22%, 5-year	N2/3→ N0 at resection; T4N0 or 1
CALGB I	No	Yes	No	No	22%, 7 (+) year	No survival advantage for complete resection or pathologic CR
CALGB II	Yes	No	Yes	No	23%, 3-year	Complete resection
Rush-Presbyterian	No	Yes	No	Yes	31%, 3-year	T3N0 or T3N1
Tufts	Yes	No	No	Yes	N2: 73%, 3-year IIIB: 32%, 3-year	Complete response

Abbreviations: as given in Tables 5.2, 5.4, 5.6; CR, complete response.
[a] References for studies given in Tables 5.2, 5.4 and 5.6; updates for SWOG 8805: Albain 1997b, K.S. Albain and J.J. Crowley 1998, personal communication; update for CALGB I: Strauss 1997. Update for the Toronto trial: RL, Burkes 1966, personal communication.

Long-term follow-up of several trials suggested that a plateau emerged on the tails of the survival curves. As shown in Table 5.8, 5–7 year survivals of 17%–34% were recently reported. The SWOG 8805 study suggested a plateau between years 4 and 6, the Toronto study between years 3 and 5, and the CALGB I study from years 5–7(+). However, indefinite plateaus are not expected due to competing causes of death in a patient population with a high rate of comorbid diseases. The SWOG 8805 investigators made an attempt to categorize the reasons for death, rather than assume all were cancer-related. Although cancer accounted for 64% of all deaths, 20% were due to late pneumonia long after the end of treatment, myocardial infarction, pulmonary embolus, cerebrovascular accidents, trauma, ulcer or second primaries (Albain et al. 1995).

5.5.2 Predictors of Favorable Outcome

The seven studies of induction chemotherapy or chemoRT shown in Table 5.8 reported analyses of predictors of long-term survival. Methods of analysis varied: univariate versus multivariate and either predictors of overall survival from registration or from time of thoracotomy. Overall, the various predictors included pathologic complete response (occurred in approximately 20% of specimens collectively across trials), complete resection, T3N0 or T3N1 disease, T4N0 or N1 disease, and pathologic clearance of mediastinal disease (nodal downstaging). These predictors varied across trials such that when significant in one study, the same variable was not predictive in the other. This variance was especially true for complete pathologic response and complete resection. For example, neither the CALGB I nor the SWOG 8805 trial found a predictive survival advantage to either complete resection or pathologic complete response, whereas one or the other of these factors was an important favorable factor in the Memorial, Toronto and CALGB II studies.

The observation regarding the favorable prognostic impact of nodal downstaging is of interest, given it was the only significant factor in a multivariate model that included complete resection rate, pathologic complete response and multiple other factors in the SWOG 8805 study (Albain et al. 1995). The survival 3 years after thoracotomy for those with uninvolved nodes at surgery was 41% versus only 11% if there was persistent mediastinal disease. This variable of nodal downstaging was not assessed in any of the other reports. Implications of this finding were that clearance of disease in the mediastinum may be a surrogate marker for eradication of distant chemotherapy-sensitive micrometastases, such that these patients may be the optimal candidates for additional postoperative chemotherapy. And, persistent N2 or N3 disease may predict the presence of distant resistant disease. These implications raised the question: Was surgery necessary if induction cleared the mediastinal disease – or – were these patients the best candidates for optimal local control? Whether molecular correlates (for example, K-Ras, p53, proliferative rate) obtained on biopsy

Table 5.9. Third generation trials of induction chemotherapy plus concurrent hyperfractionated radiotherapy followed by surgery

Group	References	No. patients	Stage subset	Chemotherapy	Radiotherapy
Boston (MGH)	Choi et al. 1997	42	All biopsy-proven stage IIIA(N2), mixed bulk	PVF × 2 concurrent with RT → surgery → FVF × 1 concurrent with RT	42 Gy split (1.5 b.i.d. × 7 → 10 day rest → 1.5 b.i.d. × 7); postoperative 12–18 Gy (1.5 b.i.d.)
West German Cancer Center	Eberhardt et al. 1997	94	All, mediastinoscopy and bulky: 6, advanced T3; 46, 2 or more N2 nodes; 42, IIIB (T4 or contralateral N3)	EP × 3 → reduced dose EP × 1 with RT → surgery	45 Gy (1–5 Gy b.i.d. over 3 weeks); PCI later in trial

Abbreviations: as given in Tables 5.2 and 5.4; PCI, prophylactic cranial irradiation.

Table 5.10. Outcome of third generation trials of induction chemotherapy plus concurrent hyperfractionated radiotherapy

Group[a]	Resection rate (of initial n)	Treatment-related mortality	Survival	Predictors of favorable outcome
Boston (MGH)	93%	7%	57%, 5-year	Five-year survival by stage at thoracotomy: Stage 0 or I 79% Stage II 42% Stage III 18%
West German Cancer Center	53% (60% IIIA, 45% IIIB)	6%	28%, 4-year (31% IIIA 26% IIIB)	N2/3 → N0 in 80%, but no difference in survival if pathologic CR or not; PCI decreased brain metastases

CR, complete remission; PCI, prophylactic cranial irradiation.
[a] References for studies given in Table 5.9.

material pre- and/or post-induction might improve identification of the optimal patients for surgical resection await the results of ongoing ancillary studies within several of these trials.

5.6 Third Generation Trials: Induction Chemotherapy plus Concurrent Hyperfractionated Radiotherapy

5.6.1 Eligibility and Trial Design

Mature results of two important pilot studies of induction chemoRT, in which the RT was given in twice daily fractions, were reported in 1997, and are detailed in Table 5.9 (Choi et al. 1997; Eberhardt et al. 1997) Forty-two patients with mixed bulk, biopsy-proven stage III(N2) disease were treated on the Massachusetts General Hospital (MGH) trial and 94 patients were enrolled on the West German Cancer Center (WGCC) study. The latter trial required mediastinoscopy and all patients had advanced disease: either bulky T3 (six patients), two or more positive N2 nodes (n = 46) or stage IIIB (n = 42, either T4 or contralateral N3 nodes). The concurrent chemotherapy plus hyperfractionated RT protocols are outlined in Table 5.9. The MGH group used split course RT, split before the surgery as well as after (with one additional cycle of chemotherapy), whereas the WGCC trial gave continuous hyperfractionated RT and all treatment was completed before the surgery. Stable disease was not resected.

5.6.2 Outcome and Predictors of Survival

The results of these two studies are summarized in Table 5.10. The resection rates differed, in that 93% of patients had a complete resection in the MGH study, whereas 60% of the stage IIIA subset and 45% of the stage IIIB group in the WGCC study were completely resected. This difference in large part may be due to a significant percentage of cases with non-bulky disease in the MGH study. Treatment-related mortality was no greater than reported in trials that tested either induction chemotherapy alone or induction chemoRT with standard single daily fractionation of RT. Sixty percent of patients in the MGH trial were able to complete the "posterior" chemoRT given after the surgery.

Sites of initial failure in the MGH study were reported in detail. Only local-regional relapse occurred in 15% of those with a recurrence, only brain in 30%, other distant site only in 45% and both local and systemic in 10%. The WGCC investigators also reported a high rate of initial brain relapses that occurred relatively early in the follow-up period. Prophylactic cranial irradiation was mandated in the latter half of the trial and significantly decreased these brain events.

Long-term survival outcomes were provocative in both studies (Table 5.10). Yet, the 5-year survival of 37% in the MGH trial was identical to that reported in the Toronto trial of induction chemotherapy alone (Table 5.8). It is not possible to determine if the hyperfractionated RT resulted in greater benefit, because both of these studies accrued patients with a mixture of bulky and minimal N2 disease and it is not clear if the percentage with high disease bulk was greater in the MGH trial than in the Toronto study. The WGCC trial clearly accrued more patients with bulky disease, which in part explains the slightly lower survival (38% overall at 4 years, with 31% of IIIA and 26% of IIIB alive at 4 years). Therefore, the intriguing results of the MGH and WGCC trials suggest that a randomized study that tests single versus twice-daily fractionation in the induction regimen is needed in identically staged patients with uniform disease bulk.

The analysis of predictors of survival in the MGH trial provides independent validation of the SWOG finding that mediastinal nodal downstaging is a critical favorable determinant for long-term survival (Choi et al. 1997; Albain et al. 1995). Patients with stage 0 or I tumors at surgery had a 79% 5-year survival after thoracotomy in the MGH trial, and those with N0 or N1 downstaging had a 41% 3-year survival in SWOG 8805. Nodal downstaging was noted in 80% of the subset with N2 or N3 disease in the WGCS study, but there was no difference in survival if pathologic complete remission was achieved or not (Eberhardt et al. 1997). An independent analysis of the impact of mediastinal nodal clearance is planned, but stable disease was not resected.

5.7 Randomized Trials of Induction Therapy in Resectable Disease

5.7.1 Study Population and Trial Design

Four small randomized trials in resectable non-small cell lung cancer were conducted in each of which the control arm of surgery alone, was compared with induction chemotherapy, with or without variably-timed RT (Pass et al. 1992; H.I. Pass 1996, personal communication; Yoneda et al. 1995; Roth et al. 1994; Rosell et al. 1994). These programs are described in Table 5.11. The first two studies are rarely discussed, whereas the latter two are debated frequently. These trials differ from many of those described in the previous sections, above, in that all four required operable disease; that is, surgery alone was deemed the acceptable standard for the control arm. However, the bulk of disease varied across the four studies. Patients with bulky disease were enrolled in the NCI (multiple N2 nodes on mediastinoscopy) and Japanese (clinically bulky) trials. The NCI trial was the most homogeneous in the stage subsets accrued. However, the M.D. Anderson and Spanish studies did not require N2 disease and mediastinal node biopsy was not mandated if the CT scan was negative. Of note, in the surgical control arm of the M.D. Anderson trial, 40% of cases were actually stage IIIB or IV at time of operation. Thus, the treatment groups of the small M.D. Anderson and Spanish studies were quite heterogeneous regarding stage subsets.

The induction chemotherapy regimens were cisplatin-based and were also variably given after surgery depending on the study (see Table 5.11). The use of RT was also different in each trial: either postoperatively only in the non-chemotherapy arm, concurrent with the induction chemotherapy, postoperatively only if residual disease, or postoperatively for all patients.

5.7.2 Outcome of the Four Randomized Trials

Three of the four trials closed prematurely. The NCI trial was stopped early due to slow accrual, whereas the M.D. Anderson and Spanish studies were halted due to survival differences (Table 5.11). In the NCI study, although there was no statistical difference between the two arms, the *P* value has continued to decrease with longer follow-up, in favor

Table 5.11. Randomized trials of surgery with or without induction therapy in resectable non-small cell lung cancer[a]

Group	References	No. patients	Stage subset(s)	Disease burden	Chemotherapy	RT	2–3 year suvival		
							No ChT	ChT	*P* value
NCI[b]	Pass et al. 1992	28	IIIA(N2) by biopsy	Bulky	EP pre- and postoperatively	Postoperatively in no-ChT arm only	21%	46%	0.12
Japan	Yoneda et al. 1995	83	Clinical IIIA and IIIB	Bulky	Vdp preoperatively	Concurrent with CT	40%	37%	NS
M.D. Anderson	Roth et al. 1994	60	IIIA(N2) not required; node biopsy not required; some IIIB	Minimal bulk	CEP pre- and postoperatively	Postoperatively only if residual disease	15%	56%	<0.05
Spain	Rosell et al. 1994	60	IIIA(N2) not required; node biopsy not required	Minimal bulk	FIM preoperatively	Postoperatively for both arms	0%	30%	<0.05

Abbreviations: as in Tables 5.2, 5.4 and 5.6; I, ifosfamide; NS, not significant; NCI, National Cancer Institute; ChT, chemotherapy.
[a] Modified from Albain 1997a.
[b] Study undated: H.I. Pass 1996, personal communication.

of the chemotherapy arm (Pass 1996, personal communication). There were differences in recurrence patterns by arm in the NCI trial: less distant but more local disease was observed in the induction chemotherapy group. The group with preoperative chemoRT had a survival identical to the surgeryalone arm in the Japanese study (Yoneda et al. 1995).

The other two randomized trials (M.D. Anderson, Spain) were closed early due to their strongly positive results in favor of the induction chemotherapy arms, as shown in Table 5.11 (Roth et al. 1994; Rosell et al. 1994). Longer follow-up data were shown for both studies at the Eighth World Lung Cancer Conference, as of this writing not yet published (Roth 1997, meeting presentation). At a median follow-up of 81 months, 32% of patients were alive in the induction chemotherapy group versus 16% in the surgery-alone arm ($P = 0.06$) in the M.D. Anderson study. The *P* value became significant if only deaths due to cancer were considered. In the Spanish trial, no patients survived in the surgery group, versus there were 16% long-term survivors in the induction chemotherapy arm.

The M.D. Anderson and Spanish trials continue to generate much discussion and debate. The consensus is that these results are provocative, but they are not definitive. There are various aspects of the design and outcome of the studies that call for confirmatory trials. As mentioned above, the major concern is that of marked substage heterogeneity within these two trials. It is not clear that the early stopping rules for these very small trials accounted for the strong potential influence of even slight substage or molecular prognostic factor imbalances between the two arms. Minor shifts between arms of these factors would have a major impact on the survival differences. Furthermore, the surgical control arms fared poorly, possibly due to substage imbalance (e.g., high rate of stage IIIB/IV in the M.D. Anderson control arm). However, in the Spanish trial the surgery-alone arm had 37% patients with N0 or N1 disease. But, more patients in the control arm had tumors with K-RAS mutations and aneuploid DNA, both potential adverse prognostic factors. Small differences in unstratified prognostic factors such as K-RAS could potentially affect the results. It is hoped that the larger ongoing and planned randomized trials that control for these factors will confirm the promising results of these small trials.

5.8 Surgical Considerations

It is beyond the scope of this chapter to review all the critical surgical issues involved in the conduct of and observed within the analyses of these studies. Nevertheless, several summary points should be made. First and foremost, a multidisciplinary team approach is mandatory from the time of diagnosis. This team should include a thoracic surgeon with expertise in the technical demands of post-induction surgery and postoperative care, medical and radiation oncologists, a pulmonologist and a radiologist. This same multidisciplinary involvement is necessary at the re-evaluation point after induction. At this time, re-staging tests should be reviewed and the optimal time for surgery decided (usually 3–5 weeks after completion of the induction before the development of fibrosis).

Although some trials were designed to offer post-induction resection only to those with a complete or partial response, it may be more important to document lack of progression. Patients with stable disease on CT scans of the chest after the induction are often found to have either minimal or no tumor in the pathology specimen and should also be offered resection. For example, in the SWOG 8805 study, there were 37 patients who had stable disease after induction. Thirty of these underwent thoracotomy, of whom 26 were resected. Of these, 12 (46%) had no residual tumor or only rare microscopic foci (Albain et al. 1995).

A more difficult and theoretical question is what should define a complete resection. Should the margins for resection encompass the original extent of disease, or must these margins be dictated by the amount of residual tumor? How extensive should search for contralateral nodal disease be conducted? These issues move from the theoretical to the practical as more experience is gained among the multidisciplinary teams and as the induction regimens become more innovative. In part, the answers to these questions will be dictated by the role surgery is eventually defined to play: a local control modality versus critical for long-term survival.

The type of surgical resection required is to a large degree determined by the initial extent and bulk of disease. At least for those trials in which patients with marginally resectable or unresectable disease were accrued, more complex operations are necessary and technical experience of the thoracic surgeon in postinduction surgery is critical (Rusch and Benfield 1993). Of the resections performed in the SWOG 8805 trimodality trial, 43% were standard lobectomies, 15% complex lobectomies (extrapleural, spine, chest wall or sleeve resections), 13% pneumonectomies and 29% intrapericardial pneumonectomies (Albain et al. 1995; Rusch et al. 1994). The acute surgical morbidities appear to be similar regardless of the type of induction, unless too much time is allowed to elapse in those patients who received RT as part of the induction and extensive fibrosis is therefore encountered.

5.9 Treatment-Related Morbidity and Mortality

The morbidity from induction chemotherapy or induction chemoRT followed by surgery is not insignificant. The most common side effects are the expected myelosuppression from chemotherapy and esophagitis, more often observed after chemoRT. Both of these toxicities are usually manageable on an outpatient basis. However, pulmonary complications, especially those observed in the postoperative period, are the greatest concern, as discussed above. This toxicity manifests as either an extensive pneumonitis, usually culture-negative, or ARDS-like picture, the latter of which has a high mortality rate. Pulmonary morbidity and mortality were reported in most studies of combined modality therapy at rates higher than expected from RT or surgery alone. It occurs after all types of induction chemotherapy regimens, with or without RT, usually in those patients who required a pneumonectomy. These pulmonary complications result from multifactorial causes (Zeldin et al. 1984; Mathru et al. 1990; Fowler et al. 1993; Roach et al. 1995). Although high dose radiation above 45 Gy has been implicated (Fowler et al. 1993), the occurrence of this severe problem in trials with no induction RT and the lack of an excess rate in other trials with high-dose RT (Law et al. 1997; Choi et al. 1997; Eberhardt et al. 1997) underscore that lymphatic sump disruption and post-pneumonectomy shunts may be less well tolerated after induction chemotherapy. The preoperative DLCO may be the most important screen for this problem, which is being studied prospectively in the current North American Intergroup phase III trial in N2 disease.

The other major morbidity experienced by many patients after induction therapy followed by surgery is a post-treatment constitutional syndrome. This consists of a constellation of symptoms including thoracotomy pain, malaise, anorexia and poor pulmonary reserve. This syndrome probably occurs at a greater frequency than with radiation or surgery alone and its rate is under-reported. It often resolves within a year after treatment, but its lingering presence is clearly discouraging to the patient and caregiver. Prospective quality of life analyses and active rehabilitation protocols for this population are sorely needed.

Finally, it must be emphasized that these combined modality programs were tested in the "fittest" patients who were fully ambulatory and had general medical conditions that permitted the rigors of this therapy. Eligibility criteria were of necessity quite strict in these trials and it may be dangerous to offer this type of treatment outside of a clinical trial, especially to patients who have a poor performance status and/or major co-morbidities. Clinical trials geared to the large group of patients ineligible for these aggressive approaches are fortunately expanding, with first reports expected shortly.

5.10 Has an Optimal Treatment Program Emerged?

It is clear that no induction program has emerged as superior to the others to date. The major reasons for no current consensus are: (a) lack of large randomized trials that address a single question in a homogeneously staged group of patients; (b) marked variability in study populations, staging methods and disease bulk across the trials reviewed in the preceding sections; and (c) difficulty in defining what constitutes a "resectable" versus an "unresectable" tumor. Thus, it is difficult to put these variations aside to strictly consider the questions of optimal chemotherapy, RT, and combinations of these modalities in the published studies. Nevertheless, some evidence is presented by a few trials, although clear answers to these questions must await ongoing and planned randomized studies.

5.10.1 Chemotherapy: Old Versus New Agents

There is no chemotherapy induction regimen that currently can be recommended as superior and no randomized trials exist that asked (or are asking) this question. All programs with published safety data and long-term follow-up employed second-generation cisplatin combinations, either alone as induction therapy or in sequence or concurrent with RT. Pilot studies of induction chemotherapy or chemoRT that used one of the taxanes, gemcitabine, vinorelbine or other newer agents in combination with cisplatin or carboplatin prior to surgery have been initiated and reported in meeting summaries or in abstract form. However, it is too early to determine if these approaches will be at least as safe and hopefully superior to the studies reviewed in this chapter. Prior to establishing their safety as presurgery induction programs, the feasibility and superiority of adding new agents within a chemoRT approach (with no surgery) in locally advanced disease should first be proven.

There are data from the chemoRT trials in unresectable stage III disease (without subsequent surgery) that provide reassurance regarding the value of continuing studies that employ second generation chemotherapy in induction regimens prior to surgery. Specifically, the role of etoposide has been questioned. In two successive phase II trials in identically staged patients conducted by the Avignon, France group, superior 3-year survival was achieved with concurrent cisplatin, etoposide and RT compared with cisplatin and RT: 38% versus 16%, $P < 0.003$ (Reboul 1996, meeting presentation). The addition of etoposide was an independent favorable predictor of survival in a multivariate analysis.

Furthermore, some have suggested that current standard of care should require replacement of the older with new agents in the induction chemotherapy or chemoRT. However, this recommendation is premature. Numerous phase II pilot studies of a platin plus a taxane, usually paclitaxel, in combination with RT but without subsequent surgery, were recently reported with encouraging early results (Choy et al. 1994; Frascl et al. 1997). However, none of these newer programs tested in carefully staged subsets have yet reported superiority in long-term follow-up. In a recent update, response rates in four successive trials of paclitaxel and RT ± carboplatin were 73%–77%, very similar to the response rates of the second and third generation induction programs reviewed herein (Choy 1997). The 3-year survivals of 15.5% and 19%, available in two of these trials, and the 2-year survival of 40% in a third study are comparable to those reported in the past for chemoRT without surgery. For example, the 2- and 3-year survivals after the combination of cisplatin, etoposide and concurrent RT without surgical resection in the SWOG 9019 stage IIIB study were 33% and 26%, respectively (Albain et al. 1997). Therefore, completion of ongoing randomized studies that employ second-generation chemotherapy in combination with RT prior to surgery can be justified.

Meanwhile, the outcomes of important randomized studies that are testing the safety and efficacy of various new agents in combination with RT (but without surgery) are eagerly awaited. These studies should be completed with a full safety analysis before surgical resection is added to the program. As these new trials mature, it will be critical to monitor the stage subset mix and substage documentation methods in order to determine if the anticipated reports of superiority may be solely attributed to the change in chemotherapy.

5.10.2 Is Radiotherapy Necessary in the Induction Regimen?

A Brazilian study stands alone as the only randomized trial to date that addressed the need for RT in the induction regimen (Fleck et al. 1994). As shown in Table 5.12, 96 patients with clinically bulky or biopsy-proven stage IIIA(N2) and T4 IIIB disease were randomized between chemoRT followed by surgery versus chemotherapy alone followed by surgery. Two programs commonly employed at the time were tested: cisplatin and 5-fluorouracil plus RT versus the MVP regimen. In the initial (and only published) report at the 1994 American Society of Clinical Oncology meeting, survival was significantly better for chemoRT than for pre- and postoperative chemotherapy in these patients with mixed stage III disease. Significantly more neutropenia and neurologic toxicity were observed in the MVP arm, whereas there was a higher rate of mucositis in the chemoRT group. Recently, updated results were made available but are not yet published: the 5-year survival is 31% in the chemoRT arm versus 15% in the MVP arm ($P = 0.05$) (Fleck 1997, personal communication).

Confirmatory studies in a homogeneously staged population are needed to validate this result, but one other hint regarding the necessity of RT came from a Japanese trial that did not include surgery (Kubota et al. 1994). Patients with stage III disease without progression after two cycles of cisplatin-containing chemotherapy were randomized to 60 Gy (2 Gy/day) or observation. The 3-year survival was 29% versus 3% in favor of the addition of RT.

The safety and efficacy of preoperative hyperfractionated RT combined with chemotherapy followed by surgery were defined in two recent trials (Sect. 5.6). A randomized study of single versus twice-daily fractionation combined with chemotherapy (but with no subsequent surgery) is ongoing by the RTOG, but no trial testing the type of induction fractionation with the addition of surgery is in progress at this writing.

5.10.3 Timing of Radiotherapy in Induction Trials with Surgery

Controversy also exists regarding the optimal timing of RT with respect to chemotherapy and surgery. The debate was that concurrent induction chemoRT was more toxic than sequential and that no data existed to support its use over RT alone in unresectable disease. A review of the toxicity profiles in the studies reviewed herein suggested they are actually quite simi-

Table 5.12. Other randomized trials that address role of various modalities within induction programs for non-small cell lung cancer

Group or study	References	No. patients	Stage subset	Question	Design	Outcome
Brazil[a]	Fleck et al. 1994	96	Stage IIIA(N2) and T4 IIIB; N2 nodes bulky on CT or biopsy-proven	Role of RT in the induction?	PF + RT vs MVP ↓ Surgery ↓ RT vs MVP (if residual disease)	five-year survival 31% vs 15% in favor of PF + RT ($P = 0.05$)
NCI Canada	Payne et al. 1997	31	Biopsy-proven stage IIIA(N2)	Induction then surgery vs RT?	PV → surgery vs RT alone	Closed early due to slow accrual; survival cuves superimposed at 2 years
RTOG 89-01	Inculet et al. 1997	71	Biopsy-proven stage IIIA(N2)	Postinduction surgery vs RT?	MVP or VP ↓ Surgery vs RT ↓ MVP or VP	Closed early due to slow accrual; $P = 0.62$ for overall survival; 4-year: 13% for surgery vs 20% for RT

Abbreviations: as in Tables 5.2, 5.4, 5.6; RTOG, Radiation Therapy Oncology Group.
[a] Update provided by J. Fleck 1997, personal communication.

lar, regardless of when the RT was given, although concurrent chemoRT regimens may have a higher rate of esophagitis or mucositis. But, operative mortality rates were no different, even if hyperfractionated RT regimens were employed. Of note, the CALGB had great difficulty completing the RT when it was given "posterior" to the surgery (SUGARBAKER et al. 1995). Furthermore, the North Central Cancer Treatment Group (NCCTG) reported that concurrent chemroRT significantly increased time to progression and lowered systemic failure rates compared to RT alone (no surgery was attempted) (MCGINNIS et al. 1995). This study was terminated early due to publication of reports of superiority of chemoRT over RT alone in unresectable disease.

While no trials have been conducted with postinduction surgery to address the concurrent versus sequential chemoRT question, an important Japanese study was recently reported in unresectable, stage III disease (FURUSE et al. 1997). There was a significant long-term survival advantage to the concurrent over the sequenced regimen. An ongoing RTOG trial directly tests this question in locally advanced disease (but without surgical resection).

5.10.4 After Induction Chemotherapy: Is Surgery Necessary?

Another question raised by the trials reported to date is whether surgery is superior to RT after induction chemotherapy. As reviewed in Sect. 5.5.2, several studies reported no prognostic impact of complete resection. For example, the CALGB I study update showed that many of the long-term survivors did not undergo a complete resection (STRAUSS 1997). Therefore, two randomized studies were designed to address this question, one by the NCI Canada (n = 31) and the other by the RTOG (n = 71) (PAYNE et al. 1997; INCULUT et al. 1997). These trials are described in Table 5.12, both of which gave induction chemotherapy followed by surgical resection in one arm versus either definitive RT alone or induction chemotherapy followed by RT in a meticulously staged, homogeneous population with stage IIIA(N2) disease. Both of these trials closed prematurely due to impaired accrual, but were recently reported for the first time. The survival curves overlap in both studies. The 4-year survival was 13% in the surgery arm and 20% for the RT group in the RTOG study. Ongoing studies are designed to definitively answer this question (see Sect. 5.11.1).

5.11 Ongoing Trials

5.11.1 Phase III Trials in Stage III(N2) Disease

There are three large randomized phase III trials ongoing worldwide in patients with biopsy-proven stage IIIA(N2) disease. The study designs are shown in Table 5.13. The current High Priority North American Intergroup Trial (RTOG, SWOG, ECOG, CALGB, NCCTG and NCI Canada) tests the trimodality program developed by the SWOG (ALBAIN et al. 1995) versus the same induction chemoRT but no surgery with full dose RT in pathologically documented, bulky N2 disease. Accrual has increased and ongoing analyses of toxicity by the Data and Safety Monitoring Committee permit continuation of this study. No unexpected toxicities or excess postoperative mortality were observed in the first 170 patients accrued (ALBAIN, RUSCH, TURRISI and SCOTT 1998, personal communication). The European Intergroup trial asks whether surgical resection or RT is optimal after three cycles of induction chemotherapy (SPLINTER et al. 1997a). At the point of accrual of 179 patients, an interim analysis showed a resection rate of 89%, 3 treatment-related deaths and downstaging in 42%. Patients were able to complete the postchemotherapy RT. The third trial is a follow-up study of the phase II West German Cancer Center trial (EBERHARDT et al. 1997). This study will test the impact of surgery after induction chemotherapy followed by more chemotherapy plus concurrent, hyperfractionated RT versus observation.

5.11.2 Ongoing Trials in Early Stage or Minimal Bulk Disease

Ongoing randomized phase II or phase III studies in early stage disease ask if preoperative chemotherapy adds to surgical resection alone. These studies, summarized in Table 5.14, all test a cisplatin-containing regimen in variable stage subsets, excluding N2 disease. The French trial met its accrual goal in March 1997 and results are awaited at this writing (DEPIERRE et al. 1994). The EORTC trial is accruing slowly and may not reach its accrual goal (SPLINTER et al. 1997b) and the other studies are very early in accrual. A phase II pilot study of carboplatin plus paclitaxel prior to resection in patients with stage T2N0, T1-2N2 or T3N0-1 disease is in progress and a

Table 5.13. Ongoing randomized phase III trials that ask if surgery is necessary in biopsy-proven stage IIIA (N2) NSCLC

Group	Projected number of patients	Design
North American Intergroup	510	EP × 2 + single fx RT, concurrent ↙ ↘ EP × 2 + Complete RT to 61 Gy with no break / Surgery ↓ EP × 2
European Intergroup	480	Any cisplatin-containing regimen ↙ ↘ Surgery / Single fx RT
West German Consortium	NA	Taxol + P → hyperfx RT + Taxol + P ↙ ↘ Surgery / Observation

Abbreviations given in other tables; fx, fraction.

Table 5.14. Ongoing randomized phase II or phase III trials that ask if induction chemotherapy is necessary

Group	Stage	Design	Status
French Phase II	T2N0, II, IIIA	Surgery vs PIM → surgery (postoperative RT in both arms if T3 or N2(+) at surgery)	Met accrual goal (n = 372) on 3/1/97
EORTC Randomized Phase II	I, II, IIIA (N0)	EP × 2 → surgery vs surgery alone	Ongoing, accrual very slow
Netherlands Phase III	T2N0, N1, T3N0	EP × 2–4 (to maximum response) → surgery vs surgery alone	Ongoing
England Phase III	"Early Stage"	Cisplatin-containing ChT × 3 → surgery vs surgery alone	Ongoing

Abbreviations as in other tables.

randomized follow-up trial is under consideration (Pisters et al. 1997).

5.12 The Two Induction Therapy Controversies: Is There a Consensus?

After considering the worldwide data reviewed herein on induction therapy followed by surgery, one can revisit the questions posed in Sect. 5.1 and Table 5.1. Should post-induction surgery become the standard of care in advanced stage III disease and, if so, for which subsets? Should surgical candidates with initially resectable disease always receive preoperative chemotherapy and, if so, which stage subgroups? Many practitioners, especially in North America, have concluded yes to both questions and routinely prescribe such treatments outside a clinical trials for many stage subsets. However, the majority Consensus Statement of the International Association for the Study of Lung Cancer (IASLC) emphasized that the data argue that it is premature to reach these conclusions in either disease group (Perry et al. 1997).

First, the IASLC Consensus Statement pointed out that while feasibility and safety were demonstrated and that some provocative outcome data were reported, post-induction surgery has not yet been proven to be superior to chemoRT or chemotherapy alone. Thus, this approach should not be routinely applied to unresectable or marginally resectable bulky N2 or stage IIIB disease, for which chemoRT remains the standard of care. Second, the Consensus Statement concluded that surgery alone is still the standard (versus preoperative chemoRT or chemotherapy) for the minimal bulk, "up front" resectable subsets. This issue remains unsettled because of the small numbers and stage subset biases in the two randomized trials with positive results (Roth et al. 1994; Rosell et al. 1994) and the superimposition of survival curves in the two (albeit incomplete) trials that tested a non-surgery arm (Payne et al. 1997; Inculet et al. 1997).

Fortunately, ongoing and planned randomized trials (Tables 5.13, 5.14) should provide definitive answers to these two questions. Yet, there are growing trends to attempt resection of disease in all patients following chemo ± RT, and/or to add new agents to induction RT ahead of published pilot safety and efficacy data in clearly defined subsets, and/or to routinely give third-generation chemotherapy prior to resection in those patients with early stage disease. These practice trends may jeopardize the worldwide accrual to the randomized trials and, if so, this debate will remain the most controversial area in the management of NSCLC. It is hoped that oncologists and thoracic surgeons will support these studies and thus allow answers to these critical questions.

References

Albain KS (1997a) Induction chemotherapy with or without radiation followed by surgery in stage III non-small cell lung cancer: update and perspectives. Oncology 11[Suppl 9]:51–57

Albain KS (1997b) Author update on: concurrent cisplatin/etoposide plus chest radiotherapy followed by surgery for stages IIIA(N2) and IIIB non-small-cell lung cancer: mature results of Southwest Oncology Group phase II study 8805. Classic Pap Curr Comm 2:145–158

Albain KS, Rusch VW, Crowley JJ et al (1995) Concurrent cisplatin/etoposide plus chest radiotherapy followed by surgery for stages IIIA(N2) and IIIB non-small cell lung cancer: mature results of Southwest Oncology Group Phase II Study 8805. J Clin Oncol 13:1880–1892

Albain KS, Crowley JJ, Turrisi AT et al (1997) Concurrent cisplatin/etoposide plus radiotherapy for pathologic stage IIIB non-small cell lung cancer: a Southwest Oncology Group phase II study (S9019). Proc Am Soc Clin Oncol 16:128a

Bitran JD, Golomb HM, Hoffman PC et al (1986) Protochemotherapy in non-small cell lung carcinoma. An attempt to increase surgical resectability and survival. A preliminary report. Cancer 57:44–53

Bloedorn FG, Cowley RA, Cuccia CA, Mercado R (1961) Combined therapy with irradiation and surgery in the treatment of bronchogenic carcinoma. Am J Roentgenol 85:875–885

Bonomi P, Gale M, Faber LP et al (1992) Is clinical stage III non-small cell lung cancer a homogeneous group? Proc Am Soc Clin Oncol 11:292

Bromley LL, Szur L (1955) Combined radiotherapy and resection for carcinoma of the bronchus: experience with 66 patients. Lancet 2:937–941

Burkes RL, Shepherd FA, Ginsberg RJ et al (1994) Blackstein ME, Goldberg ME, Todd T, Pearson FG, Jones D, Greenwood C. Induction chemotherapy with MVP in patients with stage IIIA(N2) unresectable non-small cell lung cancer: the Toronto experience. Proc Am Soc Clin Oncol 13:327

Choi NC, Carey R, Daly W et al (1997) Potential impact on survival of improved tumor downstaging and resection rate by preoperative twice-daily radiation and concurrent chemotherapy in stage IIIA non-small-cell lung cancer. J Clin Oncol 15:712–722

Choy H (1997) Author update on: phase I trial of outpatient weekly paclitaxel and concurrent radiation therapy for advanced non-small-cell lung cancer. Classic Pap Curr Comm 2:167–171

Choy H, Akerley W, Safran H et al (1994) Phase I trial of outpatient weekly paclitaxel and concurrent radiation therapy for advanced non-small-cell lung cancer. J Clin Oncol 12:2682–2686

Curran WJ, Stafford PM (1995) Lack of apparent difference in outcome between clinically staged IIIA and IIIB no-small cell lung cancer treated with radiotherapy. J Clin Oncol 8:409–415

Darwish S, Minotti V, Crino L et al (1994) Neoadjuvant cisplatin and etoposide for stage IIIA (clinical N2) non-small cell lung cancer. Am J Clin Oncol (CCT) 17: 64–67

Depierre A, Milleron B, Lebeau B et al (1994) An ongoing randomized study of neoadjuvant chemotherapy in resectable non-small cell lung cancer. Semin Oncol 21[Suppl 4]:16–19

Eagan RT, Ruud C, Lee RE et al for the Lung Cancer Study Group (1987) Pilot study of induction therapy with cyclophosphamide, doxorubicin and cisplatin (CAP) and chest irradiation prior to thoracotomy in initially inoperable stage III M0 non-small cell lung cancer. Cancer Treat Rep 71:895–900

Eberhardt W, Wilke H, Stuschke G et al (1997) Preoperative chemotherapy and concurrent chemoradiotherapy based on hyperfractionated accelerated radiotherapy followed by surgery in locally advanced inoperable non-small cell lung cancer stages IIIA and IIIB – The value of PCI. Lung Cancer 18[Suppl 1]:65

Edelman MJ, Gandara DR, Roach M III, Benfield JR (1996) Multimodality therapy in stage III non-small cell lung cancer. Ann Thorac Surg 61:1564–1572

Elias AD, Skarin AT, Gonin R et al (1994) Neoadjuvant treatment of stage IIIA non-small cell lung cancer. Am J Clin Oncol (CCT) 17:26–36

Elias AD, Skarin AT, Leong T et al (1997) Neoadjuvant therapy for surgically staged IIIAN2 non-small cell lung cancer. Lung Cancer 17:147–161

Faber LP, Kittle CK, Warren WH et al (1989) Preoperative chemotherapy and irradiation for stage III non-small cell lung cancer. Ann Thorac Surg 47:669–677

Fleck J, Camargo J, Godoy D, Teixeira P, Braga Filho A, Barletta A, Ferreira P (1994) Chemoradiation therapy versus chemotherapy alone as a neo-adjuvant treatment for stage III non-small cell lung cancer. Preliminary report of a phase III prospective randomized trial. Proc Am Soc Clin Oncol 12:333

Fowler WC, Langer CJ, Curran WJ, Keller SM (1993) Postoperative complications after combined neoadjuvant treatment of lung cancer. Ann Thorac Surg 55:986–989

Frasci G, Comella P, Scoppa G et al (1997) Weekly paclitaxel and cisplatin with concurrent radiotherapy in locally advanced non-small cell lung cancer. A phase I study. J Clin Oncol 15:1409–1417

Furuse K, Fukuoka M, Takada Y, Nishikawa H, Katagami N, Ariyosahi Y for the West Japan Lung Cancer Group (1997) A randomized phase III study of concurrent versus sequential thoracic radiotherapy in combination with mitomycin, vindesine and cisplatin in unresectable stage III non-small cell lung cancer: preliminary analysis. Proc Am Soc Clin Oncol 16:459a

Green M, Brodin O, Choi N et al (1994) Pre-operative and post-operative treatments in stage III NSCLC. Lung Cancer 10[Suppl]:S15–S17

Inculet R, Scott C, Dar AR et al (1997) Phase III study comparing chemotherapy and radiation therapy with preoperative chemotherapy and surgical resection in patients with non-small cell lung cancer with spread to mediastinal lymph nodes: a Radiation Therapy Oncology Group study (RTOG 89-01). Lung Cancer 18[Suppl 1]:65

Johnson DH, Piantadosi S (1994) Chemotherapy for resectable stage III non-small cell lung cancer – can that dog hunt? J Natl Cancer Inst 86:650–651

Kubota K, Furuse K, Kawahara M et al (1994) Role of radiotherapy in combined modality treatment of locally advanced non-small cell lung cancer. J Clin Oncol 12:1547–1552

Lad T, Wagner H, Piantadosi S for the Lung Cancer Study Group (1991) Randomized phase II evaluation of pre-operative chemotherapy alone and radiotherapy alone in stage IIIA non-small cell lung cancer. Proc Am Soc Clin Oncol 10:258

Law A, Daly B, Madsen M et al (1997) High incidence of isolated brain metastases following complete response in advanced non-small cell lung cancer: a new challenge. Lung Cancer 18[Suppl 1]:65

Martini N, Flehinger BJ (1987) The role of surgery in N2 lung cancer. Surg Clin North Am 67:1037–1049

Martini N, Flehinger BJ, Zaman M, Beattie EJ (1983) Results of resection in non-oat cell carcinoma of the lung with mediastinal lymph node metastases. Ann Surg 198:386–397

Martini N, Kris MG, Flehinger BJ et al (1993) Preoperative chemotherapy for stage IIIA(N2) lung cancer: the Sloan-Kettering experience with 136 patients. Ann Thorac Surg 55:1365–1374

Mathru M, Blakeman B, Dries DJ et al (1990) Permeability pulmonary edema following lung resection. Chest 98: 1216–1218

McGinnis WL, Shaw EG, Jung S-H et al (1995) Results of a phase III prospective randomized trial comparing standard thoracic radiation therapy (TRT) to twice-daily TRT ± concomitant etoposide-cisplatin chemotherapy in patients with unresectable stage IIIA/B non-small cell lung cancer. Proc Am Soc Clin Oncol 14:355

Mountain CF (1988) Prognostic implications of the International Staging System for lung cancer. Semin Oncol 3: 236–245

Mountain CF (1997) Revisions in the International System for Staging Lung Cancer. Chest 111:1710–1717

Pass HI, Pogrebniak H, Steinberg SM et al (1992) Randomized trial of neoadjuvant therapy for lung cancer: interim analysis. Ann Thorac Surg 53:992–1008

Payne DG (1991) Pre-operative radiation therapy in non-small cell cancer of the lung. Lung Cancer 7:47–56

Payne DG, Shepherd F, Johnston M et al for the National Cancer Institute of Canada Clinical Trials Group (1997) What is the standard therapy for stage IIIA non-small cell lung cancer? A randomized trial of combination chemotherapy and surgery versus radiotherapy alone. Lung Cancer 18[Suppl 1]:62

Perry MC, Deslauriers J, Albain KS et al (1997) Induction treatment for resectable non-small-cell lung cancer: a consensus report. Lung Cancer 17[Suppl 1]:15–18

Pisters KMW, Kris MG, Gralla RJ, Zaman MB, Heelan RT, Martini N (1993) Pathologic complete response in advanced non-small-cell lung cancer following preoperative chemotherapy: implications for the design of future non-small cell lung cancer combined modality trials. J Clin Oncol 11:1757–1762

Pisters KMW, Kris MG, Bunn PA, Crowley JJ, Ginsberg RJ for the Bimodality Lung Oncology Team (1997) Phase II trial of induction paclitaxel/carboplatin in early stage (T2N0, T1-2N1 and selected T3N0-1) non-small cell lung cancer. Lung Cancer 18[Suppl 1]:84

Roach M, Gandara DR, Yuo H-S et al (1995) Radiation pneumonitis following combined modality therapy for lung cancer: analysis of prognostic factors. J Clin Oncol 13:2606–2612

Rosell R, Gomez-Codina J, Camps C et al (1994) A randomized trial comparing preoperative chemotherapy plus surgery with surgery alone in patients with non-small-cell lung cancer. N Engl J Med 330:153–158

Roth J, Fossella F, Komaki R et al (1994) A randomized trial comparing perioperative chemotherapy and surgery with surgery alone in resectable stage III non-small cell lung cancer. J Natl Cancer Inst 86:673–680

Rusch VW, Benfield JR (1993) Neoadjuvant therapy for lung cancer: a note of caution. Ann Thorac Surg 55:820–821

Rusch VW, Albain KS, Crowley JJ et al (1994) Neoadjuvant therapy: a novel and effective treatment for stage IIIB non-small cell lung cancer. Ann Thorac Surg 58:290–295

Shields T, Higgins G, Lawton KR, Heilbrunn A, Khean RJ (1970) Preoperative x-ray therapy as an adjuvant in the treatment of bronchogenic carcinoma. J Thorac Cardiovasc Surg 59:49–61

Skarin A, Jochelson M, Sheldon T et al (1989) Neoadjuvant chemotherapy in marginally resectable stage III M0 non-small cell lung cancer: long-term follow-up in 41 patients. J Surg Oncol 40:266–274

Splinter TAW, Kirkpatrick A, Darwish S, van Meerbeeck J for the EORTC, GOIRC and VKSL (1997a) Randomized trial of surgery versus radiotherapy in patients with stage IIIA non-small cell lung cancer after a response to induction chemotherapy. Intergroup study 08941. Lung Cancer 18[Suppl 1]:62–63

Splinter TAW, Smit E, Postmus P, Kho GS, Maat APWM (1997b) A randomized phase II trial of neoadjuvant chemotherapy followed by surgery versus surgery alone in patients with stage I, II and IIIA(N0) non-small cell lung cancer. Preliminary analysis. Lung Cancer 18[Suppl 1]:66

Strauss GM (1997) Author update on: Neoadjuvant chemotherapy and radiotherapy followed by surgery in stage IIIA non-small-cell lung carcinoma of the lung: report of a Cancer and Leukemia Group B phase II study. Classic Pap Curr Comm 2:159–166

Strauss GM, Langer MP, Elias AD, Skarin AT, Sugarbaker DJ (1992a) Multimodality treatment of stage IIIA non-small cell lung carcinoma: a critical review of the literature and strategies for future research. J Clin Oncol 10:829–838

Strauss GM, Herndon JE, Sherman DD et al (1992b) Neoadjuvant chemotherapy and radiotherapy followed by surgery in stage IIIA non-small-cell lung carcinoma of the lung: report of a Cancer and Leukemia Group B phase II study. J Clin Oncol 10:1237–1244

Sugarbaker DJ, Herndon J, Kohman LJ, Krasna MJ, Green MR (1995) Results of Cancer and Leukemia Group B Protocol 8935. A multi-institutional phase II trimodality trial for stage IIIA(N2) non-small-cell lung cancer. J Thorac Cardiovasc Surg 109:473–485

Vansteenkiste JF, De Leyn PR, Deneffe GJ, Lerut TE, Demedts MG (1998) Clinical prognostic factors in surgically treated stage IIIAN2 non-small cell lung cancer: analysis of the literature. Lung Cancer 19:3–13

Warram J (1975) Preoperative irradiation of cancer of the lung: final report of a therapeutic trial. A collaborative study. Cancer 36:914–923

Weiden PL, Piantadosi S for the Lung Cancer Study Group (1991) Preoperative chemotherapy (cisplatin and fluorouracil) and radiation therapy in stage III non-small cell lung cancer: a phase II study of the LCSG. J Natl Cancer Inst 83:266–272

Yoneda S, Hibino S, Gotoh I et al (1995) A comparative trial on induction chemoradiotherapy followed by surgery or immediate surgery for stage III NSCLC. Proc Am Soc Clin Oncol 14:367

Zeldin RA, Normandin D, Landtwing D, Peters RM (1984) Post-pneumonectomy pulmonary edema. J Thorac Cardiovasc Surg 87:359–365

6 Adjuvant Therapy in Non-Small Cell Lung Cancer

S.S. LEONG, C.M.S. ROCHA LIMA, and M.R. GREEN

CONTENTS

6.1 Introduction

Complete resection of tumor is a critical component of curative treatment for patients with non-small cell lung cancer (NSCLC). This holds true for patients with early stage disease as well as more advanced local tumor (WATANABE et al. 1991; MCCAUGHAN et al. 1985; GREEN and LILENBAUM 1994). However, despite "curative resection," the long term survival of these patients is less than satisfactory. They are still at risk for local and distant relapse and the risk for disease recurrence increases with more advanced disease. Based on the 1997 revision of the International Staging System for lung cancer, the 5-year survival rates of 1910 patients managed with definitive surgical treatment were analyzed. It was greater than 65% for stage IA patients. For patients with stages IB, IIA and IIB disease, these rates ranged from 40% to 55%. In selected stage IIIA patients, the rate fell to approximately 25% (MOUNTAIN 1997). This higher than expected survival rate for IIIA disease reflects the more favorable characteristics of stage IIIA patients who were selected for immediate surgery and found amenable to complete resection of disease (Table 6.1). Patients who had clinically evident stage IIIA disease in the same database did poorly, with a 5-year survival of only 13%.

S.S. LEONG, C.M.S. ROCHA LIMA, and M.R. GREEN, Hollings Cancer Center, Medical University of South Carolina, 171 Ashley Avenue, Charleston, SC 29425-2225, USA

Immense time and effort have been put into exploring the role of adjuvant therapy in an attempt to improve survival outcome in patients with completely resected non-small cell lung cancer. Unlike breast cancer (BONADONNA et al. 1976, 1995; STEWART 1987) or colon cancer (LAURIE et al. 1989; MOERTEL et al. 1995), where adjuvant treatment postsurgery has clearly established its role in improving both disease free and overall survival, similar data in lung cancer are at present suggestive but not convincing enough to advocate adjuvant therapy as standard of care.

6.2 Immunotherapy

Early attempts at adjuvant treatment targeted the immune system. In 1976, MCKNEALLY and colleagues (1976) reported preliminary results in 60 patients randomized to instillation of intrapleural bacille Calmette-Guérin (BCG) or observation postsurgery. At a median follow-up time of 1 year, none of the 17 stage I patients given intrapleural BCG has relapsed while 9 out of 22 stage I patients in the control group developed recurrent disease. The mature results reported 4 years later, now with 169 patients on study, still showed benefit in stage I patients but not in stage II and III patients. The recurrence rate at 3 years was 33% in the BCG-treated group and 62% in the control group (MCKNEALLY et al. 1981). This small but provocative trial demanded further investigation. At the same time, the enthusiasm for adjuvant therapy in breast cancer fueled further interest in adjuvant treatment of other common malignancies including lung cancer.

In this environment, the United States National Cancer Institute funded the Lung Cancer Study Group (LCSG), a coalition of North American academic institutions committed to investigating adjuvant therapy strategies in patients with lung cancer. The first trial of the LCSG, 771, was designed to retest the BCG observations of MCKNEALLY et al. on a

Table 6.1. Five-year survival rates of patients with pathological stage I-IIIA disease (adapted from MOUNTAIN 1997)

TNM staging	Group staging	Number of patients	Five-year survival rate
T1N0M0	IA	511	67%
T2N0M0	IB	549	57%
T1N1M0	IIA	76	55%
T2N1M0		288	39%
T3N0M0	IIB	87	38%
T3N1M0		55	25%
T1–3N2M0	IIIA	344	23%

larger scale. Four hundred and seventy-three patients with completely resected T1N0, T2N0 or T1N1 NSCLC were randomized to receive either intrapleural BCG along with oral isoniazid 300 mg/day for a total of 12 weeks or intrapleural saline plus an oral placebo. Accrual began in August 1977 and ended in October 1980. Final analysis revealed no benefit in either time to recurrence or survival (MOUNTAIN and GAIL 1981; GAIL 1994). However, these data were not available to LCSG investigators until 1981 at the earliest. Beginning in 1977, while study 771 was still ongoing, they used intrapleural BCG and oral isoniazid, along with the additional oral agent levamisole, as the "control arm" of LCSG 772, their first trial of adjuvant chemotherapy in resected patients with NSCLC.

The inclusion of levamisole as part of an adjuvant immunotherapy regimen for lung cancer was based on preliminary data. In a small randomized study by VAN HOUTTE et al., 2 years of levamisole treatment following surgery and mediastinal irradiation suggested a possible benefit for patients with early stage disease (T1N0 and T2N0) with a trend towards improved disease free survival (VAN HOUTTE et al. 1980). However, subsequent work by ANTHONY et al., using levamisole both pre-operatively as well as in the early postoperative period, demonstrated increased postoperative mortality in the levamisole treated patients, postulated to be immune-mediated (ANTHONY et al. 1979). A subsequent randomized trial of adjuvant levamisole failed to show either benefit or harm (HERSKOVIC et al. 1988).

Various other adjuvant immunotherapeutic approaches have been reported in patients with resected NSCLC. These have included the use of intrapleural OK-432, systemic therapies with interferon and lymphokines, and active immunotherapy (LEE et al. 1994; TAKITA et al. 1991). While no solid data are available to support routine use of adjuvant immunotherapy, additional work is continuing. TAKITA et al. (1991) reported a median survival of 106 months in resected NSCLC patients treated with active immunotherapy of a carcinoma-associated antigen and complete Freund's adjuvant mixture. Patients given complete Freund's adjuvant alone reportedly experienced a median survival of 71 months. The median survival was 38 months for the control group (TAKITA et al. 1991). Confirmatory trials of Takita's work, done by other investigators, are not available. While ongoing studies of vaccine therapies are being pursued in a variety of malignancies, these approaches remain clearly experimental. Adjuvant immunotherapy has no current role in patients with resected non-small cell lung cancer.

6.3 Radiation Therapy

Early approaches to curative treatment for patients with NSCLC were hampered by inadequate staging techniques and a lesser appreciation of early systemic spread than is available today. This led to attempts at resection in patients with locally advanced disease who would not be current candidates for primary surgical management. Whether or not fully resected, these patients were often referred postoperatively to radiation oncologists for consolidative radiation therapy. Several retrospective series from this period reported improved survival for patients treated with postoperative adjuvant radiotherapy. In 1971 KIRSCH et al. noted that 7 out of 36 resected lung cancer patients who received postoperative radiotherapy (range 30–60 Gy) survived 5 years (19.4%) while none of 12 patients who did not receive radiotherapy survived that long. There was apparently no difference in the two groups with respect to demographics and extent of tumor. In a larger, widely cited retrospective review of 219 patients who underwent resection of lung cancer, GREEN et al. (1975) reported 31% (39/125) of patients treated by surgery and postoperative irradiation of 50–60 Gy survived 5 years compared to 16% (15/34) of patients treated by surgery alone. The apparent effect of radiation was more pronounced for patients with hilar or mediastinal lymph node involvement: with 5-year survivals of 35% (23/66) and 3% (1/30) for patients with and without postoperative radiotherapy respectively. These retrospective data established postoperative irradiation as a relatively routine standard of care in node-positive patients with resected NSCLC.

Prospective evaluation of the role of postoperative irradiation began with study 773 of the Lung Cancer Study Group. In this trial, patients with stage II or III squamous cell carcinoma who had undergone complete resection were randomized to receive postoperative adjuvant radiotherapy, postoperative radiation plus levamisole, or no adjuvant treatment (WEISENBURGER 1986). The levamisole arm was dropped due to low accrual, but a nearly contemporary study of the Radiation Therapy Oncology Group testing postoperative irradiation alone versus postoperative irradiation plus levamisole failed to show any benefit from the added immunotherapy adjuvant (HERSKOVIC et al. 1988). LCSG 773 involved 230 randomized patients. There was a dramatic decrease in local recurrence as the first site of failure, 41% in the controls versus 3% (1/32 failures at a mean analysis time of 3.5 years) among the radiated patients. While the overall hazard ratio for recurrence was 1.4, favoring the treated group, this difference was not statistically significant ($P = 0.188$, log-rank test). There was no evidence that radiotherapy improved survival. On subset analysis, overall recurrence rates were significantly reduced ($P = 0.03$) in 44 patients with N2 disease. However, even in this subset, there was no significant survival benefit. As already suggested by the retrospective data, postoperative radiotherapy seemed to have more overall impact in patients with higher nodal status.

Retrospective evaluation of postoperative irradiation in stage IIIA patients was performed by ASTUDILLO and CONILL (1990). They reviewed 146 stage IIIA (T3 or N2) NSCLC patients who had undergone surgical resection to determine if postoperative radiation therapy improved survival and decreased disease recurrence. Eighty-six patients received radiotherapy (45–50 Gy) and 60 did not. There was no overall improvement in survival with postoperative radiotherapy. For patients with N2 disease, however, the median survival in patients who received postoperative radiotherapy was 15 months, compared to 6 months for those who did not. Local recurrence rates were lower in patients with N2 disease given radiotherapy postresection (12.6% vs 20%). Interestingly, patients with T3N0 and T3N1 disease who received radiotherapy appeared to have worse median survival times than their surgery-only counterparts. This probably reflected the unfavorable nature of the local disease in patients who were offered postoperative radiotherapy in this nonrandomized retrospective series. But it may in part reflect a higher morbidity and mortality associated with adjuvant radiotherapy treatment. The causes of death were not described in detail.

Between July 1986 and October 1993, the Medical Research Council (MRC) Lung Cancer Working Party in the United Kingdom conducted a larger randomized trial to compare surgery alone with surgery plus postoperative radiotherapy in patients with pathological T1-2N1-2 NSCLC (STEPHENS et al. 1996). The MRC trial used a radiation prescription of 40 Gy in 15 fractions over 3 weeks compared to the LCSG's use of 50 Gy in 5 weeks. LCSG 773 was restricted to patients with squamous cell carcinoma. All non-small cell histologies were included in the MRC trial. Three hundred and eight patients were accrued, 154 to each group. The incidence of definite local failure (17.5% for the radiotherapy group and 29% in the controls) was decreased in the radiotherapy group and the time to local failure was prolonged. Yet there was no overall benefit in survival for the patients receiving adjuvant radiotherapy. In a subset analysis of the 106 patients with N2 disease, 29% (15/52) of patients who received radiotherapy developed local recurrence compared to 41% (22/54) in the control group. Interestingly, distant metastases were also reduced in the radiotherapy group, 46% (24/52), compared to 70% (38/54) in the control group. Conversely, in the N1 group, the short term outcome seemed possibly worse after adjuvant radiation, with 1-year survival of 60% in the radiotherapy group vs 71% in controls, and median survival of 16.3 months in the radiotherapy group vs 20.5 months in controls. By 2 years, the survival curves had come together. These results were reminiscent of the retrospective observations reported by Astudillo (Table 6.2).

Current data suggest that adjuvant postoperative radiotherapy alone does not significantly improve overall survival but decreases the rate of local recurrence as the first site of failure. There appears to be greater absolute benefit in patients with higher nodal status, consistent with the theoretically increased risk of significant local and regional microscopic residual disease in patients with pathologic evidence of

Table 6.2. Adjuvant radiotherapy after surgery

Investigators	Design	Stage	No.	Treatment	Results
Kirsh et al. 1971	Retrospective	–	36	30–50 Gy vs observation	Five-year survival 19.4% vs none
Green et al. 1975	Retrospective	–	219	50–60 Gy vs observation	Five-year survival 31% vs 16%
Weisenburger et al. 1986	Prospective randomized	II, III	230	50 Gy vs observation	Decreased local recurrence
Astudillo and Conill 1990	Retrospective	IIIA	146	45–50 Gy vs observation	Increased median survival and decreased local recurrence
Stephens et al. 1996	Prospective randomized	T1–2, N1–2	384	40 Gy vs observation	Decreased local recurrence

increased nodal involvement. The impact of adjuvant radiation on fully resected patients with earlier stages of NSCLC appears insignificant or potentially even deleterious.

These data do not exclude the possibility that adjuvant radiotherapy may have an important role in the context of multimodality adjuvant therapy. Reduction of local failure is unlikely to have a major survival impact in disease settings where distant failure predominates. This has been elegantly demonstrated in breast cancer studies. Numerous studies of adjuvant chest wall radiation, without the use of a systemic adjuvant as well, demonstrated a decrease in chest wall failure but no impact on overall survival. More recently, studies of adjuvant breast or chest wall radiation combined with systemic adjuvant therapy have shown improvements in survival compared to systemic adjuvant therapy alone (Overgaard et al. 1997; Ragaz et al. 1997). This finding supports the concern that there may be a significant residual submicroscopic tumor burden in the surgical bed and that this residual tumor remains a potential source of recurrence. Perhaps due to the relatively large number of remaining cells or as the result of changes associated with surgery and wound healing, these locoregional sites may be relative sanctuaries from the effects of systemic adjuvant therapy. If the systemic regimens decrease distant metastases, the additional benefit of local control provided by post-operative irradiation may combine to further improve outcome. This possibility is about to be tested in lung cancer in an intergroup study in the United States. Patients with resected stage IIIA NSCLC will all receive adjuvant chemotherapy with taxol and carboplatin. Following completion of drug therapy, patients who have not recurred will be randomly assigned to observation or thoracic radiation. A total of 360 patients will be entered and 240 are anticipated to be randomized. The trial should begin in late 1998.

Another broader but less specific test of adjuvant irradiation is already ongoing as part of the International Adjuvant Lung Trial (IALT). As discussed in detail later, this trial will randomize over 3000 resected stages I-III NSCLC patients to observation or cisplatin-based chemotherapy. At each institution, the investigators will decide whether or not to use thoracic radiation as part of their adjuvant therapy approach. Two rules apply: *all* patients at a given institution must either get radiation or not get it. This must be decided by the institutional investigators when they join the trial. Whether or not to use radiation cannot be decided on a case by case basis. If radiation is used, the timing of radiation in the patients randomized to chemotherapy is defined as following completion of drug treatment. For patients assigned to no chemotherapy, the radiation is initiated within 3–6 weeks following surgery. Analysis of this trial may provide additional information about the impact of adjuvant radiation with and without coordinated chemotherapy in patients with resected NSCLC.

6.4 Chemotherapy

Following complete resections of stages I-IIIA NSCLC, the large majority of first relapses are systemic, with the brain often the first metastatic site to be recognized (Feld et al. 1984; Martini and Flehinger 1987). For example, in stage I and II patients entered on LCSG 771, 70% of first relapses were extrathoracic, including 23% in the central nervous system (Gail 1994). In a carefully monitored group of 108 patients with fully resected stages II and III squamous carcinoma, 41% of first failures were local. Fifty-nine percent were systemic, including 12% of patients with brain only first recurrences (WEISENBURGER 1986). These and other similar data define the patterns of failure in patients with NSCLC after complete resection. They suggest the need for an effective systemic adjuvant approach as the critical component to further improved survival in patients with completely resected NSCLC.

The potential benefit of adjuvant systemic therapy after resection of an intrathoracic primary tumor has been recognized for decades. In the pre-cisplatin era, between the late 1950s and the mid 1970s, studies of adjuvant chemotherapy frequently evaluated single agents. These were most often alkylating agents with at best marginal activity in advanced lung cancer. HIGGINS et al. (1969) randomized 1035 patients to receive intravenous cyclophosphamide or placebo postresection, while MILLER (1971) used oral cyclophosphamide as the systemic intervention in a trial of over 500 patients. No survival benefit was seen in the treated patients in either study. SHIELDS et al. randomized 417 men with fully resected lung cancer to one of three arms: either prolonged intermittent intravenous cyclophosphamide alternating with intravenous methotrexate, intravenous cyclophosphamide alone, or an observation control. There was no improvement in outcome, compared to observation, for either of the treatment groups (SHIELDS et al. 1977). In an early Medical Research Council trial, GIRLING et al. (1985) assessed prolonged treatment with oral busulfan or cyclophosphamide compared to placebo in 726 patients. With 15 years of follow-up, 8% of patients given busulfan, 9% of patients treated with cyclophosphamide, and 10% of placebo patients remained alive.

Recently an international collaborative group of lung cancer trialists completed a meta-analysis of the role of adjuvant chemotherapy in patients with NSCLC (1995). Among 2145 patients in 5 studies which compared alkylating therapy to observation or placebo, there was a 15% increased risk of death among the alkylating agent treated patients. This translated into an absolute 5% decrement in survival at 5 years for those patients given adjuvant alkylating agent therapy. Whether these results were due to an increased rate of toxic death, an enhanced risk of second malignancy, or other causes is unclear. They clearly should raise a cautionary flag to remind all current investigators that adjuvant treatment approaches are not without risks and reinforce the maxim that therapies of marginal efficacy in the advanced disease setting are unlikely to be of substantial utility as adjuvant treatment.

Since first appearing in the mid 1970s, cisplatin-based chemotherapy has had a modest but significant positive impact on outcome for patients with advanced NSCLC. Several individual trials and two meta-analyses (NSCLC 1995; SOUQUET et al. 1993) have demonstrated a statistically significant improvement in overall survival for advanced disease patients receiving chemotherapy compared to best supportive care. The efficacy of cisplatin-based regimens in advanced disease patients provides a stronger rationale for testing these combination chemotherapy regimens in the adjuvant setting for patients with completely resected NSCLC.

In the late 1970s, the LCSG embarked on two randomized trials to ascertain the impact of postoperative adjuvant cisplatin-based chemotherapy in patients with stage II (T2N1) and stage III (any T3 or any N2) NSCLC. Beginning in 1977, LCSG 772 enrolled patients with "completely resected" adeno- or large cell carcinomas and pathologic confirmation of hilar and/or mediastinal nodal involvement (HOLMES and GAIL 1986). Patients with the highest mediastinal node involved with tumor were excluded as were individuals with exudative pleural effusions demonstrated at surgery. Two years later, an additional trial, LCSG 791, was initiated for patients with incompletely resected tumors (positive margins or involvement of highest paratracheal lymph node resected) of all cell types (LAD et al. 1988). In both trials, the adjuvant chemotherapy tested was CAP (cyclophosphamide, doxorubicin and cisplatin), repeated every 4 weeks for a total of six cycles. Drug doses were modest by today's standards: cyclophosphamide 400 mg/m^2, doxorubicin 40 mg/m^2, and cisplatin 40 mg/m^2. This regimen had been shown to produce partial responses in nearly one-fourth of patients with advanced lung cancer, certainly suggesting superiority to single alkylating agents (RUCKDESCHEL et al. 1985).

Following careful intraoperative staging and complete resection patients entered on LCSG 772 were randomized to receive either adjuvant CAP chemotherapy or immunotherapy with intrapleural BCG, oral isoniazid and levamisole, as discussed earlier. One hundred and forty-one patients were accrued with 130 eligible for analysis. Median disease free survival was significantly prolonged in the group receiving chemotherapy, 15 months, vs 9 months in the immunotherapy group. Overall disease free survival was also significantly improved in the CAP treated patients (P = 0.032, log-rank test). Patients treated with CAP also had a numerical improvement of 7 months in median survival: 22 months in the chemotherapy group vs 15 months in the immunotherapy group. However, the overall survival curves for the two treatment groups were not statistically significantly different ($P = 0.113$). While this small, initial adjuvant chemotherapy trial of the LCSG produced suggestive but not definitive data, it generated substantial interest and some controversy. Some saw it as a proof of principle (Holmes and Gail 1986; Holmes 1994). Most considered the data insufficient to warrant the use of adjuvant CAP as standard therapy for patients with completely resected stages II and III NSCLC.

In LCSG 791 (Lad et al. 1988), "incompletely resected" patients presumably at increased risk for local recurrence as well as distant metastatic disease were randomized to receive either split course radiation (20 Gy in five fractions followed by 3 weeks rest and then another course of 20 Gy in five fractions) alone or the same radiation plus CAP chemotherapy. For patients randomized to both chemotherapy and radiation, the first two courses of CAP were given concurrently with the two 5-day courses of radiation. The patients subsequently received four additional cycles of the CAP regimen. One hundred and seventy-two patients were accrued to LCSG 791 with 164 eligible for analysis. Approximately 90% of the patients had stage III disease. Again in this trial, administration of CAP chemotherapy was associated with a significant improvement in median disease free survival (14 months in the chemotherapy/radiotherapy group vs 8 months in the radiotherapy group) and a notable numerical improvement in median survival (20 months in the chemotherapy/radiotherapy group vs 13 months in the radiotherapy group) but with no statistically significant improvement in overall survival. The survival data from the 772 and 791 trials were quite similar despite the more advanced stage of disease in the 791 patients. Whether the use of radiation, the inclusion of patients with squamous cell carcinoma, improved systemic staging in the 791 patients, some combination of factors, or chance alone is responsible for this observation remains unknown.

In 1980 the LCSG initiated a third adjuvant CAP trial in NSCLC patients with completely resected T2N0 or T1N1 patients (considered stage I at the time of study). Eighty-four percent of patients had T2N0 disease. This trial used four cycles of CAP, but employed a higher dose of cisplatin (60 mg/m^2), and a shortened 3-week cycle time. Treatment with CAP was compared with an observation control (LCSG 801) (Feld et al. 1993). Two hundred and thirty-two eligible patients were randomized to chemotherapy ($n = 122$) or standard observation ($n = 110$). There were no differences in time to recurrence and time to death between treated and untreated patients. The survival curves were essentially overlapping. Enthusiasts of adjuvant chemotherapy have emphasized that there was poor compliance in the treatment group. Only 53% of patients received all four cycles of chemotherapy and only 57% of those patients received treatment on time. Nonetheless, the absence of any effect of adjuvant CAP chemotherapy in patients with what, in theory, should represent the lowest overall burden of micrometastatic disease, had a chilling impact on developing use of adjuvant chemotherapy in patients with NSCLC.

Several years following the initiation of the LCSG trials, Finnish investigators also evaluated six cycles of adjuvant CAP chemotherapy (with cisplatin 40 mg/m^2) versus observation following complete resection of mostly early stage NSCLC. One hundred and ten patients with T1-3N0 NSCLC were accrued (Nirranen et al. 1992). Ninety-nine patients (90%) had stage I disease. The 5-year survival rate was 67% in the chemotherapy group versus 56% in the control group ($P = 0.05$) and this significant survival benefit persisted at 10 years (61% vs 48%, $P = 0.05$). However, the randomized treatment groups were unbalanced relative to at least one critical prognostic feature: there were more patients who underwent pneumonectomy in the control group (22/56) than in the treatment group (11/54). Unplanned subset analysis showed no difference in survival between the two arms among pneumonectomy patients. About 72.7% from each group had died at 5 years. For patients with smaller operations, those who had chemotherapy had a 5-year survival rate of 73.5% compared to 63.7% in the control group. This difference was not statistically significant.

A somewhat larger trial testing multi-agent adjuvant chemotherapy in a heterogeneous population of resected NSCLC was reported in 1995 by Dautzenberg for a group of French investigators. Two hundred and sixty-seven patients with completely resected stage I–III disease were randomized to either immediate postoperative radiation, 60 Gy over 6 weeks ($n = 129$), alone, or to have three courses of postoperative chemotherapy with cyclophosphamide, doxorubicin, cisplatin, vincristine, and lomustine followed by the same radiation ($n = 138$). There were no differences in overall survival between the patients getting sequential chemotherapy followed by radiation and those getting radiation alone. In this study, distant metastasis occurred more frequently as first site of relapse in the radiotherapy group ($P = 0.09$), suggesting that chemotherapy had some activity against disseminated micrometastasis. Local recurrences were slightly more frequent in the chemotherapy with the delayed radiation group (26%) compared to those who received immediate radiotherapy only (19%). The disease free interval for the group randomized to chemotherapy was 16.5 months compared to 13.3 months in the arm getting radiation alone, a difference that did not reach statistical significance ($P = 0.47$, log-rank test). A subset analysis of the 137 patients who had N2 disease did demonstrate a significant benefit in overall survival ($P = 0.003$) as well as disease free survival ($P = 0.02$) favoring the chemotherapy/radiotherapy group (15.3 months vs 8.6 months). These subset data must be interpreted cautiously. They are consistent, however, with other data in stage III(N_2) patients showing that induction chemotherapy improves survival when used as part of a combined modality approach. These findings also further support the thesis, discussed earlier, that a combination of an effective systemic adjuvant plus consolidative local radiation may be the most effective eventual approach to adjuvant therapy for more advanced subsets of patients with resected NSCLC.

In a Canadian randomized trial, the combination of vindesine and cisplatin was shown to be superior to CAP chemotherapy in response rate and survival for treatment of patients with advanced NSCLC (Radd et al. 1988). These data suggested that the vindesine/cisplatin combination might also be superior to CAP as adjuvant therapy in patients with resected NSCLC. Therefore Ohta et al. randomized 209 completely resected stage III patients with T3 or N2 disease to receive postoperative vindesine and cisplatin or no further treatment (Ohta et al. 1993). Ohta's group was unable to demonstrate any difference in disease free and overall survivals between patients given adjuvant chemotherapy and the control group at a mean follow-up time of 2.6 years. Compliance was problematic. Only 41% of patients in the treatment group received all three cycles of chemotherapy.

A smaller trial of adjuvant vindesine and cisplatin plus radiation versus radiation alone for resected patients with histologically documented N2, stage IIIA NSCLC was reported by Pisters et al. (1994) from Memorial Sloan Kettering. Seventy-two patients were entered. Forty-four were completely resected. Twenty-eight were incompletely resected but treated intraoperatively with ^{125}I seed implants. All patients received 40 Gy external beam radiation postoperatively. They were then randomized to observation or 4 months of intensive vindesine and cisplatin chemotherapy. With very mature follow-up, there was no suggestion of a favorable impact of the adjuvant chemotherapy on time to progression or survival.

The 1995 meta-analysis assessed the impact of cisplatin-based adjuvant chemotherapy in 1394 patients treated on 8 separate randomized trials including the three LCSG CAP trials and 3 vindesine and cisplatin-based studies. There was an overall 13% reduction in the risk of death (hazard ratio 0.87; $P = 0.08$) in the cisplatin combination treated patients. This level of risk reduction was consistent with between a 1% decrement and a 10% improvement in 5-year survival among patients who were given the adjuvant chemotherapy. As in some of the individual studies using adjuvant cisplatin combinations, these data were provocative but not definitive. Additional, potentially larger scale trials remained necessary in order to clarify the role of adjuvant chemotherapy.

Oral UFT, a specific molar ratio combination of tegafur and uracil, has been used in patients with advanced lung cancer for more than 10 years. As a single agent it produces modest toxicity and it can be easily administered over long periods of time. In 1986, Shimizu et al. reported on a small study of daily UFT for 4 weeks or more in 13 NSCLC patients. The main toxicity was anorexia (31%). Only one patient demonstrated a partial response. However, the duration of treatment was very short. A subsequent phase II trial using UFT and cisplatin in patients with advanced NSCLC demonstrated a 35% response rate (Ichinose et al. 1995). Two randomized adjuvant chemotherapy studies by Japanese investigators using oral UFT were reported in 1995. The first trial randomized 309 completely resected patients with stage I–III NSCLC to either postoperative chemotherapy with cisplatin, doxorubicin and UFT or observation (Study Group of Adjuvant Chemotherapy for Lung Cancer 1995). Five-year disease free and overall survival data were slightly better in the treatment group. The difference did not reach statistical significance. When the data were adjusted for prognostic variables, statistical significance was achieved. The second study, a three-arm trial by Wada et al., enrolled 323 completely resected patients with stage I–III disease between December 1985 and July 1988 (Wada et al. 1996). Three hundred and ten randomized patients were eligible for analysis. Two hundred and twenty-eight had no disease. The three arms were: one cycle of cisplatin/vindesine plus oral UFT for 1 year; oral UFT alone for 1 year; or observation. The 5-year survival rates were 60.6%, 64.1% and 49%, respectively, for the three arms. A log-rank analysis of the three arms revealed a borderline overall difference ($P = 0.053$). A subset comparison of UFT alone versus the observation control arm showed a significant benefit for postoperative administration of UFT ($P = 0.022$ log-rank test) (Table 6.3).

In a retrospective analysis of 532 postresection patients, 132 were given tegafur without uracil as postoperative adjuvant therapy. A significantly higher 5-year survival was found in tegafur-treated patients with stage I disease (Tanaka et al. 1996). The Japan Lung Cancer Research Group on Postsurgical Adjuvant Chemotherapy is now conducting a comparative study of surgery versus surgery and UFT in patients with pathologic stage I adenocarcinoma.

6.4.1 Limitations of Available Data

Twenty-three randomized trials of adjuvant chemotherapy for patients with resected NSCLC were evaluated as part of the 1995 meta-analysis. Few of the individual studies were positive and the aggregate findings of the meta-analysis suggested additional randomized studies were necessary. Review of the meta-analysis database highlights the small size of individual trials and the stage-based heterogeneity of the patients treated. In earlier studies, compliance was often poor and doses of adjuvant therapy actually administered were well below those prescribed. The recent UFT studies are of interest but need confirmation before defining a new standard of care. Additional, larger scale randomized trials, modeled on recent studies in breast and colon cancer, will be necessary to carefully and convincingly test the potential efficacy of adjuvant chemotherapy in patients

Table 6.3. Adjuvant chemotherapy after surgery

Investigators	Design	Stage	No.	Treatment	Results
Niranen et al. 1992	Prospective randomized	T1–3N0 (90% stage I)	110	CAP[a] vs observation	Five-year survival 67% vs 56%
Feld et al. 1993 (LCSG)	Prospective randomized	I (T2N0, T1N1)	232	CAP[b] vs observation	No benefit
Lad et al. 1988 (LCSG)	Prospective randomized	II, III (incomplete resection, 90% stage III)	164	CAP[a]/concurrent RT vs RT	Median survival 20 months vs 13 months
Dautzenberg et al. 1995	Prospective randomized	I–III	267	COPAC[c]/RT vs RT	No benefit
Ohta et al. 1993	Prospective randomized	III(T3 or N2)	219	Vp[d] vs observation	No overall benefit
Pisters et al. 1994	Prospective randomized	III(N2)	72	RT/VP[e] vs RT	No benefit
Study Group of Adjuvant Chemotherapy for Lung Cancer 1995	Prospective randomized	I–III	309	AP/UFT[f] vs observation	Five-year survival 61.8% vs 58.1%
Wada et al. 1996	Prospective randomized	I–III	310	VP/UFT[g] vs UFT vs observation	Five-year survival 60.6% vs 64.1% vs 49%

[a] Cyclophosphamide 400 mg/m^2, doxorubicin 40 mg/m^2, cisplatin 40 mg/m^2 q4 wks × 6 cycles.
[b] Cyclophosphamide 400 mg/m^2, doxorubicin 40 mg/m^2, cisplatin 60 mg/m^2 q3 wks × 4 cycles.
[c] Cycles 1 and 3: doxorubicin 40 mg/m^2, vincristine 1.2 mg/m^2, cisplatin 75 mg/m^2 on D1, lomustine 80 mg D3,4; cycle 2: cyclophosphamide 600 mg/m^2, vincristine 1.2 mg/m^2, cisplatin 75 mg/m^2 on D1.
[d] Vindesine 3 mg/m^2 D1,8, cisplatin 80 mg/m^2 D1 q4 wks × 3 cycles.
[e] Vindesine 3 mg/m^2 wkly ×5 then 2-wkly ×8, cisplatin 120 mg/m^2 D1, 29, 71, 113.
[f] One dose of doxorubicin 26 mg/m^2, cisplatin 66 mg/m^2, plus oral UFT 8 mg/kg/day for 6 months.
[g] One dose of cisplatin 50 mg/m^2, vindesine 2–3 mg/m^2 2-wkly ×3 doses, plus oral UFT 400 mg/day for 12 months vs UFT alone for 12 months vs observation.

with completely resected NSCLC. Several new agents, including vinorelbine, the taxanes, gemcitabine, and CPT-11, with increased single agent activity against advanced NSCLC have become available over the last several years. Inclusion of these agents in adjuvant chemotherapy regimens may facilitate a clearer demonstration of efficacy for adjuvant chemotherapy in patients with resected NSCLC.

6.4.2 Ongoing Trials

Numerous larger scale, randomized, multicenter adjuvant chemotherapy trials are now underway. In North America, an Intergroup trial comparing postoperative radiotherapy combined with cisplatin and etoposide versus thoracic radiotherapy alone in stage II and IIIA patients recently completed its accrual of over 450 patients. Two additional North American Intergroup trials are ongoing. In one trial (CALGB 9633), stage IB T2N0 patients are randomized to observation or four cycles of paclitaxel and carboplatin. The accrual target for this select subgroup is 500 patients. In the second trial (BR-10), a Canadian - United States collaboration led by NCIC, T2N0 and T1-2N1 patients are randomized to observation or 16 doses of weekly vinorelbine and 4 equally spaced doses of cisplatin. The overall accrual target is 600.

Several large scale, often multinational, adjuvant trials are ongoing under the auspices of European investigators. Two adjuvant trials randomizing patients to vinorelbine alone or vinorelbine plus cisplatin versus observation postresection (ANITA 1 + 2) are being coordinated by French investigators. The total planned accrual will be 1222 (800 for vinorelbine/cisplatin versus control and 442 for vinorelbine alone versus observation). The Adjuvant Lung Project Italy (ALPI) Trial, originally started by Italian investigators but now with broader EORTC participation, is structured to accrue 1240–1840 stage I–IIIA patients. Randomization choices are three cycles of postoperative adjuvant mitomycin, vindesine, and cisplatin or no adjuvant chemotherapy. Radiation may be utilized at the discretion of individual investigators. The British Thoracic Society is assessing either preoperative or postoperative cisplatin-based chemotherapy versus observation in several groups of NSCLC patients (BLT). Four thousand patients will be randomized postresection to either observation or chemotherapy. In patients randomized to chemotherapy, investigators may select three cycles of either cisplatin, vindesine or cisplatin, ifosfamide and mitomycin. In a parallel trial, another 2500 resected patients given postoperative radiation will be randomly assigned to also receive three cycles of chemotherapy or no additional therapy. The International Adjuvant Lung Trial (IALT), projecting accrual of 3300 resected stage I–IIIA NSCLC patients, is now active worldwide. The randomization is to chemotherapy or observation. As noted earlier, each institution participating in IALT must commit to consistent use of radiation or avoidance of radiation as part of the locoregional therapy for all patients treated at their site. Physicians may choose from among four 2-drug, cisplatin-based, chemotherapy options (Table 6.4). These last two trials, BLT and IALT, are classic large simple trials. Large numbers of patients are accrued. Small differences are sought. Data acquisition is kept to a minimum. Treatment options, such as different chemotherapy regimens, are offered

Table 6.4. Current adjuvant trials

Trial	Accrual	Patient group	Treatment
INT 0115[a]	>450	II, IIIA	Etoposide/cisplatin + RT vs RT alone
CALGB 9633	500	IB (T2N0)	Taxol/carboplatin vs observation
BR 10	600	IB, II (T2N0, T1–2N1)	Navelbine/cisplatin vs observation
ANITA 1	800	I–IIIA	Navelbine/cisplatin vs observation
ANITA 2	442	I–IIIA	Navelbine vs observation
ALPI	1240–1840	I–IIIA	Mitomycin/vindesine/cisplatin vs observation (±RT)
BLT	4000	I–IIIA	Cisplatin-based chemotherapy vs observation
BLT	2500	I–IIIA	Cisplatin-based chemotherapy vs observation (after RT)
IALT	3300	I–IIIA	Cisplatin-based chemotherapy vs observation (±RT)

[a] Completed accrual.
ANITA, Adjuvant Navelbine International Trialist Association; ALPI, Adjuvant Lung Project Italy; BLT, The Big Lung Trial; IALT, International Adjuvant Lung Trial.

within the context of randomization. This approach may be the basis for future criticism of these trials if there is no evidence of an overall benefit of the adjuvant therapy. However, the impact of the relatively similar chemotherapy regimens is likely to be quite similar. The flexibility should facilitate accrual. With the large number of patients expected to be accrued to these studies both individually and collectively, a much stronger foundation for judgment about adjuvant chemotherapy for patients with resected NSCLC should be available within the next several years.

6.5 Conclusion

Available data concerning the use of adjuvant radiotherapy and/or chemotherapy in patients with completely resected NSCLC are insufficient to recommend either as standard care. Adjuvant radiotherapy decreases local recurrence but has not been shown prospectively to improve overall survival. For patients with N2 disease, retrospective data and subset analyses of randomized trials suggest benefit. A new prospectively randomized trial of chemotherapy with or without consolidative radiation for patients with N2 disease may clarify the role of adjuvant radiation.

In some studies adjuvant chemotherapy improves disease free but not overall survival. Other studies suggest a true survival benefit. There may be a differential effect based on stage of disease. In the meta-analysis, cisplatin-based chemotherapy produced a 13% decrease in the risk of recurrence, with a possible survival benefit of up to 10% at 5 years. However, the difference favoring cisplatin was insufficient to reach the traditional 0.05 level of significance. Oral UFT data are provocative and additional studies with this agent are underway. Fortunately, several very large scale adjuvant chemotherapy trials are currently accruing resected NSCLC patients. These trials should provide us with definitive information about the role of adjuvant therapies for patients with completely resected non-small cell lung cancer.

References

Anthony HM, Mearns AJ, Mason MK, Scott DG, Moghissi K, Deverall PB, Rozycki ZJ, Watson DA (1979) Levamisole and surgery in bronchial carcinoma patients: increase in death from cardiorespiratory failure. Thorax 34:4–12

Astudillo J, Conill C (1990) Role of postoperative radiation therapy in stage IIIa non-small cell lung cancer. Ann Thorac Surg 50:618–623

Bonadonna G, Brusamolino E, Valagussa P, Rossi A, Brugnatelli L, Brambilla C, De Lena M, Tancini G, Bajetta E, Musumeci R, Veronesi U (1976) Combination chemotherapy as an adjuvant treatment in operable breast cancer. N Engl J Med 294(8):405–410

Bonadonna G, Valagussa P, Moliterni A, Zambetti M, Brambilla C (1995) Adjuvant cyclophosphamide, methotrexate, and fluorouracil in node-positive breast cancer. N Engl J Med 332(14):901–906

Dautzenberg B, Chastang C, Arriagada R, Le Chevalier T, Belpomme D, Hurdebourcq M, Lebeau B, Fabre C, Charvolin P, Guerin RA (1995) Adjuvant radiotherapy versus combined sequential chemotherapy followed by radiotherapy in the treatment of resected non-small cell lung carcinoma – a randomized trial of 267 patients. Cancer 76(5):779–786

Feld R, Rubinstein LV, Weisenberger TH (1984) Sites of recurrence in resected stage I non-small-cell lung cancer: a guide for future studies. J Clin Oncol 2(12):1352–1358

Feld R, Rubinstein L, Thomas PA (1993) Adjuvant chemotherapy with cyclophosphamide, doxorubicin, and cisplatin in patients with completely resected stage I non-small-cell lung cancer. J Natl Cancer Inst 85(4):299–306

Gail MH (1994) A placebo-controlled randomized double-blind study of adjuvant intrapleural BCG in patients with resected T1N0, T1N1, or T2N0 squamous cell carcinoma, adenocarcinoma, or large cell carcinoma of the lung. Chest 106[6 Suppl]:287S–292S

Girling DJ, Stott H, Stephens RJ, Fox W (1985). Fifteen-year follow-up of all patients in a study of post-operative chemotherapy for bronchial carcinoma. Br J Cancer 52:867–873

Green MR, Lilenbaum RC (1994) Stage IIIA category of non-small-cell lung cancer: a new proposal. J Natl Cancer Inst 86(8):586–588

Green N, Kurohara SS, George FW III, Crews QE (1975) Postresection irradiation for primary lung cancer. Radiology 116:405–407

Herskovic A, Bauer M, Seydel HG, Yesner R, Doggett RL, Perez CA, Durbin LM, Zinninger M (1988) Post-operative thoracic irradiation with or without levamisole in non-small cell lung cancer: results of a radiation therapy oncology group study. Int J Rad Oncol Biol Phys 14(1):37–42

Higgins GA, Humphrey EW, Hughes FA, Keehn RJ (1969) Cytoxan as an adjuvant to surgery for lung cancer. J Surg Oncol 1(3):221–228

Holmes EC (1994) Surgical adjuvant therapy for stage II and III adenocarcinoma and large cell undifferentiated carcinoma. Chest 106[suppl]:293S–296S

Holmes EC, Gail M (1986) Surgical adjuvant therapy for stage II and stage III adenocarcinoma and large-cell undifferentiated carcinoma. J Clin Oncol 4:710–715

Ichinose Y, Takanashi N, Yano T, Asoh H, Yokoyama H, Tayama K, Hara N, Ohta M (1995) A phase II trial of oral tegafur and uracil plus cisplatin in patients with inoperable non-small cell lung cancer. Cancer 75(11):2677–2680

Kirsh MM, Kahn DR, Gago O, Lampe I, Fayos JV, Prior M, Moores WY, Haight C, Herbert S (1971) Treatment of bronchogenic carcinoma with mediastinal metastases. Ann Thorac Surg 12(1):11–18

Lad T, Rubinstein L, Sadeghi A (1988) The benefit of adjuvant treatment for resected locally advanced non-small-cell lung cancer. J Clin Oncol 6(1):9–17

Laurie JA, Moertel CG, Fleming TR, Wieand HS, Leigh JE, Rubin J, McCormack GW, Gerstner JB, Krook JE, Malliard J, Twito DI, Morton RF, Tschetter LK, Barlow JF (1989) Surgical adjuvant therapy of large-bowel carcinoma: an evaluation of levamisole and fluorouracil. J Clin Oncol 7(10):1447–1456

Lee YC, Luh SP, Wu RM, Lee CJ (1994) Adjuvant immunotherapy with intrapleural streptococcus pyogenes (OK-432) in lung cancer patients after resection. Cancer Immunol Immunother 39:269–274

Martini N, Flehinger BJ (1987) The role of surgery in N2 lung cancer. Surg Clin North Am 67(5):1037–1049

McCaughan BC, Martini N, Bains MS, McCormack PM (1985) Chest wall invasion in carcinoma of the lung – therapeutic and prognostic implications. J Thorac Cardiovasc Surg 89:836–841

McKneally MF, Maver C, Kausel HW (1976) Regional immunotherapy of lung cancer with intrapleural BCG. Lancet i:377–379

McKneally MF, Maver C, Lininger L, Kausel HW, Mclduff JB, Older TM, Foster ED, Alley RD (1981) Four-year follow-up on the Albany experience with intrapleural BCG in lung cancer. J Thorac Cardiovasc Surg 81(4):485–491

Miller AB (MRC) (1971) Study of cytotoxic chemotherapy as an adjuvant to surgery in carcinoma of the bronchus. Br Med J 2:421

Moertel CG, Fleming TR, Macdonald JS, Haller DG, Laurie JA, Tangen CM, Ungerleider JS, Emerson WA, Tormey DC, Glick J, Veeder MH, Mailliard JA (1995) Fluorouracil plus levamisole as effective adjuvant therapy after resection of stage III colon carcinoma: a final report. Ann Intern Med 122(5):321–326

Mountain CF (1997) Revisions in the international system for staging lung cancer. Chest 111:1710–1717

Mountain CF, Gail MH (1981) Surgical adjuvant intrapleural BCG treatment for stage I non-small cell lung cancer. J Thorac Cardiovasc Surg 82(5):649–656

Nirranen A, Niitamo-Korhonen S, Kouri M, Assendelft A, Mattson K, Pyrhonen S (1992) Adjuvant chemotherapy after radical surgery for non-small-cell lung cancer: a randomized study. J Clin Oncol 10(12):1927–1932

Non-Small Cell Lung Cancer Collaborative Group (NSCLC) (1995) Chemotherapy in non-small cell lung cancer: a meta-analysis using updated data on individual patients from 52 randomized trials. Br Med J 311:899–909

Ohta M, Tsuchiya R, Shimoyama M, Sawamura K, Mori T, Miyazawa N, Suemasu K, Watanabe Y, Tomita M, Terashima M (1993) Adjuvant chemotherapy for completely resected stage III non-small-cell lung cancer. J Thorac Cardiovasc Surg 106(4):703–707

Overgaard M, Hansen PS, Overgaard J et al (1997) Postoperative radiotherapy in high-risk premenopausal women with breast cancer who receive adjuvant chemotherapy. N Engl J Med 337:949–955

Pisters KM, Kris MG, Gralla RJ, Hilaris B, McCormack PM, Bains MS, Martini N (1994) Randomized trial comparing postoperative chemotherapy with vindesine and cisplatin plus thoracic irradiation with irradiation alone in stage III(N2) non-small cell lung cancer. J Surg Oncol 56(4):236–241

Ragaz J, Jackson SM, Ne N et al (1997) Adjuvant radiotherapy and chemotherapy in node-positive premenopausal women with breast cancer. N Engl J Med 337:956–962

Rapp E, Pater JL, Willan A, Cormier Y, Murray N, Evans WK, Hodson DI, Clark DA, Feld R, Arnold AM, Ayoub JI, Wilson KS, Latreille J, Wierzbicki RF, Hill DP (1988) Chemotherapy can prolong survival in patients with advanced non-small-cell lung cancer – report of a Canadian Multicenter Randomized Trial. J Clin Oncol 6(4):633–641

Ruckdeschel JC, Finkelstein DM, Mason BA, Creech RH (1985) Chemotherapy for metastatic non-small-cell bronchogenic carcinoma: EST 2575, Generation V – a randomized comparison of four cisplatin-containing regimens. J Clin Oncol 3(1):72–79

Shields TW, Humphrey EW, Eastridge CE, Keehn RJ (1977) Adjuvant cancer chemotherapy after resection of carcinoma of the lung. Cancer 40:2057–2062

Shimizu E, Kimura K, Sone S, Inoue I, Nakamura Y, Noda Y, Hojo F, Yagi M, Nakanishi S, Yamasaki K et al (1986) A phase II study of UFT in non-small cell lung cancer (in Japanese). Jpn J Cancer Chemother 13(10):2970–2973

Souquet PJ, Chauvin F, Boissel JP, Cellerino R, Cormier Y, Ganz PA, Kaasa S, Pater JL, Quoix E, Rapp E et al (1993) Polychemotherapy in advanced non-small cell lung cancer: a meta-analysis. Lancet 342:19–21

Stephens RJ, Girling DJ, Bleehen NM, Moghissi K, Yosef HMA, Machin D (1996) The role of post-operative radiotherapy in non-small cell lung cancer: a multicentre randomised trial in patients with pathologically staged T_{1-2}, N_{1-2}, M_0 disease. Br J Cancer 74:632–639

Stewart HJ (MRC) (1987) Adjuvant tamoxifen in the management of operable Breast cancer: the Scottish trial. Lancet ii:171–175

Study Group of Adjuvant Chemotherapy for Lung Cancer (Chubu, Japan) (1995) A randomized trial of postoperative adjuvant chemotherapy in non-small cell lung cancer (the Second Cooperative Study). Eur J Surg Oncol 21:69–77

Takita H, Hollinshead AC, Adler RH, Bhayana J, Ramundo M, Moskowitz R, Rao UNM, Raman S (1991) Adjuvant, specific, active immunotherapy for resectable squamous cell lung carcinoma: a 5-year survival analysis. J Surg Oncol 46:9–14

Tanaka F, Yanagihara K, Wada H, Hitomi S (1996) Advantage of post operative oral administration of tegafur (FT) for completely resected P-stage I-IIIA non-small cell lung cancer (NSCLC). Proc Am Soc Clin Oncol 393:1189

Van Houtte P, Bondue H, Rocmans P, Michel J, Wybran J, Dalesio O, Balikdjian D, Vanderhoeft P, Kenis Y (1980) Adjuvant immunotherapy by levamisole in resectable lung cancer: a control study. Eur J Cancer 16:1597–1601

Wada H, Hitomi S, Teramatsu T (1996) Adjuvant chemotherapy after complete resection in non-small-cell lung cancer. J Clin Oncol 14(4):1048–1054

Watanabe Y, Shimizu J, Oda M, Hayashi Y, Watanabe S, Iwa T (1991) Results of surgical treatment in patients with stage IIIA non-small-cell lung cancer J Thorac Cardiovasc Surg 39:44–49

Weisenburger (the Lung Cancer Study Group) (1986) Effects of postoperative mediastinal radiation on completely resected stage II and stage III epidermoid cancer of the lung. N Engl J Med 315(22):1377–1381

7 Induction or Concurrent Chemotherapy and Radiation Therapy for Locally Advanced Non-Small Cell Lung Cancer

R. KOMAKI and J.D. COX

CONTENTS

7.1 Introduction

Thoracic radiation therapy was considered to be the standard care for patients with inoperable non-small cell lung cancer (NSCLC) in the United States for many years. Although the long-term results of such treatment were far from satisfactory (a large number of investigators reported approximately 1 patient of 20 treated survived 5 years), it was the only modality that offered any possibility of cure for patients with unresectable tumors. Over the past few years, combined chemotherapy and thoracic radiation therapy (TRT) have become standard treatment for patients with unresectable NSCLC if they have good performance status and minimal or no weight loss (SHAAKE-KONIG et al. 1992; DILLMAN et al. 1990; LECHEVALIER et al. 1991; SAUSE et al. 1995).

However, the timing of chemotherapy in relation to the TRT that produces the least toxicity and the best survival is still to be determined. Although the many new cytotoxic agents that are emerging will likely change what is considered to be the best chemotherapy, one of the most fundamental strategic questions is the value of induction chemotherapy followed by TRT compared with concurrent chemotherapy with TRT. In this chapter, induction (or neoadjuvant) chemotherapy means that anticancer drugs are given several days or more likely several weeks before radiation therapy and concurrent therapy means that anticancer drugs are given simultaneously, usually within 24–72 h of initiation of radiation therapy and then usually repeated at intervals or given continuously through the entire radiation therapy course.

R. KOMAKI, Professor of Radiation Oncology, The University of Texas M.D. Anderson Cancer Center, 1515 Holcombe Blvd., Box 97, Houston, TX 77030, USA
J.D. COX, Professor and Chairman, Department of Radiation Oncology, The University of Texas M.D. Anderson Cancer Center, 1515 Holcombe Blvd., Box 97, Houston, TX 77030, USA

7.2 Rationale and Mechanisms of Induction or Concurrent Chemotherapy and Radiation Therapy

7.2.1 Induction Chemotherapy and Radiation Therapy

When radiation therapy is applied to the primary tumor and regional lymph nodes of the NSCLC, it is assumed that tumor will be eradicated within the treatment volume but that failure may occur outside of the radiation therapy ports. The more precise the treatment plan and the higher the dose of radiation therapy, the more certain the tumor control will be. If regional or distant metastasis occurs, the tumor is thought to have seeded before local radiation therapy was given. The fundamental observations relevant to combinations of chemotherapy and radiation therapy are certainly not new. In a classic description, STEEL and PECKHAM (1979) put forth a list of four potential strategies to improve the therapeutic outcome: (1) toxicity independence, (2) protection of normal tissues, (3) spatial cooperation, and (4) enhancement of tumor response. The latter two strategies are most relevant to the discussion of the relative values of induction versus concurrent chemotherapy and radiation therapy. Spatial cooperation is the most obvious and the most thoroughly evaluated. It relies upon chemotherapy to eradicate subclinical spread of the disease and on radiation therapy to eradicate the locoregional tumor that is evident from physical examination and imaging studies. Although spatial cooperation means that radiation therapy would be effective for the locoregional tumor and chemotherapy needs to be effective for the micro-metastasis, there is no way to anticipate whether spatial cooperation can best be established by sequential or concurrent chemotherapy and radiation therapy. For spatial cooperation, it is not necessary to see interaction between radiation therapy and chemotherapy, although different toxicities characterize the two modalities. Improvement of the therapeutic ratio by spatial cooperation has been convincingly demonstrated for breast cancer (EARLY BREAST CANCER TRIALS COLLABORATIVE GROUP 1992). There is beginning to be evidence that systemic chemotherapy can eradicate subclinical NSCLC metastasis (Cox et al. 1997).

To improve the outcome by combining chemotherapy and radiation therapy in a manner that enhances tumor response, but with acceptable effects on normal tissues, is the challenge that faces medical and radiation oncologists. For NSCLC, complete toxicity independence is an impossible goal since both chemotherapy and radiation therapy must be applied both to the tumor and normal tissues. On the other hand, it is not necessary to achieve true supra-additivity to find benefit in the radiation and chemotherapy combination. As noted by STEEL and PECKHAM (1979), favorable effects on the tumor population could be achieved by additive or even subadditive effects. The authors prefer the term "supra-additivity" rather than "synergism," since the use of "synergism" does not leave room for an interaction between chemotherapy and radiation that is to the left of the edge of the envelope of additivity (Fig. 7.1). When a response would be greater than would be expected from a simple sum of the chemotherapy and radiation therapy results, the term "supra-additive" will be used (a point to the left of the envelope of additivity) (Fig. 7.1). A point to the right of the envelope indicates a subadditive response, i.e., inhibition or antagonism. Between sub- and supra-additive there is an envelope of additivity to indicate enhancement of the effect from either one modality. The broken lines in Fig. 7.1 indicate that chemotherapy or radiation therapy allowed radiotherapy to be given more than its single dose level for the iso-effect; thus this broken line implies protection.

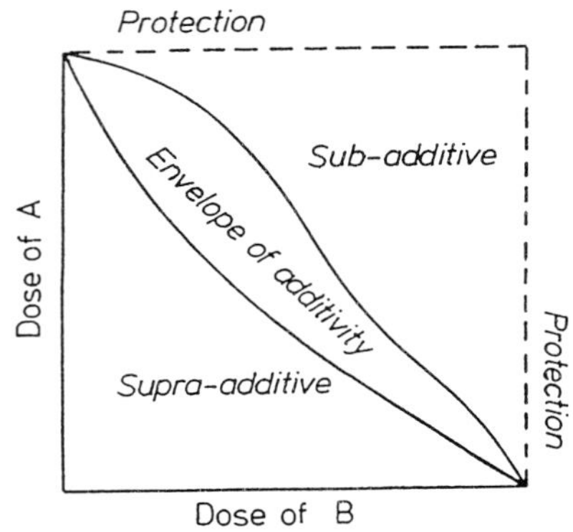

Fig. 7.1. An *isobologram* is an isoeffect plot of the doses of two agents that together give a fixed biological effect. If dose-response curves are nonlinear, there is a region of uncertainty about the existence of "additivity." (Reproduced by permission from STEEL and PECKHAM 1979)

One key to improving the therapeutic index is to minimize resistance to radiation and anti-cancer drugs. Whenever radiation or an anticancer drug is applied sequentially, subpopulations that remain viable may start to proliferate and so cause treatment failure (Fig. 7.2) (TUBIANA et al. 1968). This phenomenon of repopulation during a course of treatment is well appreciated and underlies the requirement that the cycles of chemotherapy be given at the shortest intervals permitted by hematological recovery. It also underlies choice of a course of fractionated radiation therapy. Accelerated repopulation, especially accelerated tumor cell proliferation (WITHERS et al. 1988), leads to regimens in which a greater number of radiation treatments are given within certain time periods, especially for carcinomas of the head and neck and lung. Accelerated proliferation is less fully appreciated in the chemotherapy literature as evidenced by the consistent advocacy of induction chemotherapy prior to local treatments. However, accelerated regrowth of surviving tumor cells may have great relevance to sequential versus concurrent treatments for NSCLC.

7.2.2 Concurrent Chemotherapy and Radiation Therapy

The development of the resistance of malignant cells might be reduced more effectively by the simul-

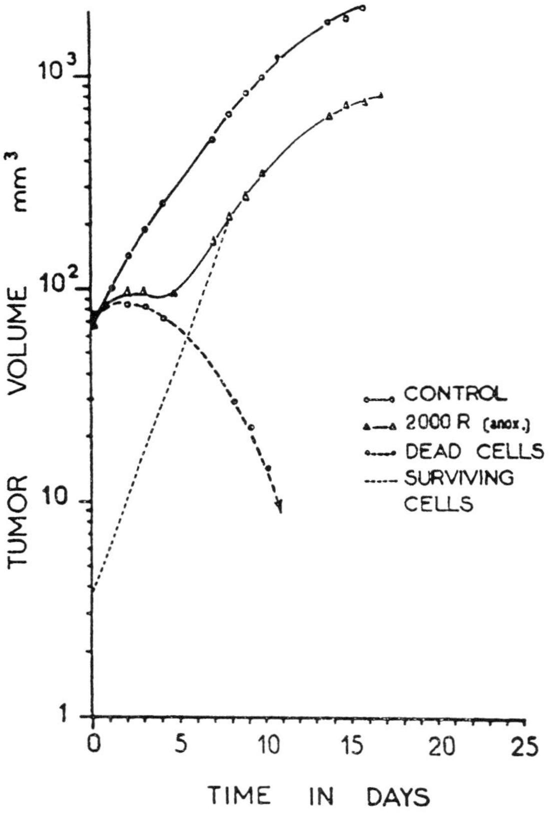

Fig. 7.2. The evolution of the size of an irradiated tumor is caused by two phenomena: the removal of nonviable cells and the proliferation of surviving cells. After 7000 cGy, all the cells are killed and the evolution of the volume of the tumor indicates the rate of elimination of dead cells. (Reproduced by permission from TUBIANA et al. 1968)

taneous use of radiation and anti-cancer drugs since repopulation time is restricted. Radiation damage depends on the formation of free radicals and fixation of the DNA damage caused by these free radicals. Oxygen is also required for free radical-induced damage to occur. Therefore, hypoxia in the tumor is one of the important factors determining resistance to radiation. The mechanisms of resistance to radiation and anti-cancer drugs are: (1) increased DNA repair, (2) binding of free radicals by glutathione and other sulfhydrils, (3) increased levels of glutathione/s transferase and other enzymes that eliminate free radicals, and (4) increased expression of Bcl-2 or other genes leading to decreased ability to undergo apoptosis (TANNOCK 1996).

Another important way to improve therapeutic index is to inhibit cell proliferation of malignant cells and not suppress those in the normal tissue. Standard radiation therapy for human beings has been fractionated radiation therapy to prevent normal tissue damage. However, fractionated radiation therapy inflicts sublethal damage to the malignant and normal cells, with the assumption that the normal tissue will have a greater capacity to repair and repopulate (Fig. 7.3A,B) (TANNOCK 1996). When induction chemotherapy is given before radiation therapy, there is some cell killing and shrinkage of the tumor, which may improve blood supply and delivery of nutrients to the tumor, which in turn would most likely lead to higher rates of cell proliferation at the time of initiation of radiation therapy (Fig. 7.3A). When anti-cancer drugs are used concurrently, there is a reduction in the repopulation that otherwise occurs between fractions, and this re duction might be sufficient to overcome the disadvantage of more rapidly repopulating cells (Fig. 7.3B). It is difficult to measure cell proliferation precisely, although BrdUrd uptake in the biopsy specimen or surgical specimen may reveal the rate of proliferation (BEGG et al. 1990).

7.3 Results of Clinical Trials in NSCLC

7.3.1 Induction Chemotherapy Followed by Radiation Therapy

The first positive randomized trial of induction chemotherapy and radiation therapy for inoperable NSCLC was conducted by the Cancer and Leukemia Group B (CALGB 8433) (DILLMAN et al. 1990, 1996) (Table 7.1). In this study of induction chemotherapy, 180 patients with stage III NSCLC, good performance status, and no more than 5% weight loss were randomly assigned to receive cisplatin (100 mg/m^2 on days 1 and 29) and vinblastine (5 mg/m^2 weekly for 5 weeks). Fifty days after the start of chemotherapy, radiation therapy was begun and a 60 Gy total dose was administered at 2.0 Gy/fraction, 5 days/week for 6 weeks. The comparison was with the same radiation therapy given alone, starting on day 1. This trial was stopped before the planned enrollment when an interim analysis revealed that the induction chemotherapy arm was so superior to the radiation therapy alone arm that it met their early-stopping rules. Long-term follow-up showed that the survival benefit of induction chemotherapy persisted. Data have not been available regarding local tumor control or failure patterns.

The second trial to show a survival benefit from induction chemotherapy was reported from France

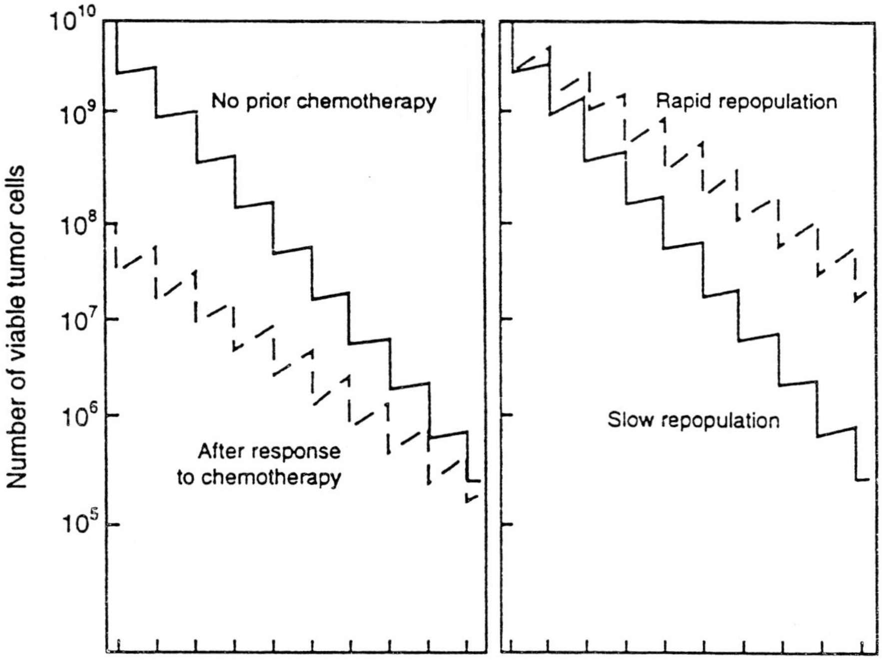

Fig. 7.3. **a** Schematic cell survival curves illustrate possible effects of neoadjuvant chemotherapy (*dashed line*). In this theoretical example, chemotherapy leads to tumor response so that there are 100-fold less viable cells at the initiation of radiotherapy. Tumor shrinkage may lead to improved nutrition of surviving cells such that their repopulation during fractionated radiotherapy is faster. This effect can lead to loss of the initial therapeutic benefit as shown schematically by the convergence of the two curves. (Reproduced by permission from TANNOCK 1996.) **b** Schematic diagram illustrates influence of repopulation of surviving cells between radiation treatments on overall survival of a cell population (e.g., a tumor or normal tissue) treated by fractionated radiation. The cell kill per fraction is assumed to be equal for the two curves, but repopulation is faster for the dashed curve than for the solid curve. Concurrent use of chemotherapy might inhibit repopulation, leading to greater cell kill, thus converting the survival curve from the dashed to the solid line. (Reproduced by permission from TANNOCK 1996)

Table 7.1. Randomized (I)induction chemotherapy followed by radiation therapy for inoperable NSCLC

Trials (year)	Chemotherapy	RT (Gy)	No. pts. analyzed	MS (m)	2 years (%)	Difference
MATTSON et al. (1988)	CAPx8	55 (sp)	119	10.6	19	NS
	–	55 (sp)	119	10.2	17	
DILLMAN et al. (1990)	VBL/DDPx2	60 (c)	78	13.8	26	$P = 0.007$
	–	60 (c)	77	9.7	13	
LECHAVALIER et al. (1992)	VCPCx6	65 (c)	176	12	21	$P = 0.02$
	–	65 (c)	177	10	14	
WOLF et al. (1994)	IVd	50 (sp)	37	13.7	24	$P = 0.016$
	–	50 (sp)	41	9	12	
SAUSE et al. (1995)	VBL/DDPx2	60 (c)	152	13.6	31	$P = 0.03$
	–	60 (c)	152	11.4	21	
		69.6 (HFX)	154	12.2	24	

CAP, cyclophosphamide, Adriamycin, platinum; VBL, vinblastine; DDP, cisplatin; VCPC, vindesine, cyclophosphamide, cisplatin, CCNU; IVd, ifosfamide, vindesine.

(ARRIAGADA et al. 1991; LECHEVALIER et al. 1991, 1992). This multi-institutional cooperative trial enrolled 353 patients in a study of 3 monthly cycles of vindesine (1.5 mg/m^2 on days 1 and 2), cyclophosphamide (200 mg/m^2 on days 2–4), cisplatin (100 mg/m^2 on day 2), and lomustine (75 mg/m^2 on day 3) followed by radiation therapy with a total dose of 65 Gy at 2.5 Gy/fraction, 4 days/week) beginning approximately 11 weeks after the start of chemotherapy compared with the same radiation therapy alone beginning on day 1. In addition to an improvement in survival with induction chemotherapy, they found a statistically significant reduction in the incidence of distant metastasis. They documented clearly through the systematic use of fiberoptic bronchoscopy and biopsy at the site of the original lesions 3 months after the start of treatment that there was no improvement in local tumor control. In fact, the rates of local persistence at the original disease sites exceeded 80% in both arms of the study.

The third trial to support the value of induction chemotherapy was conducted by the Radiation Therapy Oncology Group (RTOG 88-08) in collaboration with the Eastern Cooperative Oncology Group (ECOG 4588) (Sause et al. 1995). It had the same two arms as CALGB 8433 and a third arm of hyperfractionated radiation therapy (total dose 69.6 Gy, 1.2 Gy/fraction twice each day, 5 days/week for 6 weeks). A failure pattern analysis of this study (RTOG 88-08/ECOG 4588) by Komaki et al. (1997b) found no effect on local tumor control from the induction chemotherapy.

Two other randomized trials of induction cisplatin-based chemotherapy and radiation therapy showed no improvement in survival. Mattson et al. (1988) reported a study of 238 patients randomized to induction chemotherapy followed by split-course radiation therapy with a total dose of 55 Gy compared with the same radiation therapy and found no difference in median or 2-year survival. Another randomized comparative trial (Morton et al. 1991) that did not include cisplatin in the induction regimen also failed to show benefit from induction chemotherapy.

Trovo et al. (1990) reported a trial in which the sequence was reversed. Radiation therapy to the primary and regional lymph nodes was given with a total dose of 45 Gy in 15 fractions, 5 fractions/week, for 3 weeks. This treatment was compared with the same radiation therapy followed by CAMP (cyclophosphamide 300 mg/m^2 i.v. days 1 and 8; doxorubicin 20 mg/m^2 i.v. days 1 and 8; methotrexate 15 mg/m^2 i.v. days 1 and 8; procarbazine 100 mg/m^2 p.o. days 1–10) which was initiated 4 weeks after completion of radiation therapy. Of the 111 patients randomized, 62 were enrolled in the radiation arm and 49 were enrolled in the radiation therapy plus CAMP arm. There were no differences in time to progression, survival, or failure patterns between the two arms. It is appropriate to note that a meta-analysis of clinical trials comparing radiation therapy alone with radiation therapy plus chemotherapy has suggested that only cisplatin-based regimens have been associated with improved results (Non-small Cell Lung Cancer Collaborative Group 1995).

7.3.2 Concurrent Chemotherapy and Radiation Therapy

7.3.2.1 Single-Agent Chemotherapy and Radiation Therapy

As noted above, the potential benefit from the use of concurrent chemotherapy and radiation therapy is the improvement in local tumor control (Tannock 1996). An important study from the European Organization for Research and Treatment of Cancer (EORTC) reported by Schaake-Koning et al. (1992) supports the hypothesis that increased local tumor control can be achieved by concurrent treatments (Table 7.2). They compared radiation therapy alone with a total dose of 55 Gy (3.0 Gy/fraction, 5 frac-

Table 7.2. Randomized concurrent (±) chemotherapy and radiation therapy for inoperable NSCLC

Concurrent trials (year)	Chemotherapy		RT (Gy)	No. pts. analyzed	MS (m)	2 year (%)	Difference *P* value
Schaake-Konig et al. (1992)	DDP	daily	55 (sp)	107	10.8	26	*P* = 0.009
		weekly	55 (sp)	110	10.2	19	
		–	55 (sp)	114	9.8	13	*P* = 0.36
Trovo et al. (1992)	DDP		45/3W (c)	84	9.97	14	NS
	–		45/3W (c)	83	10.3	14	
Blanke (1995)	DDP		60 (c)	107	10	15	NS
	–		60 (c)	108	9	9	
Jeremic et al. (1996)	CBDCA/E		69.6 (HFX) (c)	65	22	43	*P* = 0.021
	–		69.6	66	14	26	

CBDCA/E, carboplatin and etoposide.

tions/week for 2 weeks, an interruption of 3–4 weeks, followed by 2.5 Gy/fraction, 5 fractions/week for 2 weeks) with the same radiation therapy and concurrent cisplatin given once weekly at 30 mg/m^2 or daily at 6 mg/m^2. More than 100 patients were enrolled in each of the three arms of this study, and both concurrent cisplatin/irradiation arms had significantly higher local control rates compared with radiation therapy alone; the survival rates in the two cisplatin arms were modestly improved. This trial made two important contributions: it confirmed the radiation-sensitizing effects of cisplatin and it supported the importance of local tumor control in survival in inoperable NSCLC. However, Trovo et al. (1992) reported a cooperative trial from Italy addressing the same hypothesis, with different results. They compared radiation therapy with a total dose of 45 Gy in 15 fractions in 3 weeks to the same radiation therapy preceded each day with an i.v. injection of cisplatin, 6 mg/m^2, approximately 1 h before treatment. A total of 173 patients were randomized. They found no differences in time to progression, survival, or failure patterns between the two arms.

7.3.2.2 Multiagent Chemotherapy and Radiation Therapy

The most intensive approach to combining chemotherapy and radiation therapy is the concurrent use of multiagent combinations with either standard or accelerated irradiation. This approach has the potential to increase local control, decrease distant metastasis, and thus to improve survival. It also has the greatest potential for acute toxicity.

The results of many single-arm pilot studies have been published, but few studies to date have compared the experimental arm with standard or even with other combined modality regimens. Komaki et al. (1997a) reported the results of RTOG Protocol 92-04. This was a randomized comparison of two regimens that had been piloted in earlier RTOG trials. One arm consisted of an induction cisplatin/vinblastine regimen similar to that found to be superior to radiation therapy alone in CALGB 8433 and RTOG 88-08/ECOG 4588, then concurrent cisplatin (75 mg/m^2) and standard radiation therapy (63 Gy in 34 fractions: 45 Gy at 1.8 Gy/fraction for 5 weeks plus a boost of 18 Gy at 2.0 Gy/fraction). The other arm used cisplatin 75 mg/m^2 i.v. on days 1 and 29 and etoposide 50 mg p.o. on days 1–5, 8–12, 29–33, and 36–40 concurrent with hyperfractionated radiation therapy (HFX) with a total dose of 69.6 Gy given as 1.2 Gy twice daily, 5 days/week for 6 weeks beginning on day 1. The results showed a lower risk of nonhematological toxicity with the induction regimen, but the HFX/chemotherapy arm had a lower in-field progression rate. The median survivals and 1-year survival rates were quite similar (15.5 months and 65% for induction followed by concurrent cisplatin vs 14.1 months and 58% for HFX/concurrent chemotherapy) (Komaki et al. 1997a).

A randomized comparative study of concurrent versus induction chemotherapy/radiation therapy has been reported (Furuse et al. 1997) in abstract form by the West Japan Lung Cancer Group (Table 7.3). Mitomycin (8 mg/m^2 days 1 and 29), cisplatin (80 mg/m^2 days 1 and 29), and vindesine (3 mg/m^2 days 1,8,29, and 36) were combined with radiation therapy. In the induction arm the chemotherapy was completed and then radiation therapy was given with a total dose of 56 Gy "in a conventional schema." In the concurrent arm, radiation therapy was started on day 2 of the MVP regimen and a split-course regimen was used with the same total dose (56 Gy given as 2.0 Gy times 14 followed by an interruption of 10 days and then another 14 fractions of 2.0 Gy). Of 314 evaluable patients, the 158 enrolled in the sequential arm had a median survival of 13.3 months and 2-year and 3-year survival rates of 25.6% and 12.5% respectively. The 156 patients enrolled in the concurrent arm had a median survival of 16.5 months and 2- and 3-year survival rates of 37% and 27% respectively.

Table 7.3. Randomized concurrent vs induction chemotherapy and radiation therapy for inoperable NSCLC

Ref (year)	Chemotherapy	RT (Gy)	No. pts. analyzed	MS (m)	2 years (%)	Difference
Komaki et al. (1997a)	PoE +	69.6 (HFX-C)	82	14.4	34	NS
	VBL/DDP → RT	63 (c) + Pld	80	15.5	35	
Furuse et al. (1997)	MVP + RT	56 (sp)	156	16.5	37	$P = 0.0473$
	MVPx2 → RT	56 (sp)	158	13.3	25.6	

PoE, cisplatin and oral etoposide; Pld, low dose of cisplatin; MVP, mitomycin, vinblastine and cisplatin.
C, continuous radiation therapy; sp, split course of radiation therapy.

There was greater hematological toxicity in the concurrent arm, but the median survival was significantly ($P = 0.0473$) longer.

A phase III comparative trial has been completed by the RTOG (Protocol 94-10), but the results are not yet available. This study compared the induction chemotherapy and radiation therapy now considered standard since the results of CALGB 8433 and RTOG 88-08/ECOG 4588 (Komaki et al. 1997b). A second arm uses the same chemotherapy but the radiation therapy is started on day 1 instead of day 50. The third arm is the HFX plus concurrent i.v. cisplatin/oral etoposide that was used in RTOG 92-04 described above. Results of the study should be available in the year 2000.

7.3.2.3
Toxicity from Combined Chemotherapy and Radiation Therapy

Whenever aggressive combined chemotherapy and radiation therapy are given to patients with inoperable lung cancer, toxicity to the lung, esophagus, and bone marrow limit the dose of chemotherapy and radiation therapy as well as duration of treatment. Because of toxicity, dose often needs to be modified and/or patients need a break to complete the prescribed treatment. Delays in completing radiation have been documented to influence the outcome negatively (Cox et al. 1993).

Toxicity to the lung from chemo- and radiation therapy manifests as acute pneumonitis, which is usually encountered toward the end of a course of radiation therapy or 1–3 months after completion of radiation therapy. Symptoms of acute pneumonitis are shortness of breath, dry cough, and low-grade fever. Late effects on the lung start around 6 months after radiation therapy and manifest as fibrosis; radiation doses higher than 25 Gy given in the conventional manner are the usual cause.

Antitumor agents known to cause dose-dependent lung fibrosis are bleomycin, busulfan, and carmusine; methotrexate causes fibrosis in hypersensitive people (Muggia et al. 1983). Cyclophosphamide, vincristine, actinomycin D, Adriamycin, bleomycin, 5-fluorouracil, cisplatin and methotrexate are non-antitumor agents to enhance the radiation effect, although 5-fluorouracil, cisplatin and methotrexate are considered as safe antitumor agents to be given with radiation (Steel 1988; van der Maase et al. 1986; van der Maase 1986). The postulate of increased radiation toxicity to the lung by Adriamycin, actinomycin D, and bleomycin has been confirmed clinically (Phillips and Fu 1976; Sadeghi 1988). According to several clinical trials, the Adriamycin-containing regimens such as cisplatin, Adriamycin and cyclophosphamide (CAP) for NSCLC have not increased lung toxicity as long as the regimen is induction (Mattson and Maasilta 1989; Trovo et al. 1990). Concurrent cisplatin–radiation therapy regimens increase local control through radiosensitizing effects (Shaake-Konig et al. 1992). According to this study, radiation therapy alone caused a 31% incidence of the lung damage, weekly cisplatin caused a 44% incidence, and daily cisplatin with concurrent radiation therapy caused a 35% incidence. Chest X-ray detected grade III and IV fibrosis (Shaake-Konig et al. 1992). The symptoms due to late damage of the lung are more related to lung volume than to dose. Acute pneumonitis is not always a predictor of late lung damage.

Usually thoracic radiation therapy given to the proximal lesion or mediastinal lymph nodes causes acute esophagitis during or shortly after completion of radiation therapy, especially if such anti-tumor agents as cisplatin or Adriamycin were given simultaneously. The late effects of radiation on the esophagus are manifest as stenosis several months after the completion of treatment or in more severe cases as necrosis leading to fistula formation. Necrosis and fistula formation are very rare complications unless there is tumor progression or mechanical damage to the esophagus (such as that caused by dilatation of the esophagus).

5-Fluorouracil (5-FU) and Adriamycin enhance radiation effects on the mucosa (Phillips and Fu 1976; Steel 1988). Lokich et al. (1989) reported severe esophagitis among patients who received continuous 5-FU with concurrent radiation therapy; late stenosis resulted. Umsawadi et al. (1985) reported a higher incidence of severe esophagitis when CAP was given concurrently with thoracic radiation: the incidence was 80% in patients who received concurrent chemo- and radiation therapy compared to 27% in patients who received induction treatment. Also, according to his report, the incidence of late stricture of the esophagus was 43% for concurrent vs 2% for the induction approach. Sadeghi et al. (1988) reported that 35% of patients who received radiation therapy alone had severe esophagitis compared to 57% of patients who received radiation with CAP. Vindesine with radiation therapy may also increase incidence of esophagitis according to Coy (1970) and Dillman et al. (1990), although the incidence might have been higher if they had given concurrent instead of induction chemotherapy. In the EORTC study, cisplatin was given as a sensitizer, which caused similar acute severe esophagitis rates by three different arms: 49% by weekly 30 mg/m^2 cisplatin alone, 49% by 6 mg/m^2 daily cisplatin, and 46% by radiation alone. They did not report any late stricture of the esophagus by radiation alone or radiation with cisplatin (Shaake-Konig et al. 1992).

Byhardt et al. (1997) reported five completed trials for stage II–III inoperable NSCLC patients who were treated by an induction regimen of chemotherapy (cisplatin and vinblastine) followed by standard radiation therapy, 60 Gy in 6 weeks (group I), by a combined induction (vinblastine and cisplatin) and concurrent regimen of cisplatin and standard radiation therapy, 60 Gy in 6 weeks (group II), or by a concurrent regimen of chemotherapy (oral etoposide and cisplatin) and hyperfractionated radiation therapy (69.6 Gy in 6 weeks) (group III). All patients had good performance status, and two of five trials required less than 5% weight loss for eligibility. The acute (within 90 days from the start of radiation therapy) and late (after 90 days from the start of radiation therapy) toxicity were reported. Grade III or higher toxicity was defined as severe. *Overall* grade IV or V acute reactions were fairly similar between groups, but the incidence of severe *nonhematologic* acute toxicity was significantly different among the three groups ($P < 0.0001$). Differences in incidence of toxicity between groups I and II were not statistically significant. Group III had a significantly higher incidence of severe acute nonhematologic toxicity (55%) compared to group I (27%) or group II (34%) ($P < 0.0001$ and $P = 0.0005$, respectively). This difference was caused primarily by differences in the incidence of severe acute esophagitis, 34% in group III vs 1.3% in group I and 6% in group II ($P < 0.0001$). Overall, grade IV or V late toxicity was not significantly different. Severe late pulmonary toxicity was more severe in group II (21%) and group III (20%) than in group I (10%) ($P = 0.035$). However, the incidence of late esophageal toxicity did not differ significantly between the three groups ($P = 0.077$) (Tables 7.4, 7.5). According to the report, group I had a significantly lower overall response rate (63%) than either group II (77%) or group III (79%) ($P = 0.03$ and 0.003, respectively) (Byhardt et al. 1998).

Table 7.4. Comparison of acute toxicity according to treatment intensity grouping

Type of acute toxicity	Group 1 Ind CT + Standard RT (88-08)	Group 2 Ind/Conc CT/Std RT (88-04, 92-04 arm 1)	Group 3 Conc CT/Hfx RT (90-15, 91-06, 92-04 arm 2)	
Overall ≥grade 4	77/152 (51%)	57/109 (52%)	95/200 (47.5%)	
Overall grade 5	4/152 (3%)	1/109 (1%)	6/200 (3%)	
Non-hematologic ≥grade 3	41/152 (27%)	37/109 (34%)	110/200 (55%)	$P < 0.0001$
Lung ≥grade 3	9/152 (6%)	4/109 (4%)	14/200 (7%)	
Esophageal ≥grade 3	2/152 (1.3%)	6/109 (6%)	68/200 (34%)	$P < 0.0001$
Hematologic ≥grade 3	107/152 (70%)	84/109 (77%)	146/200 (73%)	
Hematologic ≥grade 4	71/152 (47%)	56/109 (51%)	92/200 (46%)	
Hematologic ≥grade 5	0/152 (0%)	1/109 (1%)	5/200 (2.5%)	

Table 7.5. Comparison of late toxicity according to treatment intensity grouping

Type of late toxicity	Group 1 Ind CT + Standard RT (88-08)	Group 2 Ind/Conc CT/Std RT (88-04, 92-04 arm 1)	Group 3 Conc CT/Hfx RT (90-15, 91-06, 92-04 arm 2)	
Overall ≥grade 4	71/136 (51%)	5/82 (6%)	12/170 (7%)	
Overall grade 5	2/136 (1%)	2/82 (2%)	3/170 (2%)	
Non-hematologic ≥grade 3	19/136 (14%)	21/82 (26%)	48/170 (28%)	$P = 0.0098$
Lung ≥grade 3	14/136 (10%)	17/82 (21%)	35/170 (20%)	$P = 0.035$
Esophageal ≥grade 3	3/136 (2%)	3/82 (4%)	13/170 (8%)	$P = 0.077$
Hematologic ≥grade 3	7/136 (5%)	5/82 (6%)	6/170 (4%)	
Hematologic ≥grade 4	3/136 (2%)	1/82 (1%)	3/170 (2%)	
Hematologic ≥grade 5	1/136 (<1%)	1/82 (1%)	0/170 (0%)	

7.4 Discussion

For patients who have inoperable or unresectable NSCLC with good performance status and a less than 5% weight loss, recent data suggest that concurrent chemotherapy and radiation therapy improve local control and survival. Esophageal toxicity and late lung effects are the major treatment-related complications of concurrent chemotherapy and radiation therapy, especially for the patients with large tumors. To reduce these complications, smaller radiation volumes that spare esophagus and lung as much as possible are needed. Solutions include 3D conformal treatment, the radioprotector amifostine, and chemoprotectors of the esophagus, bone marrow, and kidney (TANNEHILL et al. 1997). MCMILLAN and HART (1986) has demonstrated enhanced experimental metatastic capacity of malignant cells when anticancer drugs were given as induction treatment. They tested the effect of in vitro pretreatment of B16 murine melanoma cells with various antitumor agents on their subsequent experimental metastatic capacity. Methotrexate, cytosine arabinoside, 5-azacytidine, and aphidicoline significantly increased the number of lung nodules following the intravenous injection of tumor cells. However, this effect was not seen with melphalan or 5-fluorouracil. The authors determined that antitumor drugs may induce mutations of malignant cells that accelerate metastasis to distant sites or shift cells into more active phases of the cell cycle. Nonetheless, there has been enough evidence that induction chemotherapy causes more mutations or resistant clonogens that future efforts to develop effective treatment should focus on concurrent chemo- and radiation therapy regimens. Induction (sequential) treatment may, however, become fruitful if we can develop systemic treatments that kill the last clonogens or overcome the accelerated proliferation of the clonogens typically induced by present induction regimens; of course, bone marrow suppression, esophagitis, or lung toxicity must be minimal as well.

In summary, concurrent chemotherapy and radiation therapy seems to be more efficacious to control unresectable NSCLC but with more acute toxicity. The RTOG 94-10 protocol is testing the effectiveness of sequential treatment, concurrent treatment, and aggressive concurrent chemo- and hyperfractionated radiation therapy by a randomized fashion. The protocol will be completed by April 1998. Survival, locoregional control, and toxicity will be reported in the year 2000.

References

Arriagada R, Le Chevalier T, Quoix E et al (1991) Effect of chemotherapy on locally advanced nonsmall cell lung carcinoma: a randomized study of 353 patients. GETCB, FNCLCC, and CEBI trialists. Int J Radiat Oncol Biol Phys 20:1183–1190

Begg AC, Hofland I, Moonen L et al (1990) The predictive value of cell kinetic measurements in a European trial of accelerated fractionation in advanced head and neck tumors: an interim report. Int J Radiat Oncol Biol Phys 19:1449–1453

Blanke C, Ansari R, Mantravadi R et al (1995) Phase III trial of thoracic irradiation with or without cisplatin for locally advanced unresectable non-small cell lung cancer: a Hoosier Oncology Group protocol. J Clin Oncol 13:1425–1429

Byhardt RW, Scott C, Sause WT et al (1998) Response, toxicity failure patterns, and survival in five Radiation Therapy Oncology Group (RTOG) trials of sequential and/or concurrent chemotherapy and radiotherapy for locally advanced non-small cell carcinoma of the lung. Int J Radiat Oncol Biol Phys 42:469–478

Cox JD, Pajak TF, Asbell S et al (1993) Interruptions of high-dose radiation therapy decrease long-term survival of favorable patients with unresectable non-small cell carcinoma of the lung: analysis of 1244 cases from 3 Radiation Therapy Oncology Group trials. Int J Radiat Oncol Biol Phys 27:493–498

Cox JD, Scott CB, Emami B et al (1997) Addition of chemotherapy to radiation therapy alters failure patterns by cell type within non-small cell carcinoma of lung (NSCCL): analysis of radiation therapy oncology group (RTOG) trials. Lung Cancer 18:126

Coy P (1970) A randomized study of irradiation and vinblastine in lung cancer. Cancer 26:803–807

Dillman RO, Seagren SL, Propert KJ et al (1990) A randomized trial of induction chemotherapy plus high-dose radiation versus radiation alone in stage III non-small-cell lung cancer. N Engl J Med 323:940–945

Dillman RO, Herndon J, Seagren SL et al (1996) Improved survival in stage III nonsmall cell lung cancer: seven-year follow-up of Cancer and Leukemia Group B (CALGB) 8433 trial. J Natl Cancer Inst 88:1210–1216

Early Breast Cancer Trials Collaborative Group (1992) Systemic treatment of early breast cancer by hormonal, cytotoxic, or immune therapy. Lancet 339:1–15, 71–85

Furuse K, Fukuoka M, Takada Y et al (1997) A randomized phase III study of concurrent versus sequential thoracic radiotherapy (TRT) in combination of mitomycin (M), vindesine (V), and cisplatin (P) in unresectable stage III non-small cell lung cancer (NSCLC): preliminary analysis. Proc Am Soc Clin Oncol 16:459a

Jeremic B, Shibamoto Y, Acimovic L, Milisavljevic S (1996) Hyperfractionated radiation therapy with or without concurrent low-dose daily carboplatin/etoposide for stage III non-small cell lung cancer: a randomized study. J Clin Oncol 14:1065–1070

Komaki R, Scott C, Ettinger D et al (1997a) Randomized study of chemotherapy/radiation therapy combinations for favorable patients with locally advanced inoperable nonsmall cell lung cancer: Radiation Therapy Oncology Group (RTOG) 92-04. Int J Radiat Oncol Biol Phys 38:149–155

Komaki R, Scott CB, Sause WT et al (1997b) Induction cisplatin/vinblastine and irradiation vs irradiation in unresectable squamous cell lung cancer: failure patterns by cell type in RTOG 88-08/ECOG 4588. Int J Radiat Oncol Biol Phys 39:537–544

LeChevalier T, Arriagada R, Quoix E et al (1991) Radiotherapy alone versus combined chemotherapy and radiotherapy in nonresectable non-small cell lung cancer. First analysis of a randomized trial in 353 patients. J Natl Cancer Inst 93:417–423

LeChevalier T, Arriagada R, Tarayre M et al (1992) Significant effect of adjuvant chemotherapy on survival in locally advanced non-small-cell lung carcinoma. J Natl Cancer Inst 84:58

Lokich J, Chaffey J, Neptune W (1989) Concomitant 5-fluorouracil infusion and high dose radiation for stage III non-small cell lung cancer. Cancer 64:1021–1025

Mattson K, Maasilta P (1989) Pulmonary toxicity. Lung Cancer 5:305–310

Mattson K, Holsti LR, Holsti P et al (1988) Inoperable non-small cell lung cancer: radiation with or without chemotherapy. Eur J Clin Oncol 3:477–482

McMillan TJ, Hart IR (1986) Enhanced experimental metastatic capacity of a murine melanoma following pretreatment with anticancer drugs. Clin Exp Metastasis 4:285–292

Morton RF, Jett JR, McGinnis I et al (1991) Thoracic radiation therapy alone compared with combined chemoradiotherapy for locally unresectable nonsmall cell lung cancer. Ann Intern Med 115:681–686

Muggia FM, Louie AC, Sikic BI (1983) Pulmonary toxicity of antitumor agents. Cancer Treat Rev 10:221–243

Non-small Cell Lung Cancer Collaborative Group (1995) Chemotherapy in non-small cell lung cancer: meta-analysis using updated data on individual patients from 52 randomized clinical trials. Br Med J 311:899–909

Phillips TL, Fu KK (1976) Quantification of combined radiation therapy and chemotherapy effects on critical normal tissues. Cancer 37:1186–1200

Sadeghi A, Payne D, Rubinstein L et al (1988) Combined modality treatment for resected advanced non-small cell lung cancer: local control and local recurrence. Int J Radiat Oncol Biol Phys 15:89–97

Sause WT, Scott CB, Taylor SG IV et al (1995) RTOG 88-08 and ECOG 4588:Preliminary results of a phase III trial in regionally advanced unresectable non-small cell lung cancer. J Natl Cancer Inst 87:198–205

Schaake-Konig C, van den Bogaert W, Dalesio O et al (1992) Effects of concomitant cisplatin and radiotherapy on inoperable non-small cell lung cancer. N Engl J Med 326:524–530

Steel GG (1988) The search for therapeutic gain in the combination of radiotherapy and chemotherapy. Radiother Oncol 11:31–53

Steel GG, Peckham MJ (1979) Exploitable mechanisms in combined radiotherapy-chemotherapy: the concept of additivity. Int J. Radiat Oncol Biol Phys 5:85–91

Tannehill SP, Mehta MP, Larson M et al (1997) Effect of amifostine on toxicities associated with sequential chemotherapy and radiation therapy for unresectable non-small-cell lung cancer: results of a phase II trial. J Clin Oncol 15:2850–2857

Tannock IF (1996) Treatment of cancer with radiation and drugs. J Clin Oncol 14:3156–3174

Trovo MG, Minatel E, Veronesi A et al (1990) Combined radiotherapy and chemotherapy versus radiotherapy alone in locally advanced epidermoid bronchogenic carcinoma. A randomized study. Cancer 65:400–404

Trovo NG, Minotel E, Fravelun G et al (1992) Radiotherapy versus radiotherapy enhanced by cisplatin in Stage III non small cell lung cancer. Int J Radiat Oncol Biol Phys 24:11–16

Tubiana M, Frindel E, Malaise E (1968) The application of radiobiologic knowledge and cellular kinetics to radiation therapy. Am J Roentgen Rad Ther Nucl Med 102:822–830

Umsawadi T, Valdivieso M, Barkley HT et al (1985) Esophageal complications from combined chemoradiotherapy (cyclophosphamide + adriamycin + cisplatin + XRT) in the treatment of non-small cell lung cancer. Int J Radiat Oncol Biol Phys 11:511–519

von der Maase H (1986) Experimental studies on interactions of radiation and cancer chemotherapeutic drugs in normal tisues and solid tumour (review). Radiother Oncol 7:47–68

von der Maase H, Overgaard J, Vaeth M (1986) Effect of cancer chemotherapeutic drugs on radiation-induced lung damage in mice. Radiother Oncol 5:245–258

Withers HR, Taylor JM, Maciejewski B (1988) The hazard of accelerated tumor clonogen repopulation during radiotherapy. Acta Oncol 27:131–146

Wolf M, Hans K, Becker H et al (1994) Radiotherapy alone versus chemotherapy with ifosfamide/vindesine followed by radiotherapy in unresectable locally advanced nonsmall cell lung cancer. Semin Oncol 21:42–47

8 Exclusive Radiotherapy for NSC Lung Cancer

H.-P. HEILMANN, F. WUERSCHMIDT, and H. BUENEMANN

CONTENTS

8.1 Historical Background

8.1.1 Survival Without Treatment

In order to evaluate the effect of radiation therapy on survival it is necessary to look at the natural course of the disease without treatment. Patients without any treatment or with symptomatic therapy have a 5-year survival rate of 0%–1.3% (BIGNALL et al. 1967; BUCHBERG et al. 1951; HYDE et al. 1965). Median survival of untreated patients varies between 2.0 and 10.6 months (BECKER et al. 1957; LANZOTTI et al. 1977). Median survival is strongly correlated with the performance status of the patient and the histologic type of the tumor (HYDE et al. 1973). Patients with a performance status of 90% had an average survival of 22 weeks, decreasing to only 4.5 weeks if the performance status was only 40% (Fig. 8.1). Patients with adenocarcinomas lived 13 weeks, and patients with small cell lung cancer only 6.76 weeks. Similar data on median survival in untreated patients were published by STANLEY (1980). Weight loss during the last 6 months is another factor influencing survival. In untreated patients with tumors confined to one side of the thorax, survival is about 4.3 months, and in patients with tumors beyond one-half of the chest only 2.1 months (HYDE et al. 1965).

8.1.2 Early Publications on Radiotherapy of Lung Cancer

Radiation therapy of lung cancer has been a problem for radiation oncologists during all periods of development of radiotherapy. In 1940, LEDDY and MOERSCH showed a 1-year survival of 20% and a 5-year survival of 4% in patients treated with radiation while all patients without radiation therapy died; nevertheless with kilovoltage equipment only palliation or treatment of superficial metastases was possible. In advanced cases, interstitial radiation treatment was tried (ORMEROD 1937). The main treatment modality remained surgery.

With the introduction of cobalt machines and the possibility of applying higher tumor doses in the 1960s, there was much enthusiasm to overcome the problem. The possibility of destroying tumor cells with external radiation treatment was demon-

H.-P. HEILMANN, F. WUERSCHMIDT, H. BUENEMANN, Hermann-Holthusen Institute of Radiotherapy, St. George's Hospital, Lohmuehlenstr. 5, D-20099 Hamburg, Germany

strated by Bromley and Szur (1955). In 40% of preoperatively irradiated patients no tumor was found during autopsy. Bloedorn (1966) reported 35% of patients without tumor after preoperative irradiation, Rissanen and coworkers (1968) 30% Eichhorn and coworkers (1972) published an average rate of 39% depending on fractionation and total doses.

A radiological documented reduction of tumor (partial remission and complete remission) in 87% of patients in correlation with total doses was shown by Pereslegin et al. (1977) and Rubin (1974). The reduction of tumor size was 70%–90% (Salazar et al. 1976). So, for some time radiotherapy with megavolt therapy (cobalt machines) was thought to be an alternative to surgical treatment. Unfortunately, very soon the limits of the new radiation techniques were obvious and, on the other hand, a deterioration of treatment results by radiotherapy was supposed because of immune suppression (Israel 1976). Consequently, there was a typical backlash: irradiation was said to be of no value in the treament of lung cancer.

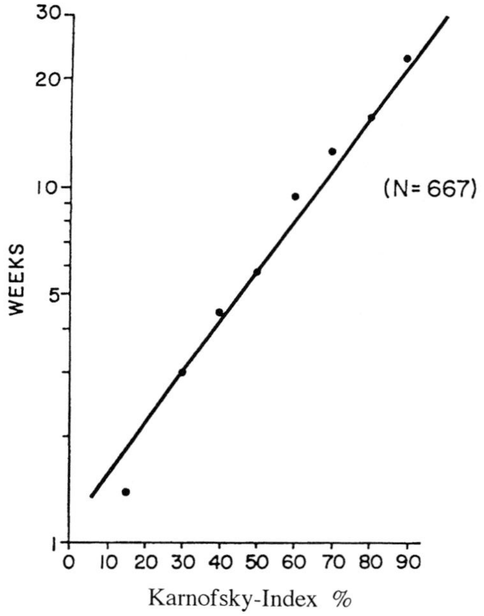

Fig. 8.1. Correlation between Karnofsky Index and median survival in untreated NSCLC patients. (From Hyde L, Wolf J, McCracken St, and Yesner R. Natural course of inoperable lung cancer. Chest 64:309–312, 1973)

Trials – randomized or not – were designed to compare radiotherapy of lung cancer with no treatment. Neglecting all biological knowledge of the relationship of tumor dose and tumor cell destruction published in the early 1930s (Holthusen 1936), radiotherapy was performed with total doses of about 4000 cGy, a dose which is too low to cure lung cancer. As a result, there was no difference in survival between patients treated by radiotherapy with 40 Gy or with no treatment at all (Durrant et al. 1971; Berry et al. 1997; Roswit et al. 1968). So even in 1978, Gross and Klein (1978) made a statement in the *Deutsches Ärzteblatt* that only surgery gives a curative chance to lung cancer patients.

In spite of this, in the late 1960s there were several publications on a small, but measurable effect of curative radiotherapy on survival of patients with non-small cell lung cancer (Guttmann 1971; Smart 1966; Schnepper and Vielberg 1967). Shehata (1977) and Coy (1978) published 5-year survival rates up to 10% with radiotherapy in non-small cell carcinoma. In 1976, Heilmann and coworkers (1976) published a multicenter retrospective evaluation of the effect of radiotherapy on non-small cell lung cancer (17 radiotherapy departments in Germany and Austria participated). A total of 3662 patients were treated with definitive radiotherapy, and follow-up was at least 5 years. The overall survival rate at 5 years was only 2% (Table 8.1), but in patients with T1-2NoMo tumors treated with higher doses a 5-year survival rate of 8.4% was seen (Table 8.2).

Table 8.1. Survival rates after definitive radiation therapy of lung cancer: all stages (Heilmann et al. 1976)

Time after treatment	No. patients, central tumors	Percentage survival	No. patients, peripheral tumors	Percentage survival
Treatment	3662	100.0	961	100.0
1 year	1142	31.2	296	30.8
2 years	394	10.8	94	9.8
3 years	161	4.4	48	5.0
4 years	91	2.5	24	2.5
5 years	73	2.0	19	2.0

As in other publications, in this study there was a clear relationship between radiation dose and survival. Patients treated with radiation doses between 5000 and 6000 cGy had higher survival rates than patients irradiated with lower doses. The relationship between total dose and survival was mentioned by PIERQUIN and coworkers even in 1965. The influence of an increasing biological dose on tumor reduction in X-rays of the lung was shown by SALAZAR (1979) (Fig. 8.2).

SHERMAN and coworkers (1981) reported a recurrence rate of 50% with doses <5000 cGy and only 5% with 5500–5900 cGy. Cox et al. (1979) demonstrated the relationship between local control and survival and the effect of increasing biologic dose levels on survival (Fig. 8.3).

In conclusion, the possibility of destroying non-small cell lung cancer (NSCLC) by radiotherapy was demonstrated by different authors. There was a clear relationship between total dose, extent of tumor reduction and survival. Doses of at least 6000 cGy were necessary to locally control NSCLC and achieve a curative effect of radiation.

8.2 Curative Radiotherapy

8.2.1 Arguments for Exclusive Radiotherapy

At a time when combined modality techniques, like neoadjuvant chemotherapy, simultaneous chemoradiotherapy and sequential chemoradio- or radiochemotherapy, are discussed, what are the arguments for exclusive radiotherapy?

- Radiotherapy alone is better tolerated than a combined modality.
- Without chemotherapy higher doses of radiation can be applied, and only high total doses give curative chances.

Table 8.2. Survival rates after definitive radiation therapy of lung cancer: T1-2 No Mo cases (HEILMANN et al. 1976)

Time after treatment	No. patients, central tumors	Percentage survival	No. patients, peripheral tumors	Percentage survival
Treatment	203	100.0	47	100.0
1 year	87	42.9	26	55
2 years	42	20.7	13	28
3 years	21	10.3	9	19
4 years	20	9.9	6	13
5 years	17	8.4	5	10

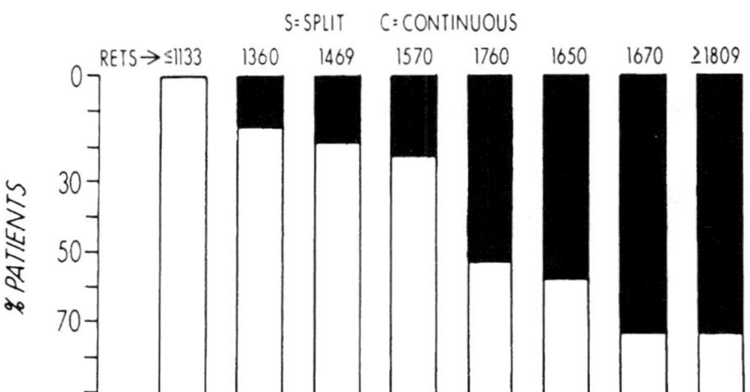

Fig. 8.2. Percent are regression of the pulmonary shadow 1 month after completion of radiotherapy for squamous cell carcinoma in relation to increasing NSD doses within each fractionation schedule employed. (From SALAZAR et al. Cancer 37:2636–2650, 1976. Copyright © (1976) American Cancer Society. Reprinted by permission of WILEY-LISS, Inc., a subsidiary of JOHN WILEY & SONS, Inc.)

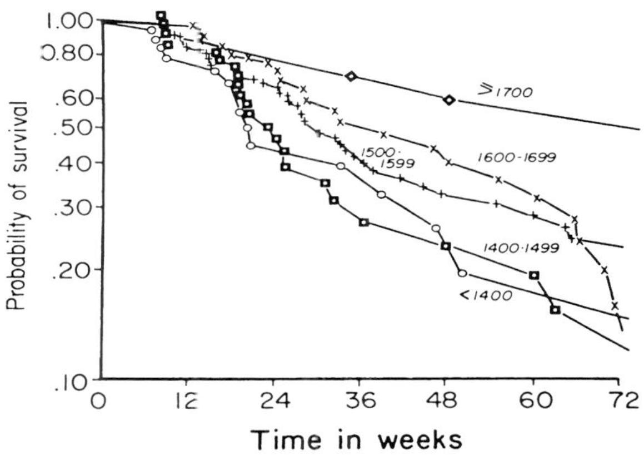

Fig. 8.3. Effect of increasing biological dose level in radiation therapy on survival in bronchopulmonary cancer. (From Cox et al. 1979)

- Last but not least, up until now it has not been proven that a combination of chemotherapy with radiotherapy gives better results than radiotherapy alone as long as high total doses are applied (Komaki et al. 1997a,b).

8.2.2 Patient Selection

The majority of patients with lung cancer present with advanced tumors and/or distant metastases at the time of diagnosis. The sites of metastases via the lymphatic system (Luomanen and Watson 1968) are most frequent into the hilar nodes, 74% (502/676), mediastinal nodes, 62% (420/676), and supraclavicular nodes, 19% (129/676). Sites of hematogenous metastases are 44% (296/676) in the adrenal glands, 43% (289/676) in the liver, 35% (234/676) in the bone and 19% (130/676) in the brain. In this entire series there were only 83/676 single metastatic sites, 16/676 to the other lung, 16/676 to the bone, 15/676 to the liver, 13/676 to the brain, 12/676 to the heart and 11/676 to the adrenals.

Curative treatment is only possible in a minority of about 30%–40% of all patients with lung cancer. Most of these are candidates for surgery. So, a relatively small part of the patient population is subject to the question whether curative radiotherapy is possible or not.

In deciding which patients are candidates for curative radiotherapy, history is one of the most important parts of the examination. Along with physical examination it indicates evidence for poor prognostic factors or suggests lines of inquiry to develop evidence for poor prognostic factors. The poor prognostic factors are

- Acute dyspnea, due to pneumonia
- Weight loss >5%
- Anorexia
- Asthenia
- Cough
- Chest pain
- Fever
- Atelectasis
- Recurrent pneumonia

Patients with acute pneumonia, weight loss, anorexia and asthenia have a median survival of only 3 months (Green et al. 1971).

In the detection of occult metastatic disease bone scans, computed tomography and magnetic resonance imaging play an important role. Recently, the value of the positron emission tomography (PET) has been repeatedly demonstrated (Schiepers 1997; Guhlmann et al. 1997; Erasmus et al. 1997; Steinert et al. 1997).

In conclusion, candidates for curative radiotherapy are patients with:

- No distant metastases
- A Karnofsky Index ≥70%
- Tumors with limited tumor volume (≤5 cm maximal diameter)

8.2.3 Differences Between Histologic Subtypes

Whether there are differences in the outcome between histologic subtypes is controversial. There is evidence that squamous cell carcinomas have a lower rate of distant metastases than adenocarcinomas and large cell carcinomas. In a series of 349 patients with adenocarcinomas and large cell carcinomas, one-third of patients with large cell carcinoma developed brain metastasis within 1 year, and patients with adenocarcinoma continued to develop brain metastasis even into the 5th year (Cox and Komaki 1986). On the other hand, patients with these histologic subtypes show better results with definitive radiotherapy than those with squamous cell carcinoma (Cox et al. 1986).

From our own experience, the differences in 5-year survival between the subtypes of NSCLC are not relevant. For indication of curative radiotherapy, we feel that histologic subtype is not an important prognostic parameter.

8.2.4 Superior Sulcus Tumors

Superior sulcus tumors, with or without Pancoast's syndrome, are a special type of NSCLC. In contrast to other tumors, preoperative irradiation is common, and radiotherapy alone often is only palliative.

8.3 Radiation Therapy Techniques

8.3.1 Target Volumes

Target volumes in curative radiotherapy of NSCLC are a topic of discussion and personal opinion.

Details are given in another chapter of this book. The standard recommendation is to include the tumor and the known lymph nodes with a safety margin of about 1 cm. The upper and middle mediastinum normally is included up to a total dose of 50 Gy, and in tumors of the lower lobes also the lower parts of the mediastinum.

In contrast, KROL and coworkers (1996) from the Netherlands treated 108 medically inoperable patients with non-small cell lung cancer (T1 and peripheral T2) with a 60-Gy split course or 65 Gy continuous treatment. The target volume included the primary tumor only, without regional lymph nodes. Of patients in complete remission, only two had a regional recurrence as the only site of relapse; an additional two patients had a locoregional recurrence. They came to the conclusion that the low regional relapse rate does not support the need for the use of large fields encompassing regional lymph nodes. Using small target volumes, higher doses could be given and better local control rates could be expected.

On the other hand, CHOI and DOUCETTE (1981) observed improved survival rates in patients with unresectable non-small cell bronchogenic carcinoma by an innovative high-dose en bloc radiotherapeutic approach encompassing the tumor, the whole mediastinum and the supraclavicular nodes.

In clinical practice, volume must be tailored individually depending on tumor location, tumor size, and involved lymph nodes. The dose-limiting factors are the volume of uninvolved lung included in the portals and the spinal cord tolerance.

8.3.2 Dose Distribution

Dose distribution in curative radiotherapy of lung cancer should be different in sequential phases of the treatment. For the first weeks, normally up to a dose of 50 Gy, a larger volume should be treated. In order to spare the spinal cord and the lungs, two- or three-field techniques are adequate. High radiation doses should be restricted to the tumor and the involved mediastinal lymph nodes. Multileaf collimators or individually constructed metal shields should be used in order to irradiate as little lung tissue as possible. Three-dimensional treatment planning is thought to give better results (NESTLE et al. 1996), but up until now there has been little experience as to whether long term outcome really is improved.

8.3.3 Total Doses

As shown previously, there is much evidence that in NSCLC higher total doses give better remission rates and, as a consequence, better long term survival. In spite of this even today in many trials total dose is restricted to 50 or 60 Gy. It is obvious that a high percentage of lung tumors can only be destroyed with doses >60 Gy, approaching 70 Gy and more. Because of the dose limiting factors, the application of high total doses is strongly correlated to a sophisticated treatment planning.

8.3.4 Fractionation

In the literature, there is a variety of fractionation schemes and single doses. Standard fractionation is 5 times weekly 2.0 Gy = 10 Gy/week. The main variations are high single doses, interruptions of treatment (split course) and hyper-/accelerated fractionation.

8.3.4.1 Single Dose

In the 1960s and 1970s, high single doses were used by several groups. SCHUMACHER (1976) treated patients with NSCLC with high energy electrons of a betatron giving single doses of 500–1000 cGy. He published 5-year survival rates of about 6% with this technique. Because of the poor technical performance of dose distribution with electrons, normal tissue damage, especially to the lungs, was severe.

EICHHORN (1981) compared standard fractionation with initial high doses controlled by autopsies. Radiation was given in daily, small fractions (200 cGy), large fractions (600 cGy) every 5th day, or a single high dose followed by daily low-dose treatment. The highest proportion of tumors free of viable cells was found in patients who had received small daily fractions in both operable and inoperable tumors.

8.3.4.2 Split-Course Radiotherapy

Before the influence of repopulation and treatment time was known, planned interruptions of radiotherapy were recommended. The so-called split-course technique was better tolerated than standard fractionation schemes, as HOLSTI and coworkers

(1976) from Finland demonstrated. In the split-course treatment there was a 2–3 weeks' interruption after 25–30 Gy. This break was compensated by a 10% increase in the total dose. With increasing radiobiological knowledge, this treatment policy was suspended.

8.3.4.3 Hyperfractionation and Accelerated Fractionation

The rationale for hyperfractionation is sparing of late normal tissue effects. The dose per fraction is decreased below 1.8 Gy and the daily dose would not exceed 2–2.4 Gy. An accelerated hyperfractionated regimen would typically apply a dose per fraction of about 1.8–2.0 Gy twice daily or 1.4–1.5 Gy three times daily (CHART). As a consequence, the overall treatment time is about the same in hyperfractionated radiotherapy whereas it is decreased in accelerated radiotherapy. However, as acute normal tissue effects are increased with accelerated radiotherapy, treatment breaks have to be introduced in most cases after 2–3 weeks. Recently the possible advantages and critical issues on hyperfractionation have been discussed by Beck-Bornholdt et al. (1997).

8.4 Results of Exclusive Curative Radiotherapy

8.4.1 Results with Conventional Fractionation

In 1981, Choi and Doucette treated 162 cases of NSCLC with two different treatment techniques. Patients treated with small volumes and tumor doses of 40–45 Gy had a 2-year survival of 10% and a 3-year survival of only 3%. With an en bloc approach and tumor doses of 60–64 Gy, 2-year survival was 36%, 3-year survival 28%. Patients treated with >50 Gy had a 5-year survival of 7.5%. Sherman and coworkers (1981) treated 348 cases. The 5-year survival rate of the whole group was 5.6%, and patients in stage I and II did better. In stage III there was a clear dose relationship: patients treated with less than 50 Gy had a recurrence rate of 50%; with higher doses recurrences were less frequent.

A similar dose relationship was published by the RTOG (Perez et al. 1987). Local failure with 40 Gy was 48%, with 50 Gy 38% and with 60 Gy 27%. Unfortunately, 75%–80% of all patients developed distant metastases.

In 43 stage I, technically operable patients, Haffty et al. (1988) achieved a 3-year survival rate of 36% and a 5-year rate of 21% with radiation doses of 5400–5900 cGy. As mentioned previously, the percentage of patients for curative radiotherapy is small. Those 43 cases were part of 1646 patients referred. A Chinese group (Zhang et al. 1989) treated 44 early cases with 55–70 Gy/6–7 weeks delivered by conventional fractionation. Survival rates at 1, 3, and 5 years were 93%, 55%, and 32% respectively. The favorable factors in this series were:

- Patients without any intercurrent disease but refused operation
- T1 lesions
- Complete regression of the lesion at the conclusion of radiotherapy
- Doses ranging from 69 to 70 Gy

Gauden and coworkers from Australia (1995) reported the results of 347 patients with T1 and T2N0M0 tumors treated at the Queensland Radium Institute during the period 1985–1992. The main reasons for not proceeding to surgery included poor performance status, old age, or refusal to submit to surgery. The median age for the group was 70 years, with the range being 34–90 years. The overall survival rate was 27% at 5 years with a median survival of 27.9 months. There was a strong correlation of survival to tumor size.

In a Greek series (Koukourakis et al. 1995), 153 patients with inoperable NSCLC were treated with radiotherapy alone. A retrospective analysis showed a 5-year disease-free survival for T1-2 N0-1 and T3 N0-1 staged patients of 30% (7/23) and 25% (4/16) respectively when the tumor normalized total dose (NTD) (alpha/beta = 10 Gy) was 56–64 Gy vs 12% (5/41) and 0% (0/10) when the NTD was 48–55 Gy. This difference was statistically significant for the squamous cell histology group. The higher doses significantly altered the patterns of death in N0, 1 staged squamous cell carcinoma and adenocarcinoma patients. Forty-five percent (22/55) and 41% (12/29) of squamous cell and adenocarcinoma patients, respectively, died from local relapse without evidence of distant metastases when NTD was less than 55 Gy vs 21% (9/42) and 13% (2/15) when the NTD delivered was 56–64 Gy ($P < 0.05$).

As mentioned previously, Krol et al. (1996) treated 108 patients with early peripheral NSCLC (stage I) with radiotherapy defined to the tumor without elective nodal irradiation. Three-year survival was 31%, 5-year survival 15%. The question of elective nodal irradiation was also raised by KUPELIAN and coworkers (1996). They treated 71 patients by radiation therapy alone (median total radiation dose 63.23 Gy) because of medical contradindications to surgery. Coverage of nodal drainage areas did not affect survival or local control. Overall survival rates at 3 and 5 years were 19% and 12%, respectively.

The importance of volume parameters for survival of NSCLC was outlined by MARTEL and coworkers (1997). Patients with tumor volumes <200 cm^2 had a better survival than patients with bigger tumor volumes. Tumor volume was also one of five prognostic factors described by WIGREN (1997). The other four were disease extent, clinical symptom score by FEINSTEIN, performance status and hemoglobin level. Patients with three or more risk factors had a 2-year survival of less than 2%, whereas patients with no risk factors had a 2-year survival of 53%!

Three-dimensional treatment planning is also used to improve results of radiotherapy of NSCLC (ROBERTSON et al. 1997; ARMSTRONG et al. 1997). Number of treated patients and follow-up time are not sufficient to give valid data on survival.

8.4.2 Results with Split-Course Radiotherapy

In the Finnish series (HOLSTI et al. 1976), for each tumor site local control and failure rates for the two treatment techniques – conventional fractionation and split-course therapy were similar. No significant differences in 5- and 10-year survivals were noted. Acute side effects were milder in all patients treated with the split course. The occurrence of late reactions was similar in both treatment groups.

However, in 1993, the RTOG published the long-term results of three trials with 1244 cases. Interruptions of high dose radiation therapy decreased long-term survival of favorable patients with unresectable NSCLC (COX et al. 1993).

8.4.3 Results with Hyperfractionation and Accelerated Fractionation

In the RTOG trial 83-11 no significant differences in the risks of acute or late effects in normal tissues were found among 848 patients analyzed in five arms with increasing radiation doses (COX et al. 1990). Comparisons with results in similar patients treated with 60 Gy in 30 fractions of 2.0 Gy 5 days/week for 6 weeks suggest a benefit from hyperfractionated radiation therapy with 69.6 Gy.

The same treatment policy – 1.2 Gy twice daily to a total dose of 69.6 Gy – was used by JEREMIC et al. (1997). Forty-nine patients in stage I NSCLC were treated with hyperfractionated radiotherapy. The median survival time was 33 months, and the 5-year survival rate was said to be 30%.

In a pilot study, BRINDLE et al. (1993) treated 21 evaluable patients with unresectable stage IIIA or B non-small cell lung cancer, using 6000 cGy in 40 fractions of 150 cGy twice daily, 6 h between fractions. Toxicity was relatively high, and results are not comparable because of the small number of patients.

The best known study with accelerated fractionation is CHART. Because of the fact that human tumor cells can proliferate rapidly, and giving radiotherapy in many small fractions may reduce long-term normal-tissue morbidity, the CHART regimen (continuous hyperfractionated accelerated radiotherapy) was designed. Thirty-six small fractions of 1.5 Gy are given three times/day to a total dose of 54 Gy in only 12 consecutive days. The long-term follow-up of a trial of CHART versus conventional radiotherapy in patients with locally advanced non-small cell lung cancer (NSCLC) has been published recently (SAUNDERS et al. 1997): 563 patients were entered by 13 centers between April 1990 and March 1995. Included were patients with NSCLC localized to the chest with a performance status of 0 or 1 in whom radical radiotherapy was chosen as the definitive management. Patients were randomly allocated in a 3:2 ratio to CHART or conventional radiotherapy. The latter was 30 fractions of 2 Gy to a total dose of 60 Gy in 6 weeks. The groups were well matched for possible prognostic factors. Overall there was a 24% reduction in the relative risk of death, which is equivalent to an absolute improvement in 2-year survival of 9% from 20% to 29% (P = 0.004, 95% CI 0.63–0.92). Subgroup analyses (predefined) suggest that the largest benefit occurred in patients with squamous cell carcinomas (82% of the cases), in whom there was a 34% reduction in the relative risk of death (an absolute improvement at 2 years of 14% from 19% to 33%). During the first 3 months, severe dysphagia occurred more often in the CHART group than in the group on conventional radiotherapy (19% vs 3%). Otherwise, there were no important differences in short-term or long-term morbidity. In this series, CHART compared with conventional radiotherapy gave a significant improvement in survival of patients with NSCLC.

8.4.4 High-LET Radiation

The results of a combined cobalt-neutron treatment were investigated in Berlin-Buch (EICHHORN and LESSEL 1976). The difference in response of human tumors to high and low LET radiation has been investigated in a series of inoperable, histologically confirmed bronchial carcinomas. One hundred and forty-nine were treated with low LET radiation alone (^{60}Co gamma rays) and 108 with a combination of gamma-rays and fast neutrons of mean energy 6 MeV, one-fifth to one-third of the effective dose being from neutrons. The response was analyzed by histological examination of the autopsy specimens. Tumor cell destruction was found to be significantly greater in the neutron-treated series. The two series were not strictly randomized but were closely similar to terms of tumor volume, histological grade and total treatment time. The sequence of treatments with neutrons and gamma-rays (N-gamma, gamma-N, gamma-N-gamma) was found to have no influence on the results.

8.5 Results of Definitive Radiotherapy in Inoperable NSCLC Patients Treated Between 1976 and the End of 1996 at the Hermann-Holthusen Institute, Hamburg

8.5.1 Patients and Treatment Modalities

Inoperable non-small cell lung cancer (NSCLC) patients were treated with irradiation alone at the Hermann-Holthusen Institute for Radiotherapy, General Hospital St. Georg, Hamburg. The results of stage I–III patients were reported recently, demonstrating 5-year survival rates of 8% for all patients (WURSCHMIDT et al. 1994). Here we present an update of the data of 397 patients suffering from inoperable NSCLC. All patients were irradiated with a total dose of 70 Gy at 2.0 Gy/fraction. The majority of patients were treated with 8–10 MeV photons but occasionally 5 MeV photons or cobalt-60 gamma-rays were used. Treatment volumes included the primary tumor with a safety margin of about 2 cm and ipsilateral hilar and mediastinal lymph nodes. The contralateral hilus and the supraclavicular fossae were not regularly irradiated. The total dose of the primary volume was 40–50 Gy. After a planned break with varying length (median 12 weeks), a restaging was performed excluding patients from further radiotherapy if distant metastases were documented, or if radiation-induced excessive normal toxicity, or no change or progress of tumor volume was observed. The boost volume comprised the primary tumor and all clinically involved lymph nodes. A boost dose of 20–30 Gy was applied. The spinal cord dose was kept below 40 Gy. None of the patients received chemotherapy.

8.5.2 Results of Curative Treatment

The overall survival was determined from start of irradiation to the date of death or last follow-up. If no information about the cause of death was achieved, death due to recurrent tumor was assumed. Estimates of survival were obtained by the product-limit method of Kaplan and Meier. In Fig. 8.4 the updated results of NSCLC stage I patients are shown. The 2- and 5-year survival rates were 32.6% and 9.6%. The median survival time (MST) was 18.5 months. In Fig. 8.5 results of NSCLC stage II are shown. Stage IIA included T1N1M0 cases and stage IIB T2N1M0 and T3N0M0 cases. The latter were formerly classified as stage IIIA, but in the latest TNM classification are staged as IIB. The 2- and 5-year survival rates were 27% and 14% for stage IIA and 39% and 11% for IIB cases. The MST was 14.9 months.

In Fig. 8.6 results are given for stage III patients. Stage IIIA included T3N1M0 and T1-3N2M0 cases. All T4 and all N3 cases were classified as stage IIIB disease. In stage IIIA, the 2- and 5-year survival rates were 26.9% and 6.7%; the MST was 14.3 months. The results of stage IIIB patients were frustrating even if they received 70 Gy total dose. The 2-year survival probability was only 5% and no patient lived longer than 29 months. The MST was 8.5 months. There were only 22 patients with IIIB disease, reflecting our policy normally not to treat patients with this advanced stage in a curative fashion. The disappointing results confirm our policy that there is no curative approach with radiotherapy alone in stage IIIB even if irradiated with high doses. We now therefore limit

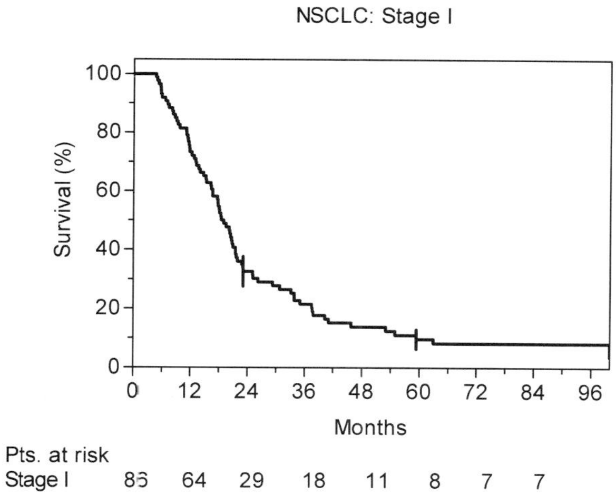

Fig. 8.4. Survival rates of inoperable NSCLC patients with stage I disease (means and SE). Actuarial survival estimates are shown from start of radiotherapy. All patients received radiotherapy alone with no addition of chemotherapy

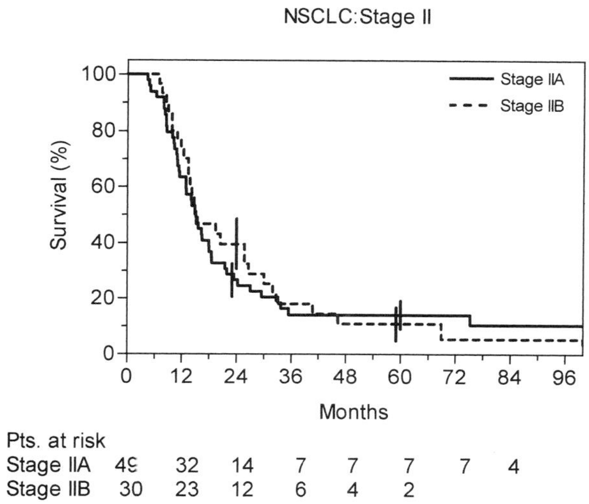

Fig. 8.5. Survival rates of inoperable NSCLC patients with stage II disease (means and SE). Actuarial survival estimates are shown from start of radiotherapy. All patients received radiotherapy alone with no addition of chemotherapy. The *solid line* denotes stage IIA disease patients; the *broken line* stage IIB. There is no significant difference between the two groups

the total dose to 50 Gy as a palliative treatment option in stage IIIB disease. A summary of the treatment results is given in Table 8.3.

As most of our patients had a planned break after 40 or 50 Gy for restaging procedures and decision about further treatment, it is interesting to look at the effect of the length of the break on treatment results. As there are accumulating reports in the literature especially in head and neck cancer but also in

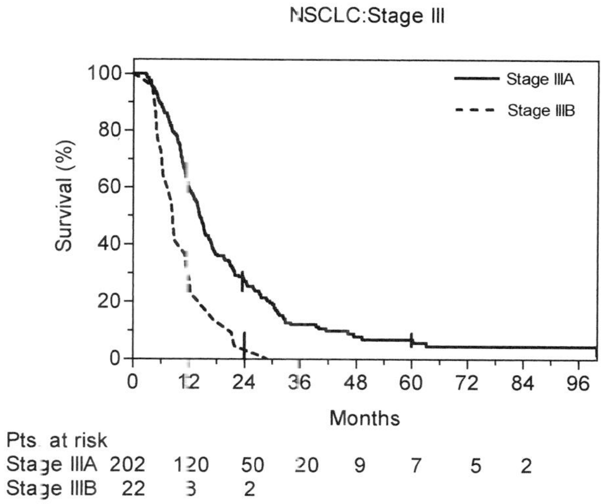

Fig. 8.6. Survival rates of inoperable NSCLC patients with stage III disease (means and SE). Actuarial survival estimates are shown from start of radiotherapy. All patients received radiotherapy alone with no addition of chemotherapy. The *solid line* denotes stage IIIA disease, the *broken line* stage IIIB. The difference is statistically significant (log rank, $P = 0.0013$)

lung cancer that extended overall treatment times can compromise results, it could be expected that survival rates decreased with increasing duration of the break. Willers et al. (1998) analyzed the data of our patients treated with 70 Gy. They found no difference in outcome whether a planned break of 7–11 weeks, 12 weeks, or >12 weeks was introduced after 40 or 50 Gy. In univariate and multivariate analysis only complete response of the tumor and sex remained as significant prognosticators. Treatment duration and length of the break were not important for prognosis.

8.5.3 Normal Tissue Toxicity

The high-dose radiotherapy was well tolerated. No treatment related death occurred. Moderate to severe pneumonitis requiring drug treatment was observed in 9%, esophagitis RTOG grade 3–4 in 11%, nausea and/or vomiting in 3% and chest pain in 2%.

8.5.4 Results of Palliative Treatment

Palliative treatment in NSCLC patients with distant metastasis is given with the aim of symptom relief.

Table 8.3. Survival rates and median survival times in non-small cell lung cancer treated with radiotherapy alone at the Hermann-Holthusen Institute for Radiotherapy, Hamburg

Stage	Survival rates (%) ± SE						
	N	1 year	2 years	3 years	4 years	5 years	MST (months)
I	86	73.3 ± 4.8	32.6 ± 5.1	21.5 ± 4.5	13.8 ± 3.8	9.6 ± 3.3	18.5
IIA	49	63 ± 7	27 ± 6	14 ± 5	14 ± 5	14 ± 5	14.9
IIB	30	73 ± 8	39 ± 9.0	18 ± 7	11 ± 6	11 ± 6	14.9
IIIA	202	59.6 ± 3.5	26.9 ± 3.2	11.9 ± 2.5	7.8 ± 2.2	6.7 ± 2.2	14.3
IIIB	22	32 ± 10	5 ± 5				8.5

Table 8.4. Patient characteristics in metastatic non-small cell lung cancer treated at the Hermann-Holthusen Institute for Radiotherapy, Hamburg

Total: 562	*n*	(%)
Age (years)		
31–55	186	(33)
56–64	155	(28)
65–71	123	(22)
72+	98	(17)
Sex		
Male	429	(76)
Female	133	(24)
Karnofsky performance status		
80–100	319	(57)
60–70	175	(31)
40–50	40	(7)
20–30	1	
Unknown	27	(5)
Metastatic site		
Brain	82	(15)
Bone	203	(36)
Liver	33	(6)
Other	13	(2)
Multiple sites	231	(41)
Symptom relief[a]		
Complete/partial improvement	149	
No change/progressive disease	94	
Not stated	319	

[a] Symptom relief after palliative radiotherapy.

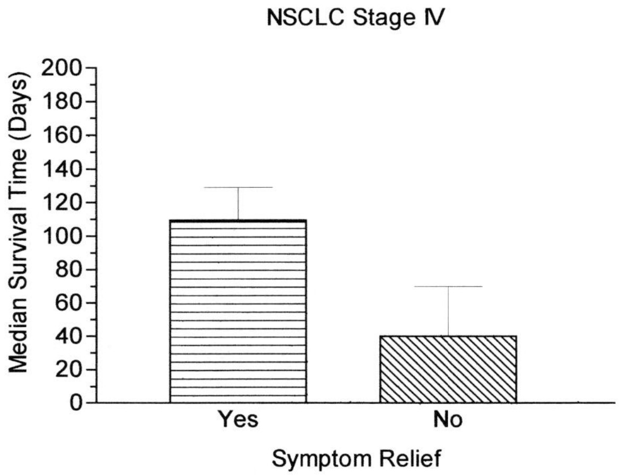

Fig. 8.7. The median survival times (in days) are shown for stage IV NSCLC patients treated with palliative radiotherapy. The two groups shown are those *with* symptom relief at the end of radiotherapy (*hatched bar*) and *without* relief (*crossed pattern*). The *error bars* denote the 95% confidence interval

At our institution we irradiate bone or brain metastases with 2.5 Gy/fraction four times weekly to 40 Gy. If the patient's general condition is very poor and his or her life expectancy short (weeks), the dose per fraction is increased to 3.0 Gy or occasionally to 4.0 Gy. Total doses are adjusted as well to about 30 Gy. If the patient is in good general condition, has a single metastatic lesion, e.g., of the brain, or a large lymph node in the supraclavicular region, the total dose would be increased to 50 Gy at 2.0-Gy fractions five times weekly. Simple treatment techniques with parallel-opposing fields are preferred. Photon irradiation with energies of 6–10 MV and an SSD of 100 cm were given in most cases; occasionally cobalt-60 was used at an SSD of 80 cm. In other institutions, even in palliative radiotherapy hyperfractionated treatment regimes are used (Okawa et al. 1988).

Characteristics of the patients are shown in Table 8.3. Fifty-seven percent were in a good general condition with a Karnofsky performance index (KPI) of >=80%. Bone metastases were treated in 36%, brain metastases in 15% and multiple sites in 41%. In 243 of 562 patients information about symptom changes was recorded (Table 8.4). Ninety-four out of 243 (40%) had no change or progressive symptoms and 149/243 (60%) had complete or partial improvement of their symptoms. If symptom relief was achieved, patients had a significantly longer median survival time (MST) of about 110 days than patients with no symptom relief (MST about 40 days) as is shown in Fig. 8.7.

In palliative irradiation of NSCLC the influence of fractionation is of minor importance. Symptom relief may be better with high single doses and short treatment time (Teo et al. 1988; Papavasiliou et al. 1987).

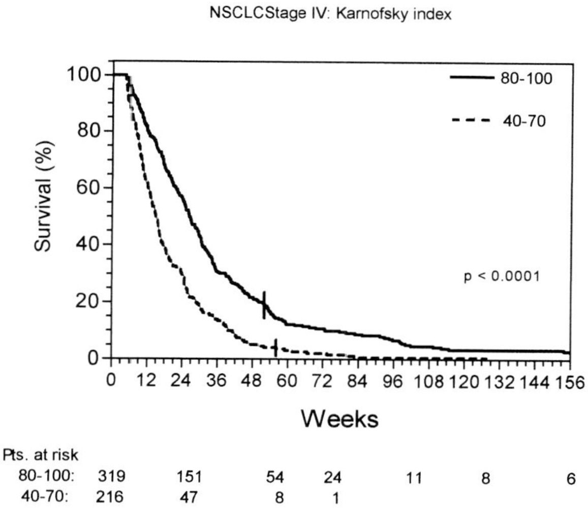

Fig. 8.8. Survival rates of stage IV NSCLC patients (means and SE) are given. Overall survival estimates are shown from start of radiotherapy. All patients received palliative radiotherapy. The *solid line* denotes patients with a Karnofsky performance index at start of radiotherapy of at least 80%. The *broken line* denotes a Karnofsky performance index of 40%–70%. The difference between the two curves is highly significant (log rank, $P < 0.0001$)

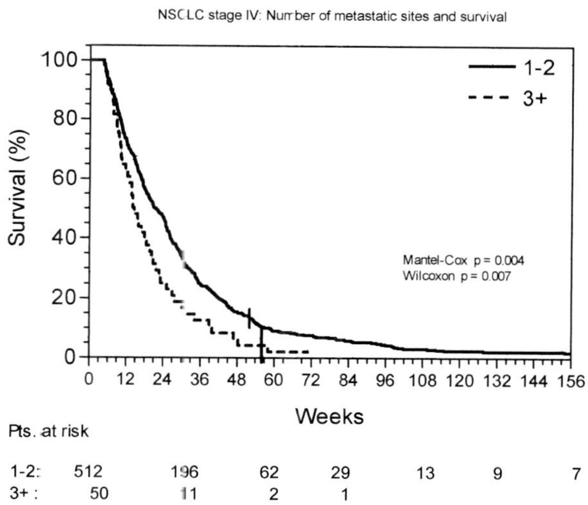

Fig. 8.9. Survival rates of stage IV NSCLC patients (means and SE) are given. Overall survival estimates are shown from start of radiotherapy. All patients received palliative radiotherapy. The *solid line* denotes patients suffering from one or two different metastatic sites; *the broken line* denotes 3 or more metastatic sites. The difference between the two curves is significant (log rank, $P < 0.004$)

Table 8.5. Survival rates and median survival times in non-small cell lung cancer with distant metastasis treated at the Hermann-Holthusen Institute for Radiotherapy, Hamburg

	6 months[a]	12 months[a]	MST (days)[b]	P^c
Age (years)				
31–55	38.0% (30.8, 45.2)	10.4% (5.8, 15)	149.5 (135, 176)	
56–64	44.0% (36, 52)	19.6% (13.1, 26.1)	157 (124, 189)	n.s.
65–71	42.6% (33.8, 51.4)	10.0% (6.6, 15.4)	137 (110, 184)	
72+	28.7% (19.3, 38.1)	8.0% (2.3, 13.7)	121 (109, 144)	
Sex				
Male	38.4% (33.7, 43.1)	12.1% (8.9, 15.3)	139 (122, 160)	
Female	41.7% (33.2, 50.2)	13.6% (7.6, 19.6)	160 (129, 183)	n.s.
KPS				
80–100	51.8% (46.1, 57.5)	18.9% (14.4, 23.4)	185 (170, 207)	
40–70	23.2% (16.7, 29)	3.9% (1.2, 6.6)	104 (92, 114)	<0.0001
Metastatic sites[b]				
1–2	40.8% (36.4, 45.2)	13.3% (10.2, 16.4)	148.5 (135, 172)	0.0035[d]
3+	23.0% (12.1, 34.9)	4.2% (0, 9.9)	99 (82, 138)	0.007[a]

[a] Survival rates (mean ± 95% confidence interval).
[b] Median survival time (95% confidence interval).
[c] Generalized Wilcoxon test (Peto-Prentice).
[d] Mantel-Cox test.

Table 8.6. Multivariate analysis. Non-small cell lung cancer with distant metastasis treated at the Hermann-Holthusen Institute for Radiotherapy, Hamburg

Variable	Risk Ratio	95% CI	Chi-square	*P* value
KPS	1.6	1.4, 1.9	33.174	<0.001
Metastatic sites	1.5	1.1, 2.1	6.779	0.009

Covariates included in the model: Karnofsky performance status (80–100 vs 40–70), number of metastatic sites (1–2 vs 3+), age (31–55 vs 56–64 vs 65–71 vs 72+), and sex.

In univariate analysis the KPI and the number of metastatic sites were of significant importance for the overall survival probability. In Fig. 8.8 results of patients with stage IV NSCLC are given stratified for their KPI. Patients with a KPI of at least 80% had 6- and 12-month survival rates of 51.8% and 18.9% and an MST of 6.1 months. Patients with a KPI below 80% had 6- and 12-month survival rates of 23.2% and 3.9% and an MST of 3.4 months. The difference is significant ($P < 0.0001$). In Fig. 8.9 survival probability and the number of metastatic sites is shown. Patients with one or two involved sites had 6- and 12-month survival rates of 40.8% and 13.3% and an MST of 4.9 months. Significantly lower ($P = 0.0035$) survival rates and MST were observed in patients with more than two sites involved. Their 6- and 12-month survival rates were 23% and 4.2% and the MST was 3.3 months. A summary of the results is given in Table 8.5. In a multivariate analysis (Cox proportional hazards model) including KPI, number of involved metastatic sites, age and sex, only KPI and number of metastatic sites were significant predictors for survival probability (Table 8.6).

8.5.5 Recommendations for Definitive Radiotherapy of NSCLC from the Experiences of the Hermann-Holthusen Institute, Hamburg

Based on our experience and data from the literature (Asco 1997), we recommend irradiating patients with inoperable NSCLC with a total dose of 70 Gy in stage I–IIIA disease if no additional concomitant chemotherapy is given. Stage IIIB disease has such a poor prognosis even after 70 Gy that we do not see an indication for curative radiotherapy. These patients should be treated with 45–50 Gy in 2.0- to 2.5-Gy fractions if irradiation is given as the sole modality.

References

ASCO (1997) Clinical practice guidelines for the treatment of unresectable non-small-cell lung cancer. J Clin Oncol 15:2996–3018

Armstrong J, Raben A, Zelefsky M, Burt M, Leibel S, Burman C, Kutcher G, Harrison L, Hahn C, Ginsberg R, Rusch V, Kris M, Fuks Z (1997) Promising survival with three-dimensional conformal radiation therapy for non-small cell lung cancer. Radiother Oncol 44:17–22

Beck-Bornholdt HP, Dubben HH, Liertz-Petersen C, Willers H (1997) Hyperfractionation: where do we stand? Radiother Oncol 43:1–21

Becker J, Werner K, Kuttig H, Scheer KE, Weitzel G (1957) Das Bronchuskarzinom in strahlenklinischer Sicht, part 2: Strahlentherapie. Strahlentherapie 103:348–367

Berry RJ, Laing AH, Newman CR, Peto J (1997) The role of radiotherapy in treatment of inoperable lung cancer. Int J Radiat Oncol Biol Phys 2:433–439

Bignall JR, Martin M, Smithers DW (1967) Survival in 6086 cases of bronchial carcinoma. Lancet I:1067–1970

Bloedorn FG (1966) Rationale and benefit of preoperative irradiation in lung cancer. JAMA 196:340–341

Brindle JS, Shaw EG, Su JQ, Mailliard JA, Frank AR, Laurie JA, McLean M, Tackett DM, Owens DT (1993) Pilot study of accelerated hyperfractionated thoracic radiation therapy in patients with unresectable stage III non-small cell lung carcinoma. Cancer 72:405–409

Bromley LL, Szur L (1955) Combined radiotherapy and resection for carcinoma of the bronchus. Lancet II:937–941

Buchberg A, Lubliner R, Rubin EH (1951) Carcinoma of the lung: duration of life of individuals not treated surgically. Diss Chest 20:257–272

Choi NC, Doucette JA (1981) Improved survival of patients with unresectable non-small-cell bronchogenic carcinoma by an innovated high-dose en-bloc radiotherapeutic approach. Cancer 48:101–109

Cox JD, Komaki R (1986) Prophylactic cranial irradiation for squamous cell carcinoma, large cell carcinoma, and adenocarcinoma of the lung: indications and techniques. Ut Md Anderson Clin Conf Cancer 28:233–237

Cox JD, Eisert DR, Komaki R, Mietlowski W, Petrovich Z (1979) Patterns of failure following treatment of apparently localized carcinoma of the lung. In: Muggia FM, Rozencweig M (eds) Lung cancer: progress in therapeutic research. Raven, New York, pp 279–288 (Progress in cancer research and therapy, vol 11)

Cox JD, Barber Derus S, Hartz AJ, Fischer M, Byhardt RW, Komaki R, Wilson JF, Greenberg M (1986) Is adenocarcinoma/large cell carcinoma the most radiocurable type of cancer of the lung? Int J Radiat Oncol Biol Phys 12:1801–1805

Cox JD, Azarnia N, Byhardt RW, Shin KH, Emami B, Pajak TF (1990) A randomized phase I/II trial of hyperfractionated radiation therapy with total doses of 60.0 Gy to 79.2 Gy: possible survival benefit with greater than or equal to 69.6 Gy in favorable patients with Radiation Therapy Oncology Group stage III non-small-cell lung carcinoma: report of Radiation Therapy Oncology Group 83-11. J Clin Oncol 8:1543–1555

Cox JD, Pajak TF, Asbell S, Russell AH, Pederson JB, Emami B, Roach MI (1993) Interruptions of high-dose radation therapy decrease long-term survival of favorable patients with unresectable non-small cell carcinoma of the lung. Analysis of 1244 cases from 3 Radiation Therapy Oncology Group (RTOG) trials. Int J Radiat Oncol Biol Phys 27:493–498

Coy P (1978) Curative radiotherapy in lung cancer. Int J Radiat Oncol Biol Phys 4[Suppl 2]:72

Durrant KR, Ellis F, Black JM, Berry RJ, Ridehalgh FR, Hamilton WS (1971) Comparison of treatment policies in inoperable bronchial caarcinoma. Lancet I:715–719

Eichhorn HJ (1981) Different fractionation schemes tested by histological examination of autopsy specimens from lung cancer patients. Br J Radiol 54:132–135

Eichhorn HJ, Lessel A (1976) A comparison between combined neutron- and telecobalt-therapy with telecobalt-therapy alone for cancer of the bronchus. Br J Radiol 49:880–882

Eichhorn H-J, Lessel A, Rotte K-H (1972) Einfluß verschiedener Bestrahlungsrhythmen auf Tumor- und Normalgewebe in vivo. Strahlentherapie 143:614–629

Erasmus JJ, Patz EF Jr, McAdams HP, Murray JG, Herndon J, Coleman RE, Goodman PC (1997) Evaluation of adrenal masses in patients with bronchogenic carcinoma using 18F-fluorodeoxyglucose positron emission tomo-graphy (see comments). AJR Am J Roentgenol 168:1357–1360

Gauden S, Ramsay J, Tripcony L (1995) The curative treatment by radiotherapy alone of stage I non-small cell carcinoma of the lung. Chest 108:1278–1282

Green N, Kurohara SS, George FW III (1971) Cancer of the lung: an in-depth analysis of prognostic factors. Cancer 28:1229–1233

Gross R, Klein O (1978) Neuere Entwicklungen auf dem Gebiet der zytostatischen Kombinationschemotherapie. Dtsch Arztebl 75:2121–2128

Guhlmann A, Storck M, Kotzerke J, Moog F, Sunder Plassmann L, Reske SN (1997) Lymph node staging in non-small cell lung cancer: evaluation by (18F) FDG positron emission tomography (PET). Thorax 52:438–441

Guttmann RJ (1971) Radical supervoltage radiotherapy in inoperable carcinoma of the lung. In: Deeley T (ed) Modern radiotherapy, carcinoma of the lung. Appleton-Century Crofts, New York

Haffty BG, Goldberg NB, Gerstley J, Fischer DB, Peschel RE (1988) Results of radical radiation therapy in clinical stage I, technically operable non-small cell lung cancer. Int J Radiat Oncol Biol Phys 15:69–73

Heilmann H-P, Doppelfeld E, Fernholz HJ, Birkner R, Schlicker H, Becker G, Gordon-Harris L, Hackl A, Sager WD, Jentsch F, Kraft W, Bünemann H, Horstmann W, Hassenstein E, Kuttig H, Wieland C, Schmidt N, Müller A, Quäck J, Buchelt L, Hess F, Koop EA, Lieven van H, Heinze HG, Castrup W, Wannenmacher M, Rey G, Voss AC, Nuse A, Eibach E, Grund W, Bohndorf W, Schindler G (1976) Ergebnisse der Strahlenbehandlung des Bronchial-karzinoms. Dtsch Med Wschemschr 101:1557–1562

Holsti LR, Mantyla M, Schumacher W (1976) Split-course versus continuous radiotherapy. Analysis of a randomized trial from 1964 to 1967. The use of high-energy electrons in the treatment of inoperable lung and bronchogenic carcinoma. Acta Oncol In 27:153–161

Holthusen H (1936) Erfahrungen über die Verträglichkeitsgrenze für Röntgenstrahlen und deren Nutzanwendung zur Verhütung von Schäden. Strahlentherapie 57:254–268

Hyde L, Yee J, Wilson R, Patno ME (1965) Cell type and the natural history of lung cancer. JAMA 193:140–142

Hyde L, Wolf J, McCracken St, Yesner R (1973) Natural course of inoperable lung cancer. Chest 64:309–312

Israel L (1976) A discussion of current strategies for limited unresectable squamous cell carcinoma and adenocarcinoma of the lung. In: Israel L, Chahinian AP (eds) Lung cancer, natural history, prognosis and therapy. Academic, New York, pp 295–299

Jeremic B, Shibamoto Y, Acimovic L, Milisavljevic S (1997) Hyperfractionated radiotherapy alone for clinical stage I nonsmall cell lung cancer. Int J Radiat Oncol Biol Phys 38:521–525

Komaki R, Scott C, Ettinger D, Lee JS, Fossella FV, Curran W, Evans RF, Rubin P, Byhardt RW (1997a) Randomized study of chemotherapy/radiation therapy combinations for favorable patients with locally advanced inoperable nonsmall cell lung cancer: Radiation Therapy Oncology Group (RTOG) 92-04. Int J Radiat Oncol Biol Phys 38: 149–155

Komaki R, Scott CB, Sause WT, Johnson DH, Taylor SG, Lee JS, Emami B, Byhardt RW, Curran WJ Jr, Dar AR, Cox JD (1997b) Induction cisplatin/vinblastine and irradiation vs. irradiation in unresectable squamous cell lung cancer: failure patterns by cell type in RTOG 88-08/ECOG 4588. Radiation Therapy Oncology Group. Eastern Cooperative Oncology Group (see comments). Int J Radiat Oncol Biol Phys 39:537–544

Koukourakis M, Skarlatos J, Kosma L, Giatromanolaki A, Yannakakis D (1995) Radiotherapy alone for non-small cell lung carcinoma. Five-year disease-free survival and patterns of failure. Acta Oncol 34:525–530

Krol AD, Aussems P, Noordijk EM, Hermans J, Leer JW (1996) Local irradiation alone for peripheral stage I lung cancer: could we omit the elective regional nodal irradiation? Int J Radiat Oncol Biol Phys 34:297–302

Kupelian PA, Komaki R, Allen P (1996) Prognostic factors in the treatment of node-negative nonsmall cell lung carcinoma with radiotherapy alone. Int J Radiat Oncol Biol Phys 36:607–613

Lanzotti VR, Thomas DR, Byle LE, Smith TL, Gehan EA, Samuels ML (1977) Survival with inoperable lung cancer. Integration of prognostic variables based on simple clinical criteria. Cancer 39:303–313

Leddy ET, Moersch HJ (1940) Roentgen therapy for bronchogenic carcinoma. JAMA 115:2239–2242

Luomanen RKJ, Watson WL (1968) Autopsy findings. In: Watson WL (ed) Lung cancer. A study of five thousand Memorial Hospital cases. Mosby, S Louis

Martel MK, Strawderman M, Hazuka MB, Turrisi AT, Fraass BA, Lichter AS (1997) Volume and dose parameters for survival of non-small cell lung cancer patients. Confirmation of a prognostic index for patients with inoperable non-small cell lung cancer. A practical prognostic index for inoperable non-small cell lung cancer. Radiother Oncol 44:23–29

Nestle U, Nieder C, Abel U, Niewald M, Ukena D, Berberich W, Schnabel K (1996) A palliative accelerated irradiation regimen (PAIR) for advanced non-small-cell lung cancer (NSCLC). Radiother Oncol 38:195–203

Okawa T, Kita M, Goto M, Nishijima H, Miyaji N (1988) Randomized prospective clinical study of small, large and twice-a-day fraction radiotherapy for painful bone metastases. Radiother Oncol 13:99–104

Ormerod FC (1937) The pathology and treatment of carcinoma of the lung. J Laryngol Otol 52:733–745

Papavasiliou C, Kouvaris J, Vasilopoulos P, Ioannou R, Riris C (1987) Effective palliation of advanced non-small cell lung cancer by short duration irradiation. Radiother Oncol 9:269–272

Pereslegin IA, Kunitsyn AG, Aleinikov GE (1977) Kombinierte Behandlung des Bronchialkarzinoms unter Einbeziehung der präoperative Bestrahlung. Med Radiol (Mosk) 22:3–8

Perez CA, Pajak TF, Rubin P, Simpson JR, Mohiuddin M, Brady LW, Perez Tamayo R, Rotman M (1987) Long term observations of the patterns of failure in patients with unresectable non-oat cell carcinoma of the lung treated with definitive radiotherapy. Report by the Radiation Oncology Group. Cancer 59:1874–1881

Pierquin B, Gravis P, Gelle X (1965) Étude de 688 cas de cancers bronchiques traités par téléradioth érapie (200 kV and 22 MV). J Radiol Electrol 46:201–216

Rissanen PM, Tikka U, Holsti LR (1968) Autopsy findings in lung cancer treated with megavoltage radiotherapy. Acta Radiol Ther 7:433–442

Robertson JM, Ten Haken RK, Hazuka MB, Turrisi AT, Martel MK, Pu AT, Littles JF, Martinez FJ, Francis IR, Quint LE, Lichter AS (1997) Dose escalation for non-small cell lung cancer using conformal radiation therapy. Int J Radiat Oncol Biol Phys 37:1079–1085

Roswit B, Patno ME, Rapp R, Veinbergs A, Feder B, Stuhlbarg J, Reid CB (1968) The survival of patients with inoperable lung cancer: a large-scale randomized study of radiation therapy versus placebo. Radiology 90:688–697

Rubin Ph (1974) Lung cancer: histopathologic analysis as related to treatment policy in radiation response. In: Vaeth J (ed) Relationship of histology to cancer treatment. Karger, Basel (Frontiers of radiation therapy and oncology, vol 9)

Salazar OM (1979) Tumor control and radiation toxicity in the treatment of lung cancer: an analysis of time-dose-volume factors. In: Muggia F, Rozencweig M (eds) Lung cancer: progress in therapeutic research. Raven, New York, pp 267–278 (Progress in cancer research and therapy, vol 11)

Salazar OM, Rubin Ph, Brown JC, Feldstein ML, Keller BE (1976) Predictors of radiation response in lung cancer. Cancer 37:2636–2650

Saunders M, Dische St, Barrett A, Harvey A, Gibson D, Parmar M, CHART Steering Committee (1997) Continuous hyperfractionated accelerated radiotherapy (CHART) versus conventional radiotherapy in non-small-cell lung cancer: a randomised multicentre trial. Lancet 350:161–165

Schiepers C (1997) Role of positron emission tomography in the staging of lung cancer. Lung Cancer 17:S29–S35

Schnepper E, Vielberg H (1967) Ergebnisse der Kobalt 60-Teletherapie des Bronchialkarzinoms. Strahlentherapie 133:176–183

Schumacher W (1976) The use of high-energy electrons in the treatment of inoperable lung and bronchogenic carcinoma. In: Kramer S et al (eds) High energy photons and electrons; clinical applications in cancer management. Wiley, New York, pp 255–284

Shehata WM (1977) Role of radiation therapy in bronchogenic carcinoma. Ohio State Med J 73:605–611

Sherman DM, Weichselbaum R, Hellman S (1981) The characteristics of long-term survivors of lung cancer treated with radiation. Cancer 47:2575–2580

Smart J (1966) Can lung cancer be cured by irradiation alone? J Am Med Assoc 159:1034–1035

Stanley K (1980) Prognostic factors for survival in patients with inoperable lung cancer. J Natl Cancer Inst 65:25–32

Steinert HC, Hauser M, Allemann F, Engel H, Berthold T, von Schulthess GK, Weder W (1997) Non-small cell lung cancer: nodal staging with FDG PET versus CT with correlative lymph node mapping and sampling. Radiology 202: 441–446

Teo P, Tai TH, Choy D, Tsui K (1988) A randomized study on palliative radiation therapy for inoperable non small cell carcinoma of the lung. Int J Radiat Oncol Biol Phys 14: 867–871

Wigren T (1997) Confirmation of a prognostic index for patients with inoperable non-small cell lung cancer. Radiother Oncol 44:9–15

Willers H, Würschmidt F, Bünemann H, Heilmann H-P (1998) High-dose radiation therapy alone for inoperable non-small cell lung cancer. Experience with prolonged overall treatment times. Acta Oncologica 37:101–105

Wurschmidt F, Buenemann H, Buenemann C, Beck-Bornholdt HP, Heilmann HP (1994) Inoperable non-small cell lung cancer: a retrospective analysis of 427 patients treated with high-dose radiotherapy. Int J Radiat Oncol Biol Phys 28:583–588

Zhang HX, Yin WB, Zhang LJ, Yang ZY, Zhang ZX, Wang M, Chen DF, Gu XZ (1989) Curative radiotherapy of early operable non-small cell lung cancer. Radiother Oncol 14:89–94

9 Three-Dimensional Conformal Radiotherapy in Treatment of Bronchogenic Carcinoma

B. Emami

CONTENTS

9.1 Introduction

Surgery is considered the initial treatment of choice for any patient with operable/resectable lung cancer. Unfortunately, only a small percentage of patients are candidates for surgery and suitable for complete resection. Approximately 40% of patients present locoregional disease, for which radiotherapy has long been considered one of the primary treatment modalities. Recent randomized studies by Dillman et al. (1996), Arriagada et al. (1991) and Komaki et al. (1997) suggest a small but definite benefit in favor of combined chemotherapy and radiotherapy over radiotherapy alone. Based on these data, combined chemoradiation is currently considered the treatment of choice for this group of patients. As pointed out by Van Houtte (1997), there are two major problems with this consideration. First, these results are largely based on a select subset of patients with favorable prognostic factors (weight loss less than 5%, performance status above 70) and after careful staging procedures. Patients included in randomized trials represent a very small proportion of all lung cancer patients treated (1%). Extending this approach to all patients may produce considerable unnecessary toxicity and morbidity, jeopardizing the small possible benefits from combining drugs and radiation, especially in less healthy or less meticulously staged patients (Van Houtte 1997). The second and probably more important problem with these studies is that even with combined modality treatment the local control rate remains unacceptably low. In a report by Arriagada et al. (1991), combined chemotherapy (platinum based) and radiation therapy (65 Gy) produced only a 10% local control rate at 2 years. If we accept the fact that local tumor control at the primary site is a prerequisite for any chance of a significant improvement in survival and cure, a rethinking of our traditional approach to this disease is definitely required.

Recent technological advances in the areas of computers, faster CT scans, and graphics during the last decade have given birth to three-dimensional conformal radiotherapy (3D CRT) (Purdy and Emami 1992, 1995; Emami et al. 1998). The enhanced capabilities 3D CRT in superior and more accurate delineation of target volumes and normal structures, along with advanced dose calculation algorithms, have allowed clinicians to increase the dose to the tumor and decrease the dose to the uninvolved normal structures. This process has created a new opportunity to search for an improved therapeutic outcome in radiotherapy of lung cancer. The specific goal of 3D CRT is to provide a mechanism for increasing the tumor dose as a means of a possible increase in tumor control.

9.2 Dose Response Relationship in Carcinoma of the Lung

One of the many principles which govern the practice of radiation oncology is the existence of a dose response relationship. The clinical dose response relationship in lung cancer is usually influenced by biological and physical factors. Analysis of theoretical dose response curves based on biological prin-

B. Emami, Department of Radiation Oncology, Loyola University Medical Center, 2160 S. First Avenue, Maywood, IL 60153, USA

ciples (EMAMI 1996) is suggestive of inadequacy of the doses currently used in clinical practice. From this hypothetical analysis it is not unreasonable to assume that to achieve a tumor control of 50%–80% for lung cancer would require doses of 100 Gy or more. Due to the fact that many factors influence local control with radiation therapy, the slope of the curve and the dose for control of a given tumor may vary significantly.

Although past studies, including the Radiation Therapy Oncology Group (RTOG) trials in the 1970s (PEREZ et al. 1987, 1993), have hinted at the existence of a clinical dose response relationship in lung cancer, there has been no convincing evidence to substantiate and unequivocally establish the relationship between dose and local control in non-small cell lung cancer. The reported local control rates of 50%–60% in early RTOG trials are not valid due to the inadequacy of assessment of tools for tumor control (EMAMI 1996). Hyperfractionated studies of RTOG during the 1980s also failed to show any substantial dose response relationships (VAN HOUTTE 1997). Recent studies using chemoradiotherapy with doses of 65 Gy and standard fractionation documented that the true tumor control level was only 10% at 2 years (ARRIAGADA et al. 1991). These results are not surprising. From the original teachings of FLETCHER (1973), it is generally accepted that for epithelial tumors the dose for eradication of microscopic disease is 50–60 Gy and for gross disease 1–3 cm in dimension it is approximately 75 Gy. On the other hand, a significant majority of patients seen with inoperable lung cancer in radiotherapy clinics have an average tumor size of 4–6 cm. Even with knowledge of the above information, it is a fact that in most centers patients with lung cancer, irrespective of their tumor size, are treated with doses of 50–60 Gy. There have been two proposed reasons for the utilization of these low doses: (1) tolerance of normal tissue and inability of the current two-dimensional technology to exceed these doses without unacceptable complications and (2) all of these patients will die of distant metastasis and therefore local control is not important. The latter argument is unsubstantiated because none of the publications on the radiotherapy of inoperable/unresectable lung cancer to date have shown an acceptable rate of local tumor control from locoregional treatment. Therefore, one does not know whether or not these patients would die of distant metastasis if there was a high rate of locoregional control to begin with. Considering the first argument, it becomes clear that one of the reasons for treating patients to the "tolerance of normal tissues" is for the irradiation of large volumes which encompass large volumes of uninvolved normal tissues (see below).

The basic physical elements of radiotherapy of lung cancer which relate to local control include volume and the technical accuracy with which the dose is delivered to the target volume. More precisely they involve the precision of target volume definition and of dose delivery, the dose given to the intended volume, and the degree to which uninvolved normal tissues are excluded from the treatment volume (DUTRIEX 1984).

9.3 Issue of Volume

Based on a high incidence of hilar and mediastinal nodal metastasis, traditional practice has been to irradiate large fields, not only encompassing the primary tumor but also the regional lymph nodes of hilum, mediastinum and supraclavical nodes, whether they are grossly involved or have the potential to be involved (so-called subclinical disease). Although this practice appears to be sound, the therapeutic benefit of treating subclinical nodal involvement (potential disease) has never been demonstrated in radiotherapy of lung cancer. Irradiation of large volumes which encompass significant volumes of uninvolved normal tissues such as lung, heart, and spinal cord is the source of potential complications. Fear of these complications has largely been responsible for the nondelivery of the required tumoricidal dose to the primary tumors of lung cancer and thus resulting in an unacceptably poor local control rate and survival.

The complex anatomy of the thorax with the proximity of the critical normal structures (e.g., spinal cord, heart, lungs) together with the practice of treating large volumes of subclinical disease with its resultant potential for unacceptable complications has set a limit on the prescription dose to between 60 and 70 Gy (DILLMAN et al. 1996; ARRIAGADA et al. 1991; KOMAKI et al. 1997).

Thus, the scenario for the current practice of radiotherapeutic treatment of lung cancer can be stated: We are unnecessarily irradiating large volumes which include significant volumes of normal tissues such as lung, esophagus, heart, and spinal cord, and the fact that we cannot exceed the tolerance of doses of these structures with current technology means we are not able to deliver the required tumoricidal dose to large size primary tumors. There is a need to rethink the rationale for the treatment of such large volumes.

Recent studies have shown that with 3D CRT it is possible to design a special dose distribution to conform to the desired target volume while reducing the dose to normal tissues (FUKS et al. 1991). This approach, therefore, has the potential to decrease the possibility of normal tissue toxicity and permit dose escalation to the tumor with the hope of improving local control rate (PURDY and EMAMI 1995; EMAMI et al. 1988; FUKS et al. 1991). Moreover, since the advent and utilization of 3D CRT in radiotherapeutic management of lung cancers, several investigators have questioned the value of inclusion of large volumes in radiotherapy of lung cancer and there are several recent prospective ongoing studies in which investigators have omitted "subclinical nodal metastatic regions" from their treatment volumes (GRAHAM et al. 1994, 1995; ARMSTRONG et al. 1993, 1998; LEIBEL et al. 1996).

9.4 Local Control Versus Survival

Current results on survival in patients with lung cancer treated with radiation therapy are disappointing (VAN HOUTTE 1997). Although past clinical experience suggests a relationship between dose/local control and survival, there has been no study to substantiate and unequivocally establish the relationship between local control and survival in non-small cell lung cancer. The report of RTOG protocol 7301 on 376 patients with carcinoma of the lung indicated a better 3-year survival with 60 Gy than with lower doses of radiation (PEREZ et al. 1987). In another analysis from the results of the same protocol, it was also suggested that there is a relationship between local control and survival (PEREZ et al. 1993). The problem with these analyses is that the assessment of local control has been based on radiographic evaluations (chest X-rays), which have proven to be unrealistic and the eventual 5-year survival is still under 10% (5%–9%) (PEREZ et al. 1987). RTOG studies of hyperfractionated regiments in the 1980s did not substantiate the above relationship either (COX et al. 1990). Among 519 patients, prognostic factors were favorable in 248 (performance status of 70–100 and weight loss <5%) and unfavorable in 271. There was no significant difference in survival in patients with unfavorable prognostic factors between the five arms. Although there was a suggestion of a benefit in survival up to a dose of 69.6 Gy in patients with favorable prognostic factors, higher doses failed to show any improvement. There was increased pulmonary toxicity, and it is thought that this may have negatively interacted and produced inferior survival. It is important to note that these patients were treated with conventional 2D (large volume followed by small volume) radiotherapy technology. Several explanations have been put forward to try to justify the absence of a benefit in utilizing hyperfractionation regiments. Discussion of this issue is beyond the scope of the current review.

9.5 Experience with Three-Dimensional Conformal Radiotherapy

The move from the 1D to the 2D technique in the 1970s (EMAMI et al. 1978) was a major improvement. Nevertheless, even after 2 decades of using 2D technology, there are also serious limitations to this technique, which are listed below:

1. Lack of realistic appreciation target volumes
2. Lack of appreciation of real volume of normal tissue/organs irradiated to various doses
3. Deficiencies in the algorithms of the computing dose
4. Failure to compute dose throughout the volume of interest
5. Unavailability of tools to compare and judge rival plans
6. Inadequate definition of geometric coverage of anatomic structures by external beams
7. Failure to provide tools for specifying and verifying the accuracy of treatment delivery

As can be seen, with the current practice of radiotherapy (simulation film and possibly one slice of CT scan), it is impossible to accurately delineate the target volumes which are needed to be spared. Moreover, there is little information on the true volumes of normal tissue at risk which are radiated to various doses of radiation therapy and how these two relate to clinical complications. Another current deficiency of 2D radiotherapy is the limitation of beam arrangements to co-planar beams. Finally, judgement of the merits of rival plans of treatment is difficult, and is secondary to the lack of information supplied by 2D plans. For these reasons, three-dimensional radiotherapy becomes a unique tool for increasing tumor dose and decreasing normal tissue complications (PURDY and EMAMI 1992, 1995; EMAMI et al. 1998; FUKS et al. 1991; GRAHAM et al.

1994, 1995; ARMSTRONG et al. 1993, 1998; LEIBEL et al. 1996).

In order to review the current status of 3D CRT in lung cancer, one has to take into consideration the various stages and procedures involved in 3D CRT (Table 9.1). It is important to note the various stages of this process utilize different tools and systems.

In order to evaluate the level of utilization of various tools in 3D CRT systems and degree of "scientific sophistication," I have done an informal survey of several institutions with claimed 3D capabilities. Institutions within the 3D conformal group of NCI protocols (United States) were not included. It was assumed that they use full 3D CRT capabilities. The list below shows the various degrees of "3D conformality" by those institutions.

Patient immobilization is usually done using an alpha cradle or thermoplast. There were a few institutions who claimed to have 3D CRT but did not immobilize their patients.

CT scanning is done either by specialized CT scans within radiotherapy departments or is carried out in diagnostic CT scans with some connections to treatment planning systems of the radiotherapy department. Scans are normally used for contouring of desired targets and normal tissue structures.

Table 9.1. Three-dimensional radiation therapy planning and conformal radiotherapy

I. Delineation of target volumes
- Evaluation of patient, tumor (staging) and normal tissue/organs
- Patient immobilization
- CT scanning
- Contouring of target volumes and normal organs
- Volumetric CT data-transfer to RTP system
- 3D dose calculations and display (DVH, dose surface, dose statistics)
- Plan evaluation-optimization of 3D beam arrangement

II. Pre-delivery preparation
- Digitally reconstructed radiograph (DRR)
- Block template
- Verification of portals
- Marking of patient
- Radiographic verification
- Blockmaking (Cerrobend) → block check
- Multileaf collimation

III. Treatment delivery

IV. Treatment verification and documentation
- Portal films
- On line imaging
- Verification systems

RTP, radiation treatment planning; CT, computed tomography.

Contouring of target volumes and normal organs is done using one of the commercially available contouring devices. For example, at Loyola University we have utilized AQSIM from Picker International, Ohio, United States. Again, I have found a variable degree of utilization of this tool. Some institutions contour only one target volume. Some institutions contour target volumes and a few but not all of the normal tissues as detailed in RTOG protocols. In contouring target volumes a few follow the ICRU-50 recommendations and most do not.

Virtual simulation and design of portals and initial beam arrangements are either done using the same contouring device (i.e., AQSIM) or after transferring data to 3D CRT systems. The survey showed varying degrees of "3D conformality" in the planning within institutions. In designing portals I have found some variability. Several community institutions outline a gross target volume only using available contouring systems. Subsequently a digitally reconstructed radiograph (DRR) is produced and portals are designed in a 2D beam arrangement format, namely AP-PA with margins as has been practiced in 2D radiotherapy. They basically use DRR with GTV on it instead of simulation film. Several institutions use the terminology of "bean-eye-view radiotherapy" and this is the extent of their involvement in 3D without full utilization 3D CRT tools. In my informal survey I have found this to be more prevalent within community radiotherapy departments. Few institutions follow the above format but selected normal tissue volumes are also depicted on DRRs. ICRU recommendations for drawing clinical target volume (CTV) and planning target volume (PTV) are not followed in most of these institutions. Even when the ICRU recommendations are followed, there are significant variations in choice of margins both for CTV and PTV.

Three-dimensional dose calculations, plan evaluations/optimization of the 3D beam arrangements using displayed tools such dose value histograms, dose cloud, and dose statistics are performed either through institutionally created or commercially available systems. For example, at Loyola University we have utilized a commercial device manufactured by CMS Corporation, St. Louis, Missouri, United States. Utilization of the full 3D CRT system is done only in selected large institutions and universities.

The volume of radiation "irradiated volume" also shows significant variations from institution to institution. The most commonly practiced routine is the inclusion of a primary tumor with an appropriate margin and potential nodal areas of mediastinum, both hilar and supraclavicular with a 1-cm margin. Although the gross tumor is usually contoured, the large volumes are usually not contoured. This volume is usually designed on DRR (simulation film) per 2D routine, and is taken to a basic dose of around 4000–4500. Subsequently, the contoured gross target volume with margins can be treated using beams-eye-view generated portals up to a desired dose of 60/65 Gy. Other institutions have omitted the contralateral hilum and contralateral supraclavicular whereas they include the ipsilateral supraclavicular, hilum and entire mediastinum. At the other end of the spectrum, there are institutions that basically follow the recommendations of the RTOG 93-11 protocol, in which the volume of radiation would include primary tumor with adequate margin, ipsilateral hilum, and the nodal regions of mediastinum whether grossly (radiographically) or biopsy proven.

The tumor dose of radiation is usually varied between 60 and 70 Gy. Most institutions utilize a 66-Gy tumor dose.

From the above informal survey it appears that there is no uniform approach for dose, technique, or conformality in using 3D CRT. Therefore, the results can hardly be meaningful except for the fact that they represent an effort at implementation of some form of 3D CRT in the treatment of bronchogenic carcinoma.

There are, however, some structured efforts in the utilization of 3D CRT in the treatment of lung cancer.

Graham et al. (1994) compared their traditional beam arrangements with 3D conformal treatment plans in ten patients with advanced bronchogenic carcinoma using full 3D technology. Evaluations were done by dose volume histograms (DVH), dose statistics, and dose surfaces. Analysis confirmed that the 3D technology produced better delineation of target volumes, better coverage of target volumes by the prescribed dose and significantly improved protection of the critical structures from high doses of radiation therapy. It was found that commonly used beam arrangements for the treatment of non-small cell lung cancer were often inadequate to safely deliver tumor doses of greater than 70 Gy. Three-dimensional conformal treatment plans with multiple beam arrangements allowed dose to gross tumor to be escalated to at least 80 Gy while maintaining acceptable or improved doses to the normal surrounding tissues. The main dose limiting structure for tumors of the lung is the surrounding lung tissue. Preliminary results were reported by Armstrong et al. (1998) on 18 patients with non-small cell lung cancer treated with 3D technology, one grade III and one grade IV pulmonary toxicity. The lung volumes most correlated with these higher grade pulmonary toxicities were 49% of the lung volume receiving >25 Gy. Martel et al. (1994) have also reported on mean lung doses on 40 lung cancer patients who were divided into groups that did or did not have pulmonary complications. She reported that the mean dose to the individual lungs and the total lung volume was on the average higher in those who developed pneumonitis (average 35 Gy and 18 Gy, respectively) compared to those who did not develop complications (29 Gy and 18 Gy, respectively).

Martel et al (1994) also evaluated normal tissue complication probability (NTCP) model and dose volume histogram (DVH) analysis in the design and implementation of dose escalation protocols for lung cancers, and reported the ability to correlate the incidence of pneumonitis with normal tissue complication probability (NTCP) calculations. This correlation was able to separate out patients at low and high risk of complications, but the exact NTCP score was not an exact percentage of the incidence of pneumonitis. Ten Haken et al. (1993) have developed and implemented a dose escalation protocol stratifying patients based on their effective volume (*^{V}effective*) as a parameter to assess the risk of the development of pneumonitis after treatment. While this protocol has escalated doses to patients up to at least 90 Gy (*and it is expected to go even higher*), the development of pneumonitis has been low and acceptable.

Martel et al. (1997) analyzed the 3D plans of a consecutive series of 76 patients with inoperable locally advanced unresectable non-small cell lung cancer. Their objective was to study the effect of tumor volume and dose factors derived from 3D treatment planning of dose distribution on survival outcome. Their results indicate that, in addition to nodal staging stage, the actual tumor volume determined by 3D treatment planning also had a significant bearing on survival. Patients with tumor volumes of <200 cm^3 and negative nodes had the best survival. From their analysis it appears that dose influences local control and survival when tumor volumes are taken into account. The authors suggest that dose prescription for lung cancer treatment might be better written based on tumor volume size.

Oetzel et al. (1995) also reported a retrospective analysis of 86 patients with lung and esophageal cancer and correlated this mean ipsilateral lung dose with NTCP calculations. They concurred with Martel et al. that there was a good correlation with the incidence of pneumonitis and a high NTCP calculation. Like Martel, their data showed the best fit when ipsilateral single lung calculations were used.

Graham et al. (1997) evaluated 70 patients who had been treated with 3D treatment planning. Patients were stratified for the development of pneumonitis by the volume of the gross tumor (*GTV in cc*), the mean ipsilateral lung dose (*in GY*), the percentage of the ipsilateral lung receiving greater than 20 Gy, the percentage of the total lung volume receiving greater than 20 Gy and the effect volume (*[v]effective*). Analysis of data for the development of ≥grade II and ≥grade III pneumonitis in the 70 patients revealed that stratifying patients by GTV or mean dose to the ipsilateral lung failed to adequately stratify the patients for the development of pneumonitis. The percentage volume of either the ipsilateral or total lung volumes and/or the effective volume appear to equally stratify the patients according to risk. The skill and technology of various institutions in being able to calculate a *[v]eff* was thought to be variable in the institutions that are expected to use this method for stratification. It was thought that the easier parameter to stratify for pneumonitis risk would be the percentage of total lung receiving a threshold dose of 20 Gy.

The Radiation Therapy Oncology Group is prospectively conducting a multi-institutional dose escalation trial in which patients are assigned one of the three treatment arms based on the dose to total lung volume as shown in Table 9.2. Within each group there is a gradual dose escalation schema. This schema is chosen to avoid an excessive rate of pneumonitis. This protocol is different in several ways from other collaborative studies in lung cancer:

Table 9.2. Proposed RTOG Dose Escalation Trial for non-small cell lung cancer (modified from EmAmi 1996)

Group 1[a] <25%	Dose level 1: 70.9 Gy/33 fx/7–8 wks
	Dose level 2: 77.4 Gy/36 fx/7–8 wks
	Dose level 3: 83.8 Gy/39 fx/8–9 wks
	Dose level 4: 90.3 Gy/42 fx/9–10 wks
Group 2[a] 25%–<37%	Dose level 5: 70.9 Gy/33 fx/7–8 wks
	Dose level 6: 77.4 Gy/36 fx/7–8 wks
	Dose level 7: 83.8 Gy/39 fx/8–9 wks
Group 3[a] > = 37%	Dose level 8: 64.5 Gy/30 fx/6–7 wks
	Dose level 9: 70.9 Gy/33 fx/7–8 wks
	Dose level 10: 77.4 Gy/36 fx/7–8 wks

[a] Initial stratification is based on percentage of the total lung volume receiving >20 Gy. Dose escalation is done within individual groups: group 1, low risk for pneumonitis; group 2, intermediate risk for pneumonitis; group 3, high risk for pneumonitis.

(1) immobilization is required, (2) the complete plan of the treatment has to be optimized and finalized before patient registration. It is the dose to 20% of the total lung volume that determines which treatment arm patient will be assigned. (3) Dose escalations are based on dose to normal tissue rather than dose to tumor. And, finally (4), institutions who wish to participate have to show their capability of performing 3D CRT by completing the prerequisite test as determined by the 3D QA Center in St. Louis, Missouri, USA.

9.6 Clinical Experience

The potential advantages of 3D treatment planning for target volume coverage and normal tissue sparing over conventional techniques when applied to patients with lung cancer were initially identified by Emami et al. (1991). In their study DVHs and a variety of dose statistics (i.e., minimum dose, maximum dose, mean dose, percentage of a specified volume receiving the prescribed dose) were identified as useful tools in evaluation and optimization of 3D plans. Three-dimensional target volumes and dose display were also important. Superiority of BEV-based radiation therapy in accurate delineation of treatment volumes and avoidance of geographic misses have been shown by Vijayakumar et al. (1991).

Improved planning and dosimetric ability of 3D CRT to increase doses to lung cancer targets have been shown by several authors (Graham et al. 1994; Armstrong et al. 1993; Ten Haken et al. 1993).

Hazuka et al. (1993) reported on 88 patients with non-small cell lung cancer on whom BEV planning was used. From their retrospective analysis, they concluded that it was feasible to deliver uncorrected tumor doses up to 74 Gy with standard fractionation using BEV display (Table 9.3).

Armstrong et al. (1993) in a preliminary analysis of 3D CRT in nine patients with unresectable non-small cell lung cancer, suggested that 3D CRT may provide superior delivery of high-dose irradiation with reduced risk to normal tissue. In their analysis the *[v]eff* (effective volume) and the percentage volume of the total lung volume exceeding 20 Gy (as a threshold dose) appeared to be the best parameters by which to stratify patients for risk of developing pneumonitis; both parameters indicated the strong volume dependence of the lungs to irradiation. Further study and a parameterization of the NTCP formula were recommended.

Table 9.3. Survival rates for non-small cell lung carcinoma: overall survival percentage

	No. of pts.	Stage	Dose (Gy)	Median survival (mos.)	2 years (%)
Hazuka et al. 1993	88	HI (19)	>60	26	62
		III-B (69)		14	35
Leibel et al. 1996	33	1-II (7)	64–72	16.5	33
		IIIA–B (28)			
Graham et al. 1995	70	All stages I–II (19)	60–74	20	44
		IIIA–B (54)			90[a]
					55[a]
Armstrong et al. 1997	45	I–II (6)	52–72	15.7	32
		IIIA–IIIB (39)			

[a] Cause-specific survival.

Leibel et al. (1996) reported results with 3D CRT of non-small cell lung cancer and compared them with published data from conventional treatments reported by cooperative groups (Table 9.3).

Armstrong et al. (1997), in an update of the Memorial Hospital Experience, reported on the results of 45 patients with non-small cell lung cancer who were treated with 3D CRT. There were 6 stage I and II and 39 stage IIIA and B. There was a dose range from 52.2 to 72 Gy with a median dose to gross tumor disease of 70.2 Gy. The results show a median survival of 15.7 months and a 2-year survival rate of 32%. A dose histogram analysis of 31 patients revealed a correlation between risk of pulmonary toxicity and indices of dose to lung parenchyma. Of eight who developed grade 3 or higher pulmonary toxicity, three developed in patients with >30% of lung volume receiving over 25 Gy. Only 1/23 patients (4%) with <30% lung receiving over 25 Gy developed pulmonary toxicity ($P = 0.04$). The authors conclude that despite adverse prognostic criteria, median survival is encouraging and may be higher than some combined modality approaches. Dose volume histogram parameters would be useful to determine the maximum dose for individual patients and thereby permit avoidance of toxicity.

Robertson et al. (1997) reported on 48 non-small cell lung cancers treated with 3D CRT. Their doses ranged from 63 to 84 Gy. Their report noted no pneumonitis in the 30 patients currently available beyond 6 months time. The authors conclude that successful dose escalation in a volume-dependent organ can be performed using 3D CRT. Using 3D CRT they have been able to treat some patients to the total dose of radiation over 50% higher than traditional doses. The important conclusion of this study is that there has been no negative effect due to exclusion of elective nodal radiation on the outcome.

Table 9.3 is a summary of reported survivals for NSCLC patients treated with 3D CRT. These results compare favorably with the results of chemoradiotherapy trials, though they have not been tested in a randomized fashion. Also the results thus far reported have used modest doses (60–74 Gy). The results of dose escalation trials are necessary to confirm the anticipated benefit of 3D CRT for lung cancer.

9.7 Future Trends

In addition to the above-mentioned ongoing clinical studies, there are other innovative efforts related to the 3D CRT of lung cancer which will have a significant impact on the future applications of this technology in treating lung cancer.

Marks et al. (1995) have utilized perfusion scans for optimization of treatment planning and beam direction in radiotherapy of lung cancer. The authors conclude that lung perfusion scans provide functional information not provided by CT scans that can be useful in designing radiation treatment beams that minimize incidental radiation of the functional regions of the lung. One important outcome of their research is that three-dimensional functional data be used to generate functional dose volume histograms (DV_fHs) that may be more predictive of physiological consequences of the radiation than conventional DVHs.

Marks et al. (1997) have also used perfusion imaging technology to understand and assist the radiation therapy induced regional lung dysfunction. The authors conclude that radiation therapy induced regional lung dysfunction occurs in a dose-dependent manner and develops within 3–6 months following radiation. In contrast to classical "sigmoid" dose response curves, derived mainly from changes following whole lung radiation, their data suggest a more gradual relationship between regional dysfunction and radiotherapy dose. Their research will have an important impact on future studies of evaluation pulmonary complications in radiotherapy of lung cancer.

Initial experimentation with Intensity Modulated Radiation Therapy (IMRT) and Gated Radiotherapy is underway in a few institutions (Derycke et al. 1997; Balter et al. 1996). Although both of the above ideas appear to be attractive, their potential utility in clinical practice is currently undetermined.

References

Armstrong JG, Burman C, Leibel SA et al (1993) Three-dimensional conformal radiation therapy may improve the therapeutic ratio of high dose radiation therapy for lung cancer. Int J Radiat Oncol Biol Phys 26:685–689

Armstrong J, Raben A, Zelefsky M, Burt M, Leibel S, Burman C, Kutcher G, Harrison L, Hahn C, Ginsberg RJ, Rusch V, Kris M, Fuks Z (1997) Promising survival with three-dimensional conformal radiation therapy for non-small cell lung cancer. Radiother Oncol 44:17–22

Armstrong J, Zelefsky M, Burt M et al (1998) Strategy for close escalation using three dimensional conformal radiation therapy for lung cancer (in press)

Arriagada R, Le Chevalier T, Quoix E et al (1991) Effect of chemotherapy on locally advanced non-small cell lung carcinoma: a randomized study of 353 patients. Int J Radiat Oncol Biol Phys 20:1183–1190

Balter JM, Ten Haken RK, Lawrence TS, Lam KL, Robertson JM (1996) Uncertainties in CT-based radiation therapy treatment planning associated with patient breathing. Int J Radiat Oncol Biol Phys 36(1):167–174

Cox JD, Azarnia N, Byhardt RW, Skin KH, Emami B, Pojak TF (1990) A randomized Phase I/II trial of hyperfractionated radiation therapy with total doses of 60.0 Gy to 79.2 Gy: possible survival benefit with ≥69.6 Gy in favorable patients with RTOG stage III non-small-cell lung carcinoma: report of RTOG 83-11. J Clin Oncol 8:1543–1555

Derycke S, Van Duyse B, De Gersem W, De Wagter C, De Neve W (1997) Non-coplanar beam intensity modulation allows large dose escalation in stage III lung cancer. Radiother Oncol 45:253–261

Dillman RO, Herndon J, Seagren SL, Eaton WL Jr, Green MR (1996) Improved survival in stage III non-small cell lung cancer: seven-year follow-up of cancer and Leukemia Group B (CALGB) 8433 Trial. JNCI 88(17):1210–1215

Dutriex A (1984) When and how can we improve precision in radiotherapy. Radiother Oncol 1:275–292

Emami B (1996) Three dimensional conformal radiation therapy in bronchogenic carcinoma. Semin Radiat Oncol 6(2):92–97

Emami B, Purdy JA, Manolis J, Barest G, Cheng E, Coia L, Doppke K, Galvin J, LoSasso T, Matthews, Munzenrider, Shank B (1991) Three-dimensional treatment planning for lung cancer. Int J Rad Oncol Biol Phys 21:217–227

Emami B, Melo A, Carter B (1978) Value of computed tomography in radiotherapy of lung cancer. Am J Radiol 131:63–67

Emami B, Graham MV, Michalski JM, Perez CA (1998) Three-dimensional conformal radiation therapy: clinical aspects. Principles and practice of radiation oncology, 3rd edn. Perez, Brady

Fletcher G (1973) Clinical dose-response curves of human malignant epithelial tumors. Br J Radiol 46:1–12

Fuks Z, Leibel S, Rutcher G, Mohan R, Ling C (1991) Three dimensional conformal treatment: a new frontier in radiation therapy. In: DeVita VJ, Hellman S, Rosenberg S (eds) Important advances in oncology

Graham MV, Matthews JW, Harms WB, Emami B, Glazer HS, Purdy JA (1994) Three-dimensional radiation treatment planning study for patients with carcinoma of the lung. Int J Radiat Oncol Biol Phys 29:1105–1117

Graham MV, Purdy JA, Emami B, Matthews JW, Harms WB (1995) Preliminary results of a prospective trial using three-dimensional radiotherapy for lung cancer. Int J Radiat Oncol Biol Phys 33:993–1000

Graham M, Purdy J, Harms W, Emami B, Drzymala R, Lockett M (1997) Clinical results of three-dimensional radiation therapy for non-small cell lung cancer: the Washington University experience. Radiother Oncol (submitted for publication)

Hazuka MB, Turrisi AT, Lutz ST et al (1993) Results of high-dose thoracic irradiation incorporating beam's eye view display in non-small cell lung cancer: a retrospective multivariate analysis. Int J Radiat Oncol Biol Phys 27:273–284

Komaki R, Scott CB, Sause WT, Johnson DH, Taylor SG, Lee JS, Emami B, Byhardt RW, Curran WJ, Dar AR, Cox JD (1997) Induction cisplatin/vinblastine and irradiation vs. irradiation in unresectable squamous cell lung cancer: failure patterns by cell type in RTOG 88-08/ECOG 4588. Int J Rad Oncol Biol Phys 39:537–544

Leibel S, Armstrong J, Kutcher G et al (1996) 3D conformal radiation therapy for non-small cell lung carcinoma: clinical experience at the Memorial Sloan-Kettering Cancer Center. Front Radiat Ther Oncol 29:199–206

Marks LB, Spencer DP, Sherouse GW, Benter G, Clough R, Vann K, Jaszczak R, Coleman RE, Prosnitz LR (1995) The role of three dimensional functional lung imaging in radiation treatment planning: the functional dose-volume histogram. Int J Radiat Oncol Biol Phys 33(1):65–75

Marks LB, Munley MT, Spencer DP, Sherouse GW, Bentel GC, Hoppenworth J, Chew M, Jaszczak RJ, Coleman RE, Prosnitz LR (1997) Quantification of radiation-induced regional lung injury with perfusion imaging. Int J Radiat Oncol Biol Phys 38(2):399–409

Martel MK, Ten Haken RK, Hazuka MB, Turrisi AT, Fraass BA, Lichter AS (1994) Dose-volume histogram and 3D treatment planning evaluation of patients with pneumonitis. Int J Radiat Oncol Biol Phys 28:575–581

Martel MK, Strawderman M, Hazuka MB, Turrisi AT, Fraass BA, Lichter AS (1997) Volume and dose parameters for survival of non-small cell lung cancer patients. Radiother Oncol 44:23–29

Oetzel D, Scraube P, Hensley F, Stoka-Perez G, Menke M, Flentje M (1995) Estimation of pneumonitis risk in 3-dimensional treatment planning using dose-volume histogram analysis. Int J Radiat Oncol Biol Phys 33:455–460

Perez C, Pajak T, Rubin P (1987) Long-term observations of the patterns of failure in patients with unresectable non-oat cell carcinoma of the lung treated with definitive radiotherapy: report by the RTOG. Cancer 59:1874–1881

Perez C, Bauer M, Edelstein S (1993) Impact of tumor control on survival in carcinoma of the lung treated with irradiation. Int J Radiat Oncol Biol Phys 12:539–547

Purdy JA, Emami B (1992) Computed tomography and three-dimensional approaches to radiation therapy. In: Levitt S (ed) Technological basis of radiation therapy: practical clinical applications. Lea and Febiger, Philadelphia, pp 56–66

Purdy JA, Emami B (eds) (1995) 3D radiation treatment planning and conformal therapy, proceedings of an international symposium

Robertson JM, Ten Haken RK, Hazuka MB, Turrisi AT, Martel MK, Pu AT, Littles JF, Martinez FJ, Francis IR, Quint LE, Lichter AS (1997) Dose escalation for non-small cell lung cancer using conformal radiation therapy. Int J Radiat Oncol Biol Phys 37(5):1079–1085

Ten Haken R, Martel M, Kessler M et al (1993) Use of V_{eff} and iso-NTCP in the implementation of dose escalation protocols. Int J Radiat Oncol Biol Phys 27:2689–2695

Van Houtte P (1997) Stage III non-small cell lung cancer: still a challenge for the radiation oncologist. Int J Radiat Oncol Biol Phys 39(3):533–536

Vijayakumar S, Myrianthopoulos L, Rosenberg I et al (1991) Optimization of radical radiotherapy with beam's eye view techniques for non-small cell lung cancer. Int J Radiat Oncol Biol Phys 21:779–788

10 Endoluminal Brachytherapy: A Curative Modality?

H. MARSIGLIA, P. BALDEYROU, and E. LARTIGAU

CONTENTS

10.1 Introduction

Lung cancer carries a poor prognosis. If radical surgery remains the treatment of choice, it is feasible only in one out of four patients, the disease being diagnosed in the majority of cases in non-operable patients (general status) or at an advanced stage (stages III, IV). Thus external beam radiotherapy and/or chemotherapy is often the exclusive treatment. The poor clinical outcome is linked to limited thoracic local control (<20% at 2 years) and to distant metastases (>50% 2 years). New therapeutic approaches need to be investigated, exploring systemic, locoregional and also purely local treatments.

High-dose rate brachytherapy (HDR) is one of the local treatments (Speiser and Spratling 1993; Khanavkar et al. 1991; Bedwinek et al. 1992; Chang et al. 1994). It has been introduced recently in Europe and can be administered on an outpatient basis for a variety of tumour sites (oesophagus, cervix, endometrium, head and neck, etc.). New tools have been developed in order to perform intraluminal treatments: high-activity miniaturised sources (iridium-192, 10 Ci), afterloading machines with total radioprotection, software with 3D dose distribution and modern imaging techniques (echoendoscopy, CT scan, MRI) for the definition of target volume. As with all the recently developed treatments, many considerations must be taken into account before implementation into clinical practice.

10.2 The Dose Rate Effect

The dose rate is one of the main factors governing the biological consequences of the dose delivered to tissues (Mazeron and Lartigau 1993). In general, the biological effect for a given dose decreases with a lowering of the dose rate and a longer overall treatment time. Two processes are responsible for this: the repair of sublethal damage and repopulation, which occurs in irradiated tissue. The therapeutic ratio (tumour control/late sequelae) will be very dependent on any modification of the dose rate and/or the dose per fraction. Low-dose rate (LDR) brachytherapy is performed with a temporary implant delivering a continuous dose rate over a few days. With HDR the radioactive source delivers a dose rate above 12 Gy/h (treatment time of a few minutes) (ROACH et al. 1990). Increasing the dose rate and the dose per fraction leads to a more elevated rate of unrepaired lesions in normal tissue with a slower renewal rate than tumour. These different parameters must be taken into account in order to obtain a compromise between the practical implementation of endobronchial brachytherapy and the radiobiological elements specific to HDR irradiation. In addition, the target volume should be calculated with a highly accurate margin so that only the tumour is treated and normal tissues are spared (BALDEYROU et al. 1995, 1996; USUDA et al. 1993).

H. MARSIGLIA, P. BALDEYROU and E. LARTIGAU, Departments of Radiotherapy and Medicine, Institut Gustave Roussy, 39, rue Camille Desmoulins, F-94805 Villejuif, France
Present address: H. MARSIGLIA, Divisione di Radioterapia, Istituto Europeo di Oncologia, Via Ripamonti, 435, I-20141, Milan, Italy

10.3
When Is HDR Brachytherapy Indicated?

HDR brachytherapy can be used in bronchial cancers for palliation in case of tumour obstruction or recurrence after previous treatments (SUTEDJA et al. 1994). In curative treatment, HDR brachytherapy could be used alone for superficial lesion or combined with external radiotherapy for limited non-operable tumours (ROACH et al. 1990; HUBER et al. 1997). Despite the large development of the technique, some questions remain unanswered. The studies which are currently being performed should evaluate treatment dose, time interval, total number of sessions and treated volumes and the improvements in local control and survival together with the incidence of late complications. In addition, a further objective is to compare the results obtained in different centres. To achieve this goal, a common language is needed for all the comparison parameters (evaluation of tumour volume, response in terms of reduction in volume but also physical or functional signs, how to express the dose during BT, complications during and after BT, etc.).

10.4
The Institut Gustave Roussy Experience

In France, brachytherapy (or curietherapy) is a traditional form of anticancer treatment. The progress achieved during the last 3 decades in LDR brachytherapy, with miniaturised sources and computerised dosimetry, has considerably widened the scope of BT. HDR brachytherapy is under rapid development in France and preliminary results show excellent tolerance and a high remission rate (TAULELLE et al. 1996; TRÉDANIEL et al. 1994; PEROL et al. 1997; HENNEQUIN et al. 1997).

The main purpose of our study was to define in which subgroups of patients endobronchial HDR brachytherapy improves local control and survival, and what were the best fractionation schedule and overall treatment time.

10.4.1
Population

Between September 1992 and June 1996, 34 patients were treated (32 males and 2 females), with a median age of 64 years (range 44–82 years). All patients were unfit for surgery or external beam radiotherapy after evaluation by a multidisciplinary team (thoracic surgeons, pneumologist, medical oncologists and radiotherapist) because of gross respiratory insufficiency ($n = 23$) and/or significantly compromised cardiac function ($n = 8$), a past history of previously treated lung cancer ($n = 11$) or a history of a non-pulmonary cancer [head and neck ($n = 7$), bladder ($n = 2$) and breast ($n = 1$)]. In three of these patients the poor prognosis associated with their previously treated cancer rendered them unfit for more aggressive treatment. The histologic diagnosis in 33 patients was squamous cell carcinoma (6 in situ) and one large-cell carcinoma. In 2 cases the tumours were located in the trachea, in 21 patients on the right side of the thorax and on the left in 11 patients. In 22 cases the tumour was found at a bifurcation, in 26 cases in the main or lobular bronchi and in 6 at the segmental or subsegmental level. Initial staging by CT scan confirmed the absence of local extension or lymph node involvement. The bronchoscopic description classified tumour shapes as either flat ($n = 12$), spherical ($n = 1$), villous ($n = 17$) or cylindrical ($n = 4$), when the tumour was partially circumferential. The average tumour volume was 0.25 cm^3 (range 0.006–6.28 cm), calculated as a function of the median length (10 mm, range 2–40 mm), median width (5 mm, range 2–20 mm) and median thickness (3 mm, range 1–20 mm). One patient received prior chemotherapy but tumour regression was not achieved and disease was found to be stable at bronchoscopic assessment. One patient presented with a carcinoma in situ which had been treated 2 years earlier by photodynamic therapy. Tumours were visualised at bronchoscopy in all the patients. In two patients the presenting symptom was haemoptysis. Written informed consent was obtained for all patients.

10.4.2
Treatment Preparation

Patients were treated on an outpatient basis. Local anaesthesia was used after preparation with codeine and hydroxidine. Catheter placement was done by the organ specialist. After defining the limits of the tumour, verifying the correct positioning of the application, its fixation and immobilisation, check films were taken for quality control. The treatment catheter was inserted under the control of an image intensifier to determine the most appropriate placement site. Dummy catheters were carefully positioned to separate the treatment catheter from the

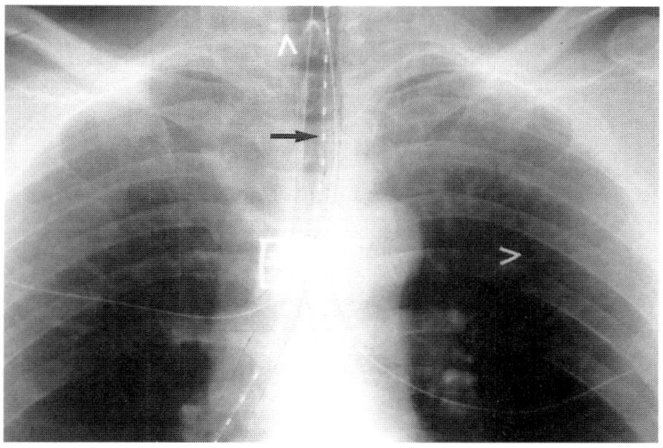

Fig. 10.1. Insertion of dummy catheters (*arrow*) between the posterior wall of the intermediate bronchus and the treatment catheters

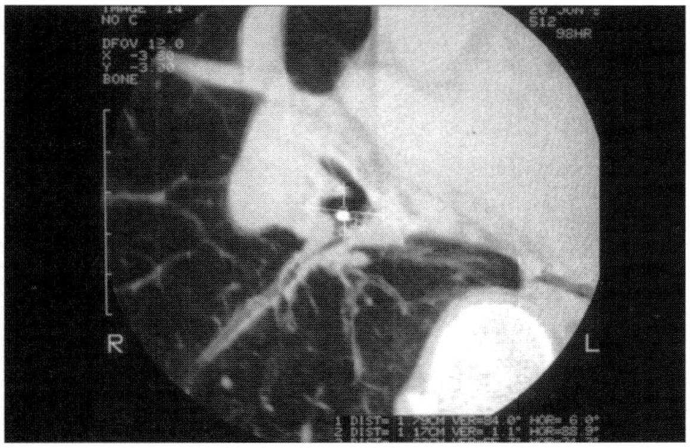

Fig. 10.2. CT scan of a treatment catheter without dummy catheters or applicator

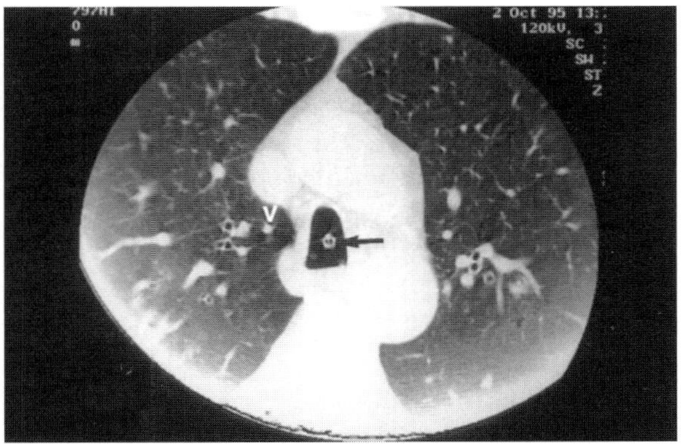

Fig. 10.3. CT scan of a treatment catheter in an applicator (*arrow*)

bronchial wall when necessary, and thus limiting overdosage of the mucosa by direct contact with the source. The number and position of the catheters were decided at the initial bronchoscopy, taking into account the site of the lesion (Fig. 1). These dummy catheters, introduced into the adjacent bronchi around the tumour, helped define the tumour site on the orthogonal films. A more recent innovation has been to use a greased silicone nasogastric tube that can be slid down over the treatment catheter in order to push away the bronchial side walls (Figs. 2, 3). This replaced the need for multiple dummy catheters, with the diameter of the tube (French 14, 16, 18) chosen to create the desired space. A graduated guidewire was placed inside the treatment catheter for the orthogonal films and the determined target volume outlined. Endobronchial irradiation was performed using an iridium-192 source with an activity of 370 Gbq (10 Ci). After dosimetry planning (computerised system with 3D reconstruction), the patient was connected to the machine.

10.4.3
Evaluation of the Tumour Source Relationship

CT scan assessment was required in half of the cases, for superficial tumours, when uncertainty persisted regarding the distance between the source and the bronchial wall, or when the proximity of an important vascular structure could not be clearly determined. CT scan studies were only generally required for the first treatment application, except in two patients in whom the dose distribution was modified after the first CT. The distance between the tumour and the catheter was determined using three methods: (1) the space between the mucosa and the sources was measured by inserting dummy catheters between them. When several dummy catheters were used, they could be visually examined and their position controlled by bronchoscopy; (2) direct CT measurements; and (3) the diameter of the silicon sleeve slid along the treatment catheter.

10.4.4
Prescription

The total dose delivered was 30 Gy in six weekly fractions of 5 Gy. The prescription point for treatment could vary according to the tumour volume, but it never exceeded a distance of 10 mm from the catheter. The delivered dose specified at 10 mm was always measured and reported. As uncertainty persisted regarding the extent of the target volume, some safety margins may have been overestimated.

10.4.5 Follow-up and Results

All patients had a clinical and bronchoscopic examination at each follow-up visit along with chest X-rays, at 2 months post-treatment and then every 6 months. CT scans were not performed routinely. A biopsy specimen was obtained from the original tumour site and analysed histologically at each control visit. Survival rates were estimated using Kaplan-Meier methods, and the 95% confidence intervals by the method described by Rothman (1978). Of the 34 patients, 27 completed the 6 planned applications, 1 patient stopped treatment after 3 fractions and 6 had between 5 and 8 fractions in order to optimise the computerised treatment planning. The median time between applications was 7 days with a minimum of 2 and a maximum of 21 days. In 27 patients, only 1 treatment catheter was used, 2 catheters were needed in 6 patients, and 3 in 1 case, to ensure adequate tumour coverage, especially when the tumour was at a bronchial bifurcation. In 68% of cases (n = 23) one or multiple dummy catheters or a silicon nasogastric tube was used to separate the treatment catheter from the bronchial wall. One catheter was used in 12 cases, 2 in 10 cases, and 3 on 1 occasion. The silicon tube was used in the five most recent cases. The prescription point was 5 mm in 3 patients, 6 mm in 2, 7 mm in 8, 8 mm in 3, 9 mm in 1 and 10 mm in 17 patients. This point was modified in nine patients during treatment. The median prescription point was 9.6 mm (range 5–10) and the average 8.4 mm. The specified dose at 10 mm was calculated to be 4 Gy on the inside of the curve and 3.8 Gy on the outside of the curve. The median volume that received the prescribed dose was 12.3 cm^3 (2–20 cm^3). The median volume which received the highest dose, i.e., twice the prescribed dose, was 3.9 cm^3. The median volume which received the specified dose was 14.1 cm^3 (7–26 cm^3) and the volume which received twice the specified dose was 4.5 cm^3 (2–8 cm^3).

Treatment was well tolerated. One patient stopped his treatment after three fractions and is still in complete remission. A complete response, evaluated at bronchoscopy and at histology, was achieved in 32 of 34 patients at the first follow-up visit 2 months post-treatment. At that time, two patients had local progression. One of these early failures was attributable to an underestimation of the initial tumour volume. In the second case, the safety margins had been tight because of an anticipated risk of bronchial and vascular haemorrhage which was overestimated.

The local relapse rate was 15% at 1 year (CI 6–33%), and 27% at 3 years (CI 10–55%). Two of these patients had dose prescription points at 5 mm and 10 mm, respectively. The third patient had a centrally located relapse with no signs of local recurrence. This new lesion was considered more likely to come from his previous T2N1 lung cancer, which had been treated surgically 4 years earlier. A second primary was diagnosed in two patients. Both of these patients remain in complete remission after further definitive treatment by brachytherapy.

No patients were lost to follow-up. One patient died suddenly at home from an unknown cause. All of the other causes of death were obtained from the family or the general practitioner. Of the 11 deaths, 4 were considered to be due to non-related medical causes, one to a late complication (haemoptysiae), 3 to second cancers and 3 to the primary bronchial cancer. Overall survival was 78% at 2 years (61–89% confidence interval), with a median follow-up of 29 months (CI 5–50 months).

10.4.6 Complications

One unexpected pneumothorax occurred and was the only adverse event with the 462 catheter insertions. The patient required transthoracic drainage for 2 days and no further problems were encountered. One patient died of haemoptysis after a bronchial biopsy performed 24 months after treatment, even though he was in complete remission and had no signs of necrosis. No acute ulceration of the bronchus was seen and no debridement of an ulcer or insertion of a prosthesis was required. In six cases, the previously obstructed or stenosed lumen was reopened as a result of brachytherapy.

10.5 Discussion

The detection of small, centrally located bronchial cancers is not rare. Thirty-four percent of patients treated for stage I lung cancer will develop a second lung primary within 3 years (Martini et al. 1995).

Saito estimated that there was a risk of a third cancer in 47% of those already treated for two (Saito et al. 1994). Regular bronchial endoscopy may be useful in patients undergoing follow-up treatment for head and neck or oesophageal cancers. Many patients at high risk of developing lung cancer are suffering from cardiac or respiratory insufficiency. In our group of selected patients, the therapeutic alternatives are limited to other endoluminal techniques such as laser, cryotherapy and photodynamic therapy (Cavaliere et al. 1996). Published data show 13 responses among 21 cases treated by cryotherapy (Homasson et al. 1986), and 13 complete responses among 18 laser treatments and 100% among cases of carcinoma in situ (Brutinel et al. 1984). These studies are subject to criticism since the size, volume, shape and stage of the initial lesions were not described in detail, nor was precise information provided about follow-up. Only the in situ disease is likely to benefit from photodynamic therapy. Sutedja obtained 10 out of 11 remissions while treating stage 1 disease (Sutedja et al. 1992), and Edell reported 14 out of 28 remissions for superficial tumours (Edell and Cortese 1992). Hayata reported from 72% to 77% of complete responses according to whether the mucosa was more nodular or superficial (Hayata et al. 1993).

All of these treatments are effective if the tumour is superficial, but they are unable to treat thick tumours. As it is practically impossible to be totally certain that a bronchial lesion is indeed an in situ carcinoma, brachytherapy offers an advantage since, in theory, it will reduce the likelihood of undertreatment. Patients with small cancers, which are detected early and considered as being operable, have a 5-year survival rate between 63% and 76% (Flehinger et al. 1992). However, in subjects with limited cardiorespiratory reserve, an operative procedure may be hazardous given the central position of these lesions. Patients with small tumours treated exclusively by external beam radiation have a more dismal survival rate of 36–40% at 3 years and 38% at 5 years depending on the tumour size (Rafty et al. 1988; Noordjik et al. 1988).

The survival rate of the patients in our series was 78% at 2 years and 43% at 3 years as other factors (age, general medical, second cancer, etc.) must be taken into consideration. The number of surviving patients is also too small to allow sufficient power for an analysis of survival at 3 years. Consequently this survival rate of 43% cannot be considered a true reflection of local control. Our patient population had favourable prognostic factors with small and relatively superficial cancers. Usuda showed that tumours of less than 1 cm had an insignificant risk of metastases, and that the risk rose to 9% for tumours measuring between 10 and 20 mm (Choi et al. 1985). A well-circumscribed tumour which has not penetrated the bronchial wall, as depicted on CT scan and measuring less than 1 cm, is curable with brachytherapy, provided the dose prescription point is carefully chosen. If a spacer is used to maintain the treatment catheter as central as possible within the bronchus and avoid direct contact with the wall, and if its dimensions are defined precisely, then endo luminal brachytherapy can be established as a practical effective and safe treatment.

The optimal minimum dose appears to be 30 Gy. The fractionation schedule chosen in our study, delivering weekly treatments of 5 Gy, is a compromise between practical, clinical, biological and ethical considerations. Our experience indicates that the two early failures can be due to the non-respect of adequate safety margins. The three local failures have also been examined retrospectively focusing on the tumour and the volume treated, including the safety margin. The tumour volume in the right bronchus was probably underestimated in one patient. The second relapse occurred in the patient who had also failed locally at the same site with photodynamic therapy. The third recurrence occurred just at the upper limit of the radiation field. In our opinion, the problems encountered with these patients are probably related to the difficulties of defining tumour volume and the distance between the source and the bronchial wall or the vessels. This may have led to an overestimation of the risk of necrosis, and thus to an excessively cautious choice of the prescription depth. This seems to be less problematic with the new technique using the silicon sleeve, which may be particularly useful for tumours situated on the curve of the bronchus, the site of failure in two of our patients. Dummy catheters will not guarantee that the treatment catheter is absolutely parallel to the bronchial orifice at all times, particularly when there is a curvature. The data published on radical HDR brachytherapy are scanty and conflicting (Taulelle et al. 1996; Trédaniel et al. 1994; Perol et al. 1997; Hennequin et al. 1997; Ono 1995; Herf et al. 1977; Speiser 1993). In particular, a high rate of haemorrhage has been reported in many studies. This is almost certainly because the dose prescription point is systematically 10 mm, with no attempts to protect the bronchial wall from direct contact with the radiation source. Improvements should be possible in the future for optimal dose distribution. In Ono's series (1995), the population was not selected on the basis of cardiorespiratory criteria, the prescription point was not indicated and complications were not reported for this group of patients.

The morbidity has been low in our study. Apart from one pneumothorax, which was directly related to the number of catheters used, no other cardiac or respiratory complications occurred. The most comparable procedure is transbronchial biopsy, and according to the literature, the pneumothorax rate is 5.5% when four to five parenchymal biopsy specimens are obtained (Herf et al. 1977). No radiation damage to the bronchial mucosa necessitated interventions such as stenting in our study. This is in contrast with that reported by Speiser, who described a 9–13% chance of this happening in his series, according to the dose prescription point (Speiser 1993), some of the patients, however, having also undergone external beam radiotherapy. Perol published his results on a more comparable group in which 10 out of 18 patients developed fibrotic stenosis without external radiation. By careful technical evaluation, by avoiding direct mucosal contact and by prescribing doses per fraction <7 Gy, it is possible to treat limited bronchial tumours with a very low complication rate. Due to treatment tolerance and in order to decrease failure rate, a new study is starting with the same total dose prescribed, with a treatment schedule delivering twice weekly fractions for a total treatment time of 3 weeks.

10.6 Conclusion

High-dose rate brachytherapy is a safe and effective treatment for small central bronchial tumours and is particularly useful in patients with poor general condition contraindicating classic definitive treatment. The two most important parameters are the depth of the dose prescription (treated volume) and avoiding direct contact with the normal surrounding mucosa. With such precautions and adequate source positioning for optimal dose distribution, a good quality application can be achieved, with minimal long-term morbidity.

References

Baldeyrou P, Strauss C, Chatel A, Marsiglia H, Albano M, Gerbaulet A (1995) Endobronchial brachytherapy: CT-scan to evaluate the depth of dose prescription. In: Proceedings of the 78th Annual Meeting. American Radium Society, Paris, 1995

Baldeyrou P, Marsiglia H, Strauss C, Chatel A, Palau R, Lartigau E, Grunenwald D (1996) Endobronchial markage of tumours for a better localisation of small-sized endobronchial carcinoma; an essay with injection of Lipiodol. In: Proceedings of the 9th Combined Meeting of the World Congress of Bronchology and World Congress of Broncho-esophagology, Taiwan, 1996

Bedwinek J, Petty A, Bruton C, Sofield J, Lee L (1992) The use of high-dose rate endobronchial brachytherapy to palliate symptomatic endobronchial recurrence of previously irradiated bronchogenic carcinoma. Int J Radiat Oncol Biol Phys 22:23–30

Brutinel WM, Cortese DA, McDougall JC (1984) Bronchoscopic phototherapy with the Neodynium Yag laser. Chest 86:158–159

Cavaliere S, Venuta F, Foccoli PF, Toninelli C, La Face B (1996) Endoscopic treatment of malignant airway obstruction in 2008 patients. Chest 110:1536–1542

Chang LL, Horvath J, Peyton W, Ling SS (1994) High dose rate afterloading intraluminal brachytherapy in malignant airway obstruction of lung cancer. Int J Radiat Oncol Biol Phys 28:589–596

Choi NC, Kanarek DJ, Kazemi H (1985) Physiologic changes in pulmonary function after thoracic radiotherapy for patients with lung cancer and role of regional pulmonary function studies in predicting postradiotherapy pulmonary function before radiotherapy. Cancer Treatment Symposia 2:119–129

Edell S, Cortese DA (1992) Photodynamic therapy in the management of early superficial squamous cell carcinoma as an alternative to surgical resection. Chest 102:1319–1322

Flehinger BJ, Kimmel M, Melamed MR (1992) The effect of surgical treatment on survival from early lung cancer. Chest 101:1013–1018

Hayata Y, Kato H, Konaka C, Okunaka T (1993) Photodynamic therapy in early stage lung cancer. Lung Cancer 9:287–294

Hennequin C, Tredaniel J, Durdux C, Zalcman G, Dray M, Manoux D, Perret M, Housset M, Hirsch A, Maylin C (1997) Curiethérapie endobronchique: l'expérience de Saint-Louis. Cancer/Radiotherapie 1:159–164

Herf SM, Suratt PM, Arora NS (1977) Deaths and complications associated with transbronchial lung biopsy. AM Rev Resp Dis 115:708–711

Homasson JP, Renault P, Angebault M, Bonniot JP, Bell NJ (1986) Bronchoscopic cryotherapy for airway strictures caused by tumours. Chest 90:159–164

Huber RM, Fischer R, Hautmann H, Pollinger B, Haussinger K, Wendt T (1997) Does additional brachytherapy improve the effect of external irradiation? A prospective, randomized study in central lung tumors. Int J Radiat Oncol Biol Phys 38:533–540

Khanavkar B, Stern P, Albert W, Nakhosteen JA (1991) Complications associated with brachytherapy alone or with laser in lung cancer. Chest 99:1062–1065

Martini N, Bains NS, Burt ME et al (1995) Incidence of local recurrence and second primary tumours in resected stage I lung cancer. J Thorac Cardiovasc Surg 109:120–129

Mazeron JJ, Lartigau E (1993) Curiethérapie à Haut débit de dose: aspects radiobiologiques. Bull Cancer/Radiotherapie 80:511–513

Noordijk EM, Poest Clement EVD, Hermans J, Wever AMJ, Leer JWH (1988) Radiotherapy as an alternative to surgery in elderly patients with resectable lung cancer. Radiother Oncol 13:83–89

Ono R (1995) Brachytherapy. Nakayama-Shoten (ed), pp 80–81

Perol M, Caliandro R, Pommier P, Malet C, Montbarbon X, Carrie C, Ardiet JM (1997) Curative irradiation of limited endobronchial carcinomas with high-dose-rate brachytherapy. Chest 111:1417–1423

Rafty BG, Goldberg NB, Gerstley J, Fischer DB, Peschel RE (1988) Results of radical radiation therapy on clinical stage I, technically operable non-small cell lung cancer. Int J Radiat Oncol Biol Phys 15:69–73

Roach M, Leidholdt EM, Tatera BS, Joseph J (1990) Endobronchial radiation therapy (EBRT) in the management of lung cancer. Int J Radiat Oncol Biol Phys 18:1449–1454

Rothman KJ (1978) Estimation of confidence limits for the cumulative probability of survival in life; table analysis. J Chron Dis 31:557–560

Saito Y, Sato M, Sagawa M, Kanma K, Takahashi S, Usuda K, Nagamoto N, Endo C, Chen Y, Sakurada A, Aikawa H, Fujimura S (1994) Multicentricity in resected occult bronchogenic squamous cell carcinoma. Ann Thor Surg 57:1200–1205

Speiser BL, Spratling L (1993) Remote afterloading brachytherapy for the local control of endobronchial carcinoma. Int J Radiat Oncol Biol Phys 25:579–587

Speiser BL (1993) Radiation bronchitis and stenosis secondary to high-dose rate endobronchial irradiation. Int J Radiation Oncol Biol Phys 25:589–597

Sutedja T, Baas P, Stewart F, Zandwijk N Van (1992) A pilot study of photodynamic therapy in patients with inoperable non-small cell lung cancer. Eur J Cancer 28A:1370–1373

Sutedja G, Baris G Zandwijk N Van, Postmus PE (1994) High dose rate brachytherapy has a curative potential in patients with intraluminal squamous cell lung cancer. Respiration 61:167–168

Taulelle M, Chauvet B, Vincent P, Félix-Faure C, Bucciarelli B, Garcia R, Reboul F (1996) Curiethérapie endobronchique à haut débit de dose: résultats et complications chez 139 patients. Bull Cancer/Radiotherapie 83:127–134

Trédaniel J, Hennequin C, Zalcman G, Walter S, Homasson JP, Maylin C, Hirsch A (1994) Prolonged survival after high-dose rate endobronchial radiation for malignant airway obstruction. Chest 105:767–772

Usuda K, Saito Y, Nagamoto N, Sato M, Sagawa M, Kanma K, Takahasi S, Endo C, Fujimura S (1993) Relation between bronchoscopic findings and tumour size of roentgenographically occult bronchogenic squamous cell carcinoma. J Thorac Cardiovasc Surg 106:1098–1103

11 Integration of Radiation Therapy and Chemotherapy for Small Cell Lung Cancer

H. WAGNER

CONTENTS

11.1 Introduction

Lung cancer currently afflicts about 180 000 persons per year in the United States and, with present treatments, will be fatal to about 85% of them (PARKER et al. 1997). Small cell lung cancer (SCLC) makes up about 25% of these patients, of whom about 20%–30% of these are staged as having "limited" disease at presentation. With the infrequent exception of the patients found following excision of an undiagnosed pulmonary nodule to have AJCC stage group I or II SCLC, the vast majority of patients with limited SCLC (L-SCLC) have stage III disease at presentation (SHEPHERD et al. 1993). It has been quite clear for several decades, learned from the rapid systemic progression of patients treated only with loco-regional therapies, that the "limited" in this system refers to bulk of disease rather than to its anatomic extent. Thus L-SCLC is rightly seen as a disease with two components, a detectable one in the chest (lung and mediastinum) and a present but not yet visible one elsewhere. (This model ignores for the moment the question of "sanctuary" systemic sites such as the CNS.)

H. WAGNER, Thoracic Oncology Program & Division of Radiation Oncology, H. Lee Moffitt Cancer Center, 12902 Magnolia Drive Tampa, FL 33612-9416, USA

This bimodal distribution of disease as well as its observed responsiveness to ionizing radiation and chemotherapeutic agents have led to decades of clinical investigation of combined modality therapy for L-SCLC. It has been demonstrated time and time again that approaches which include both systemic chemotherapy and thoracic radiation therapy (TRT) have yielded survivals superior to those seen with either single modality (WARDE and PAYNE 1993; PIGNON et al. 1992). Yet it has been difficult to optimize these combinations, or in all cases to apply lessons learned in other malignancies such as breast cancer, malignant lymphomas, or pediatric tumors such as Wilms' tumor or Ewing's sarcoma. This may reflect the biologic behavior of SCLC but may also serve to remind us that differences in host populations may make it hard to generalize tumor biology.

This chapter will address several current questions in the optimal integration of radiation and chemotherapy for patients with L-SCLC, questions whose answers lead to distinct clinical actions with definable outcomes and costs. These questions pertain to the traditional radiation therapy parameters of dose, fractionation, and volume, as well as the permutations of radiation and chemotherapy timing and sequencing. These "details" have historically been considered of marginal relevance and often settled more by oncopolitics than by careful clinical trial. The fact that we remain unable to provide these answers with great certainty measures the length that clinical research has to go in this disease. Lack of demonstration of differences in outcome as a function of radiation dose or radiation-chemotherapy sequence based on non-randomized comparisons within large meta-analyses, or in small and underpowered phase III trials, or in trials where the particular regimen used (e.g., doxorubicin containing chemotherapy) may bias against a particular treatment sequence (e.g., concurrent chemoradiation) should not confuse us into thinking that important and clinically useful differences do not exist. Some have speculated that advances in the molecular understanding of cancer biology will soon lead to new therapies which will so supplant out current ones that such optimization will be irrelevant. Unless such therapies are absolutely non-toxic and independent of tumor burden, we should be cautious of such promises. We ought not rest hoping that the next therapeutic paradigm will entirely remove these questions.

In addition to these considerations regarding the integration of thoracic radiation therapy and chemotherapy, brief attention will be paid to the continuing question of prophylactic cranial irradiation, its indications, results, and toxicity, and, finally, a proposal about a possible role for radiation therapy in the management of a subset of patients with extensive SCLC.

11.2 Chemotherapeutic Agents and Their Dose and Scheduling

Many chemotherapeutic agents of differing mechanism of action have substantial single agent activity against SCLC (Elias 1997). The combination of these to produce effective treatment regimens has been constrained in part by common toxicities such as myelosuppression, overlapping resistance mechanisms such as those mediated by p-glycoprotein and multidrug resistance protein, as well as possible resistance to apoptosis by absent p53 function. Several highly active regimens have, however, been developed. One group is based on cyclophosphamide and doxorubicin, with vincristine (Oncovin) (COD) or etoposide (CED) commonly used as an additional agent. The other group is based on cisplatin (or carboplatin) and etoposide (PE). These two regimens produce similar response rates and survival when compared in patients with limited or extensive disease. There is evidence for limited cross activity in relapsing patients, but early alternation of the two regimens has not shown convincing superiority to use of only one as initial therapy with the option of using the other at relapse (Wagner 1994). Myelosuppression is more severe with COD or CED than with PE. Of greatest concern for treatment of patients with limited disease is the difficulty in combining thoracic radiation therapy with COD or CED. Both acute toxicities such as myelosuppression and esophagitis and late cardiac and pulmonary effects are more severe with CED or COD than combined with concurrent or closely alternated TRT than they are with similar combinations using PE as the chemotherapeutic regimen. When therapy is reduced or delayed to allow tolerable toxicity in these settings, the benefits of closely combining TRT and chemotherapy may be compromised.

There is no consistent evidence that increases in chemotherapy dose, certainly to doses requiring stem cell support, are beneficial in SCLC. Several prospective trials have failed to show any benefit overall, although they have not excluded a small effect in patients with limited disease. As these trials in general did not integrate early TRT in the treatment plan for patients with limited disease, they may have not evaluated high-dose chemotherapy in an optimal setting. There are suggestions of survival benefit in selected patients receiving high dose chemotherapy and stem cell support after they have responded to induction chemotherapy (Elias 1997). These patients subsequently also received TRT and prophylactic cranial irradiation (PCI), which would reduce the risk of failure in non-CNS systemic sites and thus increase the sensitivity of detecting a benefit from high-dose chemotherapy. Two trials have suggested benefit for a dose increase in the initial cycles of chemotherapy in patients with limited disease. There are also little data to suggest that prolongation of chemotherapy for more than four to six courses, the use of alternating non-cross resistant regimens, or dose intense weekly regimens are of benefit. All of these approaches had appeared promising in phase II studies, which were not verified in larger phase III trials (Wagner 1994).

11.3 Radiation Dose and Fractionation

Data on dose control in SCLC are relatively sparse and their interpretation is made difficult by the variation in chemotherapy regimens accompanying the radiation. Without effective chemotherapy, most patients die within 1 year, usually of systemic disease, and may not live long enough for locoregional relapse to become manifest. Survival is poor, but local control may appear good. With more effective systemic therapy, survival and thus time at risk for local failure lengthen, and the observed frequency of locoregional relapse may increase unless the chemotherapy controls local disease at least as well as systemic disease. However, if chemotherapy given concurrently with TRT acts as a radiation sensitizer (whether or not this is selective for tumor over normal tissue), it may directly improve local control. The direct effects and indirect effects mediated by observation time may be in opposite directions. ARRIAGADA has lucidly discussed the need for careful calculation of rates of relapse in local as well as systemic sites to better understand these relationships (ARRIAGADA et al. 1992).

Recent series report that locoregional relapse occurs in about 50% of patients treated with tumor doses in the range of 40–50 Gy using conventional daily fractions of 1.8–2.5 Gy. It is not clear whether there is a disadvantage to split course irradiation as is usually the case in the absence of effective chemotherapy. It is also not clear that dose escalation with single daily fractionation and thus lengthening of the overall treatment period is very effective in improving control. CHOI et al. reported data from several sequential treatment regimens at the Massachusetts General Hospital and showed improvement in local control as doses increased from 30 Gy to 50 Gy (CHOI and CAREY 1989). He also noted that all local control rates were substantially less at 3 years than at 1 year. Even at this higher dose, local failure at 2 years was seen in 40% of patients. Data from the Gustav-Roussy Institute show similar local control for 45 Gy, 55 Gy, and 65 Gy (all split course interdigitated with chemotherapy) (ARRIAGADA et al. 1991). The one trial which randomized patients to two dose levels was reported by COY et al. for the National Cancer Institute of Canada (NCIC) (COY et al. 1994). Patients were randomized between two relatively low dose arms, 25 Gy/10 fractions and 37.5 Gy/15 fractions. The higher dose showed improved local control at early time points (2 years) but this decreased with time, indicating the inadequacy of both of these dose levels in producing durable local control.

The convention of daily fractionation five times per week is clearly based more on sociology than radiation biology. Recognition of this has led to a wide variety of alternate fractionation regimens, whose scientific rationale is based in part on the rapid proliferative rate of untreated SCLC and the lack of a significant shoulder on its in vitro radiation cell survival curve (CARNEY et al. 1983, 1985). One appealing approach has been to deliver TRT in an accelerated fashion with modestly reduced fraction size, e.g., 1.5 Gy b.i.d. After phase I–II trials showed that this regimen was tolerable and gave survival rates apparently superior to chemotherapy and concurrent conventionally fractionated TRT to 45 Gy, the ECOG coordinated a US Intergroup trial which randomized patients with L-SCLC to two radiation fractionations, 45 Gy/25 fractions/5 weeks (q.d. fractionation) or 45 Gy/30 fractions/3 weeks (b.i.d. fractionation). Radiation therapy began on the 1st day of chemotherapy, which consisted of four cycles of PE. Treatment was not to be interrupted for acute toxicities such as esophagitis or myelosuppression (unless complicated by sepsis). Between 1988 and 1993 417 patients were entered on the study. Mature results of this trial now demonstrate a statistically significant improvement in survival for the b.i.d. arm, with a 5-year actual (not actuarial) survival of 28% vs 21% ($P = 0.047$). A component of local failure after complete response was seen in 75% of q.d. patients and 42% of b.i.d. patients ($P = 0.006$). Grade 3 acute esophagitis was twice as common in the b.i.d. arm but other toxicities did not differ (JOHNSON et al. 1996; TURRISI 1998).

While this trial establishes the superiority of this b.i.d. regimen to this q.d. regimen, it does not mandate that only b.i.d. irradiation be used in treating patients with L-SCLC. Rather it demonstrates that improvements in local control can translate to improvements in survival, and encourages efforts to improve local control still further. The CALGB has attempted to increase total dose with both q.d. and b.i.d. fractionation, and, using a frequency of 33% grade 3 esophagitis as a limiting toxicity, established 45 Gy when treating b.i.d. or 70 Gy when given with both induction and concurrent PEO, as maximal tolerated doses (CHOI et al. 1995). There is presently consideration among several US cooperative groups to prospectively compare these two regimens, using PE chemotherapy and beginning TRT with cycle 1 (Fig. 11.1).

11.4 Sequencing and Timing of Radiation and Chemotherapy

When combining radiation and chemotherapy, these modalities may be given either in sequence, concurrently, or in an alternating or interdigitated fashion. Radiation may also be given either early or at the end of a series of cycles of chemotherapy. These options give rise to a great number of permutations of sequencing and timing, even for the same total radiation dose and the same chemotherapeutic regimen (Table 11.1).

Recognition of the systemic nature of SCLC has discouraged investigation of strategies in which RT is given first followed by chemotherapy. The majority of approaches have either given several cycles of chemotherapy followed by TRT or given TRT concurrently with chemotherapy from the outset. There has also been investigation of alternated or

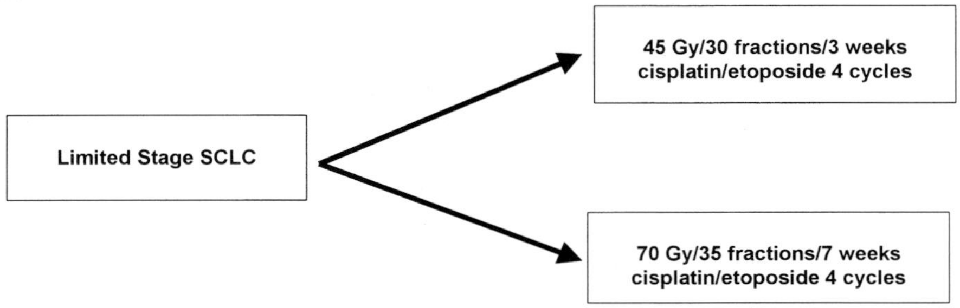

Fig. 11.1. Proposed ECOG/CALGB Intergroup Trial for Patients with Limited SCLC. An alternative proposal would give two cycles of initial chemotherapy with PE or another regimen and follow with concurrent chemoradiation, using the postchemotherapy target volume

Table 11.1. Possible timing and sequencing of radiation and chemotherapy

Sequential
  CT → RT
  RT → CT
Concurrent
  For example, CT and RT given during the same time period and often on the same day. If concurrent treatment is given and the overall duration of RT is less than that of CT (which is almost always the case), several timing options are possible:
    Early CT/RT → CT → CT → CT
    Mid CT → CT → CT/RT → CT
    Late CT → CT → CT → CT/RT
Alternating (Interdigitated)
  For example, CT → RT → CT → RT → CT → RT → CT

interdigitated cycles of chemotherapy and TRT, based on results in animal model systems suggesting superior efficacy and less toxicity with this approach than either sequential or concurrent combinations (Looney and Hopkins 1986). While logistically more complicated and less popular than either the sequential or concurrent approaches, this sequence has been investigated by several institutions, notably the Gustav-Roussy Institut, without suggestion that it was more effective or less toxic than concurrent approaches (Arriagada et al. 1991, 1994). In ECOG the combination of PE and 45 Gy/30 fractions (1.5 Gy/ fraction b.i.d.) was tested both concurrently and as an alternating combination with the TRT given as three courses of 15 Gy/10 fractions interspersed between the first four cycles of chemotherapy (Turrisi et al. 1990; Johnson et al. 1993). Although these two phase II trials were not compared prospectively, they were conducted sequentially and had identical entry requirements and patient characteristics. Neither outcome (median or 3 year survival) nor toxicity was different between the two arms. This would suggest that much of the apparent benefit of concurrent chemoradiation may come from the early use of both modalities without delay of either rather than from specific radiosensitization.

Several theoretical and practical factors are involved in the choice of timing and concurrence. Starting treatment with concurrent radiation and chemotherapy provides maximal treatment intensity both locally and systemically, and takes advantage of possible radiosensitization by the chemotherapeutic agents. But use of both modalities simultaneously increases acute toxicities, particularly esophagitis, and to some degree myelosuppression and possibly pneumonitis. This is less of a problem with chemotherapeutic regimens now in common use such as PE compared with earlier ones such as COD, but can be an issue for some patients, particularly those of more advanced age, borderline performance status, or gastro-esophageal reflux. Unless the radiosensitzation produced by chemotherapeutic agents is selective for tumor cells, concurrent radiation and chemotherapy may be intolerably toxic. These considerations limit the use of active agents such as doxorubicin or gemcitabine concurrently with TRT. Starting radiation therapy after several cycles of chemotherapy may allow treating a smaller target volume if the tumor regresses substantially during chemotherapy, but poses the risk of allowing both proliferation and metastasis of tumor cells which may be radiation sensitive but drug resistant.

Few published trials have addressed prospectively the issues of the timing and sequencing of radiation and chemotherapy in LSCLC. Those which have been reported vary in important details and it is not surprising that they reach different conclusions (Table 11.2).

The Cancer and Leukemia Group B (CALGB) conducted a three arm trial randomizing patients to chemotherapy alone or combined with TRT (50 Gy/6

Table 11.2. Randomized trials of timing and fractionation of TRT in patients with limited SCLC

Trial	RT (Gy/Fr/week)	CT	MST (months)	% 2-year survival	% 5-Year survival	% local failure
CALGB	50/25/6 d1	COE/COD	13	15	6.6	~50
	50/25/6 d42	COE/COD	14.5	25	12.8	~50
NCIC	45 d22	PE/COD	20	40	20	-
	45 d106	PE/COD	15	34	11	-
INT 0096	45/25/5 d1	PE × 4	18.6	40.1	21	75
	45/30/3 d1	PE × 4	22.6	46.5	29	42
Shultz	40/22/4.5 or 45/22 S d1	PE/COD	10.7	-	-	-
	40/22/4.5 or 45/22 S d120	PE/COD	12.9	-	-	-
Takada	45/30/3 d1	PE	31.3	-	-	-
	45/30/3 d85	PE	20.8	-	-	-
Lebeau	50/20/4 d22	CED	13.5	-	-	-
	50/20/12 ALT	CED	14.2	-	-	-
Work	40-45/20-22/7 S d1	PE/COD	10.5	20	11	72
	40-45/20-22/7 S d126	PE/COD	12	19	12	68
Gregor	50/20/4 d106	CED	15	26	15 (3 year)	60
	50/20/12 ALT	CED	14	23	12 (3 year)	60
Jeremic	54/28/4 d1	CPE/PE	34	71	30	42
	54/28/4 d42	PE/cPE/PE	26	53	15	63

ALT, alternating with chemotherapy; S, split course; PE, cisplatin/etoposide; cPE, carboplatin/etoposide; COD, cyclophosphamide/vincristine/doxorubicin; CED, cyclophosphamide/etoposide/doxorubicin.

weeks) begun either on day 1 or day 64 of chemotherapy and given concurrently with it (Perry et al. 1987) Both arms including TRT were superior to the chemotherapy only regimen for local control and survival, and there was a trend favoring the delayed TRT arm (2-year survival 25% vs 15%). At last update the 5-year survival continues to favor delayed TRT, 3% for chemotherapy alone, 6.6% for early TRT and 12.8% for delayed TRT (Perry et al. 1996). In this trial the dose intensity of chemotherapy (using a non-cisplatin based regimen) was deliberately reduced in the early TRT arm, which may have adversely biased it. Two prospective trials have suggested that such early drug dose intensity is an important determinant of survival in SCLC, at least for patients with limited disease.

The NCIC randomized patients receiving alternating cycles of COD and EP to receive TRT (40 Gy/15 fractions/3 weeks) concurrent with either the first or third cycle of PE (Murray et al. 1993). Survival was significantly superior for patients receiving early TRT (median 21.2 vs 16 months, 4-year 25% vs 15%). Surprisingly, the main difference in patterns of relapse was in the incidence of CNS rather than control of intrathoracic disease.

Shultz et al. treated patients with limited SCLC using alternating cycles of EP and COD and randomized them between TRT (40 Gy/22 fractions/4½ weeks or 45 Gy/22 fractions by split course) starting on day 1 or day 120 (Shultz et al. 1988). There was a non-significant difference in median survival favoring delayed TRT (10.7 vs 12.9 months). Long term survival and local control have not been reported. Both arms of this trial used rather low total radiation doses.

Takada reported preliminary results of a phase III trial conducted by the Japanese Clinical Oncology Group (JCOG) in which patients with L-SCLC were treated with four cycles of PE chemotherapy and randomized to receive TRT (45 Gy/30 fractions/3 weeks) starting either concurrent with the first or following the fourth cycle of chemotherapy (Takada et al. 1996). With a median follow-up time of 18.6 months, median survival was 20.8 months for the late sequential TRT and 31.3 months for early concurrent TRT. It should be kept in mind that two comparisons were made in this trial, early vs late TRT and concurrent vs sequential chemoradiation and that neither question on its own will be unambiguously answered.

Gregor has reported the results of an EORTC trial comparing alternating versus sequential chemoradiotherapy for patients with L-SCLC (Gregor et al. 1997). Chemotherapy was with CED. Radiation therapy was given either interspersed between cycles of chemotherapy (1000 cGy/4 fractions/1 week) for four courses or at completion of all chemotherapy. Overall median survival was 15 months and 2-year survival 25%. There were no survival differences between the two treatment arms. There was significantly more hematologic (but not other acute) toxicity in the alternated arm which led to a reduced dose delivery of both chemotherapy and radiotherapy in this arm compared with the sequential arm. Local failure was a major problem in both arms, with local failure the site of first relapse in 60% of all patients. This trial exemplifies some of the difficulties of trying to answer questions about optimal radiation therapy scheduling outside the context of the chemotherapy used. The CDE regimen as used in this study is more myelosuppressive than PE and conclusions which apply to the combination of radiation therapy with one may not apply to the other. Work has reported results of a randomized prospective trial conducted in Denmark which was designed to compare early with late TRT. The actual treatment regimen used was rather unusual, with, in the early TRT arm, the first half of a split course radiotherapy regimen preceding any chemotherapy. The late TRT arm also used split course irradiation. In neither arm was TRT given concurrently with chemotherapy, which in both arms consisted of three cycles of PE and six cycles of COD. The timing of TRT in this trial had no significant effect on 2-year survival or 2-year in-field recurrence rate. However, the 2-year survivals reported in this trial were 20% for early and 19% for late TRT, markedly inferior to what has been reported by several groups for early TRT concurrent with chemotherapy (Wagner 1997a). Either the patients in this trial had more advanced disease or poorer performance status than those in recent North American and Japanese trials or the overall treatment was sufficiently inactive as to make the timing of TRT a moot point.

Lebeau et al. reported a randomized trial comparing concurrent RT starting with the second cycle of chemotherapy (50 Gy/20 fractions) with alternating treatment between cycles 2-3-4-5 (Lebeau et al. 1996). In the alternating regimen the radiation dose for the first two courses was 20 Gy/8 fractions and was 15 Gy/6 fractions for the third course. Chemotherapy was CED in both arms. Median survival was 407 days for the concurrent arm and 426 days for the alternating arm. More severe lung fibrosis was noted with concurrent therapy, and compliance with the schedule of radiotherapy was poor, particularly for the alternating treatment arm.

Jeremic et al. conducted a phase III trial in which 107 patients with L-SCLC were randomized to receive TRT starting at week 1 or week 6 of therapy (Jeremic et al. 1997). RT was given with 1.5 Gy fractions b.i.d. to a total dose of 54 Gy with concurrent daily carboplatin/etoposide (cPE). A total of four cycles of PE were also given, either all following the concurrent chemoradiation or for one cycle prior to TRT and three cycles following. Median and 2-year survivals for early and delayed TRT were 34 and 26 months and 30% vs 15% respectively, which was significant on multivariate analysis. Local recurrence-free survival was also significantly better in the early TRT arm, 58% vs 37% at 5 years. Murray has reported a meta-analysis of trials which have used both TRT and chemotherapy for L-SCLC, using 3-year disease free survival as an outcome measure as a function of the interval from the start of chemotherapy to the start of TRT (Murray et al. 1993). Results were significantly better for those regimens beginning TRT not more than 6 weeks from the start of chemotherapy. With long delays (20 weeks or more) results were little better than without TRT.

11.5 Volume

The appropriate target volume for TRT has not been defined. Several separate questions may be raised:

- What amount of elective nodal irradiation is appropriate?
- What margins are required for ill-defined primary lesions with extensions into lung parenchyma and/or atelectasis?
- If several cycles or chemotherapy are given prior to TRT, should the target volume be based on pre- or postchemotherapy tumor volume?

Prospective trials have not adequately addressed the issues of margins, ill-defined tumors, or elective nodal volume. Many older trials recommended that portals cover all known primary disease with 2-cm margins and include bilateral hilar, mediastinal, and supraclavicular nodes. While retrospective analysis of patients on a SECSG trial showed a higher rate of local failure (69 vs 32%) in those not adhering to these requirements than those who did, it was not stated that the excess failures occurred in the areas which would have been irradiated had the protocol been adhered to. It may simply be that the failure rates were higher in larger tumors and that these portals were often kept "tight" to avoid excessive lung irradiation. This trial was also conducted prior to the use of CT-based treatment planning and target volumes were approximate at best. More recent trials in which routine irradiation of the contralateral hilum or any supraclavicular nodes were eliminated have not reported high failure rates in these sites and have excellent survivals (WILLIAMS and TURRISI 1997).

Deferring TRT until completion of all chemotherapy, typically four to six cycles, is not an effective way to combine these modalities. One trial conducted by the SWOG which prospectively compared pre- vs. post-treatment tumor volumes as TRT target volumes used such an approach, and was limited to patients who had a partial rather than complete response to their initial chemotherapy. The lack of a difference in this trial is not convincing evidence of the adequacy of post-treatment volumes. More persuasive is the report from the Mayo Clinic where, over a period of several years, treatment philosophy shifted from treating pre-chemotherapy to postchemotherapy volumes after two or three cycles of chemotherapy. In an analysis by LIENGSWANGSWONG, local failure rates were not different in the two arms (LIENGSWANGSWONG et al. (1994). Those local failures seen in the group treated to the post-chemotherapy volumes were central rather than peripheral, suggesting that they would not have been prevented with larger treatment volumes.

If it is correct that postchemotherapy volumes are adequate, and also that a delay of two or three cycles before starting radiation (particularly if it is given concurrently with remaining cycles of chemotherapy) is not harmful, two possible advantages may arise from the use of the smaller volumes:

- Reduced toxicities if treating to the same total doses as presently used.
- The ability to use higher total doses without necessarily increasing toxicity over present levels. While some normal tissue doses, such as that to the esophagus adjacent to bulky subcarinal nodes, will not likely be reduced by treating postchemotherapy volumes, the length of esophagus treated to significant dose, as well as the volume of lung, should be significantly spared (KUMAR 1997).

Treatment volume may be an issue worth addressing prospectively. Such a trial would logically require three arms (early TRT to the initial tumor volume, delayed TRT to the initial tumor volume, and delayed TRT to the postchemotherapy volume) in order to resolve both the timing and volume issues, and a large sample size to detect or exclude small differences.

11.6 Prophylactic Cranial Irradiation

Brain metastases are common in SCLC, both at initial presentation and as a site of progression following treatment. Treatment of patients with radiographically demonstrable CNS disease, whether initially symptomatic or not, is often successful on a short term basis, but long term disease control and survival is rare. It was initially believed that chemotherapy was ineffective against established brain metastases and that radiation therapy was the only effective treatment, but more recent studies have shown that brain metastases can respond to a number of chemotherapeutic agents, such as VM-26 (Vumon) and Topotecan (Hycamtin) with a frequency similar to that of extracranial metastatic disease, and with similar response frequency and duration to whole brain radiotherapy (BRAHMER and ETTINGER 1998; WAGNER 1997). Unfortunately, these response rates are modest and durations brief.

It was proposed by HANSEN that we consider prophylactic treatment of the brain with radiation or chemotherapy in patients without evidence of disease in this site (HANSEN 1980). Reasoning by analogy with acute lymphoblastic leukemia, he posited that there was a relatively intact blood-brain barrier (at least early in the development of brain metastases) so that although tumor cells could gain access to the brain, the tissue concentrations of most (non-lipophilic) chemotherapy agents was low and insufficient to eradicate disease. While the blood-brain barrier might be disrupted later in the growth of the tumor, as evidenced by the enhancement seen with CT or MRI contrast, its presence earlier in the course of disease rendered the CNS a "pharmacologic sanctuary" for tumor cells.

It became clear in the 1980s that prophylactic cranial irradiation (PCI) to modest doses, typically 25–30 Gy in 8–10 fractions, was markedly effective in reducing the CNS failure rate but did not have a dramatic effect (WAGNER 1997b). This lack of a demonstrable survival gain plus reports of major neurotoxicity in some series led to a reaction against PCI by many oncologists (CATANE et al. 1981; LEE et al. 1986; JOHNSON et al. 1985, 1990; LISHNER et al.

1990). Although a number of randomized trials were conducted, several of these included patients not in systemic response, for whom it would not be expected that PCI would give a survival gain. Even in those prospective trials limited to patients who had achieved a complete response (or very good partial response, with minor residual radiographic abnormalities which might represent only fibrosis), the small benefits seen in several trials did not achieve statistical significance. In retrospect, all of these trials were underpowered statistically to detect the relatively small increment in long term survival which might be expected if truly isolated CNS failure occurred in 10%–15% of those patients achieving CR. Several larger randomized trials conducted in the late 1980s and 1990s which were restricted to patients achieving CR strongly suggested such a survival benefit but did not individually reach statistical significance (Arriagada et al. 1995; Gregor et al. 1996). When all randomized trials of PCI in complete responders were combined in a meta-analysis using individual patient data, however, the improvement in 3-year survival was highly significant, increasing from 15.3% in the control group to 20.7% in those patients receiving PCI (Arriagada et al. 1998). The relative risk of death for patients receiving PCI was 0.84 (95% CI 0.73–0.97). There was a trend to increasing benefit as the PCI dose was increased but this was not a randomized variable. The benefits of PCI were seen independent of patient age, performance status, disease extent or type of induction treatment.

One past reason for the reluctance to recommend PCI was concern that neurologic function would be impaired by this treatment, leading to a poor quality of life for both cured patients and those dying of extracranial systemic metastases. It was noted in the early 1980s that some long term survivors of SCLC, most of whom had received PCI, developed deterioration of psychomotor function several years after completing treatment (Catane et al. 1981; Lee et al. 1986; Johnson et al. 1985, 1990; Lishner et al. 1990). Both the frequency and severity of these symptoms varied considerably among series. In addition, there has been no standardization of reporting of these late effects, with some investigators reporting impairment in daily living, others abnormalities on detailed neuropsychiatric testing, and still others asymptomatic changes on MR imaging of the brain. While the picture was by no means clear, it served as a powerful counter-argument to those advocating PCI, especially if there was no benefit of PCI for long term survival.

More careful analysis has suggested that these early alarms were both exaggerated and somewhat misdirected. First, several of the series reporting a high incidence of CNS dysfunction following PCI used large fractions (3–4 Gy) often with concurrent or subsequent chemotherapy. In several series chemotherapeutic agents with known access to the CNS and known neurotoxicity, such as methotrexate and the nitrosoureas, were used. Such "dangerous liaisons" may well have contributed to the high rates of toxicity seen (Turrisi 1990; Crossen et al. 1994). Second, the early studies were retrospective and lacked good baseline data on neurologic function of patients prior to PCI. More recent studies have tested patients before and after PCI and found little or no deterioration in overall neurological or psychological functioning following PCI to moderate dose (e.g., 25–30 Gy/10–12 fractions) when this is given after most or all chemotherapy (Arriagada et al. 1995; Gregor et al. 1996). A somewhat surprising finding of several of these studies, however, was that a large proportion of patients with SCLC have significant baseline neuropsychiatric impairment prior to PCI (Cull et al. 1994; Komaki et al. 1995; van Osterhout et al. 1996). Some of this may be due to chemotherapy but many patients are abnormal prior to any therapy, when compared with age- and sex-matched controls. Studies are currently underway to compare patients with SCLC with those with NSCLC and squamous cell carcinoma of the head and neck. These should help to identify the relative roles of toxic exposures (e.g., tobacco, alcohol) and possible paraneoplastic syndromes specific to SCLC. Several such syndromes, such as Eaton Lambert syndrome and optic neuropathy, are well characterized in SCLC, and it is possible that at least part of what was formerly considered radiation toxicity may instead be a manifestation of the disease process itself.

11.7 Should Patients with Extensive SCLC Receive Radiation Therapy as Part of Their Initial Treatment?

When combined radiation and chemotherapy were first being explored in SCLC, several trials looked at this approach in patients with extensive as well as limited disease. These trials, now over a decade old, generally used cyclophosphamide and nitrosourea based chemotherapy, and radiation therapy to modest doses (40–40 Gy) now recognized to be inadequate to obtain local control. That these trials uniformly failed to show any survival benefit for radiation to the thorax and other sites of disease in these patients should come as no surprise (Wagner 1994). More recently, the group in Vancouver has included thoracic radiation in their treatment of patients with extensive chemotherapy with an intense weekly chemotherapy regimen called CODE (cisplatin/Oncovin/doxorubicin/etoposide). Patients having good response of their extrathoracic disease received thoracic radiation therapy after completion of the 12-week course of induction chemotherapy. Dose was 25 Gy in 10 fractions. The reported survival of these patients appeared quite favorable, with suggestion of a plateau of long-term survivors, and local failure seemed reduced even with this modest dose of radiation. Unfortunately, attempts to confirm these encouraging results in a prospective trial by the NCIC and SWOG were stopped because of excessive toxicity with this regimen, with about 10% treatment related deaths compared with 3% in a more conventional chemotherapy alone regimen of alternating PE and CED.

These negative trials may have suffered from poor systemic regimens and poor selection of patients. It is unlikely that modest doses of radiation therapy (30 Gy) will be useful in controlling SCLC at sites of initially bulky extrathoracic disease, even after a good response to chemotherapy. The experience in treating intrathoracic disease would argue against this approach. On the other hand, there exists a subset of patients with extensive SCLC whose extrathoracic disease is limited to a single detectable site which can be irradiated to reasonably high dose (45 Gy or more), e.g., those with disease limited to the brain, or solitary bone or adrenal metastases. The prognosis of these patients, particularly those with only metastases to the brain, is more favorable than that of other patients with extensive disease (Giannone et al. 1987; Kochhar et al. 1997). It would seem logical in these patients to consider a treatment regimen of initial chemotherapy for two cycles, then, in responders, two further cycles of chemotherapy with concurrent radiation therapy to sites of thoracic and extrathoracic disease. Radiation to the brain might be withheld until after completion of chemotherapy to reduce neurotoxicity. Whether this approach would be superior to chemotherapy alone will require prospective trials, which are currently being planned.

11.8 Conclusions and Future Directions

This is not a time to conclude that one of our current ways of combining radiation and chemotherapy for L-SCLC is "good enough," pick your favorite, and retreat to the endless horizon of "rationally targeted" therapies as the sole hope for therapeutic progress. The last decade has shown that modest changes in dose and sequencing of radiation and chemotherapy can have modest but significant impacts on long term survival in this disease. For the moment, it appears that the best results are obtained when both radiation and chemotherapy are given early, usually concurrently, although the reason(s) for the benefit of concurrent treatment (sensitization rather than lack of delay) are not clear. The use of agents which will reduce acute toxicity (myelosuppression, esophagitis) will make such aggressive treatment more tolerable, while, with improved long term survival, more attention will have to be paid to late complications and the development of second primary tumors. PCI has been shown to be effective in reducing CNS relapse and improving survival, but the most effective dose has not been defined. While we work to better understand the molecular peculiarities of SCLC and exploit these therapeutically, further fine tuning of radiation and chemotherapy should further improve the therapeutic outcome for our patients.

References

Arriagada R, Pellae-Cosset B, Cueto Ladron de Guevera J et al (1991) Alternating radiotherapy and chemotherapy schedules in limited small cell lung cancer: analysis of local chest recurrences. Radiother Oncol 20:91–98

Arriagada R et al (1992) Competing events determining relapse-free survival in limited small-cell lung carcinoma. J Clin Oncol 10:447–451

Arriagada R et al (1994) Alternating radiotherapy and chemotherapy in limited small cell lung cancer: the IGR protocols. French FNCLCC Lung Cancer Study Group. Lung Cancer 10(1)

Arriagada R et al (1995) Prophylactic cranial irradiation for patients with small-cell lung cancer in complete remission. J Natl Cancer Inst 87:183–190

Arriagada R, Auperin A, Pignon JP et al (1998) Prophylactic cranial irradiation overview (PCIO) in patients with small cell lung cancer (SCLC) in complete remission (CR). Proc ASCO 17:Abstract 1758

Brahmer HR, Ettinger DS (1998) The role of topotecan in the treatment of small cell lung cancer. The Oncologist 3:11–14

Carney D, Mitchell J, Kinsella T (1983) In vitro radiation and chemotherapy sensitivity of established cell lines of human small cell lung cancer and its large cell morphological variant. Cancer Res 43:2806–2811

Carney DN, Gazdar AF, Bepler G et al (1985) Establishment and characterization of SCLC cell lines having classic and variant features. Cancer Res 45:2913–2923

Catane R et al (1981) Follow-up neurological evaluation in patients with small cell lung carcinoma treated with prophylactic cranial irradiation and chemotherapy. Int J Radiation Oncology Biol Phys 7:105–109

Choi N, Carey N (1989) Importance of radiation dose in achieving improved loco-regional tumor control in limited stage small-cell lung carcinoma: an update. Int J Radiat Oncol Biol Phys 17:307–310

Choi N, Herndon J, Rosenman J et al (1995) Phase I study to determine the maximum tolerated dose of radiation in standard daily and accelerated twice daily radiation schedules with concurrent chemotherapy for limited stage small cell lung cancer: CALGB 8837 (Abstract 1113). Proc Am Soc Clin Oncol 14:363

Coy P et al (1994) Patterns of failure following loco-regional radiotherapy in the treatment of limited stage small cell lung cancer. Int J Radiat Oncol Biol Phys 28:355–362

Crossen J et al (1994) Neurobehavioral sequelae of cranial irradiation in adults: a review of radiation-induced encephalopathy. J Clin Oncol 12:627–642

Cull A et al (1994) Neurological and cognitive impairment in long-term survivors of small cell lung cancer. Eur J Cancer 30A:1067–1074

Elias AD (1997) Small cell lung cancer: state of the art therapy in 1996. Chest 112:251s–258s

Giannone L, Johnson DH, Hande KR, Greco FA (1987) Favorable prognosis of brain metastases in small cell lung cancer. Ann Int Med 106:386–389

Gregor A. et al (1996) Effects of prophylactic cranial irradiation (PCI) in small cell lung cancer (SCLC); results of UKCCCR/EORTC randomised trial. Proc ASCO 15:1139 (Abstract)

Gregor A, Drings P, Burghouts J et al (1997) Randomized trial of alternating versus sequential radiotherapy/chemotherapy in limited-disease patients with small cell lung cancer: a European Organization for Research and Treatment of Cancer lung cancer cooperative group study. J Clin Oncol 15:2840–2849

Hansen H et al (1980) Prophylactic irradiation in bronchogenic small cell anaplastic carcinoma: a comparative trial of localized versus extensive radiotherapy including prophylactic brain irradiation in patients receiving combination chemotherapy. Cancer 46:279–284

Jeremic B, Shibamoto Y, Acimovic L, Milisavljevic S (1997) Initial versus delayed accelerated hyperfractionated radiation therapy and concurrent chemotherapy in limited small-cell lung cancer: a randomized study. J Clin Oncol 15:893–900

Johnson B et al (1985) Neurologic, neuropsychologic, and cranial computed tomography scan abnormalities in 2–10 year survivors of small cell lung cancer. J Clin Oncol 3:1659–1667

Johnson B et al (1990) Neurologic, computed cranial tomographic, and magnetic resonance imaging abnormalities in patients with small cell lung cancer: further follow-up of 6- to 13-year survivors. J Clin Oncol 8:46–56

Johnson D, Turrisi AT, Kim K et al (1993) Alternating chemotherapy and twice-daily radiotherapy in limited-stage small-cell lung cancer: a pilot study of the Eastern Cooperative Oncology Group. J Clin Oncol 11:879–884

Johnson D et al (1996) Cisplatin (P) & etoposide (E) + thoracic radiotherapy (TRT) administered once or twice daily (BID) in limited stage (LS) small cell lung cancer (SCLC): final results of Intergroup trial 0096. Proc ASCO 15: Abstract 1113

Kochhar R, Frytak S, Shaw EG (1997) Survival of patients with extensive small-cell lung cancer who have only brain metastases at initial diagnosis. Am J Clin Oncol 20:125–127

Komaki R et al (1995) Evaluation of cognitive function in patients with limited small cell lung cancer prior to and shortly following prophylactic cranial irradiation. Int J Radiat Oncol Biol Phys 33:179–182

Kumar P (1997) The role of thoracic radiotherapy in the management of limited-stage small cell lung cancer. Chest 112:259s–265s

LeBeau B et al (1996) A randomized clinical trial comparing concurrent and alternated thoracic irradiation in limited small cell lung cancer (SCLC). Proc ASCO 15:Abstract 1148

Lee J et al (1986) Neurotoxicity in long-term survivors of small cell lung cancer. Int J Radiat Oncol Biol Phys 12:313–321

Liengswangwong V, Bonner J, Shaw E et al (1994) Limited stage small cell lung cancer: patterns of recurrence and implications for thoracic radiotherapy. J Clin Oncol 2:496–502

Lishner M et al (1990) Late neurologic complications after prophylactic cranial irradiation in patients with small cell lung cancer: the Toronto experience. J Clin Oncol 8:215–221

Looney WB, Hopkins HA (1986) Alternation of chemotherapy and radiotherapy in cancer management. III. Results in experimental solid tumor systems and their relationship to clinical studies. Can Treatment Rep 70:141–162

Murray N et al (1993) Importance of timing for thoracic irradiation in the combined modality treatment of limited-stage small-cell lung cancer. J Clin Oncol 11:336–344

Parker SL, Tong T, Bolden S et al (1997) Cancer statistics. CA Cancer J Clin 47:5–27

Perry M et al (1987) Chemotherapy with or without radiation therapy in limited small-cell carcinoma of the lung. N Engl J Med 316:912–918

Perry M et al (1996) Thoracic radiation therapy added to chemotherapy in limited small cell lung cancer: an update of Cancer & Leukemia Group B (CALGB) study 8083. Proc ASCO: Abstract 1150

Pignon J-P et al (1992) A meta-analysis of thoracic radiotherapy for small-cell lung cancer. N Engl J Med 327:1618–1624

Schultz H et al (1988) Timing of chest irradiation with respect to combination chemotherapy in small cell lung cancer, limited disease. Lung Cancer 4:153(Abstract)

Shepherd FA, Ginsberg RJ, Haddad R et al (1993) Importance of clinical staging in limited small-cell ling cancer: a valuable system to separate prognostic subgroups. J Clin Oncol 11:1592–1597

Takada M, Fukuoka M, Furuse K et al (1996) Phase III study of concurrent versus sequential thoracic radiotherapy (TRT) in combination with cisplatin (C) and etoposide (E) for limited-stage (LS) small cell lung cancer: preliminary results of the Japanese Clinical Oncology Group. Proc ASCO 15:Abstract 1103

Turrisi A (1990) Brain irradiation and systemic chemotherapy for small-cell lung cancer: dangerous liaisons? J Clin Oncol [Editorial] 8:196–199

Turrisi AT, Wagner H et al (1990) Limited small cell lung cancer: concurrent BID thoracic radiotherapy with platinum-etoposide:an ECOG study. Proc ASCO 9:230 (Abstract)

Turrisi A, Kim K, Sause W et al (1998) Observations after 5 year follow-up of Intergroup trial 0096: 4 cycles of cisplatin(P) etoposide(E) and concurrent 45 Gy thoracic radiotherapy (TRT) given in daily (QD) or twice-daily (BID) fractions followed by 25 Gy PCI. Survival difference and patterns of failure. Proc ASCO 17:Abstract 1757

van Oosterhout A et al (1996) Neurologic disorders in 203 consecutive patients with small cell lung cancer. Results of a longitudinal study. Cancer 77:1434–1441

Wagner H (1994) Limited small cell lung cancer: current treatment and clinical trials. Cancer Control 1:485–497

Wagner H (1997a) Thoracic irradiation of limited small cell lung cancer: have we defined optimal dose, time, and fractionation? Lung Cancer: 17(Suppl 1):137s–148s

Wagner H (1997b) Prophylactic cranial irradiation for patients with small cell lung cancer: an enduring controversy. Chest Surg Clin N Am 7:151–166

Warde P, Payne D (1992) Does thoracic irradiation improve survival and local control in limited-stage small-cell carcinoma of the lung? J Clin Oncol 10:890–895

Williams TE, Turrisi AT 3rd (1997) Role of radiotherapy in the treatment of small cell lung carcinoma. Chest Surg Clin N Am 7:135–149

Work E, Nielsen OS, Bentzen SM et al (1997) Randomized study of initial versus late chest irradiation combined with chemotherapy in limited stage small-cell lung cancer. J Clin Oncol 15:3030–3037

12 Role of Prophylactic Cranial Irradiation: Benefits and Late Effects

A. GREGOR and A. CULL

CONTENTS

12.1 Introduction

Small cell lung cancer (SCLC) represents a common and serious burden of disease and accounts for about 20% of all the histological subtypes of lung cancer (JENSON et al. 1990). SCLC has many biological and clinical characteristics which make it distinct from other histological varieties of bronchial carcinoma. Amongst them is a high propensity to brain metastases. The frequency of brain involvement in SCLC rises with time. About 20% of SCLC patients present with brain metastases at the time of diagnosis and despite good systemic tumour control up to 50% will fail in the brain by 2 years of follow-up (BUNN and ROSEN 1985). Postmortem evidence of tumour involvement of the brain can be seen in more than 80% of patients. In more than half of all these patients the brain will be the first and often the only site of failure (PEDERSON 1986).

Brain metastases cause significant clinical and psychosocial morbidity and have a profound negative impact on quality of life (FELLETTI et al. 1985). Patients relapsing in the brain are likely to spend a greater proportion of their remaining lives in hospital than patients relapsing elsewhere, e.g. in the liver (FELLETTI et al. 1985). Treatment of established brain metastases is far from satisfactory and only half of these patients will achieve satisfactory palliation by either radiotherapy (LUCAS et al. 1986; CARMICHAEL et al. 1988) or chemotherapy (POSTMUS et al. 1989).

Experience from other clinical settings in which prevention of CNS involvement by prophylactic irradiation conferred significant survival benefits (BLEYER and POPLACK 1985) has led to the introduction of prophylactic cranial irradiation (PCI) into this clinical setting. PCI has now been used sporadically for more than 2 decades. Satisfactory data for meaningful evaluation of its benefits and side effects have only been accrued more recently.

12.2 History of PCI

The first wave of clinical trials testing the concept of PCI in SCLC was completed in the late 1970s and early 1980s. The majority of these studies were positive and confirmed that low dose PCI significantly decreases the rate of occurrence of brain metastases (Table 12.1). This local effect was not translated into demonstrable survival benefit.

There was a variable distribution, within and between the individual studies, of crucial factors such as disease extent and response to induction chemotherapy. As any survival advantage which could have been offered by PCI was likely to be numerically very small, it could have been diluted by these much more powerful determinants of outcome. The ability to detect small survival differences would have been further impaired by small sample size in all of these studies. The patient numbers in individual trials varied from 30 to 250 and only 3 studies had more than 100 randomised patients.

The safety of PCI was also questioned at this time largely based on CT abnormalities seen in children

A. GREGOR, Department of Clinical Oncology, Western General Hospital NHS Trust, Crewe Road, Edinburgh, EH4 2XU, UK

A. CULL, Imperial Cancer Research Fund Psychology Research Group, Western General Hospital NHS Trust, Edinburgh, EH4 2XU, UK

receiving PCI and chemotherapy for acute lymphocytic leukaemia (Bleyer and Poplack 1985). To clarify the significance of these findings for PCI in the management of SCLC, Catane et al. (1981) examined a series of 16 long term survivors of SCLC. They found CT abnormalities in 9 of the 13 patients who had had PCI and in 2 of the 3 patients who had not. In the absence of clinically significant changes associated with these findings they concluded there was no contraindication to the use of PCI in adults with SCLC.

There followed throughout the 1980s a stream of retrospective evaluations of SCLC patients which reported evidence of serious neurotoxicity which was attributed to PCI (Ellison et al. 1982; Looper et al. 1984; Johnson et al. 1985; Lee et al. 1986; Twinjstra et al. 1987; Laukannen et al. 1988).

These studies have been reviewed in greater detail elsewhere (Crossen et al. 1994; Gregor et al. 1996). The studies varied in the neurological functions tested, in the methods of assessment used and in the timing of the assessments. There were also crucial differences in treatment parameters (e.g. neurotoxic chemotherapy, radiation schedule, timing of PCI relative to chemotherapy). Not surprisingly then, these early studies varied widely in the prevalence and severity of the abnormalities reported. Typically the investigators had access to only small numbers of long term survivors – the largest sample size was 38 (Lee et al. 1986) – the majority of whom had received PCI. Pederson et al. (1988) summarised the data from 8 studies with a total of 123 patients of whom 102 had received PCI. They concluded 45% had severe clinical side effects the clinical features of which were cognitive impairment and ataxic gait.

The failure to demonstrate improved survival with PCI and these growing concerns about its toxicity proved powerful arguments against its use and PCI was abandoned as a treatment approach in many centres. However, the continuing controversy was epitomised in 1990 by the simultaneous publication of two retrospective reviews drawing diametrically opposed conclusions. Fleck et al. (1990) reported the outcome for 58 SCLC patients achieving complete response to induction therapy in Indiana. Eleven of the 38 patients treated with PCI survived >30 months but 7 of them were reported to have clinically significant neurotoxicity although the exact nature of this was not specified. Set against this, the incidence of CNS relapse was low among those not exposed to PCI, leading the authors to challenge the value of PCI.

Lishner et al. (1990) reported the Toronto experience based on the case note review of 58 long term survivors of SCLC (>2 years). CNS metastases occurred significantly less often among the 48 patients who had had PCI. Although nine of them had neurological problems the authors attributed the majority of these to side effects of chemotherapy or other comorbidity. They concluded that PCI had an adverse effect on the daily life of only a small minority of patients and argued for the use of PCI in the management of patients with SCLC.

The clinical problem of brain metastases persisted despite improvements in the effectiveness of systemic chemotherapy and the introduction of a combined modality approach in which the addition of thoracic irradiation produced significant survival benefit (Pignon et al. 1992). With longer median survival and larger numbers of patient surviving 2 or more years from diagnosis there was a substantial increase in the absolute numbers of patients at risk from brain relapse. The true magnitude of this problem is better appreciated by using actuarial rather than absolute calculations of risk. Using this approach the observation period can be taken into account reflecting more truly the clinical significance of the risk.

It was clear then that the risks and benefits of PCI needed to be assessed in a prospective randomised trial and this view was echoed in the retrospective reviews which continued to appear from around the

Table 12.1. Early trials of PCI in SCLC

Sample size (n)	Radiation dose	% brain relapse		Reference
		PCI+	PCI−	
45	20 Gy/5 Fr	17	20	Cox et al. (1978)
217	30 Gy/10 Fr	5	22	Seydel et al. (1985)
54	24 Gy/8 Fr	0	16	Bieler et al. (1979)
163	30 Gy/10 Fr	4	18	Maurer et al. (1980)
110	40 Gy/20 Fr	9	12	Hansen et al. (1980)
30	36 Gy/10 Fr	13	73	Eagan et al. (1981)
35	40 Gy/10 Fr	12	44	Katensis et al. (1982)
29	30 Gy/10 Fr	0	27	Jackson et al. (1983)
51	40 Gy/20 Fr	0	27	Niiranen et al. (1989)

world in the early 1990s (ROSENSTEIN et al. 1992; OHONOSHI et al. 1993; SHAW et al. 1994).

12.3 Recent Evidence

The methodological shortcomings of the early reports and growing concern about the continuing clinical dilemma over the cost vs benefits of PCI led to the design and launch of a new wave of randomised trials in the early 1990s. These have now been completed and together have recruited over 1000 patients (OHONOSHI et al. 1993; WAGNER et al. 1996; ARRIAGADA et al. 1995a,b; GREGOR et al. 1997). Patient eligibility criteria reflected the aim of selecting patients with good prospects of long term survival and included as the main determinant "complete" response to induction chemotherapy (Table 12.2). The stage of disease at diagnosis was felt to be less important and only one trial limited entry to patients with no clinical evidence of extra thoracic spread (GREGOR et al. 1997). As detection of small volume metastatic disease closely reflects the staging methodology used, it may be a less important prognostic factor in practice.

Patients were randomised and PCI delivered at the time of achieving clinical remission. This procedure allowed the selection of appropriate patients for entry to the trial and avoided prolonged periods of postradiation chemotherapy, which is thought to potentiate neurotoxicity. The PCI doses were between 20 and 36 Gy in 2–3 Gy fractions. The three large studies (approximately 300 patients each) have reported remarkably consistent results (ARRIAGADA et al. 1995a,b; GREGOR et al. 1997). Two of these incorporated prospective neurological or neurofunctional assessment in their design CPH (ARRIAGADA et al. 1995a) and UK02 (GREGOR et al. 1997).

Table 12.2. Randomised trials of PCI in patients achieving complete response to induction chemotherapy

n	Stage	Induction	PCI dose	Reference
32	LD+ED	CT	30 Gy/10 Fr	ARONEY et al. (1983)
54	LD+ED	CT	24 Gy/8 Fr	HANSEN (personal communication)
46	LD+ED	CT	24 Gy/8 Fr	OHONOSHI et al. (1993)
32	LD+ED	CT+RT	25 Gy/10 Fr	WAGNER et al. (1996)
300	LD+ED	CT+RT	24 Gy/8 Fr	ARRIAGADA et al. (1995a)
211	LD+ED	CT+RT	24–30 Gy/ 8–10 Fr	ARRIAGADA et al. (1995b)
314	LD	CT+-RT	8–36 Gy/ 1–18 Fr	GREGOR et al. (1997)

LD, limited disease; ED, extensive disease; CT, chemotherapy; RT, radiotherapy.

The two French studies CPH = PCI 85 (ARRIAGADA et al. 1995a) and PCI 88 (ARRIAGADA et al. 1995b) ran in parallel. Both randomised PCI against control. PCI 85 had a prescribed dose of 24 Gy in eight fractions, PCI 88 had allowed a choice of radiation schedules but the majority of patients received either the PCI 85 schedule or 30 Gy in ten fractions (Table 12.2). Both trials have shown a highly significant reduction in brain metastases rate – overall from 59% to 40% ($P < 0.0001$) and isolated from 57% to 39% ($P < 0.0001$) in favour of the arm receiving radiation (ARRIAGADA et al. 1995a,b). The prospective radiological and neurological evaluation of the PCI 85 trial demonstrated a low and clinically insignificant rate of radiological abnormalities on CT, and no evidence of dementia or serious clinical CNS morbidity (ARRIAGADA et al. 1995a).

The UK02 (GREGOR et al. 1997) trial was initially designed as a three arm randomisation between control and two dose levels of PCI (24 Gy and 36 Gy in 2 Gy fractions). In the first 3 years it recruited only 100 patients and was therefore re-launched as a two arm study allowing institutional choice of PCI from a selection of schedules. This trial incorporated prospective neuropsychometric assessment for all the patients recruited in three of the participating institutions. The trial closed in 1995 exceeding its planned target with 314 randomised patients. The eligibility criteria remained the same throughout and only patients with limited disease (LTD) and achieving remission following induction chemotherapy were included. A number of different induction regimens were used in this international multicentre study, but all patients had to be randomised within 4 weeks of response assessment. No planned concurrent or post PCI chemotherapy was allowed although concurrent chest irradiation could be given with PCI.

The trial confirmed the effectiveness of PCI in reducing the rate of brain metastases (Fig. 12.1). At 2 years postrandomisation 52% of controls and 29% of PCI patients relapsed in the brain: hazard ratio (HR) = 0.44 (95% CI: 0.27–0.70; $P = 0.0002$). Interest-

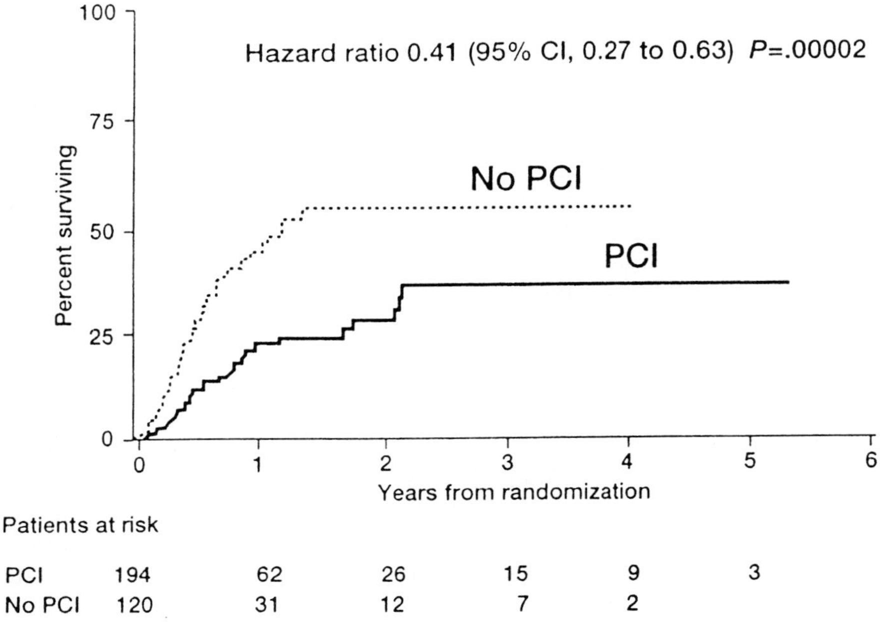

Fig. 12.1. Percentage of patients with brain metastases from randomisation (GREGOR et al. 1997)

ingly in the first 100 patients randomised in a three arm study, the significant advantage of PCI was seen only in the higher dose level (HR = 0.16; 95% CI: 0.07–0.36). The low dose PCI (24 Gy in 12 fractions; 2 Gy per fraction) behaved like the control, i.e. HR = 0.71 (95% CI: 0.36–1.43). The total dose of 24 Gy in the PCI 85 trial, which was significantly better than control (HR = 0.45), was delivered in 8, rather than the 12, fractions. It is possible that larger individual fraction size may increase the effectiveness of radiation schedules with low total doses. This supposition has not been tested and may have the disadvantage of increasing long term morbidity levels. One institutional cohort of patients in the UK02 trial was treated with 8 Gy in a single fraction and did not appear to suffer an increase in late morbidity, although the numbers were too small for a definitive assessment.

The relationship between risk of brain relapse and the different PCI schedules in the UK02 trial can be seen in Fig. 12.2. The radiation schedules have been converted into a biologically equivalent dose (BED) at 2 Gy using a linear quadratic coefficient for acutely reacting tissues or tumour (FOWLER 1989). The confidence intervals of some of the schedules RR are large, as only a few patients received them. For the randomised comparisons (24 Gy in 12 and 36 Gy in 18 fractions) and the large number of patients who were treated with 30 Gy in 10 fractions, the relationship appears linear.

This demonstration of radiation dose response is one of the few clinical examples in SCLC and is a useful contribution to the overall body of evidence governing the use of radiation in this disease. It is also the first time that a relationship between radiation dose and local control could be seen in the setting of brain metastases. The practical implications of this finding need to be confirmed in a larger trial testing formally the question of radiation dose. This is now in preparation.

12.4 Toxicity of Cranial Irradiation and Its Functional Relevance

The effects of therapeutic levels of ionising irradiation on the brain have been well described (SHELINE et al. 1980; LEIBEL and SHELINE 1987; GREGOR et al. 1996). Factors that contribute to the severity and frequency of clinically detectable abnormalities, i.e. radiation dose, fraction size and the volume of brain irradiated, are well recognised. The side effects of brain irradiation with their characteristically delayed time course have been most frequently studied in

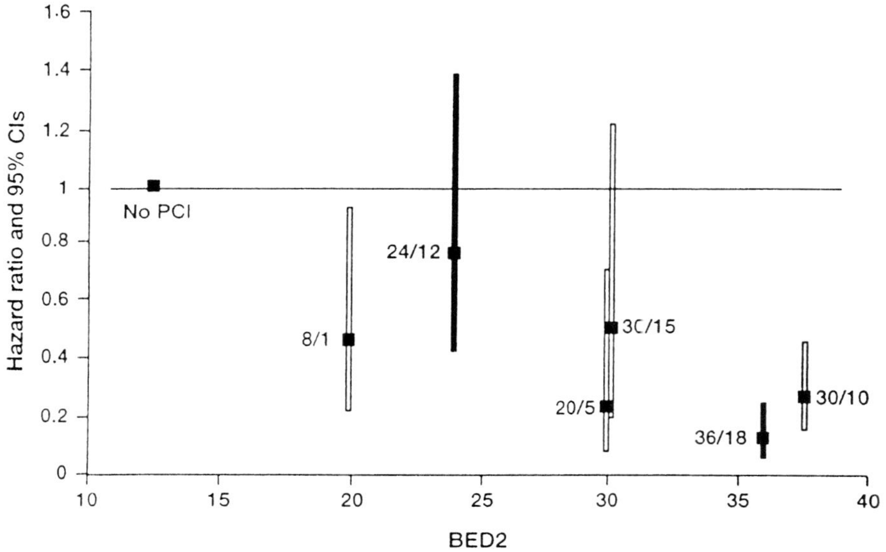

Fig. 12.2. PCI schedules and risk of brain metastases

long term survivors of brain tumours (Gregor et al. 1996; Lishner et al. 1990) particularly children (Ellenberg et al. 1987). The additional insults that chemotherapy can impose on the CNS whether given systemically or intrathecally and with or without cranial irradiation are also well known (Allen et al. 1980; Kaplan and Wiemick 1982; Jellinger 1983; Leff et al. 1988).

Subclinical abnormalities in intellectual functioning can occur following very low doses of cranial irradiation (Mulhern et al. 1988) as has been seen in randomised studies of CNS prophylaxis in paediatric ALL.

Thus the scene was set for potentially serious morbidity when PCI was introduced often without any consideration for these effects in the elderly population of patients with SCLC. They were often treated with concurrent and postirradiation chemotherapy and large individual radiation fractions even in the face of coexisting vascular morbidity.

Early reports of CNS toxicity in long term survivors of SCLC (Catane et al. 1981; Ellison et al. 1982; Looper et al. 1984; Johnson et al. 1985; Lee et al. 1986; Twijnstra et al. 1987) have described the well known and characteristic clinical and radiological features of radiation leucoencephalopathy. These were often reports of institutional or intergroup experiences collected over long periods of time, without any indications of levels of pre-morbid or pre-treatment neurological status. Most of these early patients received PCI as a part of their induction process.

12.4.1 Neuropsychological Morbidity

Clearly the impact of PCI on the higher mental function of long term survivors has remained a matter of major clinical concern. Obtaining adequate assessments of the extent and degree of neuropsychological morbidity following PCI has been problematic.

Clinical examination of mental state is not reliably carried out or systematically documented in routine oncology practice and uncontrolled clinical observations are clearly inadequate as a the sole basis for evaluating neuropsychological morbidity following PCI. Available neurotoxicity rating systems tend to focus on peripheral and sensory functions and provide inadequate coverage of higher mental functions (Castellanos and Fields 1986). Cognitive screening instruments, e.g. the Mini Mental State Examination (Folstein et al. 1975), typically have a high false negative rate (Nelson et al. 1986) and are not sensitive enough to be useful in this research setting.

Objective testing using standardised neuropsychometric assessment procedures offers a non-invasive and sensitive method of obtaining information about higher mental function. Neuropsychological assessment has increasingly been seen as an important adjuvant to clinical and imaging data in the outcome evaluation of PCI.

Three of the early reports included neuropsychometric testing as an outcome measure (JOHNSON et al. 1985; TWIJNSTRA et al. 1987; LAUKKANEN et al. 1988). Among other limitations, these retrospective studies were all restricted in sample size. The larger samples needed could be derived by multicentre collaboration but this poses the problem of the feasibility of administering neuropsychological measures in centres where no psychologist is available.

This problem was addressed in an international collaboration to review the outcome for 64 SCLC patients, surviving for ≥2 years after their induction treatment (CULL et al. 1994). A trained psychologist prepared detailed instructions for the use of four standard neuropsychological tests which were then administered by non-psychologists in the clinic setting. The assessment methods chosen proved acceptable to patients and feasible for clinic staff to administer. Testing, which took about 20 min, proved sensitive to otherwise undetected deficits of cognitive function and 54% of the sample were found to be impaired on two or more of the tests used.

Neuropsychological testing was also included in a study of the outcome for long term survivors (>2 years) of SCLC in the Netherlands (VAN OOSTERHOUT et al. 1996). The cognitive functioning of three groups of patients was assessed: those who had (a) no PCI, (b) PCI after chemotherapy or (c) PCI concurrent with/sandwiched by chemotherapy; and compared with a control group of healthy subjects matched for age and educational level. A comprehensive assessment battery was used, administered by a psychologist. All the patient groups performed significantly worse than the controls but no significant differences were found between the three patient groups, i.e. there was no evidence for additional neurotoxicity of treatment with PCI. No other treatment variables relating to the chemotherapy or radiation schedules were shown to have an effect on individual cognitive function. The authors concluded their findings were disease related rather than treatment related, although they offered no positive evidence for this.

The obvious and acknowledged limitations of these studies which lack a baseline (pre-PCI) assessment were further reinforced by data suggesting that a high proportion of SCLC patients have cognitive dysfunction prior to PCI (KOMAKI et al. 1995; MEYERS et al. 1995). This group used a comprehensive battery of neuropsychological measures to assess 30 patients with limited SCLC, before and after PCI. Of 21 patients with no prior history of neurological disorder or substance abuse, 20 showed comparable levels of impairment to the remaining 9 patients who did have such a prior history. Deficits in verbal memory were the most commonly occurring impairment followed by frontal lobe dysfunction and fine motor in-coordination. The short term (6–20 months) follow-up data available after PCI showed no significant deterioration in patients' performance from pre-PCI levels.

A further study from the same group (MEYERS et al. 1995) attempted to assess whether these deficits were related to chemoradiation treatment. The authors compared the performance of newly diagnosed, untreated patients with that of patients who had achieved a complete response to induction therapy assessed before PCI. They found no significant difference between the groups on any of the neuropsychological tests used and suggested further studies should focus on characterising the aetiology of these deficits. Rejecting the role of chemotherapy, microscopic brain metastases and mood disturbance in the cognitive impairment they observed, MEYERS et al. (1995) proposed that paraneoplastic phenomena should be studied further in this context.

The first randomised trial of PCI to include prospective assessment of neurological morbidity (ARRIAGADA et al. 1995a) reported 59% (of 229 patients) showed some abnormality at baseline. The data were not reported in detail and the abnormalities which were specifically referred to (i.e. in taste, smell and hearing) were attributed to chemotherapy. Within the first 5 years of follow-up no significant differences in neuropsychological function were found between those who had and those who had not had PCI.

The UK02 trial (GREGOR et al. 1997) was the first to include a prospective formal evaluation of patients' neuropsychological functioning. At baseline, i.e. pre-PCI, 78% of patients ($n = 125$) showed impairment on ≥1 of the 4 tests used. Although there was some evidence of new impairment on retest at 6 months and 1 year, the sample size was limited in these follow-up assessments. There was no evidence of sustained deterioration over time and no significant difference between the PCI and no PCI groups at these relatively early follow-up points.

Although neuropsychological assessment offers the most sensitive means of calibrating impairment in higher mental function, there are some practical and organisational difficulties in employing this approach in multicentre trials in this setting, particularly in an international context.

It is characteristic of psychometric assessment that the procedures to be followed in administering performance tests are standardised. However, international trials require that the tests used have been validated in translation in the appropriate languages for the participating centres. This may limit the choice of suitable measures. It has been demonstrated that some assessment tools are suitable for cross-cultural use and can be satisfactorily administered by non-psychologists in the clinic (CULL et al. 1994). Some centres may nonetheless be unable to identify personnel to take on this extra work. Computer-administered assessment systems are available for neuropsychometric testing but they are expensive and may not be a priority in the clinical setting in which SCLC patients are treated. Where outcome data are derived from only a proportion of centres participating in a trial, there is always the danger that the data will be seriously biased in some way, particularly if the selection of that subset of contributing centres is non-random.

Experience of published studies to date suggest that many centres have the capacity to organise a single neuropsychological assessment whether for a single follow-up of long term survivors of PCI (CULL et al. 1994) or a pre-treatment baseline (GREGOR et al. 1997). What is problematic is obtaining good quality data over repeated time points. High levels of attrition are to be expected as patients become too ill to be assessed or die. With small numbers of survivors these assessment procedures do not become routine for the participating centres. Furthermore, clinical follow-up may occur at a different location from the pre-treatment assessment. It has proved difficult in longitudinal studies to ensure that the staff who have been trained to do the neuropsychological assessments are available when the long term survivors present for follow-up. Thus further data are commonly lost through system failures.

Future large scale studies may find it more practical to evaluate the outcome of PCI in terms of its impact on patients' capacity to function in their everyday lives.

12.4.2 Quality of Life Assessment

There are several advantages to including quality of life (QL) assessment in the outcome of evaluation of PCI. By definition health related QL is a multidimensional concept requiring subjective evaluation. The patient self-report instruments which have been developed to measure QL typically include aspects of patients' experience that would otherwise be ignored yet which may be highly relevant to their cognitive efficiency. For example, fatigue and sleeping difficulties are commonly reported by newly diagnosed lung cancer patients (SILBERFARB et al. 1993; HOPWOOD et al. 1995) and long term survivors of SCLC (CULL et al. 1994). Similarly it may be relevant to screen for anxiety and depression. Using a standard screening questionnaire – the Hospital Anxiety and Depression Scale – HOPWOOD and THATCHER (1990) found 36% of their sample of 283 cancer patients scored as probable cases of anxiety and depression. Among cancer patients generally those who report concentration and memory difficulties have been found to have significantly higher scores on measures of anxiety depression and fatigue (CULL et al. 1996).

The value of quality of life data as an outcome measure is increasingly recognised in lung cancer clinical trials. There are undoubted advantages in collecting such data in having an assessment strategy which allows some commonality of measurement across trials and hence a means of comparing or combining data. Quality of life measurement initiated at the start of induction chemotherapy could then continue, using essentially the same approach, for monitoring the progress of patients proceeding to PCI. Supplementary questions, specific to each treatment setting, could be added to this generic core database as required.

There are currently two quality of life instruments which offer this approach – the EORTC QLQ-C30 (AARONSON et al. 1993) and the Functional Assessment of Cancer Therapy – FACT (CELLA et al. 1993). Both of these are multidimensional quality of life questionnaires designed for generic use with cancer patients and both have supplementary modules for lung cancer patients (CELLA 1992; BERGMAN et al. 1994). Validated translations of these instruments are available in a wide range of languages. As yet no supplementary questionnaire has been validated to assess the specific side effects which may arise from PCI. The ad hoc questionnaire developed by LISHNER et al. (1990) may be a useful starting point, but the best developed is probably the module designed to supplement the EORTC QLQ-C30 in evaluating the outcome of treatment for brain cancer (OSOBA et al. 1996). The EORTC QLQ-C30 has a two item scale assessing concentration/memory. The brain cancer module assesses disturbances in visual and motor functions and in communication together with a number of other relevant symptoms but it does not ask supplementary questions about higher mental function. Although questionnaires have been developed to assess memory failures in everyday life (e.g. BROADBENT et al. 1981; SUNDERLAND et al. 1984), there is clearly a problem in seeking a reliable valid account of memory failure by patient self-report alone. Self-report data have generally been found to correlate poorly with performance on objective testing (CULL et al. 1996).

Whether neuropsychological morbidity following PCI is objectively tested or subjectively reported, the clinically important issue is to assess the impact of those side effects on the patient's capacity to function in everyday life. Only two studies of PCI outcomes have attempted to include systematic quality of life assessment (CULL et al. 1994; GREGOR et al. 1997). Both these studies experienced system failures in data collection in some centres. In both, the assessment strategy included both QL assessment and neuropsychological testing. It may be more realistic in future to think of restricting outcome evaluation to QL assessment. There is well documented evidence from the NCI – Canada that where clinicians are motivated to participate in QL studies excellent quality data can be collected in multicentre trials even from patients with advanced disease (SADURA et al. 1992).

12.5 Summary and Practical Recommendations

1. PCI is effective in significantly reducing brain metastases with no significant evidence of serious morbidity for the majority of patients treated.

2. The benefit of a significant reduction in the rate of appearance of brain metastases appears to be greatest in patients achieving good response to induction chemotherapy. Patients with limited and extensive disease can benefit, but the advantage is larger for those surviving longest.

3. All three of the large recent trials (ARRIAGADA et al. 1995a,b; GREGOR et al. 1995) have shown a small but consistent survival benefit which is being quantified in a meta-analysis. The largest benefit is likely to be seen in patients with good and durable systemic disease control.

4. The optimal radiation dose has not been determined, but on the current evidence 36 Gy in 18 fractions appears to be most effective. Doses below 30 Gy in 2-Gy fractions are probably suboptimal, but their effectiveness could be increased by larger fraction size. Regimens such as 24 Gy in eight fractions or 30 Gy in ten fractions have been most commonly used in practice.

5. In addition to dose and fractionation in a radiation schedule, the timing of the administration of PCI is a key variable. The wish is to introduce PCI as early as possible in the course of treatment, having established chemotherapy response to aid the selection of appropriate patients. It is also important to avoid concurrent administration (and to lesser degree subsequent prolonged courses) of chemotherapy. It is those two features which have characterised some of the earlier treatment regimens associated with serious neurotoxicity (CATANE et al. 1981; JOHNSON et al. 1985).

Brain irradiation disrupts the blood brain barrier and thus can potentiate serious toxicity by allowing chemotherapy access to otherwise protected areas of the brain (DAVELLA et al. 1992). Delaying administration of PCI beyond 6 months from diagnosis appears to compromise its effectiveness although no randomised comparisons of timing of PCI are available. A pragmatic and practical solution consistent with the current approach of aiming to intensify and shorten the overall treatment duration in SCLC will be to introduce PCI at the end of induction therapy, within the window of the first 3–5 months from diagnosis and start of treatment.

6. Objective testing remains the method of choice for assessing neuropsychometric morbidity. It is vital that baseline assessment, pre PCI, is undertaken and further research is needed to understand the aetiology of cognitive impairment in patients with SCLC from their first presentation. There is a continuing need for longer periods of follow-up in larger samples of long term survivors to provide a clearer evaluation of the prevalence and extent of neuropsychological morbidity for SCLC patients receiving PCI according to contemporary protocols.

7. The current research agenda requires large scale international multicentre collaboration. In practice, neuropsychological assessment is unlikely to be feasible in all the centres which could participate in the next generation of PCI trials. A pragmatic clinically valuable solution would be to concentrate instead on obtaining good data on QL outcomes using an instrument such as the EORTC QLQ-C30, which has been well validated for use in international clinical trials in oncology.

12.6 Future Developments

The challenge is to determine the optimal radiation schedule. The first test will be a straightforward dose escalation which can be performed easily in a multicentre and international multigroup setting. This will set out to confirm the dose response findings of previous trials (GREGOR et al. 1995) and test a new set of functional and QL measures. The endpoints will be brain metastases free survival and QL.

The issue of timing of PCI administration does not lend itself easily to such a global setting and may need to be taken up by smaller research networks willing to use a single chemotherapy induction regimen and prescriptive combined modality treatment schedules. The use of hyperfractionated radiation schedules is interesting for the potential to reduce CNS toxicity. Acceleration would allow shorter treatment times with increased therapeutic intensity. These may need to wait for a third generation of PCI trials. As the relationships between benefit and toxicity become even more complex, it is important that any moves from classical schedules are conducted in carefully controlled and evaluated settings. Otherwise we risk once again creating a pool of patients with potentially devastating late morbidity.

We must assess the contribution that PCI could make to palliation of patients with poor prognosis SCLC. Their rate of brain metastases is similar. Prevention by using a simple schedule of irradiation at the time of chemotherapy response may be helpful. This would need a randomised comparison between PCI and control with a suitable endpoint such as functional independence.

As concern grows about the need to find a rational basis for resource allocation in health care, there is likely to be an increased effort made to develop and refine methods of combining quality of life and survival time into a simple index to facilitate evaluation. The Q-Twist, (GELBER et al. 1993), which considers quality adjusted time without symptoms or toxicity, may be one such promising approach which could be adapted for use in this setting.

In the balance that determines the overall indications for, and benefit of, any therapeutic intervention it is necessary to critically evaluate the evidence critically, to identify its shortcomings and gaps and be prepared to move forward step by step building the picture for clinical use. The story of PCI is an example of what is possible by adopting this approach. Future studies will address the unknowns in a systematic and collaborative manner speeding up the process of assessment and bringing practical benefits as well as increasing our understanding of this disease and its various treatments.

References

Aaronson NK, Ahmedzai S, Bergman B (1993) The European Organization for Research and Treatment of Cancer QLQ-C30: a quality of life instrument for use in international clinical trials in oncology. J Nat Cancer Inst 85(5):365–376

Allen JC, Rosen G, Mehta BM, Horten B (1980) Leukoencephalopathy following high dose IV methotrexate chemotherapy with leukovorin rescue. Cancer Treat Rep 64:1261–1273

Aroney RS, Aisner J, Wesley MN, Whiteacre MY, Van Echo DA, Slawson RG, Wiernik PH (1983) Value of prophylactic cranial irradiation given at complete remission in small cell lung carcinoma Cancer Treat Rep 1983:675–682

Arriagada R, Le Chavalier T, Borie F et al (1995a) Prophylactic cranial irradiation for patients with small cell lung cancer in complete remission. J Natl Cancer Inst 87:183–190

Arriagada R, Monnet I, Riviére A, Santos-Maranda JA, Laplanche A, the PCI85–PCI88 trialists (1995b) Prophylactic cranial irradiation (PCI) for patients (pts) with small cell lung cancer (SCLC) in complete response (CR) (abstract) Eur J Cancer 31A[Suppl 5]:S19

Beiker DD, Kane RC, Bernath AM, Cashdollar MR (1979) Low dose elective brain irradiation in small cell carcinoma of the lung. Int J Radiat Oncol Biol Phys 5:941–945

Bergman B, Aaronson NK, Ahmedzai S, Kaasa S, Sullivan M for the EORTC QL Study Group (1994) The EORTC QLQ-LC13: a modular supplement to the EORTC Core Quality of Life Questionnaire (QLQ-C30) for use in lung cancer clinical trials. Eur J Cancer 30A(5):635–642

Bleyer WA, Poplack DG (1985) Prophylaxis and treatment of leukaemia in the central nervous system and other sanctuaries. Semin Oncol 12:131–148

Broadbent DE, Cooper PF, fitzgerald P, Parkes KR (1981) The Cognitive Failures Questionnaire and its correlates. Br J Clin Psychol 21:1–16

Bunn PA, Rosen ST (1985) Central nervous system manifestations of small cell lung cancer. In: Aisner J (ed) Lung cancer. Churchill Livingstone, New York, pp 287–305

Carmichael J, Crane JM, Bunn PA, Glastein E, Ihde DC (1988) Results of therapeutic cranial irradiation in small cell lung cancer. Int J Radiat Oncol Biol Phys 14:455–459

Castellanos AM, Fields WS (1986) Grading of neurotoxicity in cancer therapy J Clin Oncol 4:1277–1278

Catane R, Schwade JG, Yarr I (1981) Follow-up neurological evaluation in patients with small cell lung carcinoma treated with prophylactic cranial irradiation and chemotherapy. Int J Radiat Oncol Biol Phys 7:105–109

Cella D (1992) Functional Assessment of Cancer Therapy (FACT) Scales: Manual, Center on Outcomes Research and Education, Evanston, Illinois

Cella DF, Tulsky DS, Gray G et al (1993) The functional Assessment of Cancer Therapy Scale: development and validation of the general measure. J Clin Oncol 11:570–579

Cox JD, Petrovich Z, Paig C, Stanley K (1978) Prophylactic cranial irradiation in patients with inoperable carcinoma of the lung. Cancer 42:1135–1140

Crossen JR, Garwood D, Glatstein E, Neuwelt EA (1994) Neurobehavioural sequelae of cranial irradiation in adults: a review of radiation induced encephalopathy. J Clin Oncol 12:627–642

Cull A, Gregor A, Hopwood P et al (1994) Neurological and cognitive impairment in long-term survivors of small-cell lung cancer. Eur J Cancer 30A:8:1067–1074

Cull A, Hay C, Love SB, Mackie M, Smets E, Stewart M (1996) What do cancer patients mean when they complain of concentration and memory problems? Br J Cancer 74:1674–79

Davella D, Cicciarello R, Albiero F, Mesiti M, Gogliardi ME, Daquino A (1992) Quantitative study of blood brain barrier permeability changes after experimental whole brain irradiation. Neurosurgery 30:30–34

Eagan RT, Frytak S, Lee RE, Creagan ET, Ingle JN, Nichols WC (1981) A case for preplanned thoracic and prophylactic whole brain radiation therapy in limited small cell lung cancer. Cancer Clin Trials 4:261–266

Ellenberg L, McComb JG, Siegel SE, Stowe S (1987) Factors affecting intellectual outcome in paediatric brain tumour patients. Neurosurgery 21(5):638–644

Ellison N, Bernath A, Kane R, Porter P (1982) Disturbing problems of success: clinical status of long term survivors of small cell lung cancer (SCLC) ASCO abstracts, C-579 149

Felletti R, Souhami RL, Spiro SG (1985) Social consequences of brain or liver relapse in small cell carcinomas of the bronchus. Radiother Oncol 4:335–339

Fleck JF, Ginhorn LH, Lauer RC, Schultz SM, Miller ME (1990) Is prophylactic cranial irradiation indicated in small cell lung cancer? J Clin Oncol 8:209–214

Folstein MF, Folstein SE, McHugh PR (1975) Mini mental state: a practical method for grading the cognitive state of patients for the clinician. J Psychiatr Res 12:189–198

Fowler JF (1989) The linear-quadratic formula and progress in fractionated radiotherapy. Br J Radiol 62:679–694

Gelber RD, Goldhirsch A, Cole BF (1993) Evaluation of effectiveness: Q-Twist. Cancer Treat Rev 19[Suppl A]:73–84

Gregor A, Cull A, Traynor E, Stewart M, Lander F, Love S (1996) Neuropsychometric evaluation of longterm survivors of adult brain tumours: relationship with tumour and treatment parameters. Radiother Oncol 41:55–59

Gregor A, Cull A, Stephens RJ, Kirkpatrick JA, Yarnold JR, Girling DJ, Macbeth FR, Stout R, Machin D (1997) Prophylactic cranial irradiation is indicated following complete response to induction therapy in small cell lung cancer: results of a multicentre randomised trial. Eur J Cancer 33(11):1752–1758

Hansen HH, Dombernowsky P, Hirsch FR et al (1980) Prophylactic irradiation in bronchogenic small cell anaplastic carcinoma. A comparative trial of localized versus extensive radiotherapy including prophylactic brain irradiation in patients receiving combination chemotherapy. Cancer 46:279–284

Hopwood P, Thatcher N (1990) Preliminary experience with quality of life evaluation in patients with lung cancer. Oncology 4:158–162

Hopwood P, Stephens R for the Medical Research Council Lung Cancer Working Party (1995) Symptoms at presentation in patients with lung cancer: implications for the evaluation of palliative treatment. Br J Cancer 71(3):633–636

Jackson DV, Richards F II, Cooper MR et al (1983) Prophylactic cranial irradiation in small 237(25):2730–2733

Jellinger K (1983) Pathologic effects of chemotherapy. In: Walker MD (ed) Oncology of the nervous system. Nijhoff, Boston, pp 285–340

Jenson OM, Estéve J, Moller H, Renard H (1990) Cancer in the European Community and its member states. Eur J Cancer 26:1167–1256

Johnson BE, Becker B, Goff WB et al (1985) Neurologic neuropsychologic and computer cranial tomography scan abnormalities in 2 to 10 year survivors of small cell lung cancer. J Clin Oncol 3:1659–1667

Kaplan RS, Wiemick PH (1982) Neurotoxicity of anti-neoplastic drugs. Semin Oncol 9:103–120

Katensis AT, Karpastis N, Giannakakis D et al (1982) Elective brain irradiation in patients with small cell carcinoma of the lung: a preliminary report. Excerpta Medica, Amsterdam, pp 277–284 (Lung Cancer International Congress series no 558)

Komaki R, Meyers CA, Shin DM et al (1995) Evaluation of cognitive function in patients with limited small cell lung cancer prior to and shortly following prophylactic cranial irradiation. Int J Radiat Oncol Biol Phys 33(1):179–182

Laukkanen E, Klonoff H, Allan B, Graeb D, Murray N (1988) The role of prophylactic brain irradiation in limited stage small cell lung cancer: clinical neuropsychological and CT sequelae. Int J Radiat Oncol Biol Phys 14:1109–1117

Lee JS, Umswardi T, Lee YY, Barkley HT, Murphy WK, Welch S et al (1986) Neurotoxicity in long term survivors of small cell lung cancer. Int J Radiat Oncol Biol Phys 12:313–321

Leff RS, Thompson JM, Daly MB, Johnson DB, Harden EA, Mercier RJ, Messerschmidt GL (1988) Acute neurologic dysfunction after high-dose etoposide therapy for malignant glioma. Cancer 62:32–35

Leibel SA, Sheline GE (1987) Tolerance of the central and peripheral nervous system to therapeutic irradiation. In: Lett JT, Altman KI (eds) Advances in radiation biology. Academic, New York, pp 257–288

Lishner M, Feld R, Payne DG et al (1990) Late neurological complications after prophylactic cranial irradiation in patients with small cell lung cancer: the Toronto experience. J Clin Oncol 8:215–221

Looper JD, Ginhom LH, Carcia SA, Homback NB, Vincent B, Williams SD (1984) Severe neurological problems following successful therapy for small cell lung cancer. ASCO abstracts C-903

Lucas CF, Robinson B, Hoskin PJ, Yarnold JR, Smith IE, Ford HT (1986) Morbidity of cranial relapse in small cell lung cancer and the impact of radiation therapy. Cancer Treat Rep 70:565–570

Maurer LH, Tulloh M, Weiss RB, Blom J, Leone L, Glidwell O, Pajak TF (1980) A randomized combined modality trail in small cell carcinoma of the lung: comparison of combination chemotherapy-radiation therapy versus cyclophosphamide-radiation therapy effects of maintenance chemotherapy and prophylactic whole brain irradiation. Cancer 45:30–39

Meyers CA, Byrne KS, Komaki R (1995) Cognitive deficits in patients with small cell lung cancer before and after chemotherapy. Lung Cancer 12(3):231–235

Mulhern RK, Wasserman AL, Fairclough D, Ochs J (1988) Memory function in disease-free survivors of childhood acute lymphocytic leukaemia given CNS prophylaxis with or without 1800 cGy cranial irradiation. J Clinical Oncology 6:315–320

Nelson A, Fogel S, Faust D (1986) Bedside cognitive screening instruments. J Nerv Ment Dis 2:73–83

Niiranen A, Holsti P, Salmo M (1989) Treatment of small cell lung cancer. Two-drug versus four-drug chemotherapy and loco-regional irradiation with or without prophylactic cranial irradiation. Acta Oncol 28:501–505

Ohonoshi T, Ueoka H, Kawahara S et al (1993) Comparative study of prophylactic cranial irradiation in patients with small cell lung cancer achieving a complete response. Lung Cancer 10:47–54

Osoba D, Aaronson NK, Muller M et al (1996) The development and psychometric validation of a brain cancer quality of life questionniare for use in combination with general cancer specific questionnaires. Qual Life Res 5:139–150

Pedersen AG (1986) Diagnosis of CNS-metastases from SCLC. In: Hansen HH (ed) Lung Cancer: basic and clinical aspects. Nijhoff, Boston, pp 153–182

Pedersen AG, Kristjansen PEG, Hansen HH (1988) Prophylactic Cranial Irradition and Small Cell Lung Cancer. Cancer Treat. Rev. 15:85–103.

Pignon JP, Arriagada R, Ihde D et al (1992) A meta-analysis of thoracic radiotherapy for small cell lung cancer. N Engl J Med 327:1618–1624

Postmus PE, Sleijfer DT, Haasma-Rieche H (1989) Chemotherapy for central nervous system metastases from SCLC. A review. Lung Cancer 5:254–263

Rosenstein M, Armstrong J, Kris M et al (1992) A reappraisal of the role of prophylactic cranial irradiation in limited small cell lung cancer. Int J Radiat Oncol Biol Phys 24:43–48

Sadura A, Pater J, Osoba D et al (1992) Quality of life assessment: patient compliance with questionnaire completion. J Nat Cancer Inst 84:1023–1026

Seydel HG, Creech R, Pagano M (1985) Prophylactic versus no brain irradiation in regional small cell lung carcinoma. Am J Clin Oncol 8:218–223

Shaw EG, Su JQ, Eagan RT, Jeff JR, Makysmik AW, Deigert FA (1994) Prophylactic cranial irradiation in complete responders with small cell lung cancer: analysis of the Mayo Clinic and North Central Cancer Treatment Group data bases. J Clin Oncol 12:2327–2332

Sheline GE, Wara WM, Smith V (1980) Therapeutic irradiation and brain injury. Int J Radiat Oncol Biol Phys 6(9):1215–1228

Silberfarb PM, Hauri PJ, Oxman TE, Schnurr P (1993) Assessment of sleep in patients with lung cancer and breast cancer. J Clin Oncol 11:997–1004

Sunderland A, Harris HE, Gleave J (1984) Memory failures in everyday life following severe head injury. J Clin Neuropychol 6:127–142

Twijnstra A, Boon PJ, Lormans ACM, Ten Velde GPN (1987) Neurotoxicity of prophylactic cranial irradiation in patients with small cell carcinoma of the lung. Eur J Cancer Clin Oncol 23(7):983–986

Van Oosterhout AG, Ganzevles PG, Wilmink JT, De Gues BW, Van Vonderen RG, Twijnstra A (1996) Sequelae in long terms survivors of small cell lung cancer. J Rad Oncol Biol Phys 34(5):1037–1044

Wagner H Jr, Kim K, Turrisi II A et al for the Eastern Cooperative Oncology Group and Radiation Therapy Oncology Group (1996) A randomized Phase III Study of prophylactic cranial irradiation (PCI) vs observation (OBS) in patients (Pts) with small cell lung cancer (SCLC) achieving a complete response: final report of an incomplete trial by Eastern Cooperative Oncology Group and Radiation Therapy Oncology Group (E3589/R92-01) (abstract). Proc Am Soc Clin Oncol 15:376

13 Fractionation as a Biological Dose Modifier

M.I. Saunders

CONTENTS

13.1 Introduction

Non-small cell lung cancer remains the commonest cause of cancer death in men, and the second in women. Disease often presents late, with inoperable tumour in the chest and a high chance of occult distant metastases. Despite radical treatment with radiotherapy and chemotherapy, it is estimated that over 80% of patients die with disease in their chest (Cox 1991) As control of the primary tumour is a pre-requisite for long term survival, radiation oncologists have concentrated on novel fractionation schedules as a method of altering the biological effect of the irradiation given, attempting to improve local tumour control with reduced long term side-effects.

Throughout Europe and southern England, radical radiotherapy in non-small cell lung cancer involves the use of daily fractionated radiotherapy, given Monday to Friday, over 6–7 weeks; 2 Gy is given per day to a total dose of 60–70 Gy. In Canada and in northern England, routine radical radiotherapy employs a different schedule: once again daily fractionation is given Monday to Friday, but the overall time is shortened to 3–4 weeks, the dose per fraction raised to enable a total dose of 50–55 Gy to be achieved.

When modifying fractionation schedules, the ultimate goal is to improve local tumour control, reduce morbidity and thus have the possibility of improving overall survival. Two strategies will be discussed: (1) hyperfractionation and (2) accelerated fractionation – both of these approaches aim to increase the biological effect of the radiotherapy, the first by modifying its effect on normal tissues, and the second by attempting to control tumour cell proliferation more effectively than previously. These studies highlight the interfraction interval as an important modifier of the effect of radiation. As will be seen, some of the aspects of hyperfractionation are incorporated into accelerated fractionation schedules.

M.I. Saunders, Marie Curie Research Wing, Mount Vernon Hospital, Northwood, Middlesex HA6 2RN, UK

13.2 Hyperfractionation

In treating non-small cell lung cancer, many normal tissues are encompassed in the field of irradiation: the early reacting tissues include the skin and mucosa of the aero-digestive tract; the late reacting tissues, lung, spinal cord and soft tissues of the mediastinum. In the early 1970s, it was postulated that there was a difference in response to changes in dose per fraction between early and late responding tissues: the early responding tissues react to an increase in dose per fraction in a linear fashion (the alpha effect α), as does tumour, but late responding tissues react differently with a greater increase in cell kill as the dose per fraction was raised (the quadratic or beta effect β) (Fig. 13.1). These hypotheses were embodied in the linear quadratic formula, championed by Barendsen and Fowler, $E = nd\ (1 + d/\alpha/\beta)$ (where E = effect, n = number of fractions, d = dose given per fraction and α and β are the linear and quadratic coefficients) (Barendsen 1982; Fowler 1984a, 1989). If, therefore, the dose per fraction is decreased, and the total dose maintained, there should be a reduction in late morbidity. This gave a therapeutic window whereby the total dose could be raised to give equal late morbidity with the possibility of an increase in local tumour control. Thus in hyperfractionated schedules, the dose per fraction is less than 1.8–2.0 Gy, more than one fraction is given

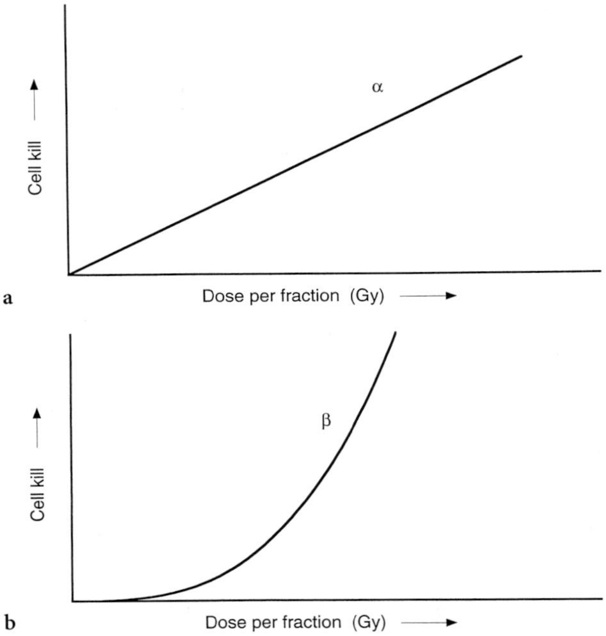

Fig. 13.1 a,b. Relationship of cell kill to dose per fraction. **a** Early reacting tissues and tumour α and **b** late reacting tissues β

per day (a necessity to achieve the total dose), the overall time is kept relatively constant and the total dose is raised.

When giving more than one fraction per day, the interfraction interval has to be carefully considered to allow for as much repair of sublethal injury as possible in normal tissues. The proportion of recoverable damage is less in tumours and acutely responding tissues than in the late responding tissues (Fowler 1984; Thames 1985). Moreover, the time for repair of sublethal injury also varies from tissue to tissue and in each, more than one process with differing time courses may be involved. The half times of repair were thought generally to be in the range of 30–120 min. In a compromise between gaining the maximum amount of repair and the practical considerations of organisation within a department, interfraction intervals of 4 h were often employed.

The RTOG carried out extensive studies of hyperfractionation. In the late 1970s, a pilot study designed to identify the appropriate fraction size in twice daily treatment in squamous cell carcinoma of the head and neck revealed that 1.5 Gy per fraction, twice daily, produced acute severe mucositis requiring treatment interruption, whereas 1.25 Gy twice per day was tolerated to 60 Gy without a break (Marks et al. 1978). In 1983, phase I and II trials were instituted in locally advanced non-small cell lung cancer. Based on the pilot studies in head and neck cancer, a dose of 1.2 Gy twice per day with a 4–8 h interfraction interval was selected. A randomised dose escalation trial was designed to allow the dose limiting effects of normal tissues to be taken into account during the study. Concurrent randomisation to the initial three dose arms of 60 Gy, 64.8 Gy and 69.6 Gy gave acceptable toxicity and the dose was raised to 74.4 Gy and 79.2 Gy. Treatment was given 5 days/week: 50.4 Gy was given to the primary tumour and regional lymphatics after which known tumour only was boosted to the total dose assigned at randomisation. All pre-treatment characteristics were well balanced amongst the five dose groups. There was no significant difference in the incidence of acute or late toxicity despite a 30% difference in total dose. The response rates were not assessed and all deaths were recorded as treatment failures. Despite the increase in dose, there was no difference in survival with dose escalation (Cox et al. 1990) (Fig. 13.2). This result could mean that maximum local control was achieved with 69.6 Gy or that treatment related toxicity mimicking tumour progression may have been scored as tumour related deaths and not toxicity (Byhardt 1995).

At the time of publication of these results, the Cancer and Leukaemia Group B (CALGB) published their results of a randomised controlled trial of conventional radiotherapy versus conventional radiotherapy with chemotherapy, which gave a survival advantage to the chemotherapy arm (Dillman et al. 1990). The RTOG re-analysed their data and found that if they used the same selection criteria as the CALGB, namely good performance status, stage III patients with <5% weight loss, then the 12- and 24-month survival rates were higher with the 69.6-Gy dose than with the lower doses ($P = 0.02$), with no survival differences between the two highest doses. Moreover, the 1- and 2-year survivals of this group were equivalent to that of the chemotherapy study: 56% and 29% for hyperfractionation to 69.6 Gy, compared with 55% and 24% for the combined modality treatment respectively (Cox et al. 1990).

These results established 69.6 Gy as the most desirable dose to achieve in the treatment of non-small cell lung cancer with hyperfractionated radiotherapy. Subsequently the RTOG has focused on the addition of chemotherapy to hyperfractionated and conventional treatment. The combined regimes were tolerable and indeed gave results comparable to that of conventional radiotherapy with chemotherapy

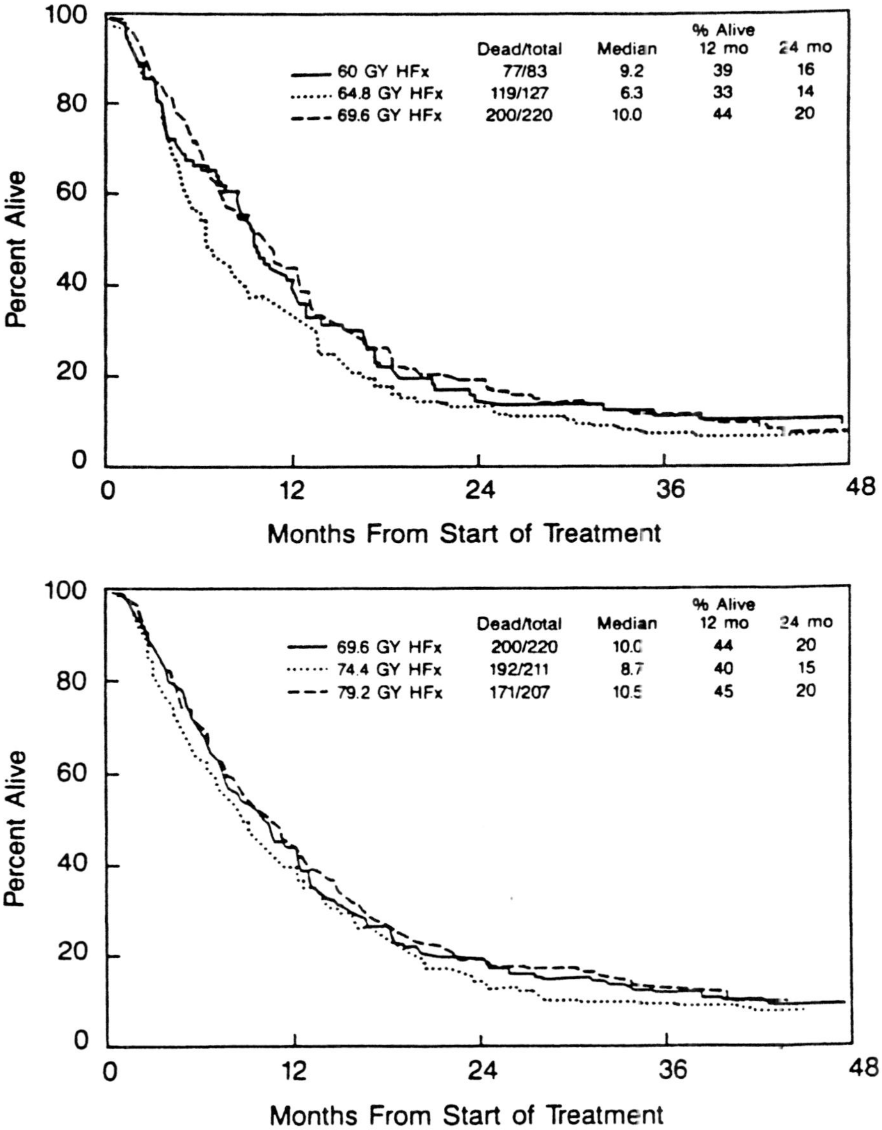

Fig. 13.2 a,b. NSCLC survival based on assigned treatment groups in RTOG 83-11. **a** Lower three doses. **b** Higher three doses. (Cox et al. 1990)

(Byhardt et al. 1995). In Europe, JEREMIC and his colleagues instituted a randomised study of hyperfractionated radiotherapy 1.2 Gy twice daily to a total dose of 69.6 Gy with or without chemotherapy consisting of carboplatin and etoposide given daily. The study showed the combination of hyperfractionated radiotherapy and low dose chemotherapy was tolerable and improved the survival of patients with stage III non-small cell lung cancer as a result of improved local tumour control (Jeremic et al. 1996).

Thus future research is now focusing on the scheduling of chemotherapy to hyperfractionated radiotherapy without any further developments of these radiation schedules.

13.3 Accelerated Radiotherapy

Volume doubling times of tumours are slow and have been estimated for non-small cell lung cancer to extend over many months (Steel 1977). When, however, the cell kinetics of individual tumour cells was studied, it was demonstrated that they were in fact dividing rapidly (Wilson et al. 1988). Bromodeoxyuridine (BrdUrd) is a chemotherapeutic drug which is incorporated into the S phase (Ts) of the cell cycle. If a low dose of BrdUrd is given to a patient, and a biopsy performed immediately, the number of cells in S phase, that is the labelling index (LI), can be estimated. If a gap of 4–6 h is allowed to pass between injection and biopsy, then using flow cytometry and immunohistochemistry, the passage of BrdUrd labelled cells through the cell cycle can be followed and the time of S phase (Ts) estimated (BEGG et al. 1985). From this the potential doubling time (Tpot) can be calculated from the formula Tpot = α LI/Ts. The mean Tpot for non-small cell lung cancer is 7.3 days. Rapid potential doubling times were also found in other tumours - head and neck, cervix, oesophagus and bowel - and led to the hypothesis that tumours could repopulate during a course of radiotherapy (BENNETT et al. 1992).

In an unperturbed tumour, 90% of the progeny of each cell division dies, giving a high cell loss factor which accounts for the difference between the volume doubling time and potential doubling time of human tumours (DENEKAMP 1982). This high cell loss factor is thought to be due to the tumour cells being deprived of oxygen and nutrients as the size of the tumour increases. When, however, an effective treatment is given and a large number of tumour cells are killed, blood supply to the tumour is restored and the progeny of each cell division could survive, reducing the cell loss factor and leading to an effective repopulation of the tumour during the treatment course.

To overcome this repopulation, shortened or accelerated forms of radiotherapy were devised. When treatment is accelerated, multiple doses are given on some (concomitant boost) or all treatment days. The dose per fraction may remain at 1.8–2.0 Gy (pure accelerated radiotherapy), or be reduced (hyperfractionated, accelerated radiotherapy). In all situations, the dose intensity of irradiation is increased and acute reactions will be more severe and dose limiting. Indeed, in some accelerated schedules the total dose has been reduced. If radiotherapy is hyperfractionated, decreased late morbidity may be expected particularly if the total dose is also reduced and the interfraction interval kept as long as possible.

1. Pure accelerated radiotherapy. BALL et al. carried out a study of pure accelerated radiotherapy, with or without chemotherapy, in locally advanced non-small cell lung cancer (BALL et al. 1995). Sixty gray was given in 2-Gy fractions over 6 weeks and was compared to 60 Gy given in 2-Gy fractions twice per day over 3 weeks with an interfraction interval of 6 h. Chemotherapy using concurrent low dose carboplatin was added to both arms of the study, giving a four arm trial. This study gave no benefit to the accelerated arm but did show benefit to the addition of chemotherapy (BALL et al. 1996).

As expected the number of patients who developed oesophagitis grade 3/4 and the length of time of oesophagitis was significantly increased. If all patients treated with accelerated or conventional radiotherapy with or without chemotherapy were analysed, there was a statistically significant increase in the time to relief of oesophagitis, $P = <0.0001$ (Fig. 13.3). Nevertheless, consequential necrosis was not reported although in follow-up seven patients developed an oesophageal stricture requiring dilatation,

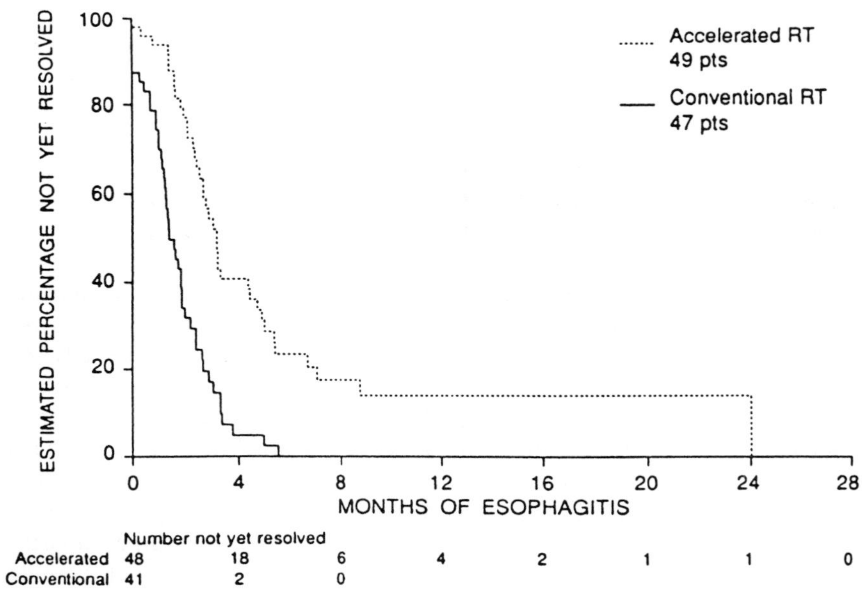

Fig. 13.3. Duration of oesophagitis in 96 patients randomised to conventional radiotherapy or accelerated radiotherapy ($P < 0.0001$, Mantel-Cox log rank test). Four patients who received little or no radiotherapy were excluded. (BALL et al. 1995)

six out of seven being in the accelerated radiotherapy arm. There was no reported increase in pulmonary or spinal cord toxicity.

2. The concomitant boost – with this technique the planning methods were used to advantage. In normal circumstances, the large volume is irradiated to encompass the tumour and mediastinum and then a small volume to include the tumour only to a high dose. The large and small volumes follow each other sequentially but in the concomitant boost, the small volume is interdigitated as a second fraction during the large volume treatment and thus the overall time is reduced by almost 2 weeks with maintenance of the total dose. Once again, the interfraction interval is important and was usually 4–6 h.

The concomitant boost was extensively studied by the RTOG, 350 patients being entered into a study in which three fractionation schedules were investigated. The large field received 1.8 Gy, followed 4–6 h later by 1.8 Gy 2–3 times weekly to the small volume boost fields. The first 61 patients received a total of 63 Gy in 5 weeks – 45 Gy to the large field and 18 Gy to the boost field; morbidity was acceptable and the next 180 patients received a total dose of 70.2 Gy in 5½ weeks – 50.4 Gy to the large field and 19.8 Gy to the boost. Once again, toxicity was acceptable and the last 114 patients received 70.2 Gy in 5 weeks – 45 Gy to the large field and 25.2 Gy to the boost. Acute toxicity was somewhat increased in the group receiving 70.2 Gy in 5 weeks but there was no difference in late toxicity among the three groups. There was also no difference in overall survival, 2-year survivals ranging from 16% (63 Gy) to 21% (70.2 Gy). It was concluded that further phase I/II testing was necessary before the concomitant boost could be taken into phase III trials (Byhardt et al. 1993).

3. Accelerated, hyperfractionated radiotherapy. Continuous, hyperfractionated, accelerated radiotherapy (CHART) is the most accelerated form of radiotherapy. The overall duration of treatment is reduced from 42 days to 12 days, by giving three fractions of 1.5 Gy/day for 12 consecutive days inclusive of Saturdays and Sundays, to a total dose of 54 Gy. The interfraction interval is 6 h during the day and 12 h overnight. With this schedule, it was hoped to improve local tumour control by reducing the time during which tumour proliferation could take place and to reduce late morbidity by using a low dose per fraction and lower than usual total dose (Dische and Saunders 1990).

Initial pilot studies in non-small cell lung cancer were carried out at Mount Vernon Hospital between 1985 and 1990 and gave evidence for improved local tumour control and survival (Saunders et al. 1991, 1993). In the light of these promising pilot studies, the CHART Steering Committee was set up under the auspices of the Medical Research Council to organise multicentre randomised controlled trials comparing CHART to conventional radiotherapy to a total dose of 60 Gy.

The randomised controlled trials commenced in April 1990 and were completed in March 1995. Thirteen co-operating centres entered 563 patients with non-small cell lung cancer, confined to the chest, performance status 0 or 1, where the definitive treatment was to be by radiotherapy. The end-points of the study were survival, local tumour control and morbidity. At completion of the trials an interim report was published showing an increase in survival to the CHART arm (Saunders et al. 1996). The database was updated in February 1997 and a further report published (Saunders et al. 1997), which showed a significant survival advantage to the CHART arm of 9% at 2 years (from 20% to 29%, $P = 0.004$) Fig. 13.4a and a significant improvement in local tumour control of 8% ($P = 0.027$). Considering the 82% of patients who had squamous cell carcinoma of the lung, the improvement in survival at 2 years was 14% (19%–33%, $P = 0.0002$) (Fig. 13.4b). This was achieved by a significant improvement in local tumour control and a reduction in distant metastases at 2 years of 11% ($P = 0.006$) and 9% ($P = 0.02$) respectively.

Acute and late morbidity were carefully monitored in the study. The acute side-effects due to treatment were confined to the oesophagus, where dysphagia occurred sooner and was more severe in the CHART arm. However, in both arms, the symptom of dysphagia settled satisfactorily, with only 9% of the CHART patients and 7% of the conventional cases reporting some persistent dysphagia at 12 weeks. In all patients, the radiation oesophagitis settled and there was no incidence of consequential necrosis. The frequency and severity of radiation pneumonitis as assessed by chest X-ray at 3 months was marginally greater in the conventionally treated cases, which was also reflected in a slightly higher incidence of symptomatic radiation pneumonitis (19% compared to 10% respectively).

Lhermitte's sign occurred in eight patients, all treated with CHART. The Lhermitte's sign occurred 3–16 months after treatment, with a mean time of occurrence of 9.1 months. In later follow-up the symptoms settled and there was no incidence of radiation myelitis.

Late morbidity was assessed in terms of pulmonary fibrosis, radiation myelitis and oesophageal strictures. In all assessments the incidence of late

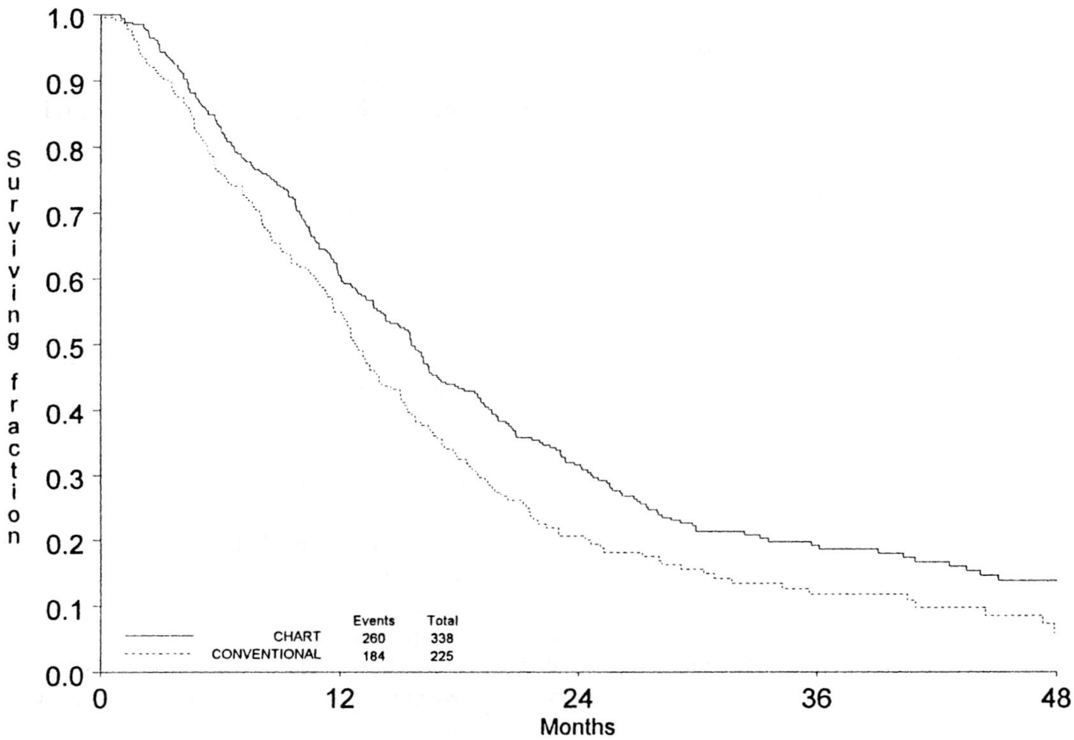

Patients at risk

	0	12	24	36	48
CHART	338	193	83	34	18
CONVENTIONAL	225	114	33	13	4

a

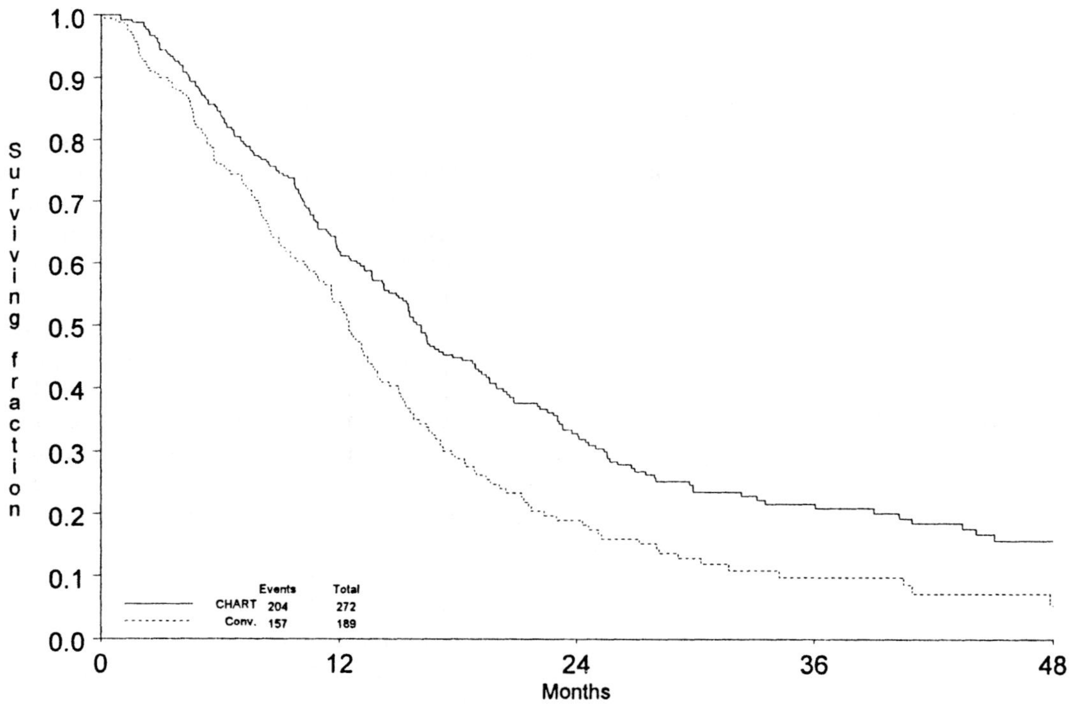

Patients at risk

	0	12	24	36	48
CHART	272	159	68	30	16
Conv.	189	93	25	8	3

b

morbidity was low and there was no difference between the two arms of the study.

In conclusion, the CHART trial gave increased local tumour control and survival with equal morbidity.

The RTOG has tested an Americanised version of CHART in 25 patients: the schedule was modified so that the three times a day radiotherapy could be accomplished within an 8-h day, 5-day week. Here 1.1 Gy three times per day with a 4-h interfraction interval was given to a total of 79.2 Gy. Acute reactions have been reported as less than that of conventional radiotherapy and early responses are favourable (HERSKOVIC et al. 1991).

In an attempt to dose escalate the CHART regimen, and in addition to make it more acceptable to a larger number of departments, CHARTWEL (CHART-Week-End-Less) has been piloted. With this, 1.5 Gy/fraction, three times per day has been given on 5 working days of the week. A total of 54 Gy was achieved in 16 days and the dose has been escalated to 60 Gy by increasing the number of fractions without any significant increase in acute morbidity. CHARTWEL to 60 Gy has been taken into randomised controlled trial in Germany comparing it to conventional radiotherapy.

In the United States a true CHARTWEL regime has been piloted by WAGNER, where 57.6 Gy is given in 36 fractions, over 16 days, by giving 1.5 Gy in the morning and evening and 1.8 Gy at midday when the small volume is treated. This regime has proved tolerable and is now being taken forward by the European Cancer Oncology Group into randomised controlled trial with the addition of neoadjuvant chemotherapy with carboplatin and Taxol (MEHTA et al. 1997). The results of this study are eagerly awaited.

13.4 Interfraction Interval

As clinical experience was gained in the treatment of tumours of the upper aero-digestive tract with more than one fraction per day, it became apparent that the interfraction interval was extremely important. In the CHART studies an interfraction interval of 6 h was chosen. Despite this, radiation myelitis was recorded in five patients with head and neck cancer at doses between 44 and 49 Gy (DISCHE and SAUNDERS 1989). This was an unexpected finding at the low dose per fraction, which should have given an opportunity for dose escalation. Subsequent animal studies showed that the increased morbidity was due to a slow component of half-time of repair in neurological tissues (ANG et al. 1992; LANDUYT et al. 1997; GUTTENBERGER et al. 1992; RUIFROK et al. 1992). Care must therefore be taken when devising regimes, such that the interfraction interval is as long as is practically possible and the dose to the spinal cord is limited.

During the CHART randomised controlled trials in which 559 patients with head and neck cancer, in addition to 338 with NSCLC, received CHART, there has been no incidence of radiation myelitis but the dose to the spinal cord in the CHART arm was limited to 40 Gy in normal circumstances, with a maximum of 44 Gy.

In the RTOG study of twice daily treatments, it was noted that those cases in which the interfraction interval was less than 4.5 h showed a higher late morbidity than those in which it was longer (MARCIAL et al. 1987). These findings were confirmed in a further review of the data reported by Cox, when once again late morbidity was increased in those in whom the interfraction interval was less than 4.5 h (COX et al. 1991).

On the other hand, JEREMIC et al. reported on the interfraction interval as regards local tumour control and survival. He analysed the effects of the interfraction interval in the study of hyperfractionated radiotherapy with or without concurrent chemotherapy in stage III non-small cell lung cancer. He showed that patients treated with shorter interfraction intervals (4.5–5 h) had a better prognosis than those treated with longer intervals (5.5–6 h), giving median survivals of 22 vs 7 months and 5-year survival rates of 27% vs 0%. Considering all the prognostic factors, multivariate analysis showed that the interfraction interval was an independent prognostic factor and he concluded that further prospective randomised controlled trials are warranted to further investigate these effects (JEREMIC and SHIBAMOTO 1996).

◀

Fig. 13.4 a,b. Kaplan-Meier curves: **a** overall survival and **b** overall survival by treatment allocated to the 461 patients with squamous cell carcinous by treatment allocated for all 563 patients randomised into the CHART trial in NSCLC. (SAUNDERS et al. 1997)

13.5 Overall Time

It was Withers and Maciejewski who first reported the effect of overall time on the outcome in terms of local tumour control in patients with head and neck cancer (Withers et al. 1988). They showed that after a lag period of 2–2½ weeks the dose had to be increased with increasing time if local tumour control was to be maintained. The lag period of 2½ weeks was subsequently challenged by Bentzen in a review of the literature but the fact that tumour repopulation may lead to decreased control with increasing overall times has not been challenged (Bentzen and Thames 1991).

A review of data at many sites has confirmed this finding. Cox et al. reviewed the effect of interruptions in radical radiotherapy in favourable patients with non-small cell lung cancer. They also found that prolongation of overall time adversely affects long term survival, which was associated with delays to completion of the planned total dose (Cox et al. 1993). In many of these studies, poor general condition, advanced tumours or unexpected acute morbidity could have led to the increase in overall time and poor survival, rather than the overall time alone. If one, however, considers studies of split course treatment, particularly if they were randomised, then the results are more reliable. In Denmark and the United States, conventional and split course radiotherapy in head and neck was compared and gave evidence for a reduction in local tumour control with prolonged overall time (Overgaard et al. 1988; Parsons et al. 1980).

These findings have implications for the management of patients with non-small cell lung cancer. Fowler et al. have estimated that a week's increase in overall time can lead to a reduction in control of 14% (Fowler and Lindstrom 1992). This must lead us to re-evaluate not only altered fractionation schemes but also conventional radiotherapy and reconsider the increase in overall time caused by bank holidays and machine servicing. At my own institution, treatment is given over such holidays, if the overall time is to be increased by more than 2–3 days.

13.6 Conclusion

The clinical regimes described have been devised in an effort to improve the therapeutic benefit in the radiotherapy of non-small cell lung cancer. The studies have shown that a low dose per fraction preferentially spares late reacting tissues and that cellular proliferation is an important cause of failure of local tumour control. Data has been presented to show that the interfraction interval and overall time are important in outcome and supports the fact that in devising future research protocols, gaps in treatment – whether that be between surgery, radiotherapy or chemotherapy – should be kept to a minimum. Care will need to be taken when combining chemotherapy with radiotherapy concurrently, as it is anticipated that there will be an increase in normal reactions and this must be kept within reasonable levels whilst completing all treatment in the shortest possible time.

References

Ang KK, Jiang GL, Guttenberger R et al (1992) Impact of spinal cord repair kinetics on the practice of altered fractionation schedules. Radiother Oncol 25:287–294

Ball D, Bishop J, Smith J et al (1995) A phase III study of accelerated radiotherapy with and without carboplatin in nonsmall cell lung cancer: an interim toxicity analysis of the first 100 patients. Int J Radiat Oncol Biol Phys 31:267–272

Ball D, Bishop J, Smith J et al (1996) A phase III study of conventional and accelerated radiotherapy (RT) with and without carboplatin in unresectable non small cell lung cancer (NSCLS). Radiother Oncol 40 [Suppl 1]:S61 (S231)

Barendsen GW (1982) Dose fractionation, dose rate and isoeffect relationships for normal tissue responses. Int Radiat Oncol Biol Phys 8:1981–1997

Begg AC, McNally NJ, Shrieve DC et al (1985) A method to measure the duration of DNA synthesis and the potential doubling time from a single sample. Cytometry 6:620–626

Bennett MH, Wilson GD, Dische S et al (1992) Tumour proliferation assessed by combined histological and flow cytometric analysis: implications for therapy in squamous cell carcinoma in the head and neck. Br J Cancer 65:870–878

Bentzen SM, Thames HD (1991) Clinical evidence for tumor clonogen regeneration: interpretations of the data. Radiother Oncol 22:161–166

Byhardt RW (1995) The evolution of Radiation Therapy Oncology Group (RTOG) protocols for non-small cell lung cancer. Int J Radiat Oncol Biol Phys 2(5):1513–1525

Byhardt RW, Pajak TF, Emami B et al (1993) A phase I/II study to evaluate accelerated fractionation via concomitant boost for squamous, adeno, and large cell carcinoma of the lung: report of Radiation Therapy Oncology Group 84-07. Int Radiat Oncol Biol Phys 26:459–468

Byhardt RW, Scott CB, Ettinger DS et al (1995) Concurrent hyperfractionated irradiation and chemotherapy for unresectable non-small cell lung cancer: results of Radiation Therapy Oncology Group (RTOG) 90–145. Cancer 75:2337–2344

Cox JD (1991) Induction chemotherapy for non-small cell carcinoma of the lung: limitations and lessons. Int J Radiat Oncol Biol Phys 20:1375–1376

Cox JD, Azarnia N, Byhardt RW et al (1990) A randomized phase I/II trial of hyperfractionated radiation therapy with total doses of 60.0 Gy to 79.2 Gy: possible survival benefit with ≥69.6 Gy in favourable patients with Radiation Therapy Oncology Group stage III non-small-cell lung carcinoma. Report of Radiation Oncology Group 83–11. J Clin Oncol 8:1543–1555

Cox JD, Pajak TF, Marcial VA et al (1991) ASTRO plenary: interfraction interval is a major determinant of late effects, with hyperfractionated radiation of carcinomas of upper respiratory and digestive tracts: results from Radiation Therapy Oncology Group Protocol 8313. Int J Radiat Oncol Biol Phys 20:1191–1195

Cox JD, Pajak TF, Asbell S et al (1993) Interruptions of high dose radiation therapy decrease long term survival of favourable patients with unresectable non small cell carcinoma of the lung: analysis of 1244 cases from 3 Radiation Therapy Oncology Group (RTOG) Trials. Int J Radiat Oncol Biol Phys 27:493–498

Denekamp J (1982) Cell kinetics and cancer therapy. Thomas, Springfield

Dillman RO, Seagren SL, Propert KJ et al (1990) A randomized trial of induction chemotherapy plus high-dose radiation versus radiation alone in stage III non-small cell lung cancer. N Engl J Med 323:940–945

Dische S, Saunders MI (1989) Continuous, hyperfractionated, accelerated radiotherapy (CHART). An interim report upon late morbidity. Radiother Oncol 16:67–74

Dische S, Saunders MI (1990) The rationale for continuous, hyperfractionated, accelerated radiotherapy (CHART). Int J Radiat Oncol Biol Phys 19:1317–1320

Fowler JF (1984a) Total doses in fractionated radiotherapy. Implications of new radiobiological data (Review). Int J Radiat Oncol Biol Phys 46:103–120

Fowler JF (1984b) What next in fractionated radiotherapy? Br J Cancer 49 [Suppl 6]:285–300

Fowler JF (1989) The linear quadratic formula for progress in fractionated radiotherapy. Br J Radiol 62:679–694

Fowler JF, Lindstrom MJ (1992) Loss of local control with prolongation of radiotherapy. Int J Radiat Oncol Biol Phys 23:457–467

Guttenberger R, Thames HD, Ang KK et al (1992) Is the experience with CHART compatible with experimental data? A new model of repair kinetics and computer simulations. Radiother Oncol 25:280–286

Herskovic A, Orton C, Seyedsadr M et al (1991) Initial experience with a practical hyperfractionated accelerated radiotherapy regime. Int J Radiat Oncol Biol Phys 21:1275–1281

Jeremic B, Shibamoto Y (1996) Effect of interfraction interval in hyperfractionated radiotherapy with or without concurrent chemotherapy for stage II nonsmall cell lung cancer. Int J Radiat Oncol Biol Phys 34:303–308

Jeremic B, Shibamoto Y, Acimovic L et al (1996) Hyperfractionated radiation therapy with or without concurrent low-dose daily carboplatin/etoposide for stage III non-small-cell lung cancer: a randomized study. J Clin Oncol 14:1065–1070

Landuyt W, Fowler J, Ruifrok A et al (1997) Kinetics of repair in the spinal cord of the rat. Radiother Oncol 45:55–62

Marcial VA, Pajak TF, Chang C et al (1987) Hyperfractionated photon radiation therapy in the treatment of advanced squamous cell carcinoma of the oral cavity, pharynx, larynx and sinuses, using radiation therapy as the only planned modality: (preliminary report) by the Radiation Therapy Oncology Group (RTOG). Int J Radiat Oncol Biol Phys 13:41–47

Marks R, Witherspoon B, Davis L et al (1978) Hyperfractionation: where we stand. A preliminary RTOG report. Proc Am Soc Ther Radiol 4:139–140

Mehta M, Tannehill S, Martin L et al (1997) ECOG 4593: Phase II hyperfractionated, accelerated radiotherapy (HART) for non-small cell lung cancer (NSCLC). Early results and RT quality assurance. Lung Cancer 18 [Suppl 1]:123 (418)

Overgaard J, Hjelm-Hansen M, Johansen LV et al (1988) Comparison of conventional and split course radiotherapy as primary treatment in carcinoma of the larynx. Acta Oncol 27:147–152

Parsons JT, Bova FJ, Million RR et al (1980) A re-evaluation of split course techniques for squamous cell carcinoma of the head and neck. Int J Radiat Oncol Biol Phys 6:1645–1652

Ruifrok ACC, Kleiber BJ, van der Kogel AJ et al (1992) Fractionation sensitivity of rat cervical spinal cord during radiation treatment. Radiother Oncol 25:295–300

Saunders MI, Dische S, Grosch E et al (1991) Experience with CHART. Int J Radiat Oncol Biol Phys 21:871–878

Saunders MI, Lyn B, Dische S (1993) Continuous, hyperfractionated, accelerated radiotherapy (CHART) in non-small cell lung cancer. Lung Cancer 9:221–228

Saunders MI, Dische S, Barrett A et al (1996) Randomised multicentre trials of CHART vs conventional radiotherapy in head and neck and non-small-cell lung cancer: an interim report. Br J Cancer 73:1455–1462

Saunders MI, Dische S, Barrett A et al (1997) Continuous hyperfractionated accelerated radiotherapy (CHART) versus conventional radiotherapy in non-small-cell lung cancer: a randomised multicentre trial. The Lancet 350:161–165

Steel GG (1977) Growth kinetics of tumours: cell population kinetics in relation to the growth and treatment of cancer. Clarendon Press, Oxford, pp 86–261

Thames HD (1985) An incomplete repair model for survival after fractionated and continuous irradiation. Int J Radiat Oncol Biol Phys 47:319–339

Wilson GD, McNally NJ, Dische S et al (1988) Measurement of cell kinetics in human tumours *in vivo*. Br J Cancer 58:423–431

Withers HR, Taylor JMG, Maciejewski B et al (1988) The hazard of accelerated tumour clonogen repopulation during radiotherapy. Acta Oncol 27:131–146

14 Biochemical and Biological Dose Modifiers for Irradiation of Lung Cancers

R.O. MIRIMANOFF

CONTENTS

14.1 Introduction

Lung cancer is one of the leading causes of cancer mortality in the world. While surgery can produce up to 40%–50% cure rates in patients with stage I and II non-small cell lung cancers (NSCLC) (SCHOTTENFELD et al. 1996), a majority of patients present with stage III or IV disease. Of these, stage IIIa and IIIb, or locally advanced disease, represent 40%–50% of all cases. In this important category, surgery alone has a very limited role and radiation therapy alone produces only about 5% long term survival. Platinum-based chemotherapy, when combined with radiotherapy, increases the survival but the overall gain is still quite modest (MIRIMANOFF 1994). Even if a majority of patients treated with radiotherapy succumb from distant metastases, it has been consistently demonstrated that the local control in locally advanced cases is quite low, somewhere between 20% and 50%. It seems that combination chemotherapy given prior to, or after radiotherapy, little alters the local failure rate (LECHEVALIER et al. 1991). It is also recognized now that in small cell lung cancer (SCLC), a disease category in which almost all patients will develop haematological metastases, there is still a significant percentage of patients who will die with uncontrolled intrathoracic disease, in spite of the fact that radiotherapy has an impact on local control and even on survival (PIGNON et al. 1992). It appears then that to improve the local control of lung cancer, and thus hopefully its survival, radiotherapy should be rendered more efficacious.

A number of means exist to ameliorate the effects of radiotherapy. These include dose escalation via conformal radiotherapy, endoluminal brachytherapy, intraoperative radiotherapy, increment of dose by unconventionally fractionated schedules, the combination of radiotherapy with newer and hopefully more efficient chemotherapies, and radiation modifiers. The former are described in other parts of the book, and the current chapter will focus on the latter.

R.O. MIRIMANOFF, Department of Radiation Oncology, Centre Hospitalier Universitaire Vaudois, CHUV, CH-1011 Lausanne, Switzerland

14.2 Definition of Modifiers

For lung cancer as for many human cancers treated with curative intent, the radiation dose is limited by the tolerance of normal critical tissues in close proximity to the tumor (TANNEHILL and METHA 1996). The distance between the well known sigmoid-shaped radiation dose-response curves of tumor and normal tissues represents the therapeutic index. Unfortunately in NSCLC the therapeutic index is not very favorable, since a dose required to obtain a probability of, say, 90% of tumor control would result, with current methods and most of the time, in unacceptable normal tissue toxicity. Separating the two dose-response curves using a radiation modifier is one particular means of improving the therapeutic index.

Chemical or biological modifiers of radiation comprise radiation sensitizers and radiation protectors. By definition, modifiers should not have an *intrinsic* therapeutic value but should be clinically active only when used in combination with irradiation. When administered alone, a true sensitizer should have no effect whatsoever on tumor cells and a true protector no effect on normal tissue. Furthermore, an ideal radiation sensitizer should not increase the damage of radiation to normal tissues, and conversely an ideal protector should not protect the tumor from irradiation.

Radiation sensitizers can be divided into several categories, including hypoxic cell sensitizers and non-hypoxic cell sensitizers. The latter family can be further subdivided into biochemical and biological sensitizers, such as the interferons. This distinction between the various categories of radiation sensitizers is practical but not always so clear-cut, since, for example, some compounds can sometimes act both as hypoxic cell sensitizers and as cytotoxic agents.

14.2.1 Hypoxic Cell Sensitizers

Hypoxia is only one of the many conditions related to microenvironmental alterations which occur in most cancers. Interestingly, the key paper by Thomlinson and Gray over 40 years ago, in which these authors described a steep fall in oxygen tension at a distance from tumor capillaries, was made following a study of the histological pattern seen in bronchial carcinomas (Thomlinson and Gray 1955).

Since these observations were made, a large body of animal and human data have demonstrated that hypoxia is present in many tumors (Rojas 1991; Vaupel et al. 1991; Höckel et al. 1991; Nordsmark et al. 1994).

Vaupel et al., using the Eppendorf oxygen electrode system, have assessed the oxygenation of various human cancers and their surrounding tissues (Vaupel et al. 1991; Höckel et al. 1991; Vaupel 1994) and have shown a very wide range of oxygen content values, which were on average lower in tumors than in their normal tissue counterpart. Gatenby, using similar techniques, correlated the degree of hypoxia with the treatment outcome, which was significantly worse in tumors with the lowest intratumoral oxygen content (Gatenby et al. 1988).

In order to understand the main strategies used to counteract radioresistance due to tumor hypoxia, a few basic related mechanisms are briefly mentioned here. There are two particular situations in which tumor cells can become hypoxic. The first, chronic hypoxia, is due to a limitation of the capacity of oxygen to diffuse beyond about 150 µm from a tumor capillary, caused by the consumption of oxygen by the cells closest to the vessel. The second, acute or intermittent hypoxia, results from intermittent opening and closure of tumor vessels (Coleman et al. 1988; Chaplin et al. 1986; Brown 1979). Whatever the cause, in hypoxic conditions it requires two to three times the radiation dose to produce the same fraction of cell killing as obtained in room air (Hall 1994a). The oxygen enhancement ratio (OER) or the sensitizer enhancement ratio (SER) represents the ratio of radiation dose required to kill the same fraction of cells under hypoxia compared to oxygen conditions (OER) or to when a sensitizer was added (SER) (Coleman et al. 1994). The presence of oxygen is of paramount importance for cell killing: oxygen is said to "fix" the DNA damage caused by free radicals induced by ionizing radiation. This process competes with the restoration of damage, in which reducing agents such as the thiols play a major role (Coleman et al. 1994). Thiol depletion could, for example, be used to increase tumor radiosensitivity. Hypoxia has many other consequences, as shown by a number of experiments using cellular or molecular biology techniques. Of the many examples, hypoxia can lead to accumulation in G_1 phase of the cell, leading to treatment resistance (Shrieve et al. 1983). Cells under hypoxia can also undergo gene amplification, which may be involved in drug resistance and metastatic potential (Luk et al. 1990; Young and Hill 1990).

The most commonly used means to overcome radioresistance induced by hypoxia are shown on Table 14.1.

The most simple and most logical strategy to counteract hypoxia is to augment oxygen delivery to tumors (Coleman et al. 1994). This can be done by using pure oxygen, hyperbaric oxygen, blood transfusion, perfluorocarbons, and carbogen (Dische 1991a,b; Overgaard and Horsman 1996; Guichard 1991; Coleman et al. 1994). Carbogen enhances tumor blood flow and shifts the hemoglobin dissociation curve to the right, thus depressing the affinity of hemoglobin for oxygen (Kruuv et al. 1967). While hyperbaric oxygen and carbogen are probably mostly active against chronic hypoxia, some chemical compounds, such as nicotinamide,

Table 14.1. Strategies to overcome radioresistance due to hypoxia

Increase in oxygen delivery
• Carbogen breathing
• Hyperbaric oxygen
• Perfluorocarbons
• Blood transfusions
• Drugs to counteract intermittent hypoxia
Hypoxic cell sensitizers
• Nitroimidazoles
• GSH depletion (BSO)
Bioreductive agents
• Mitomycin C
• Porfiromycin
• Tirapazamine

Table 14.2. Non-hypoxic cell sensitizers

Halogenated pyrimidines
• BUdR
• IUdR
• FUdR
Hydroxyurea
Lonidamide
Metoclopramide
Chemotherapeutic agents as sensitizers
• Platinum compounds
• Etoposide
• Taxanes
• Topotecan
• Vinorelbin

an amide derivative of niacin, were shown to counteract acute or intermittent hypoxia (Horsman et al. 1989). The combination of carbogen and nicotinamide led in animal models to enhancement ratios of 1.8, a major radiosensitization (Kjellen et al. 1991).

The use of hypoxic cell sensitizers represents another strategy to overcome hypoxia-induced radioresistance. The nitromidazoles are a class of widely studied compounds with so-called oxygen-mimetic properties. The early drugs metronidazole and misonidazole showed experimental SERs of 1.3–1.6, but were abandoned in the late 1980s because of their gastrointestinal and neurological toxicity. Etanidazole, and nimorazole seem to be better tolerated and have been the subject of intensive investigations (Coleman et al. 1992; Overgaard et al. 1991).

Another group of drugs, represented by mitomycin C and porfiromycin (Sartorelli 1988), were developed as bioreductive agents, that is chemotherapeutic agents activated under the hypoxic state. SR 4233 or tirapazamine is a more recent product, which was shown to enhance markedly radiation-induced tumor killing (Baker et al. 1988; Bailey et al. 1992). In contrast to mitomycin C, the enhancement ratio by tirapazamine does not decrease with the number of fractions (Brown and Siim 1996). Bioreductive drugs differ from oxygen-mimetic sensitizers, as the latter do not require metabolic activation.

Lastly, thiol depletion could be used to decrease the protection from radiation: buthionine-sulfoximine (BSO) was shown to decrease glutathione (GSH) synthesis and to sensitize hypoxic cells to radiation (Bump and Brown 1990).

As will be seen later in this chapter, clinical experience using strategies overcoming hypoxia is still limited in lung cancer.

14.2.2 Non-hypoxic Cell Sensitizers

Many drugs, sometimes referred to as aerobic radiation sensitizers, have been identified in the past 30 years. They were developed to enhance the radiosensitivity of intrinsically radioresistant oxic tumor cells. Unfortunately, the large majority of these compounds were found to be non-specific, and the almost parallel increase in normal tissue toxicity wiped out any therapeutic gain.

However, a differential sensitization is seen in a few drugs. Some of the most studied non-hypoxic cell sensitizers are shown in Table 14.2.

The halogenated pyrimidines 5-bromodeoxyuridine (BUdR) 5-iododeoxyuridine (IUdR) and fluorodeoxyuridine (FUdR) act on proliferating cells and may preferentially sensitize rapidly dividing tumor cells, rather than the more slowly proliferating surrounding normal tissue cells. BUdR and IUdR are incorporated into the DNA, and initial radiation damage by single strand break and double strand break can be increased as much as twofold (Kinsella et al. 1987). After drug exposure, the cellular repair process appears to be saturated. Analysis of the linear quadratic model shows that halogenated pyrimidines have an effect on the α-component of the radiation survival curve, which is again consistent with an increase in the DNA damage process (Miller et al. 1992).

Hydroxyurea, an antineoplastic drug used for more than 40 years, was shown in proliferating cells to induce a block in the G_1-S phase of the cell cycle, and to cause cell synchronization (Sinclair 1968). It was also demonstrated to inhibit potentially lethal damage repair after irradiation (Phillips and Tolmach 1966).

Lonidamine, a modulator of cellular energy metabolism, has a significant antineoplastic effect when combined with radiotherapy (Kim et al. 1986) or alkylating agents (Teicher et al. 1991). It does not act as an electron-affinic sensitizer, and produces a greater enhancement of radiation with fractionated schemes (Kim et al. 1986). The main mechanism of action seems to be the inhibition of potentially lethal damage repair of radiation.

Metoclopramide (MCA), a drug widely used as an antiemetic, can increase the cytotoxic effect of cisplatin and irradiation in experimental tumor models without an increase in normal tissue damage (Kjellen et al. 1989). Its mechanism of action is not completely known, but it was shown to increase the level of DNA damage and inhibit DNA repair after irradiation (Lybak and Pero 1991).

In addition to mitomycin C and hydroxyurea, many other chemotherapeutic agents can act as radiation modifiers, although in a majority of cases the specificity of their sensitizing property is of doubtful significance.

In too many experimental or clinical studies there is no clear definition of the rationale for the combination of cytotoxic drugs with radiotherapy. The association can take advantage of their spatial cooperation, their additive cytotoxic effect, or the drug can be used mainly as a radiosensitizer. A few drugs are sometimes used for this latter purpose only, and if so, they are generally used in daily small doses or in continuous infusions concurrently with daily radiotherapy, rather than in cycles.

Platinum compounds have been extensively studied for their interaction with radiation (Dewit 1987). These drugs impair radiation-induced potentially lethal damage repair of DNA and act also by free radical-related mechanisms.

Etoposide seems to fix rapidly repairable radiation-induced DNA damage; in addition cells arrested in G_2 by radiation are very sensitive to this drug (Lallev et al. 1993).

Taxol at low dose alone did not perturb the cell cycle, but when combined with irradiation it produced a prolonged block in G_2M (Steren et al. 1993), a very radiosensitive phase of the cell cycle.

Vinorelbine, a semisynthetic vinca alcaloid, is a potent inhibitor of mitotic microtubule polymerisation. It was shown to be very active against human bronchial epidermoid carcinoma (Edelstein et al. 1996). In vitro, exposure of NCI-H460 cell line to vinorelbine, followed by radiotherapy, dislosed a dose-dependent sensitivization. Ratios of fractional survival ranged from 1.7:1 at 1 Gy to 5.5.1 at 6 Gy. The greatest potential was seen after cells had plateaued in the G_2M phase of the cycle (Edelstein et al. 1996).

Topotecan can produce an important enhancement of the radioresponse, by cell cycle synchronization mechanisms and by inhibition of potentially lethal damage repair (Del Bino et al. 1992; Boothman et al. 1992).

The combination of multidrug chemotherapy and ionizing radiation will not be discussed here and will be presented in another chapter.

14.2.3 Cytokines and Interferons

The interactions between radiation and the various cytokines are very complex. Many cytokines are radiation inducible, and when released after exposure to ionizing radiation they can produce a number of autocrine or paracrine effects. Tumor necrosis factor (TNF), interleukin 1 (IL-1), platelet-derived growth factor (PDGF-β) and transforming growth factor (TGF-β) are released by irradiated cells and bind to their respective receptors to produce further biologic response (Hallahan et al. 1993). For example, TGF-β production can result in endothelial cell proliferation and is thought to be associated with the pathologic changes of late radiation injury. Conversely, IL-1 and IL-6 were shown to act as radioprotectors on the bone marrow (Hallahan et al. 1993).

Looking more specifically at the induction of cytokines by ionizing radiations on normal lung tissue, Rubin and his group conducted a series of experiments in animal models (Rubin et al. 1995). Radiation fibrosis-prone mice received thoracic irradiation at 5 and 12.5 Gy. At various times after exposure, expression of cytokine and extracellular matrix mRNA abundance was evaluated by slot-blot analysis and cellular localization by in situ hybridization and immunochemistry. These investigators showed the pattern of IL-1α and TGF-β elevation and decline, and in parallel the correlation with the elevation of the fibrogenic markers for collagen genes. The authors conclude that the temporal relationship between the elevation of specific cytokines and the histological and biochemical evidence of fibrosis serves to illustrate a continuum of response and underlies pulmonary radiation reactions (Rubin et al. 1995).

Interferons are glycoproteins produced by several cell types in response to foreign aggressions and tumors. Interferon-α (INF-α) is produced by leukocytes, interferon-β (IFN-β) by fibroblasts, macrophages and epithelial cells and interferon-γ (IFN-γ) by activated T-lymphocytes and natural killer cells. They interact with their target by binding to specific cell surface receptors, one for IFN-α and IFN-β (class I) and one for IFN-γ (class II) (Petska et al. 1987). Interferons may be cytostatic or cytotoxic. For example, INF-α causes cells to accumulate in G_0/G_1, which could be responsible for its antiproliferative effect (Tamm et al. 1987).

All three interferons augment the expression of cell surface antigens such as MHC antigens or TNF receptors, making cells more recognizable by cytotoxic lymphocytes or TNF. Interferons have also been demonstrated to enhance the effect of ionizing radiation.

Recombinant IFN-α-2b was shown to increase the sensitivity of SCLC cell lines to radiation (Kardamakis et al. 1989). In another study, IFN-β sensitized another human bronchogenic carcinoma cell line, whereas IFN-α did not (Gould et al. 1984). In a hypernephroma cell line, compared with IFN-α and IFN-γ, IFN-β had the most significant effect on repair of sublethal damage (Chang and Keng 1987). flow cytometry analysis demonstrated accumulation of cells in the radiosensitive G_2-M phase of the cell cycle (Chang and Keng 1987).

The increased antiproliferative activity with IFN-β plus radiation over either agent alone suggested synergism in two human glioma and lung cancer lines (Witt et al. 1993). Overall, there are several indications that of all IFNs, IFN-β possesses the greatest radiation killing enhancing effect.

In animal models and in clinical experiments, both radioprotection and enhancement of radiation effects were observed on normal tissues, depending on the type of interferons. IFN-β can provide radiation protection in radiation-induced fibrosis in mice (McDonald et al. 1993a). On the molecular level, there is some evidence that interferons can inhibit the release of some growth factors ultimately responsible for late radiation damage.

14.2.4 Radioprotectors

To decrease the normal tissue complication probability (NTCP) after irradiation, the most current approach consists of excluding as much normal tissue as possible from the irradiated volume, by using sophisticated three dimensional planning and conformal radiotherapy. However, in many situations, even with the best available techniques including proton-beam radiotherapy, it is impossible to spare enough critical normal tissue when the latter is totally encompassed or infiltrated to a great extent by the tumor. Thus, another method to decrease NTCP is to render normal tissue more resistant to the effects of radiation, without causing tumor protection.

Several thousands of agents defined as radioprotectors have been developed, and the most remarkable group are the sulfhydryl compounds. Cysteine was shown in the late 1940s to protect the bone marrow of rodents from total body irradiation (Patt et al. 1949). The mechanism of action involves the scavenging of free radicals produced by ionizing radiation (Hall 1994b). Sulfhydryl compounds block the process leading to the breaking of chemical bonds within the DNA by reacting with the free radicals in competition with oxygen (Hall 1994b). It is estimated that effective scavenging to the largest possible value would equal the OER with a value of 2.5–3.0. Amifostine (WR 2721) is the most effective aminothiol identified so far; the active form of the drug is WR-1065. Preclinical studies in animal and human tumor xenograft systems have shown that amifostine does not cause significant *tumor* protection (Milas et al. 1984). As seen before, the mechanisms of protection are those inherent in aminothiols; however, amifostine normal tissue selectivity is also likely to be due to additional factors (Calabro-Jones et al. 1985; Yuhas 1980). The generally inferior blood supply in tumors may result in a lower amifostine concentration in tumor cells. The conversion of amifostine to WR-1065 is dependent on capillary membrane-bound pH-dependent alkaline phosphatase, which is present in a lower concentration in neoplastic tissues than in normal tissues. Finally cellular uptake of the drug is a passive process in tumors and an active transport mechanism in normal tissues, resulting in a higher concentration in normal cells (Yuhas 1980).

14.3 Clinical Experience

It is fair to say that overall, radiation modifiers have not been studied as extensively in lung cancer as in other tumor sites. A literature review indicates that radiation sensitizers or protectors have been mainly tested in cancer types with a dominant local or locoregional pattern of extent, typically head and neck cancers, uterine cervix cancer and brain tumors. Experience with NSCLC is more limited, perhaps because this kind of tumor was not felt to be an interesting target for the study of radiation modifiers. However, and as already emphasized in the "Introduction," local failure rates after curative radiation are still quite high and it is reasonable to assume that an increment in local control can lead to improved survival, at least in a subgroup of patients.

14.3.1 Clinical Experience in Counteracting Hypoxia

An overall review was made by OVERGAARD and HORSMAN to look at all human trials designed to correct hypoxia before and/or during radiotherapy (OVERGAARD and HORSMAN 1996). Various procedures were used, including high oxygen-content gas breathing, nitroaromatic radiation sensitizers, blood transfusions, hemoglobin-affinic modifiers and nicotinamide. A total of 83 randomized trials using one or another of these procedures were identified, in which a total of over 10 000 patients were enrolled. Although a number of these trials yielded no benefit, an overview analysis of the different cancer types showed that modification of tumor hypoxia significantly improved the locoregional tumor control after radiotherapy, with an odd ratio of 1.21 (OVERGAARD and HORSMAN 1996). Indirect support for the influence of hypoxia on radioresponse comes from observations showing a correlation between tumor control and hemoglobin concentration (OVERGAARD and HORSMAN 1996; DISCHE 1991a). In this respect only two papers have shown that in lung cancer, hemoglobin level seems to have an impact on the outcome after iradiation (DISCHE 1991a). However, direct evidence of a benefit in correcting hypoxia is lacking in lung cancer from any of the eight randomized trials concerning this tumor type, as reviewed by OVERGAARD and HORSMAN. In these 8 randomized trials, 624 patients were accrued. Overall local control was 36.5% in the groups of patients treated with radiotherapy and a hypoxic modifier, versus 32.6% with radiation alone. This difference was not significant ($P = 0.32$) and the odd radio was 1.19 (±0.33) (OVERGAARD and HORSMAN 1996).

Among these randomized trials, two of the ROTGs tested misonidazole in stage III NSCLC. A first phase III study compared 53 patients treated with 6 Gy, twice weekly, for a total dose of 36 Gy with misonidazole at 1.75 gm/m^2 prior to each radiation, to a radiation of the same type alone (SIMPSON et al. 1987). This hypofractionated scheme had substantial toxicity; furthermore, no improvement in local control was seen with misonidazole. In this study, the overall median survival was particularly poor, at 7 months regardless of treatment.

Another RTOG trial compared 123 patients who received irradiation alone to 116 who were given radiation and misonidazole (SIMPSON et al. 1989). Radiotherapy was a standard fractionation regime of 60 Gy at 2 Gy per fraction in 30 fractions, and misonidazole was prescribed at 400 mg/m^2 daily, prior to each fraction. Results in the 239 eligible patients showed no improvement in response rate, local control and survival for those who received misonidazole (SIMPSON et al. 1989). As in the previous study, the median survival, 8 months for the control arm, and 7.4 months for the experimental arm, was particularly poor.

Fluosol, a perfluorochemical emulsion, has been tried as an adjuvant to radiation in the treatment of unresectable non-small cell carcinoma of the lung, and was shown to be safely administrable. Of 49 patients with locally advanced NSCLC treated with fluosol and 0_2 breathing in addition to radiotherapy, 22 experienced mild to moderate side effects, including flushing, dyspnea, hypertension and fever or chills. Radiotherapy dose was 59.4–68 Gy. Thirty-four completed the treatment, and 17 achieved a complete response. The median survival of patients completing the protocol was 15.5 months, but for the entire group of patients median survival was only 9.2 months (LUSTIG et al. 1990).

ARCON, or the administration of accelerated radiotherapy, carbogen and nicotinamide, in an attempt to overcome rapid cell proliferation, chronic and intermittent hypoxia (KJELLEN et al. 1991) has been tested in an EORTC phase I-II trial (BERNIER 1998). Thirty-nine patients with NSCLC were enrolled: 10 in the step with carbogen, 12 in the step with nicotinamide, and 17 in the carbogen and nicotinamide arm. Preliminary results indicate a moderate toxicity, with 9% grade 3 lung reactions, 11% grade 3 and 34% grade 2 gastrointestinal toxicity, and in 7% nicotinamide had to be stopped. The response rate was similar in the three arms and was 63% overall (BERNIER 1998). It is still too early to make an assessment regarding survival.

In conclusion, in spite of the fact that there is good evidence that hypoxia is present in lung cancer, there are no consistent data at this time to demonstrate that the various means of correcting hypoxia improve local control or survival in this cancer category. Further data on ARCON and on newer methods of overcoming hypoxia are awaited with interest, to see if similar strategies should be pursued.

14.3.2 Clinical Experience with Non-hypoxic Cell Sensitizers

So far, there have been no available data in the literature concerning the use of the halogenated pyrimidines IUdR and BUdR in association with radiotherapy in lung cancer.

Lonidamine with irradiation was evaluated in a prospective randomized study (SCARANTINO et al. 1994). A total of 310 patients with locally advanced lung cancer were enlisted on this study: 152 were on the placebo arm and 158 on the lonidamine arm. The radiotherapy dose was 55–60 Gy at 1.8 Gy/fraction and the lonidamine was prescribed at 256 mg/m^2 in three daily doses. The study failed to demonstrate any significant advantage in the lonidamine-treated population in overall survival, progression-free survival or median duration of local control (SCARANTINO et al. 1994).

Metoclopramide (MCA) was tested in a phase I/II study in conjunction with radiotherapy in patients with inoperable squamous cell carcinoma of the lung (KJELLEN et al. 1995). MCA was tested at two dose levels: 1 mg/kg 5 days/week or 2 mg/kg three times a week. The radiotherapy dose was 40–60 Gy with conventional fractionation. The 50% response rate, the median survival of 15 months, and the correlation between various endpoints and the total MCA doses were interpreted by the authors as favorable enough to justify the initiation of a phase II/III randomized study (KJELLEN et al. 1995).

The large majority of programs using chemotherapy and radiotherapy in locally advanced lung cancer were not conceived primarily as using cytotoxic agents as radiosensitizers. A combination of radiotherapy and chemotherapy will be dealt with in another chapter. However, in the past 15–20 years, some single agents were used concomitantly with radiation to improve its efficacy.

Continuous 5-fluorouracil (5-FU) at 300–1000 mg/m^2 was reported to be feasible but the results of two phase II studies were unconvincing (KELLY et al. 1989; LOKICH et al. 1989) and no phase III trials were undertaken.

Low dose, daily cisplatin at 3–6 mg/m^2 was tested in a series of phase II trials, showing a good feasibility and rather high response rates (VAN HARSKAMP et al. 1987; TOBIAS et al. 1987; ELLEBROCK et al. 1991; TROVO et al. 1992a). Two randomized studies were conducted to confirm these results (TROVO et al. 1992b; SCHAAKE-KONING et al. 1992). The Italian trial, in which patients were randomized between radiotherapy alone and radiotherapy with 6 mg/m^2 cisplatin daily, failed to demonstrate any difference between the two arms in median survival and in local control (TROVO et al. 1992b). The EORTC trial randomized patients between (1) no chemotherapy, (2) cisplatin 70 mg/m^2 every week and (3) cisplatin 6 mg/m^2 daily. The radiotherapy for all patients was a split-course regime with a total dose of 55 Gy, in 20 fractions. The results were positive, the arm with daily cisplatin having a significantly better local control and survival compared to the control arm (SCHAAKE-KONING et al. 1992).

Carboplatin was also tested in NSCLC in continuous infusions of 20 mg/m^2 (GROEN et al. 1994) or daily doses of 70 mg/m^2 during 5 days on weeks 1 and 5 (BALL et al. 1991) in various phase I-II trials, generally with an acceptable toxicity and relatively high response rates. The latter regime is currently being tested in a three-arm randomized trial (BISHOP et al. 1994).

Paclitaxel and radiotherapy was tested in two different phase I trials. In one of the trials, the dose of paclitaxel could be pushed to 55 mg/m^2 weekly concomitantly with a radiotherapy of 59.4 Gy (VOGT et al. 1996). In the second one, doses to 70 mg/m^2 could be administered with a dose of 50 Gy (MARANGOLO et al. 1996).In both studies it was felt that toxicity was acceptable and the response rate high. Other drugs, such as vinorelbine and CPT-11 are being investigated concurrently as radiosensitizers in NSCLC.

To sum up, there is clinical evidence that certain drugs used daily with radiotherapy act as radiosensitizers. To date, only daily cisplatin was demonstrated to improve the effect of radiotherapy on local control and survival in a large-scale randomized study, but other compounds such as metoclopramide and carboplatin are currently being investigated as radiosensitizers in phase III studies. Other drugs such as paclitaxel, CPT-11 and vinorelbine are also being subjected to intensive research.

14.3.3 Clinical Experience with Interferons

A combination of the various interferons (IFN) with radiotherapy in NSCLC was tested in a limited number of phase I and II studies, as shown in Table 14.3. MAASLITA et al. randomized 20 patients to

Table 14.3. IFN associated with RT in locally advanced NSCLC

IF	Type	Product	Authors	No. of patients	RT	IF dose	RR	Median Survival (months)	3-year survival	Toxicity
α	I	Natural leukocytes	MAASILTA et al. 1992 (FIN)	20 random	60/1.25 b.i.d.	0 3×10^6 i.m. + 3×10^6 neb.	5/10 6/10	NA	NA	Increased esophagitis in IF dose, decreased in 8/10
β	I	Recombinant *E. coli* betaseron	MCDONALD et al. 1993b	39 phase I escalating (26 stage III)	Escalating 54 or 59.4	Escalating 10 30, 60 or 90 × 10^6 i.v. days 1–3 weeks 1–3–5	CR 44% PR 38%	19.7	31% (3 and 5 years)	Decreased lung toxicity
β	I	Recombinant mammary cell Rebif.	BYHARD et al. 1996	15	60/6 w	Escalating 1.5, 3, 6 12,24 MIU/m^2	1/15 CR 6/15 PR	11		Grade IV in 5; 1/3 pts. with 24 MIU died of ARDS MTD = ~12 MIU
γ	II	Recombinant *E. coli*	SHAW et al. 1995	18	60/4 w (b.i.d.)	0.2 mg/day s.c.	CR 6% PR 33%	7.8		9/18 = 50% severe toxicity, 8/17 pneumonitis, 2/17 esophagitis, 2 toxic deaths

Rebif., recombinant beta inferferon.

hyperfractionated radiotherapy, 1.25 Gy b.i.d. to a total dose of 60 Gy, either alone or with IFN-α. IFN-α was administered both intramuscularly at $3 \cdot 10^6$ IU and by inhalation of $1.5 \cdot 10^6$ IU. This treatment proved to be laborious, the response rate being almost identical and toxicity was substantial with possible early deaths in the experimental arm (MAASLITA et al. 1992).

MCDONALD et al. conducted a phase I/II study with escalating doses of recombinant IFN-β from 10 to $90 \cdot 10^6$ IU given i.v., the first 3 days of weeks 1, 3 and 5, while concurrent radiotherapy consisted of 54 Gy–59.4 Gy at 1.8 Gy/fraction (MCDONALD et al. 1993b). For the 32 evaluable patients, the response rate was 81% with 44% achieving a complete response. An amazing median survival of 19.7 months and 5-year survival of 31% was observed, with minimal toxicity (MCDONALD et al. 1993b).

Also using recombinant human IFN-β, BYHARDT et al. conducted another phase I study in stage II, III_A and III_B, NSCLC (BYHARDT et al. 1996). Patients received a radiotherapy dose of 60 Gy at 2 Gy/fraction, and IFN-β was given subcutaneously at escalating doses of 1.5, 3, 6, 12 and 24 MIU/m^2 per treatment dose. Fifteen patients were enrolled, and 14 experienced grade 1–3 toxicity, which was primarily gastrointestinal. One patient at 24 MIU/m^2 died from sepsis and radiation pneumonitis. MTD was estimated to be at 12 MIU/m^2. One complete and six partial responses were recorded, and the median survival was 11 months (BYHARDT et al. 1996).

Recombinant IFN-γ was the subject of a pilot study carried out by SHAW et al. (1995). Eighteen patients with unresectable stge III_A and III_B NSCLC were treated with daily gamma interferon (0.2 mg subcutaneously) concomitant with accelerated radiotherapy of 60 Gy at 1.5 Gy b.i.d. Nine patients experienced severe, life-threatening or fatal complications. Eight had significant pneumonitis, which was severe in six and fatal in two. Median survival time and 1-year survival rates were 7.8 months and 38%, respectively (SHAW et al. 1995).

Other studies with recombinant IF-β are currently being carried out. RTOG 93-04 is the logical follow-up of MCDONALD et al.'s phase I/II. Patients are randomized between radiation alone, 60 Gy at 2 Gy/fraction, versus radiation with IFN-β at weeks 1,3 and 5 (BYHARDT 1995). Results are not available at this time.

GF 8540 is a multicenter European phase I trial, in which patients receive a fixed dose of radiotherapy of 64 Gy with escalating doses of IFN-β of 3, 6, 9, 12 and 18 MIU/m^2 given intravenously with daily radiotherapy (REBIF 1996). Eighteen patients have been enrolled so far, and the maximum tolerated dose has not yet been reached.

In summary, the various interferons have been recently investigated in conjunction with radiotherapy in NSCLC. Early results indicate that IFN-α and IFN-γ do not have an interesting therapeutic index and should probably be abandoned. IFN-β seemed to be very promising in a limited phase II study, with the suggestion of an increased therapeutic index. It is now currently the subject of at least two clinical investigations in the United States and Europe.

14.3.4 Clinical Experience with Radioprotectors

As for radiosensitizers, the majority of clinical studies with radioprotectors (essentially amifostine) deal with cancer types other than lung cancers (Tannehill and Mehta 1996). In previous studies, the maximal tolerated dose was found to be 340 mg/m^2 4 days/week for 5 weeks: emesis, malaise and hypotension being the main side effects (Klingermann et al. 1988; Constine et al. 1986).

In patients with stage III$_A$ and III$_B$ NSCLC, Tannehill et al. conducted a phase II study using amifostine with induction chemotherapy (cisplatin and vinblastine) followed by amifostine with radiation therapy of 60 Gy (Tannehill et al. 1997). Twenty-six patients were enrolled. Chemotherapy doses were higher than in other induction regimes. Amifostine at 340 mg/m^2, 4 days/week, or 200 mg/m^2 5 days/week was given immediately prior to radiation. Overall response rate was 60%; median survival was 13 months. Interestingly, overall toxicity, including esophagitis, was minimal with no grade 3 or 4 cases (Tannehill et al. 1997). The authors conclude that an appropriately designed randomized trial is necessary to validate these observations.

14.4 Conclusions

There are a number of potential or recognized ways to improve the therapeutic effect of ionizing radiations, and many biochemical or biological compounds have radiosensitizing or radioprotective properties, which are in many cases supported by sound radiobiological data. In contrast, only a minority of known radiosensitizers and protectors were tested in patients with NSCLC, and only very few were unequivocally shown to be active and to have an exploitable therapeutic index. In this regard, platinum compounds, the newer class of chemotherapeutic agents, IFN-β and amifostine seem to be the most promising, but this warrants further studies. This combination with other modalities to improve the efficacy of irradiation, such as conformal radiotherapy, could be the target of innovative investigations.

References

Bailey SM, Suggett N, Walton MI, Workman P (1992) Structure-activity relationships for DT-diaphorase reduction of hypoxic cell directed agents: indoloquinones and diaziridinyl benzoquinones. Int J Radiat Oncol Biol Phys 22:649–653

Baker MA, Zeman EM, Hirst VK, Brown JM (1988) Metabolism of SR 4233 by Chinese hamster ovary cells: basis of selective hypoxia cytotoxicity. Cancer Res 48:5947–5952

Ball D, Bishop J, Crennan E (1991) Concurrent radiotherapy and carboplatin in non-small cell lung cancer: a pilot study using conventional and accelerated fractionation. Austr Radiol 35:66–67

Bernier J (1998) Accelerated radiotherapy with carbogen and nicotinamide. A phase I-II study: personal communication, EORTC RT Group meeting, Milan, April 1998

Bishop JF, Ball D, Creunan E, Ryan G, Davis S, Toner GO, Brian P, Olver I (1994) Radiation and carboplatin combined-modality therapy in non-small cell lung cancer. Semin Oncol 3(S6):91–96

Boothman DA, Wang M, Schea RA, Barrows HL, Strickfaden S, Owens J (1992) Posttreatment exposure to camptothecin enhances the lethal effects of X-rays on radioresistance human malignant melanoma cells. Int J Radiat Oncol Biol Phys 24:939–948

Brown JM (1979) Evidence for acutely hypoxic cells in mouse tumors, and a possible mechanism of reoxygenation. Br J Radiol 52:650–656

Brown JM, Siim EG (1996) Hypoxia-specific cytotoxins in cancer therapy. Semin Radiat Oncol 6:22–36

Bump EA, Brown JM (1990) Role of glutathione in the radiation response of mammalian cells *in vitro* and *in vivo*. Pharmacol Ther 47:117–120

Byhardt RW (1995) The evolution of radiation therapy oncology group (RTOG) protocols for non-small cell lung cancer. Int J Radiat Oncol Biol Phys 32:1513–1525

Byhardt RW, Vaickus L, Witt PL, Chang AY, McAuliffe T, Wilson JF, Lawton CA, Breitmeyer J, Alger ME, Borden EC (1996) Recombinant human interferon-β (rHuIFN-β) and radiation therapy for inoperable non-small cell lung cancer. J Interferon Cytokine Res 16:891–902

Calabro-Jones PM, Fahey RC, Smoluk GD (1985) Alkaline phosphatase promotes radioprotection and accumulation of WR-1065 in V79–171 cells incubated in medium containing amifostine. Int J Radiat Oncol Biol Phys 47:23–27

Chang AYC, Keng PC (1987) Potentiation of radiation cytotoxicity by recombinant interferons, a phenomenon associated with increased blockage in G_2-M phase of the cell cycle. Cancer Res 47:4338–4341

Chaplin DJ, Durand RE, Olive PE (1986) Acute hypoxia in tumors: implications for modifiers of radiation effects. Int J Radiat Oncol Biol Phys 12:1279–1282

Coleman CN, Bump EA, Kramer RA (1988) Chemical modifiers of cancer treatment. J Clin Oncol 6:709–733

Coleman CN, Noll LN, Riese N, Buswell L, Howes AE, Loeffler JS, Alexander E Wen P, Harris J, Kramer RA, Hurwitz SJ,

Neben TY, Grigsby P (1992) final report of the phase I trial of continuous infusion etanidazole (SR 2508): a Radiation Therapy Oncology group Study. Int J Radiat Oncol Biol Phys 22:577–580

Coleman CN, Beard CJ, Hlatky L, Kwok TT, Bump E (1994) Biochemical modifiers: hypoxic cell sensitizers. In: Mauch PM, Loeffler JS (eds) Radiation oncology: technology and biology. Saunders, Philadelphia, pp 56–89

Constine LS, Zagars G, Rubin P, Kligerman M (1986) Protection by WR-2721 of human bone marrow function following irradiation. Int J Radiat Oncol Biol Phys 12:1505–1508

Del Bino G, Bruno S, Yi PN, Darzynkiewicz Z (1992) Apoptotic cell death triggered by camptothecin or teniposide. Cell Prolif 25:537–548

Dewit L (1987) Combined treatment of radiation and cisplatin: a review of experimental and clinical data. Int J Radiat Oncol Biol Phys 13:403–426

Dische S (1991a) What have we learnt from hyperbaric oxygen? Radiother Oncol S 20:71–74

Dische S (1991b) Radiotherapy and anemia – the clinical experience. Radiother Oncol S 20:35–40

Edelstein MP, Wolfe LA III, Duch DS (1996) Potentiation of radiation therapy by Vinorelbine (Navelbine) in non-small cell lung cancer. Semin Oncol 23(S2):S41–47

Ellebrock NA, Fossella F, Rich TA, Ajani JA, Komaki R, Roth JA, Holoye PY (1991) Low-dose continuous infusion cisplatin combined with external beam irradiation for advanced colorectal adenocarcinoma and unresectable non-small cell lung carcinoma. Int J Radiat Oncol Biol Phys 20:351–355

Gatenby RA, Kessler HB, Rosenblum JS, Coia LR, Moldorfski PJ, Hurtz WH, Broder GY (1988) Oxygen distribution in squamous cell carcinoma metastases and its relationship to outcome of radiation therapy. Int J Radiat Oncol Biol Phys 14:831–838

Gould MN, Kakrin RC, Olson S, Borden S (1984) Radiosensitization of human bronchogenic carcinoma cells by interferon beta. J Interferon Res 4:123–128

Groen HJM, van den Leest A, de Vries EGE, Uges DRA, Szabo BG, Smit EF, Mulder NH (1994) Continuous infusion of carboplatin during 6 weeks of radiotherapy in locally inoperable non-small cell lung cancer: a phase I and pharmacokinetic study. ASCO Proc J C O 13:343

Guichard M (1991) The use of fluorocarbon emulsions in cancer radiotherapy. Radiother Oncol S20:S59–64

Hall EJ (1994a) The oxygen effect and reoxygenation. In: Hall EJ (ed) Radiobiology for the radiologist. Lippincott, Philadelphia, pp 133–152

Hall EJ (1994b) Radioprotectors. In: Hall EJ (ed) Radiobiology for the radiologist. Lippincott, Philadephia, pp 183–190

Hallahan DE, Haimovitz-Friedman A, Kufe DW, Fuks Z, Weichselbaum RR (1993) The role of cytokines in radiation oncology. In: De Vita VT, Hellman S, Rosenberg SA (eds) Important advances in oncology. Lippincott, Philadelphia, pp 71–80

Höckel M, Schlenger K, Knoop C, Vaupel P (1991) Oxygenation of carcinomas of uterine cervix: evaluation by computerized 0_2 tension measurements. Cancer Res 51:6098–7003

Horsman MR, Chaplin DJ, Brown JM (1989) Tumor radiosensitization by nicotinamide: a result of improved perfusion and oxygenation. Radiat Res 118:139–150

Kardamakis D, Gillies NE, Souhami RL, Bewerley PCL (1989) Recombinant human interferon alpha-2b enhances the radiosensitivity of small cell lung cancer *in vitro*. Anticancer Res 9:1041–1044

Kelly SA, McLead PM, Ash DV (1989) The use of simultaneous radiotherapy and 5-fluorouracil in patients with inoperable squamous cell lung cancer. Clin Radiother 40:311–313

Kim JH, Alfieri AA, Kim SH, Young SW (1986) Potentiation of radiation effects on two murine tumors by lonidamine. Cancer Res 46:120–123

Kinsella TJ, Dobson PP, Mitchell JB, Fornace AJ (1987) Enhancement of x-ray induced DNA damage by pretreatment with halogenated pyrimidine analogs. Int J Radiat Oncol Biol Phys 13:733–739

Kjellen E, Wennerberg E, Pero RW (1989) Metoclopramide enhances the effect of cisplatin on xenografted squamous cell carcinoma of the head and neck. Br J Cancer 59:247–250

Kjellen E, Joiner MC, Collier JM, Johns H, Rojas AM (1991) A therapeutic benefit from combining normobaric carbogen or oxygen with nicotinamide in fractionated X-ray treatments. Radiother Oncol 22:81–91

Kjellen E, Pero RW, Brun E, Ewers SB, Jarlman O, Knöös T, Malmström P, Tennvall J, Killander D, Olsson A, Sheng Y, Wennerberg J (1995) A phase I/II evaluation of metoclopramide as radio-sensitizer in patients with inoperable squamous cell carcinoma of the lung. Eur J Cancer 31 A:2196–2202

Klingermann MM, Turrisi AT, Urtasun RC, Norfleet AL, Phillips TL, Barteloy T, Rubin P (1988) final report on phase I trial of WR-2721 before protracted fractionated radiation therapy. Int J Radiat Oncol Biol Physics 14:1119–1122

Kruuv JA, Inch WR, McCredie JA (1967) Blood flow and oxygenation of tumors in mice. Cancer 20:51–59

Lallev A, Anachkova B, Russev G (1993) Effect of ionizing radiation and topoisomerate II inhibitors on DNA synthesis in mammalian cells. Eur J Biochem 216:177–181

Le Chevalier T, Arriagada R, Quoix E, Ruffie P, Martin M, Douillard JY, Tarayse M, Lacombe-Terrier MJ, Laplanche A (1991) Radiotherapy alone versus combined chemotherapy and radiotherapy in non-resectable non-small cell lung cancer – first analysis of a randomized trial in 353 patients. J Natl Cancer Inst 83:417–423

Lokich J, Chaffey J, Neptune W (1989) Concomitant 5-fluorouracil infusion and high dose radiation for stage III non-small cell lung cancer. Cancer 64:1021–1025

Luk LK, Veinot-Drebot L, Tjan E, Tannock IF (1990) Effect of transient hypoxia on sensitivity to doxorubicin in human and murine cell lines. J Natl Cancer Inst 82:684–692

Lustig R, Loewe N, Prosnitz L, Spaulding M, Cohen M, Stilt Y, Brannon R (1990) fluosol and oxygen breathing as an adjuvant to radiation therapy in the treatment of locally advanced non-small cell carcinoma of the lung: results of a phase I/II study. Int J Radiat Oncol Biol Phys 19:97–102

Lyback S, Pero RW (1991) The benzamide derivative metoclopramide causes DNA damage and inhibition of DNA repair in human peripheral mononuclear leucocytes at clinically relevant doses. Carcinogenesis 12:1613–1617

Maaslita P, Holsti LR, Halme M, Kivisaari L, Cantell K, Mattson K (1992) Natural alpha-interferon in combination with hyperfractionated radiotherapy in the treatment of non-small cell lung cancer. Int J Radiat Oncol Biol Phys 23:863–868

Marangolo M, Emiliani E, Rosti G, Giannini M, Vertogen B, Zumaglini F (1996) Phase I/II study of Paclitaxel and Radiotherapy in non-small cell lung cancer. Semin Oncol 23 (S6):124–127

McDonald S, Rubin P, Chang A, Penney D, finkelstein J, Grossberg S, Gregory P (1993a) Pulmonary changes induced by combined mouse β-interferon and radiation in normal mice – toxic versus protective effects. Radiother Oncol 26:212–218

McDonald S, Chang AY, Rubin P, Wallenberg J, Kim IS, Sobel S, Smith J, Keng P, Muhs A (1993b) Combined betaseron R (recombinant human interferon beta) and radiation for inoperable non-small cell lung cancer. Int J Radiat Oncol Biol Phys 27:613–619

Milas L, Hunter N, Ito H, Peters LY (1984) Effect of tumor type, size and endpoints on tumor radioprotection by WR-2721. Int J Radiat Oncol Biol Phys 10:41–48

Miller EM, Fowler JF, Kinsella TJ (1992) Linear quadratic analysis of radiosensitization by halogenated pyrimidines: I. Radiosensitization of human colon cancer cells by IUdR. Radiat Res 131:81–89

Mirimanoff RO (1994) Concurrent chemotherapy and radiotherapy in locally advanced non-small cell lung cancer: a review. Lung Cancer 11:S79–99

Nordsmark M, Bentzen SM, Overgaard J (1994) Measurement of human tumor oxygenation status by a polarographic needle electrode. Acta Oncol 33:383–389

Overgaard J, Horsman MR (1996) Modification of hypoxia-induced radioresistance in tumors by the use of oxygen and sensitizers. Semin Radiat Oncol 6:10–21

Overgaard J, Sand Hansen H, Lindelov B, Overgaard M, Jorgensen K, Rasmussen B, Berthelsen A (1991) Nimorazole as a hypoxic cell radiosensitizer in the treatment of supraglottic larynx and pharynx carcinoma: first report from the Danish Head and Neck Cancer (DAHANCA) protocol 5-85. Radiother Oncol 20:143–149

Patt HN, Tyree S, Straube RL (1949) Cysteine protection against irradiation. Science 110:213–214

Pestka S, Langer JA, Zoon KC, Samnel CE (1987) Interferons and their actions. Annu Rev Biochem 56:727–777

Phillips RA, Tolmach LJ (1966) Repair of potentially lethal damage in x-irradiated HeLa cells. Radiat Res 29:413–432

Pignon JP, Arriagada R, Ihde DC, Johnson DH, Perry MC, Souhami RL, Brodin O, Joss RA, Kies MS, Lebeau B, Onoshi T, Osterlind K, Tattersall M, Wagner H (1992) A meta-analysis of thoracic radiotherapy for small-cell lung cancer. N Engl J Med 327:1618–1624

Rebif in NSCLC (1996) Study 8540: recombinant human interferon-beta (RHuIFN-beta). Investigator's Brochure. Ares-Serono

Rojas A (1991) Radiosensitization with normobaric oxygen and carbogen. Radiother Oncol 20:S65–S70

Rubin P, Johnston CJ, Williams JP, McDonald S, finkelstein JN (1995) A perpetual cascade of cytokines postirradiation leads to pulmonary fibrosis. Int J Radiat Oncol Biol Phys 33:99–109

Sartorelli AC (1988) Therapeutic attack of hypoxic cells of solid tumors: presidential address. Cancer Res 48:775–778

Scarantino CW, McCunniff AJ, Evans G, Young CW, Paggiarino DA (1994) A prospective randomized comparison of radiation therapy plus Ionidamine versus radiation therapy plus placebo as initial treatment of clinically localized but non resectable non-small cell lung cancer. Int J Radiat Oncol Biol Phys 29:999–1004

Schaake-Koning C, Van den Bogaert W, Dalesio O, Festen Y, Hoogenhout J, van Houtte P, Kirkpatrick A, Koolen M, Maat B (1992) Effects of concomitant cisplatin and radiotherapy on inoperable non-small cell lung cancer. N Engl J Med 326:524–530

Schottenfeld D, Pass HI, Mitchell JB, Johnson DH, Turrisi AT (1996) Epidemiology of lung cancer. In: Lung cancer, principles and practice, 1st edn. Lippincott-Raven, Philadelphia, pp 305–340

Schottenfeld D (1996) Epidemiology of lung cancer. In: Pass HI, Mitchell JB, Johnson DH, Turrisi AT (eds) Lung cancer, principles and practice, 1st edn. Lippincott-Raven, Philadelphia, pp 305–340

Shaw EG, Deming RL, Creagan ET, Nair S, Su JQ, Levitt R, Steen PD, Wiesenfeld M, Mailliard JA (1995) Pilot study of human recombinant interferon gamma and accelerated hyperfractionated thoracic radiotherapy in patients with unresectable stage III A/B non small cell lung cancer. Int J Radiat Oncol Biol Phys 31:827–831

Shrieve DC, Deen DF, Harris JW (1983) Effects of extreme hypoxia on the growth and viability of EMT6/SF mouse tumor cells in vitro. Cancer Res 43:3521–3527

Simpson JR, Bauer M, Wasserman TH, Perez CA, Emami BE, Wiegensberg I, Zinninger M, Martin Durbin L (1987) Large fraction irradiation with or without misonidazole in advanced non-oat cell carcinoma of the lung: a phase III randomized trial of the RTOG. Int J Radiat Oncol Biol Phys 13:861–867

Simpson JR, Bauer M, Perez CA, Wasserman TH, Emami B, Scott Doggett EL, Byhardt RW, Phillipps TL, Mowry PA (1989) Radiotherapy alone or combined with misonidazole in the treatment of locally advanced non-oat cell lung cancer: report of an RTOG prospective randomized trial. Int J Radiat Oncol Biol Phys 16:1483–1491

Sinclair WK (1968) The combined effect of hydroxyurea and x-rays on Chinese hamster cells in vitro. Cancer Res 28:198–206

Steren A, Sevin Bu, Perras J, Ramus R, Angioli R, Nguyen H, Koechli O, Averette HE (1993) Taxol as a radiation sensitizer: a flow cytometric study. Gynecol Oncol 50:89–93

Tamm L, Jasny BR Pfeffer LM (1987) Antiproliferative action of interferons. In: Pfeffer LM (ed) Mechanisms of interferon action. CRC Press, Bota Raton, pp 25–58

Tannehill SP, Mehta MP (1996) Amifostine and radiation therapy: past, present and future. Semin Oncol 29:S69–S77

Tannehill SP, Mehta MP, Larson M, Storer B, Pellet Y, Kinsella TJ, Schiller JH (1997) Effect of amifostine on toxicities associated with sequential chemotherapy and radiation therapy for unresectable non-small lung cancer: results of a phase II trial. J Clin Oncol 15:2850–2857

Teicher BA, Herman TS, Holden SA, Epelbaum R, Liu S, Frei E III (1991) Lonidamine as a modulator of alkylating agents activity *in vitro* and *in vivo*. Cancer Res 51:780–784

Thomlinson RH, Gray LH (1955) The histological structure of some human lung cancers and the possible implications for radiotherapy. Br J Cancer 9:539–549

Tobias JS, Smith BJ, Blackman G, finn G (1987) Concurrent daily cisplatin and radiotherapy in locally advanced squamous cell carcinoma of the head and neck and bronchus. Radiother Oncol 9:263–268

Trovo M, Minatel E, Franchin G, Gobitti C, Roncardin M, De Paoli A, Arcicasa M, Boz G, Bortolus R (1992a) Radiotherapy enhanced by cisplatinum in stage III non-small cell lung cancer: a phase II study. Radiother Oncol 23:241–244

Trovo M, Minatel E, Franchin G, Boccieri MG, Nascimben O, Bolzicco G, Pizzi G, Torretta A, Veronesi A, Gobitti C (1992b) Radiotherapy versus radiotherapy enhanced by cisplatin in stage III non-small cell lung cancer. Int J Radiat Oncol Biol Phys 24:11–15

Van Harskamp G, Boven E, Vermorken J, Van Dentekom H, Stam J, Hian Njo K, Karim AB, Tierie AH, Golding R, Pinedo HM (1987) Phase II trial of continued radiotherapy and daily low-dose cisplatin for inoperable, locally advanced non-small cell lung cancer. Int J Radiat Oncol Biol Phys 13:1735–1738

Vaupel P (1994) Blood flow and metabolic microenvironment of brain tumors. J Neuro Oncol 22:261–267

Vaupel P, Schlenger K, Knoop C, Hockel M (1991) Oxygenation of human tumors: evaluation of tissue oxygen distribution in breast cancers by computerized 0_2 tension measurements. Cancer Res 51:3316–3320

Vogt HG, Kolotas C, Martin T, Schneider LV, Neeb A, Mitrou PS, Diergarten K, Dornoff W, Zamboglou N (1996) Simultaneous radiochemotherapy with paclitaxel in non-small cell lung cancer: a clinical phase I study. Semin Oncol 23(S6):26–30

Witt PL, McAuliffe TL, Shadley JD (1993) Increased cytotoxicity in human lung but not glioma tumor lines by the combination of radiation and interferon-β. Proc Am Assoc Cancer 34:84

Young SD, Hill RP (1990) Effects of reoxygenation on cells from hypoxic regions of solid tumors: an anticancer drug sensitivity and metastatic potential. J Natl Cancer Inst 82:371–380

Yuhas JM (1980) Active versus passive absorption. Kinetics as the basis for selective protection of normal tissue by S-2 [3-aminopropylamino]-ethylphosphorothioic acid. Cancer Res 40:1519–1524

15 Intraoperative Radiotherapy for Lung Cancer

F.A. Calvo, J.J. Aristu, M. Moreno, M. Santos, and S.A. Fisher

CONTENTS

15.1 Introduction

15.1.1 Intraoperative Radiotherapy (IOERT) in Clinical Oncology

IOERT is an attractive radiotherapy technique able to deliver a high-quality electron radiation boost to most regions of the human anatomy (Fig. 15.1). Its feasibility is well proven during cancer surgery (Calvo et al. 1992b). Local tumor control rates in radical treatment programs combining a single-dose IOERT boost (10–20 Gy), external beam fractionated irradiation (45–50 Gy), minimal postsurgical cancer residue and chemotherapy (when indicated) have been consistently reported in the range of 85%–100%. Results in association with palliative surgery (no resection or atypical resections with macroscopic tumor residue) are modest in terms of long-term survival, but local control rates are described in the range of 40%–60% (Calvo et al. 1993). Tolerance of normal tissues to the combination of IOERT boost single high-dose (10–20 Gy) and fractionated radiotherapy (45–50 Gy) are better understood in the 1990s and with the appropriate dose prescription restrictions there is no compromise of the therapeutic index, in terms of excessive severe toxicity of clinical relevance (Shaw et al. 1990).

Interest in IOERT in modern clinical oncology is focused on the investigation of improvement in local cancer therapy. IOERT is a simple technique, but requires a complex institutional program to ensure a successful and clinically relevant implantation. The development of viable prospective multi-institutional trials is still a pending challenge for IOERT scientists and qualified institutions in the international scenario (Calvo and Hanks 1988; Gunderson 1994).

15.1.2 Local Control in Contemporary Lung Cancer Treatment

The rationale to intensify locoregional treatment is based on the observation that 30%–40% of patients die with active locoregional disease (Pérez et al. 1986, 1987; Cox 1983; Emami and Graham 1998), and it is likely that the incidence of local failure is underestimated because most published series did not utilize CT or bronchoscopy for treatment planning and/or restaging following external beam radiation therapy (EBRT). Histologic examination of bronchoscopic biopsy specimens in patients treated with irradiation or combined chemoradiation documented a local failure rate of almost 80% (Le Chevalier et al. 1991). Another reason for the

F.A. Calvo, Department of Oncology, Hospital General Universitario Gregorio Marañón, Dr. Esquerdo 46, E-28007 Madrid, Spain
J.J. Aristu, M. Moreno, Department of Oncology, Clínica Universitaria de Navarra, E-31080 Pamplona, Spain
M. Santos, Instituto Madrileño de Oncología, Emilio Vargas 16, E-28043 Madrid, Spain
S.A. Fisher, Department of Radiation Oncology, Allegheny University Hospitals, Graduate, 1800 Lombard St., Philadelphia, PA 19146, USA

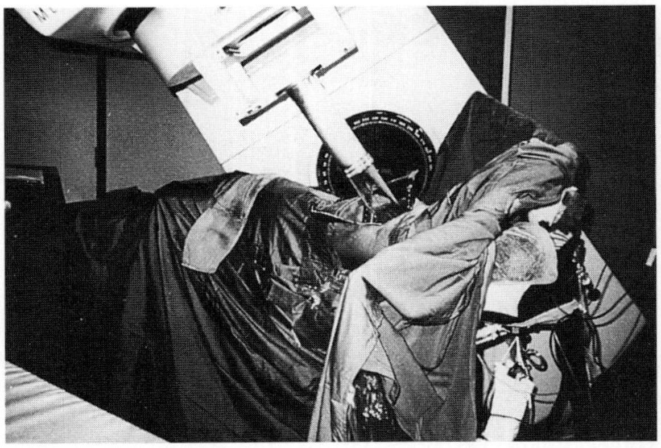

Fig. 15.1. General view of an IOERT procedure during thoracotomy for lung cancer resection in the left pulmonary apex

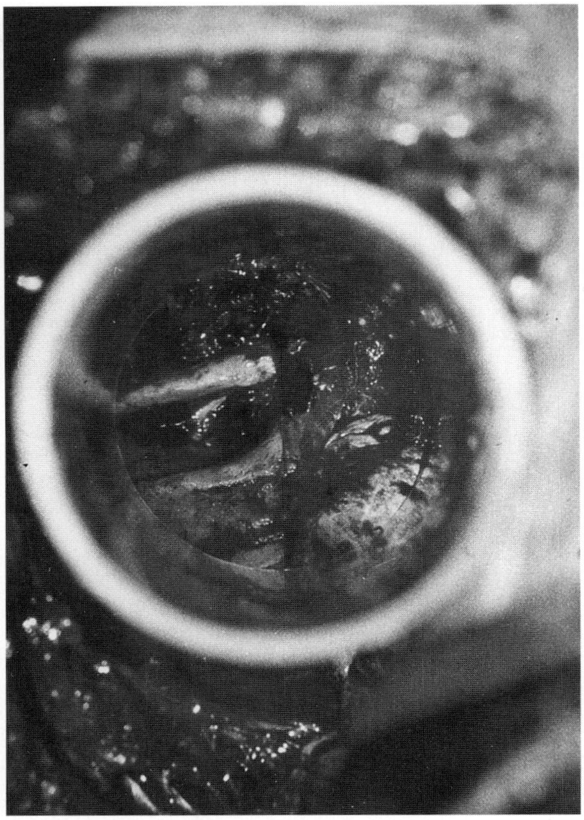

Fig. 15.2. Target volume following resection of a Pancoast tumor with involvement of the chest wall

understimation of local failure rate in patients with NSCLC is the development of distant metastases in the early follow-up period: local control is uncertain when assessed in patients surviving less than 1 year.

Expert radiotherapy opinions suggest that thoracic control in lung cancer is dose-related but radiosensitive organs such as the lung, spinal cord, and heart often limit the dose of EBRT to 45–60 Gy, a dose usually inadequate to sterilize large masses of NSCLC. In an effort to improve local control and survival, new treatment strategies have been explored, such as hyperfractionated (Cox et al. 1990, 1991) or accelerated fractionation (Byhart et al. 1993), chemoradiotherapy (Sause et al. 1995), radiation dose-escalation using three-dimensional planning and conformal irradiation (Emani et al. 1991; Armstrong et al. 1993) or intraoperative irradiation (IOERT).

Intraoperative electron radiation therapy (IOERT) is a modality able to deliver a high single dose of fast electron irradiation in a surgically defined area, while normal uninvolved and mobile tissues and organs are retracted for protection from the electron beam by surgical displacement (Fig. 15.2). Clinical experiences using IOERT in lung cancer patients have rarely been published (Pass et al. 1987; Juettner et al. 1990; Calvo et al. 1990). Methodology and clinical results, in the context of expert institutional experiences, are presented.

15.2 IOERT in Thoracic Oncology

IOERT using electrons has been explored as a radiation boosting technique in lung cancer (resectable and unresectable) (Smolle-Juettner et al. 1994; Calvo et al. 1992a), mediastinal tumors (thymoma and recurrent Hodgkin's disease) (Calvo et al. 1991) and mesothelioma (Jablons et al. 1997), after a surgical approach to the intrathoracic anatomy. In extrathoracic (external chest wall) surgery, IOERT has been successfully used in the combined treatment of soft tissue sarcomas (Calvo et al. 1995).

15.2.1 Technical Considerations

IOERT requires the adaptation of a linear accelerator with multienergetic electron beam capability (energies recommended from 6 to 20 MeV), through the development of specially designed applicators for electron beam conformation (cone sizes recommended from 5 to 12 cm diameter). The clinical program combines the efforts of surgeons, anesthesiologists, physicists and radiation oncologists to adequately select patients for IOERT indications, perform the surgical procedure (tumor resection plus normal tissue protection), transport and monitor the patient for and during intraoperative irradiation and finally decide the radiotherapeutic parameters for treatment prescription. In general, IOERT during lung cancer surgery involves the coordination of 10–15 health professionals, prolongs the surgical time approximately 30–45 min (depending upon transportation time) and induces a 2 h gap of time availability in the linear accelerator for outpatient treatment.

15.2.2 Clinical Indications

IOERT at the time of thoracotomy for a surgical approach to lung cancer has been employed in three different situations:

- Treatment of unresectable hilar and/or mediastinal disease
- Treatment of postresected residual disease (chest wall, mediastinum and/or bronchial stump)
- Adjuvant treatment of mediastinum

Conceptual indications for IOERT in thoracic surgery have been the treatment of residual disease at the primary site and/or nodal regions, or adjuvant treatment of high risk of recurrence without proven cancer residue after induction therapy and surgery. IOERT is a superselective radiation boost component available for integration in conventional radiotherapy programs for lung cancer. Lung parenchyma is the normal tissue that may benefit the most from protection from IOERT (Fig. 15.3).

Esophagus, trachea aorta and heart are difficult to displace from the IOERT beam, particularly in the treatment of mediastinal regions or left lower chest cavity. In the case that the bronchial stump is included in the IOERT field, tissue coverage with a vascularized pleural or pericardial flap is recommended to promote bronchial healing.

15.2.3 Treatment Protocols

IOERT, as an accurate radiation boost technique during lung cancer surgery, has been actively explored by investigators at the University Clinic of Navarra, Pamplona, the Madrid Institute of Oncology, Madrid, and the Graduate Hospital, Philadelphia. Treatment strategies have included the use of IOERT in the following modality sequences:

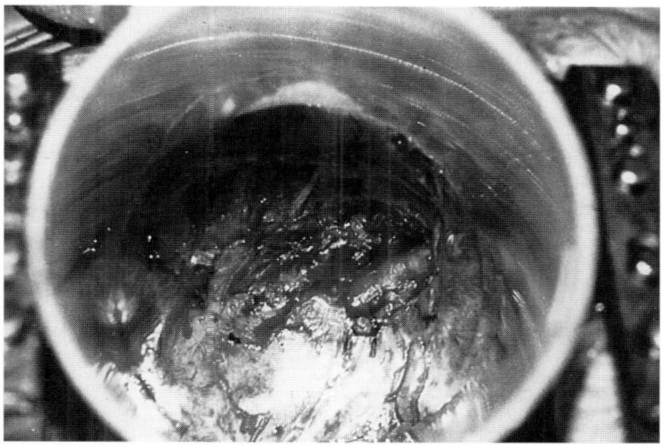

Fig. 15.3. Target volume in the right mediastinal space following lobectomy and nodal sampling

- Surgery + IOERT/EBRT (with or without resection)
- Neoadjuvant chemotherapy/surgery + IOERT/EBRT
- Preoperative chemoradiation/surgery + IOERT

Surgery consisted in general of lateral thoracotomies, modifying the intercostal site of incision depending upon tumor location. Primary lesion tumor resection was attempted (lobectomy and/or atypical resections were elected when feasible over pneumonectomy) together with ipsilateral nodal sampling. At the University Clinic of Navarra, induction chemotherapy consisted of the combination of cisplatin, mitomycin C and vindesine (three cycles), and chemoradiation included either the simultaneous administration of the described chemotherapy and 45 Gy (conventional fractionation) or a combination of cisplatin and 5-flurouracil continuous i.v. infusion during the 1 and last week of EBRT 45–50 Gy (this regimen was predominantly used in Pancoast tumors). IOERT boosted postresection tumor beds (chest wall, mediastinum, hilar, etc.) using either one single field (60% of cases) or multiple non overlapping fields (40% of cases) to encompass residual or risk areas in different sites of the thoracic anatomy. The electron energy beam was selected depending on tumor (or risk tissue) thickness, ranging from 6 to 20 MeV. The IOERT single dose was in the range of 10 (90%) to 15 Gy (10%), prescribed at the 90% isodose line. IOERT target volume definition considered the tumor resection margins, macroscopic residual disease and/or unresected palpable primary (Fig. 15.4). Attempts to protect normal uninvolved lung parenchyma were made at the time of IOERT applicator set-up for treatment, while heart, trachea, esophagus and other mediastinal

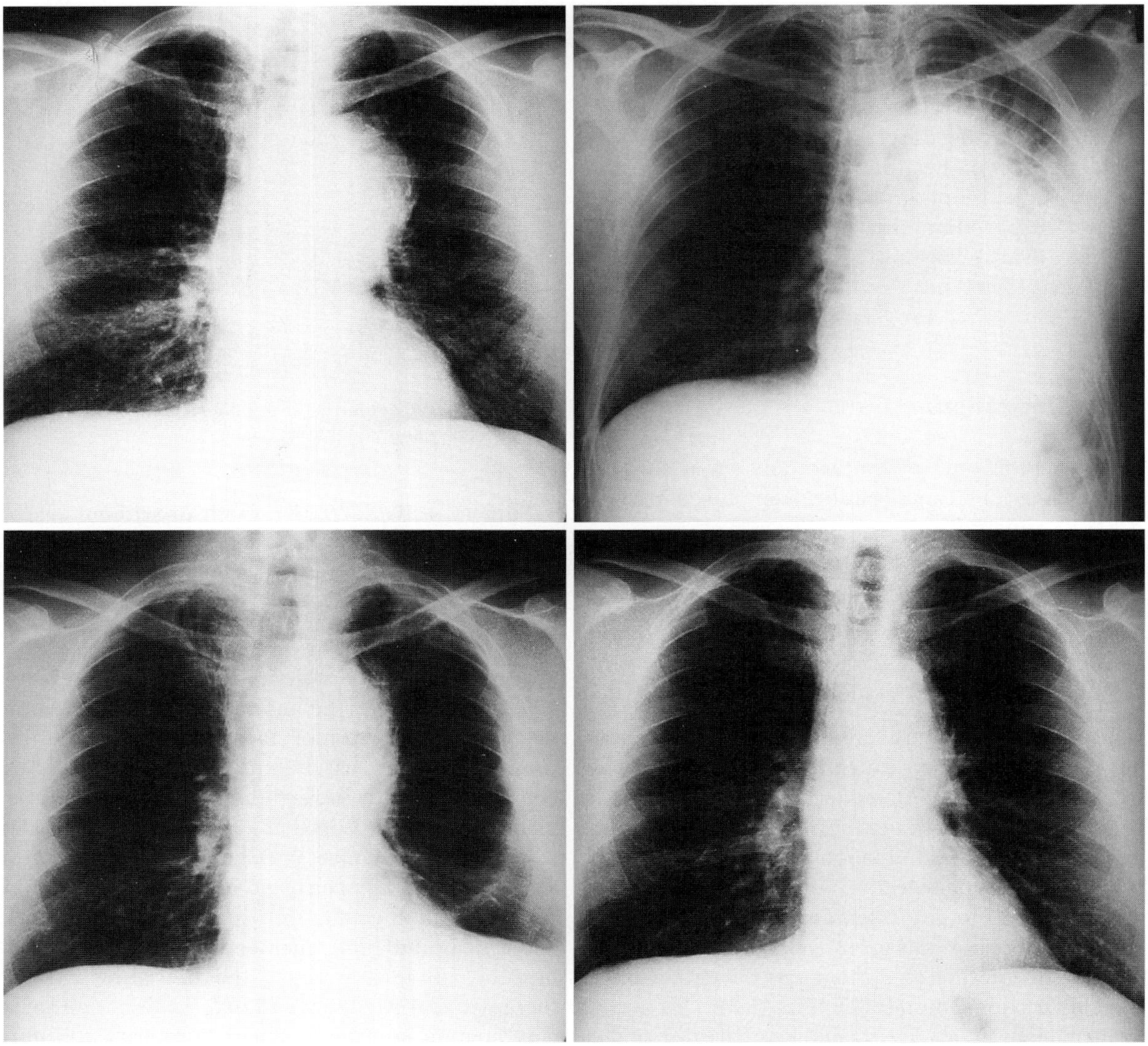

a b c d

Fig. 15.4 a–d. Chest X-ray evolution of a radiological remission of a large cell undifferentiated and unresectable left upper lobe lung cancer treated exclusively with IOERT (15 Gy) and external beam radiotherapy (46 Gy/23 fractions/5 weeks): **a** before thoracotomy; **b** pneumonitis 15 days after IOERT; **c** 4 months after external irradiation; **d** 20 months following IOERT

structures (nerve) were not displaced from their normal anatomical situation.

15.2.4 IOERT Tissue Tolerance Studies

The tolerance of mediastinal structures to IOERT has been prospectively analyzed in experimental animal studies. In a dose escalation study (Barnes et al. 1987) delivering up to 40 Gy to two separate intrathoracic IOERT fields which included collapsed right upper lobe, esophagus, trachea, phrenic nerve, right atrium, and blood vessels, pathologic changes were observed at 30 Gy in the trachea and esophagus, with severe ulceration and peribronchial and perivascular chronic inflammation in the normal lung. A dose of 20 Gy produced minimal changes in the esophagus, trachea, and phrenic nerve, but major vessels and the atrium showed medial and adventitial fibrosis, obliterative endarteritis of the vasa sarum, and severe coagulative necrosis. Acute pneumonitis was seen at all doses, and changes in the contralateral lung were detected using 12 MeV electrons.

De Boer et al. (1989) studied the effects on mediastinal structures of 20, 25, and 30 Gy. The bronchial stump healed in all dogs. Severe tissue damage was seen at all doses and included bronchovascular and esophagoaortic fistulas and esophageal stenosis.

At the National Cancer Institute (Pass et al. 1987), an experimental program evaluated the tolerance of surgically manipulated mediastinal structures to IOERT in 49 adult foxhounds and in a limited phase I clinical trial (4 patients with stage II or III NSCLC). Normal healing of the bronchial stump was found after pneumonectomy at IOERT doses of 20, 30, and 40 Gy, but there were late changes with tracheobronchial irradiation damage at all doses (5–10 months after treatment). Two out of four receiving 20 Gy developed esophageal ulceration at 6 months without late stricture. In dogs given 30 and 40 Gy, esophageal damage was severe (esophagoaortic fistula and stenosis) and one dog developed carinal necrosis. The same institution reported the results of five dogs reserved for long term studies and one stage II NSCLC patient alive at 5 years. They conclude that IOERT in the mediastinum may be safe at dose levels that do not exceed 20 Gy (Tochner et al. 1992).

Additionally experimental analysis of canine esophagus tolerance to IOERT has been reported by the NCI investigators (Sindelar et al. 1988). After right thoracotomy with mobilization of the intrathoracic esophagus, IOERT was delivered to include a 6-cm esophageal segment using a 9-MeV electron beam with escalating single doses of 0, 20, and 30 Gy. Dogs were followed clinically with endoscopic and radiologic studies and were electively sacrificed at 6 weeks or 3, 12 or 60 months after treatment. Transient mild dysphagia and mild esophagitis was observed in all dogs receiving 20 Gy, without major clinical or pathological sequelae except in one dog that developed achalasia requiring a liquid diet. At a dose of 30 Gy, changes in the esophagus were pronounced, with ulcerative esophagitis and chronic ulcerative esophagitis inducing gross stenosis after 9 months. Acute mediastinal tissue changes have also been studied (Zhon et al. 1992).

15.3 Results of IOERT in the Multidisciplinary Treatment of Stage III Non-Small Cell Lung Cancer: International Institutional Experiences

The IOERT clinical experience in lung cancer is still limited and the available data regarding treatment of NSCLC were obtained in phase I–II oriented trials in small series of patients. Abe and collegues in the initial Japanese experience questioned the value of IOERT in lung neoplasms due the early systemic dissemination of disease (Abe et al. 1977; Abe and Takahashi 1981).

15.3.1 University Clinic of Navarra, Pamplona

The IOERT methodology used has been reported in detail in previously published articles (Calvo et al. 1992a; Martínez-Monge et al. 1994; Aristu et al. 1997). Macroscopic residual surgical masses, especially in Pancoast's tumors treated with preoperative chemoradiation, may not contain viable tumor at the definitive pathology report. To select IOERT doses and electron energies, a biopsy of the surgical bed is informative. An IOERT boost to the medial aspect of the thoracic cavity apex in superior pulmonary sulcus tumors is frequently difficult to achieve but, through a Trendelenberg position of the surgical coach, it can be accomplished (Fig. 15.1).

From 1984 to 1993, 160 patients with intrathoracic tumors were treated with an IOERT component; among them 104 patients had a diagnosis of stage III NSCLC lung cancer. Age ranged from 27 to 79 years (median 61 years). There were 101 males and 3 females. Karnofsky performance status ranged from 50% to 90% (median 80%). Integral treatment strategies varied through the decade and results will be analyzed with regard to treatment intensity in multimodality management.

A description of IOERT technique characteristics in the stage III lung cancer experience includes the use of a single field to encompass the target volume in 79 procedures (76%), an applicator size ranging from 5 to 12 cm in diameter (most commonly used 7–9 cm, 66%), electron energies ranging from 6 to 20 MeV (9–12 MeV used in 100 IOERT fields, 76%) and total single doses ranging from 10 to 20 Gy (10 Gy, 80, 62%; 12.5 Gy, 7, 5%; 15 Gy, 20, 16%; >15 Gy, 22, 17%). The IOERT target volume corresponded to the following intrathoracic anatomic sites: pulmonary hilum ± mediastinum (73, 41% mediastinum), mediastinum only (15, 8%), lung parenchyma (8, 4%), and chest wall (32, 18%). Normal dose-sensitive tissues included in the IOERT field due to known tumor involvement or at high risk were: cardiac regions (10, 6%), brachial plexus (24, 14%) and esophagus (15, 8%). Severe postoperative complications were seen in 16 patients, including 10 postoperative deaths (2 bronchopleural fistulae, 2 intrathoracic hemorrhage, 1 massive pulmonary embolism and 5 sepsis). Acute reversible toxicity related to the IOERT component were: 26 episodes of grade 3–4 esophagitis III–IV, 6 symptomatic pneumonitis and 1 broncho-pleural fistulae. Late IOERT possibly related events included brachial neuropathy (6 patients), lung fibrosis (7) and bronchopleural fistulae (1).

15.3.1.1 IOERT Without a Chemotherapy Component

In 22 patients the treatment program did not include chemotherapy (early time of the experience from 1984 to 1989). Surgery consisted of pneumonectomy (1), atypical resection (3), lobectomy (8) and exploratory thoracotomy without resection (10). Ten patients had stage IIIA (5N0) and 12IIIB. Local control was observed in nine patients (50%). One patient (stage IIIA,N0) is alive and free from disease 11 years after treatment (Fig. 15.5).

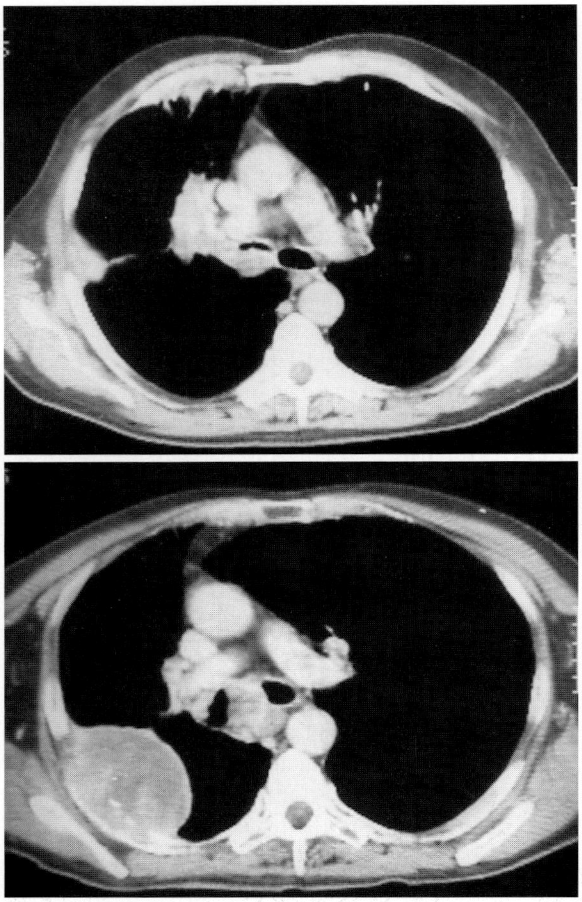

a

b

Fig. 15.5 a,b. Unusual chest wall thoracic recurrence in a patient treated with IOERT (no resection) over the primary tumor (right hilum): **a** pre-IOERT CT scan unresectable hilar mass; **b** remission and apparent tumor control in the IOERT boosted hilar region, while tumor recurrence is evident in the chest wall not treated with IOERT 10 months after surgery

15.3.1.2 IOERT with a Chemotherapy Component

The clinical experience at the University Clinic of Navarra in the treatment of stage III NSCLC incorporated at an early stage (1989) the administration of chemotherapy both intravenous and intra-arterially delivered, in a neoadjuvant fashion (Aristu et al. 1997). Surgery and external beam fractionated irradiation were always combined in the following strategy: responding patients to neoadjuvant chemotherapy were approached by surgery plus IOERT and postoperative radiotherapy, while nonresponders were treated with preoperative external irradiation followed by programmed surgery plus IOERT. Additionally patients meeting the Pancoast lesion criteria were treated with preoperative chemoradiation (Martínez-Monge et al. 1994). Results are described with regard to the integral treatment strategy.

15.3.1.2.1 Responders to Neoadjuvant Chemotherapy

In 46 patients an objective response by imaging techniques was identified following intravenous (20) or a combination of intravenous and intra-arterial chemotherapy (26). There were 24 stage IIIA (6N0) and 22 IIIB patients. Surgery achieved tumor resection in 24 patients (22 lobectomies and 2 atypical resections). Local control was achieved in 44% of patients (63% IIIA and 27% IIIB). Five patients are long term survivors 4 years or more after treatment.

15.3.1.2.2 Nonresponders to Neoadjuvant Chemotherapy

In 17 patients neoadjuvant chemotherapy (13 intravenous and 4 intravenous plus intra-arterial) did not achieve an objective tumor response: 50% had no changes and 50% less than a partial response. Preoperative chemoradiation (7 patients given radiotherapy alone) followed in the treatment strategy and produced a response 88% of the resection rate (14 lobectomies and 1 segmentectomy), together with a pT0-pTmic downstaging in the resected surgical specimen of 35%. Initial clinical stages included 5 IIIA (1N0) and 12 stage IIIB. Local control was 31%. Two patients are long term survivors with no evidence of disease (NED) 4 years after treatment.

15.3.1.2.3
PANCOAST TUMORS
In 19 patients the primary tumor involved the thoracic apex with additional clinico-radiological criteria of Pancoast lesion. Histological subtypes were: squamous cell (8), adenocarcinoma (9), and large cell anaplastic (2). Clinical stages induded 9 IIIA and 10 IIIB. Primary tumor size ranged from 4 to 14 cm maximum diameter (median diameter 7 cm). Evident chest wall involvement was established in seven patients. All patients received preoperative chemoradiation (7 i.v. and 12 i.v. + i.a.). Thoracotomy achieved resection in all cases: three atypical, seven segmentectomies and nine lobectomies. Macroscopic residual disease was left in the surgical field in five procedures. Pathologic downstaging was pT0-pTmic in 68% of the resected surgical specimens (11 pT0). Local control was 88% and 8 patients are alive NED 4 years after treatment.

15.3.2
Madrid Institute of Oncology

From February 1992 to July 1997 18 patients with stage III NSCLC were treated with an IOERT component. There were 12 males and 6 females. All patients were over 70% on the KPS scale. Age ranged from 41 to 77 years (median 62 years). Histological subtypes included: adenocarcinoma (6) and undifferentiated large cell (2) and squamous cell carcinoma (10). Primary tumor site involved the pulmonary apex (Pancoast lesions) in 11 cases, right hilum (3), left hilum (1), lingula (1) and right inferior lobe (2). Clinical tumor stages were: 11 IIIA and 7 IIIB. The IOERT surgical component was introduced in the radical multidisciplinary management of 17 previously untreated patients and in 1 case for treatment salvage of a localized recurrence in the chest wall. Surgical treatment characteristics included 16 patients resected (6 with macroscopic and 10 with microscopic tumor residue). External beam thoracic irradiation was administered to 14 patients (7 preoperatively). Neoadjuvant chemotherapy was used in 13 patients. The IOERT total dose was 10 Gy in 14 fields and 15 Gy in 6. In 16 IOERT procedures a single field was used (2 in 2 procedures). Electron energies were: 6 MeV (2), 8 MeV (1), 10 MeV (5), 12 MeV (7), 15 MeV (4), and 18 MeV (1). Applicator size ranged from 6 to 10 cm in diameter: 6 cm (1), 7 cm (7), 9 cm (7), 10 cm (5) [beveled 30° (15), 15° (2), 45° (1)]. Severe toxicities observed and possibly related to the IOERT component were: esophagitis (two cases), peripheral neuropathy (one case), thoracic abscess (one case) and bronchopleural fistula (one case).

The median follow-up time for the entire experience is 15+ months (range 3–20+). Patterns of disease recurrence identified as site of first progression were: one local relapse, one regional relapse and five patients with systemic metastasis. Overall survival is projected to be 62% and 22% at 1 and 3 years follow-up, respectively. Cause-specific survival is projected to be 33% at 3 years. Actuarial local-control rate is projected to be 85% at 3 years following IOERT.

15.3.3
Allegheny University Hospitals, Graduate

Between June 1992 and September 1997, 21 patients with non-small cell carcinoma of the lung received IOERT as part of their management. The age range was 39.4–72.5 years at the time of diagnosis (median 59.5 years). Histological tumor subtypes were: nine squamous, two adenocarcinoma, three large cell undifferentiated and seven mixed NSCLC.

All patients had a complete staging work-up prior to initiating definitive therapy. This included chest X-ray, CT scans of the chest, abdomen and pelvis, CT or MRI of the brain, liver function studies and in most cases bone scan. Pathological stages were: 1 I (T2N0) 2 II (T2N1), 15 IIIA (4 T2N2, 7 T3N0, 2 T3N1, 2 T3N2), and 3 IIIB (1 T2 N3, 2 T4 N1).

Sixteen patients received preoperative radiation therapy (5040 cGy in 14 patients and 4500 cGy in 2 patients). The treatment volume included the primary tumor and the ipsilateral hilar, mediastinal and supraclavicular lymph nodes. Neoadjuvant chemotherapy was given to all of these patients. In the early part of this series, chemotherapy consisted of two to three cycles of cisplatinum and etoposide, or in the latter part Taxol. Preoperative radiation therapy began with cycle #2 or #3 of chemotherapy depending on the pathological response. Five patients received postoperative radiation therapy (5040 cGy in three patients, 5940 cGy in two patients). Definitive surgery was performed in all cases, with either pneumonectomy (8) or lobectomy (13).

The IOERT was delivered using 7.0–9.5 cm circular cones with bevel angles of 0°, 15°, and 30°. The prescribed dose was 1000 cGy to the 90% line in all cases. Twenty-three sites were treated with 6 MeV electrons and two sites with 9 MeV electrons. Appropriate lead shielding was used to protect uninvolved structures, including lung. The IOERT target volume was located in the chest wall (10), left hilum (6), left hilum + mediastinum (1), right hilum (4), and right hilum + mediastinum (4).

The overall actuarial survival at 2, 4 and 6 years was 65%, 33% and 33% respectively. Eleven patients were alive at the time of analysis, with a median survival of 33.6 months. Eleven out of 21 patients failed locally or distantly with an NED rate of 48% and with a median survival of 30 months. The local failure rate was 14% (3 out of 21 patients, 2 patients in the IOERT field). Brain metastasis (five patients) were the most common finding of first relapse.

Complications have been rare. One patient developed pneumonitis which might be attributable to IOERT. Another patient developed posterior chest wall pain within the IOERT field. It is difficult to determine if this is related to the IOERT, the surgery or the fact that the tumor presented with chest wall involvement. The bronchial stump healed without difficulty in all cases. This may be related to several factors including the IOERT dose and meticulous surgical closure of the stump.

This early experience demonstrates that IOERT can be safely used as part of a multidisciplinary management of non-small cell lung cancer. The current recommendation in this expert group for stage III NSCLC patients is neoadjuvant chemotherapy, preoperative external beam radiation therapy followed by surgical resection and IOERT when possible.

15.4 Future Developments

An overview of the results in expert IOERT institutions confirms the initially reported feasibility of IOERT during lung cancer surgery (Arian-Shad et al. 1990; Calvo et al. 1990; Dubois et al. 1993; Fisher et al. 1994). Anatomic regions not amenable to adequate treatment by IOERT (uncertain dosimetric conditions) are the anterior chest wall spaces and the diaphragmatic domes. Tolerance to the IOERT component of therapy is modulated by the integral treatment toxicity on normal tissues (type of

Table 15.1. Patients, tumors, treatments and results in the clinical experience generated with IOERT in the treatment of lung cancer by the University Clinic of Navarra, Pamplona (CUN), the Madrid Institute of Oncology (IMO) and The Allegheny Graduate Hospital (GH)

Characteristics	CUN	IMO	GH
No. patients	104	18	21
Period	1984–1993	1993–1997	1992–1997
Tumor histology			
- Squamous cell	65	10	9
- Adenocarcinoma	26	6	2
- Other	13	2	10
Tumor stage			
- IIIA	48	11	15
- IIIB	56	7	3
Surgery			
- Resection	90	16	21
- No resection	14	2	–
External beam radiotherapy			
- Preoperative	36	7	16
- Postoperative	68	7	5
Chemotherapy			
- Neoadjuvant	53	9	16
- Neoadjuvant + simultaneous RT	29	3	5
Local recurrence			
- Resected	36	1	3
- Unresected	9	1	–
Survival (5 years)	20%	22%	33%

RT, radiotherapy.

chemotherapy, surgical manipulation, etc). IOERT specific toxicity has been identified as esophagitis (mediastinal fields), pneumonitis (unresectable tumor including collapsed normal lung in the IOERT application) and dehiscence of bronchial suture (following lobectomy or pneumonectomy). Thoracic tumor control and survival rates estimated in the present analysis do confirm preliminary reported data in clinical experiences with IOERT (Martínez-Monge et al. 1994). Further institutional expansion of IOERT and its integration in multidisciplinary protocols for lung cancer treatment, with high risk of thoracic recurrence, will test the reproducibility of this technique. Table 15.1 describes the international results published with IOERT in lung cancer trials in the present decade.

In conclusion, IOERT electrons during lung cancer surgery have proven to be feasible, tolerable and to promote high local control rates. Survival is modulated by the integral treatment intensity and disease stage at the time of initial diagnosis (Kumar et al. 1996; Rosell et al. 1994; Roth et al. 1994; Choi et al. 1997; Dilman et al. 1996). IOERT is a reliable radiation boosting technique to intensify local treatment in lung cancer patients with high risk of thoracic tumor recurrence: probably the best conformal radiation boost available in contemporary clinical radiotherapy.

References

Abe M, Takahashi M (1981). Intraoperative radiotherapy: The Japanese experience. Int J Radiat Oncol Biol Phys 7:863–868

Abe M, Yabumoto E, Nishidait et al (1977) Trials of new forms of radiotherapy for locally advanced bronchogenic carcinoma. Strahlentherapie 153:149–158

Arian-Shad, Juellner FM, Ratzenhofer B, Leitner, Porsch G, Pinter H, Ebner F, Hackl AG, Griehs (1990) Intraoperative plus external beam irradiation in nonresectable lung cancer: assessment of local response and therapy-related side effects Radiother Oncol 19:137–144

Aristu J, Martínez-Monge R, Aranmendía JM, Viera JC, Azinovic I et al (1997) Cisplatin, mitomycin, and vindesine followed by intraoperative and postoperative radiotherapy for stage III non-small cell lung cancer: final results of a phase II study. Am J Clin Oncol 20:276–281

Armstrong JG, Burman C, Leibel S, Fontenla D, Kutcher G, Zelefsky M et al (1993) Three-dimensional conformal radiation therapy may improve the therapeutic radio of high dose radiation therapy for lung cancer. Int J Radiat Oncol Biol Phys 26:685–689

Barnes M, Pass H, De Luca A, Tochner Z, Potter D, Terril R et al (1987) Response of mediastinal and thoracic viscera of the dog to intraoperative radiation therapy (IOERT). Int J Radiat Biol Phys 13:371–378

Byhardt RW, Pajak TF, Emami B, Herskovic A, Dogget RS, Olsen LA (1993) A phase I/II study to evaluate accelerated fractionation via concomitant boost for squamous, adeno, and large cell carcinoma of the lung: report of Radiation Therapy Oncology Group 84-07. Int J Radiat Biol Phys 26:459–468

Calvo FA, Hanks GE (1988) International clinical trials in intraoperative radiation therapy. Int J Radiat Oncol Biol Phys 14[Suppl 1]:5111–5117

Calvo FA, Ortíz DE Urbina D, Abuchaibe O et al (1990) Intraoperative radiotherapy during lung cancer surgery: technical description and early clinical results. Int J Radiat Oncol Biol Phys 19:103–109

Calvo FA, Santos M, Ortíz DE Urbina D et al (1991) Intraoperative radiotherapy in thoracic tumors. Front Radiat Ther Oncol 25:307–316

Calvo FA, Ortí DE Urbina D, Herreros J, Llorens R (1992a) Lung cancer. In: Calvo FA, Santos M, Brady LW (eds) Intraoperative radiotherapy, clinical experiences and results. Springer, Berlin Heidelberg New York, pp 43–50

Calvo FA, Santos M, Brady LW (1992b) Intraoperative radiotherapy. Clinical experiences and results. Springer, Berlin Heidelberg New York

Calvo FA, Micaily B, Brady LW (1993) Intraoperative radiotherapy: a positive view. Am J Clin Oncol 16:418–423

Calvo FA, Azinovic I, Martínez R, Aristu J, Abuchaibe O, Pardo F, Álvarez-Cienfuegos J, Berian JM, Cañadell J (1995) Intraoperative radiotherapy for the treatment of soft tissue sarcomas of central anatomical sites. Radiat Oncol Invest 3:90–96

Choi NC, Carey RW, Daly W et al (1997) Potential impact on survival of improved tumor downstaging and resection rate by preoperative twice-daily radiation and concurrent chemotherapy in stage IIIA non-small-cell lung cancer. J Clin Oncol 15 712–722

Cox JD (1983) Failure analysis of inoperable carcinoma of the lung of all histopathologic types and squamous cell carcinoma of the esopagus. Cancer Treat Symp 2:77–86

Cox JD, Azarnia N, Byhardt RW, Shin KH, Emami B, Pajak TF (1990) A randomized phase I/II trial of hyperfractionated radiation therapy with total dose of 60.0 to 79.2 Gy. Possible survival benefit with >69.6 Gy in favorable patients with RTOG stage III non-small cell lung carcinoma. Report of Radiation Therapy Oncology Group 83-11. J Clin Oncol 8:1543–1555

Cox JD, Pajak TF, Herskovic A, Urtasun R, Podolsky WI, Seydel HG, et al (1991) Five year survival after hyperfractionated radiation therapy for non-small cell lung carcinoma of the lung (NSCLC): results of RTOG protocol 81-08. Am J Clin Oncol 2:280–284

De Boer WJ, Mehta DM, Oosterhius JW et al (1989) Tolerance of mediastinal structures to intraoperative radiotherapy after pneunonectomy in dogs. Strahlenther Onkol 165:768

Dilman RO, Herndon J, Seagren SL et al (1996) Improved survival in stage III non-small cell lung cancer: seven year follow-up of cancer and leukemia group 13 (CALGB) 8433 trial. J Natl Cancer Inst 88:1210–1215

Dubois JB, Hay MH, Gely S et al (1993) Intraoperative radiotherapy (IOERT) in non-small cell lung carcinoma. In: Schildberg FW, Willich N, Krämling H-J (eds). Intraoperative radiation therapy. Blane Eule, Essen, pp 212–216

Emami B, Graham MV (1998) Lung. In: Pérez CA, Brady LW (eds) Principles and practice of radiation oncology. Lippincott, Philadelphia, pp 1181–1220

Emami B, Purdy JA, Manolis J, Barest G, Cheng E, Coia L et al (1991) Three-dimensional treatment planning for lung cancer. Int J Radiat Oncol Biol Phys 21:217–227

Fisher S, Fallahnejad M, Lisker S, Mason B, Swartz M, Epstein P, Adams R, Wolferth C (1994) Role of intraoperative radiation therapy (IOERT) for stage III non small cell lung cancer. Hepato Gastroenterol 41:15

Gunderson LL (1994) Rationale and results of intraoperative radiation therapy. Cancer 74:537–541

Jablons DM, Roach MIII, Jahan TH, Cameron RB (1997) Resection and IOERT followed by three-dimensional conformal radiotherapy with or without adjuvant chemotherapy for malignant mesothelioma. Front Radiat Ther Oncol 31:140–146

Juettner FM, Arian-Schad K, Porsch G et al (1990) Intraoperative megavolt radiation therapy combined with external radiation in nonresectable non-small cell lung cancer: preliminary report. Int J Radiat Oncol Biol Phys 18:1143–1150

Kumar P, Herndon II J, Langer M, Kohman LJ, Elias AD, Kass FC et al (1996) Patterns of disease failure after trimodality therapy of nonsmall cell lung carcinoma pathologic stage IIIA (N2) Analysis of Cancer and Leukemia Group B Protocol 8935. Cancer 77:2393–2399

Le Chevalier T, Arriagada R, Quoix E, Ruffie P, Martín M, Tarayre M (1991) Radiotherapy alone versus combined chemotherapy and radiotherapy in nonresectable non-small-cell lung cancer: first analysis of a randomized trial in 353 patients. J Natl Cancer Inst 83:417–423

Martínez-Monge R, Herreros J, Aristu JJ et al (1994) Combined treatment in superior sulcus tumors. Am J Clin Oncol 17:317–322

Pass HI, Sinderlar WF, Kinsella TJ et al (1987) Delivery of intraoperative radiation therapy after pneumonectomy: experimental observations and early clinical results. Ann Thorac Surg 44:14–20

Pérez CA, Baver M, Edelstein S et al (1986) Impact of tumor control on survival in carcinoma of the lung treated with irradiation. Int J Radiat Oncol Biol Phys 12:539–547

Pérez CA, Pajak TF, Rubin P, Simpson JR, Mohiuddin M, Brady LW et al (1987) Long-term observations of the patterns of failure in patients with unresectable non-oat cell carcinoma of the lung treated with definitive radiotherapy. Report by the Radiation Therapy Oncology Group. Cancer 59:1874–1881

Rosell R, Gómez-Codina J, Camps C, Maestre J, Padille J, Canto A et al (1994) A randomized trial comparing preoperative chemotherapy plus surgery alone in patients with non-small cell lung cancer. N Engl J Med 330–153

Roth JA, Fossella F, Komaki R, Ryan MB, Putnam JB Jr, Lee JS et al (1994) A randomized trial comparing perioperative chemotherapy and surgery with surgery alone in resectable stage III non-small cell lung cancer. J Natl Cancer Inst 86:673–680

Sause WT, Scott C, Taylor S, Johnson D, Livingston R, Komaki R et al (1995) Radiation Therapy Oncology Group (RTOG) 88-08 and Eastern Cooperative Oncology Group (ECOG) 4588: preliminary results of a phase III trial in regionally advanced, unresectable non-small-cell lung cancer. J Natl Cancer Inst 87(3):198–205

Shaw E, Gunderson LL, Martín J, Beart RW, Nagorney DM, Podratz KC (1990) Peripheral and ureteral tolerance of intraoperative radiation therapy: clinical and dose response analysis. Radiat Oncol 18:247–255

Sindelar WF, Hoekstra HJ, Kinsella TJ Barnes M, DeLuca AM, Tochner Z et al (1988) Response of the canine esophagus to intraoperative electron beam radiotherapy. Int J Radiat Oncol Biol Phys 15:663–669

Smolle-Juettner FM, Geyer E, Kapp KS et al. (1994) Evaluating intraoperative radiation therapy (IOERT) and external beam radiation therapy (EBRT) in non-small cell lung cancer (NSCLL) Eur J Cardiothorac Surg 8:511–516

Tochner ZA, Pass HI, Sindelar WF, DeLuca AM, Griselldl, Bacher JD, Kinsella TJ (1992) Long term tolerance of thoracic organs to intraoperative radiotherapy. Int J Radiat Oncol Biol Phys 22:65–69

Zhou GX, Zeng DW, Li WH (1992) Acute responses of the mediastinal and thoracic viscera of canine to intraoperative irradiation. In: Schildberg FW, Willich N, Kramling HJ (eds) Intraoperative radiation therapy. Proccedings of the 4th international symposium, Munich, pp 50–52

16 Should all Stage IV Non-Small Cell Lung Cancer Be Treated Palliatively?

F. CAPPUZZO, A. ZAPPALA, and T. LE CHEVALIER

CONTENTS

16.1 Introduction

Non-small cell lung cancer (NSCLC) remains a major public health problem worldwide and, during the last 30 years, therapeutic advances, even if tangible, have had only a modest impact on overall survival. At the time of diagnosis, approximately 70% of patients present with either locally advanced or metastatic disease, and cure is anecdotal particularly in metastatic disease. For patients with advanced NSCLC, the best available treatment is only palliative, and median survival rarely exceeds 10 months, with the vast majority of patients generally dying before 18–24 months from diagnosis. Chemotherapy is the most frequent option used for stage IV NSCLC, but surgery, radiotherapy and the best supportive care may also be useful for tumor management. This chapter describes the standard treatment of stage IV NSCLC and is devoted to patients with metastatic disease who are candidates for curative therapy.

F. CAPPUZZO, A. ZAPPALA, and T. LE CHEVALIER, Department of Medicine, Institut Gustave Roussy, 39, rue Camille Desmoulins, F-94805 Villejuif, France

16.2 Chemotherapy of Metastatic Non-Small Cell Lung Cancer

Even if NSCLC has traditionally been considered a chemoresistant malignancy, several cytotoxic drugs have demonstrated activity in patients with advanced disease. In this subset of patients, chemotherapy is administered not to cure disease, but to palliate symptoms and prolong survival while improving the quality of life. Although responders to chemotherapy survive longer, the net impact of this modality on survival remains modest. Median survival for untreated patients with metastatic disease is approximately 4 months and the survival advantage gained with chemotherapy ranges from 1 to 5 months. Since the late 1960s, the activity of a variety of drugs has been evaluated in NSCLC. Activity is defined as an overall response rate of at least 15%. In 1985 only five drugs were able to demonstrate such activity as single agents: cisplatin (CDDP), ifosfamide (IFO), mitomycin (MMC), vinblastine (VBL), and vindesine (VDS). The median survival obtained was 4–8 months, with anecdotal long-term survivors. CDDP was generally considered the most active single agent in NSCLC, with an overall response rate of 20% in a compilation of ten phase II trials. At the same time combination chemotherapy was also investigated to determine whether it could improve the duration of survival, response and the quality of life. One of the first chemotherapy regimens evaluated was the CAMP combination, consisting of cyclophosphamide (CTX), doxorubicin (ADM), methotrexate (MTX) and procarbazine (PCZ), which demonstrated a response rate of 26%, but most responses were brief with no impact on survival. In the 1980s most chemotherapy regimens incorporated CDDP: the combinations most frequently used included CDDP plus etoposide (VP16), CDDP plus VDS, and CDDP plus VBL, CDDP plus MMC plus VDS, and CDDP plus MMC plus IFO (Table 16.1). These combinations yielded response rates of up to 50%, with median response rates of

25%–35%, but a median duration of survival of 6–8 months and substantial toxicity. For these reasons, the balance might appear negative for several investigators and may be influenced by cultural bias. A number of randomized studies were therefore initiated to compare the best supportive care with chemotherapy (Table 16.2). The first study was conducted by CORMIER et al. (1982) and, although chemotherapy was recommended, the number of patients included in this trial was insufficient to allow definitive conclusions. Between 1985 and 1988, QUOIX et al. (1991) conducted a prospective randomized trial comparing the best supportive care versus VDS-CDDP. Of 46 patients, 24 were treated with chemotherapy (CT), 22 with supportive care (SC). The overall response rate in the CT group was 41.7% with a median survival of 199 days, compared to 73 days in the SC group ($P < 0.001$). Such favorable results were not observed in a trial performed by WOODS et al. (1990) in which median survival for the CT group was 27 weeks compared to 17 weeks for the SC group, but this difference was not statistically significant. KAASA et al. (1991) performed a randomized trial, comparing the combination CDDP plus VP16 versus SC. Median survival was 21.6 weeks in the CT group versus 16 weeks in the SC group, with a nonstatistically significant survival benefit in favor of chemotherapy. CARTEI et al. (1993) designed a randomized trial comparing the effect on survival of a chemotherapy regimen consisting of CDDP plus CTX plus MMC, versus SC. In the combined modality group, median survival was 8.5 months, compared to only 4 months in the SC group but the difference in survival was statistically significant ($P = 0.0001$). CELLERINO et al. (1991) randomly assigned 123 patients to CT (CTX plus CDDP plus epirubicin alternating with MTX plus VP16 plus lomustine) or SC. Median survival for the CT group was 34.4 weeks, versus 21.1 weeks for the SC group, with no significant differences. The trial conducted by RAPP et al. (1988) in Canada is one of the largest and the most frequently referenced. This randomized study showed that the combination of VDS and high-dose CDDP is superior to the CAP regimen (CTX, ADM, and low-dose CDDP) and that CT offers a significant advantage in terms of overall survival compared to SC ($P = 0.01$). JAAKKIMAINEN et al. (1990), having evaluated the costs of chemotherapy and supportive care reported in this trial, concluded that CT permits a reduction in cost, at least with the less expensive combination. The results of these trials are too heterogeneous to clarify the exact role of chemotherapy, but three recent analyses of these published data emphasized its importance in the management of advanced NSCLC. More convincing is the meta-analysis performed by the NON-SMALL CELL LUNG CANCER COLLABORATIVE GROUP (1995), in which individual patient data were obtained from 52 randomized trials that enrolled a total of 9387 patients. For the subgroup of patients with advanced disease, in whom CT was compared to SC, data were available

Table 16.1. Chemotherapy regimens for NSCLC

Regimen	Response rate (%)
CTX-ADM-CDDP	15–25
CDDP-VBL	15–30
CBDCA-VP16	10–30
MMC-VBL-CDDP	30–60
IFO-MMC	25–30
IFO-VP16	27
IFO-CDDP	18–35
MMC-IFO-CDDP	35–50
IFO-CBDCA-VP16	43
IFO-CDDP-VP16	25–40

Table 16.2. Randomized trials of chemotherapy (CT) versus best supportive care (BSC) in advanced NSCLC

Reference	Patients	Overall response (%)	Median survival (months)		One-year survival (%)		P
			CT	BSC	CT	BSC	
RAPP et al. 1988	150	15–25	6.1 8.1	4.2	21–22	10	0.01
QUOIX et al. 1991	49	42	7.1	2.6	NR	NR	<0.001
WOODS et al. 1990	201	28	6.8	4.3	NR	NR	NS
KAASA et al. 1991	87	11	5.0	3.8	NR	NR	NS
CARTEI et al. 1993	102	25	8.5	4.0	39	12	0.0001
CELLERINO et al. 1991	128	21	8.5	5.0	32	23	NS

NR, not reported; NS, not significant.

from 11 trials for a total of 1190 patients. Two trials used alkylating agents, one used VP16 as a single agent, and the remaining eight trials used CDDP-based chemotherapy. The results of the trials using long-term alkylating agents suggest a detrimental effect of chemotherapy, with a hazard ratio of 1.26, but the confidence interval is wide (0.96–1.66) and the result does not attain significance (P = 0.095). Meta-analysis of CDDP based trials shows that CT is beneficial, with a hazard ratio of 0.73 (P = 0.0001), and a reduction in the risk of death of 27%, which is equivalent to an absolute improvement in survival of 10% at 1 year. The results of this study also indicate that CDDP-based chemotherapy improves median survival by 6 weeks for this subset of patients. As a result, many physicians consider using CT as standard treatment for stage IV NSCLC. If CDDP-based chemotherapy is considered the standard treatment, the best platinum-based regimen is not well defined. In a European randomized trial including 612 patients, the combination of CDDP and vinorelbine (NVB), a new semi-synthetic vinca alkaloid, was compared to VDS-CDDP and to NVB alone. Neurotoxicity was more frequent in the VDS-CDDP group, even if neutropenia was significantly higher in the NVB-CDDP group. The median duration of survival was 40 weeks in the NVB-CDDP arm, 32 weeks in the VDS-CDDP arm and 31 weeks in the NVB alone arm, with a significant advantage for survival in the NVB-CDDP arm (P = 0.02 and 0.04, respectively). An objective response rate was demonstrated in 30% of patients treated with NVB-CDDP versus 19% in the VDS-CDDP arm (P = 0.02) and 14% in the NVB arm (P < 0.001). Survival rates at 1 and 2 years were 33% and 15% in the CDDP-NVB arm, 30% and 9% in the NVB arm, and 27% and 9% in the CDDP-VDS arm. Both the high response rate and the survival benefit observed with the NVB-CDDP regimen in this study suggest that this combination can be considered a reference treatment in patients with advanced NSCLC. In addition, the authors suggest that NVB alone can be proposed as an alternative treatment for patients who are unable to receive CDDP. It is noteworthy that four patients with stage IV disease on entry and treated with CDDP-NVB were still alive after 5 years. Survival adjusted by center continues to be in favor of CDDP-NVB compared to CDDP-VDS (P = 0.016) and to NVB alone (P = 0.02), with a gain in survival in both stage III and IV disease. Recently, Bonomi et al. (1996) conducted a randomized trial in which the combination of CDDP and paclitaxel was compared to that of CDDP and VP16 in 560 patients with advanced NSCLC. This ECOG study showed an advantage for the CDDP-paclitaxel regimen in terms of response (32.1% vs 12%, P < 0.001), median survival time (9.99 vs 7.69 months) and 1-year survival (39.1% vs 31.6%). Giaccone et al. (1997) have published the data on a phase III randomized trial comparing paclitaxel-CDDP to teniposide-CDDP in a mixture of advanced NSCLC patients. This study showed that the paclitaxel-CDDP combination is superior to teniposide-CDDP in terms of response, side effects and quality of life. Although median survival does not seem to have improved, the CDDP-paclitaxel combination offers better palliation than the CDDP-teniposide regimen. The results of these randomized trials indicate that new drugs such as NVB and paclitaxel in combination with CDDP can improve survival beyond that achieved with more traditional regimens such as CDDP-VDS or CDDP-VP16. Based on these data, the American Society of Clinical Oncology (ASCO) recommends CDDP-NVB, CDDP-paclitaxel or CDDP-VBL as first line treatment for metastatic NSCLC. There are no studies directly comparing CDDP and carboplatin (CBDCA), but uncontrolled phase II trials suggest that CDDP and CBDCA may be equally efficient against NSCLC. The only randomized trial comparing these two drugs in combined regimens was conducted by Klastersky et al. (1990). This study showed that CDDP-based chemotherapy may provide a higher response rate than CBDCA-based chemotherapy but no advantage in terms of survival and increased toxicity. Randomized studies comparing very high-dose CDDP (up to 200 mg/m^2), high-dose CDDP (100–120 mg/m^2) and low-dose CDDP (50–60 mg/m^2) have failed to demonstrate a significant survival benefit with higher doses despite a higher response rate but increased toxicity. New agents such as taxanes, gemcitabine and TPI inhibitors have also produced promising results used alone or in combination and are currently under investigation in phase III trials.

16.3 Treatment of Solitary Metastasis

Although chemotherapy is the standard treatment of stage IV NSCLC, this approach is only palliative. In selected cases, surgery and/or radiotherapy can play a major role in disease management, especially for single brain, adrenal or lung metastases. No data have been reported on combined resection of a primary lung tumor and a solitary liver or bone metastasis.

16.3.1
Metastasis to the Brain

The incidence of brain metastases from lung cancer is reported to be 34% in an autopsy series. Other clinical studies show that about 20% of patients with resected NSCLC have a clinically diagnosed brain lesion during the course of their disease, but it is the sole site of first recurrence in only 6.4% of patients. The majority of patients develop metachronous brain metastases predominantly in the supratentorial compartment. Without any treatment, the natural history of the disease in such patients is progressive neurologic deterioration, with a median survival of 1–3 months. Up to the 1980s, whole brain radiation therapy (WBRT) was considered the standard treatment of cerebral metastases, but patients treated with radiotherapy alone had a median survival of only 3–6 months. Several more recent studies have reported a more aggressive treatment of single brain metastases. Most centers have been recommending the resection of brain metastases in patients with a good performance status, and have demonstrated an improvement of survival, the quality of life, and a reduction in recurrence at the original site of metastasis in patients who underwent brain tumor resection (Table 16.3). In 1990, one randomized study demonstrated a significant advantage in survival at 1 year for patients undergoing surgical resection of a single brain metastasis and WBRT compared with WBRT alone. Another recent randomized trial confirmed an improvement of survival, especially in younger patients, free of extracranial disease. In patients with a poor medical condition or recurrent or unresectable brain metastases, or who refuse craniotomy, stereotaxic radiosurgery can be proposed as an alternative to surgery. It is a relatively non-invasive method delivering a single high-dose fraction of irradiation to treat a well-defined intracranial target. This technique can be adopted to treat small lesions with a diameter of less than 3.5 cm. Better tumor control rates have been reported after stereotaxic radiosurgery of brain metastasis, either at presentation (in this case, combined with classic fractionated radiotherapy), or for recurrent tumors. Between 1986 and 1995, Haprole et al. (1996) treated 260 patients with brain metastases from NSCLC, of whom 113 had an isolated brain metastasis. Fifty-two patients were treated by surgical resection and 61 by stereotaxic radiosurgery and all patients also received WBRT. The overall survival at 2 years was 33% and there was no significant difference in survival between the two groups. Thus, according to this report, stereotaxic radiosurgery and surgical treatment of brain metastasis appear to be equally efficient. In 1997, ASCO recommended resection followed by WBRT in patients with controlled extracranial disease who have an isolated cerebral metastasis in an area amenable to surgery.

Table 16.3. Survival after surgical resection of brain metastasis from NSCLC

References	Patients	Median survival (months)
Burt et al. 1994	185	14
Macchiarini et al. 1991	37	27
Wronski et al. 1995	231	11
Mussi et al. 1985	52	19

16.3.2
Metastasis to the Adrenal Gland

Stage IV NSCLC can also be treated with a curative intent for patients with both a resectable primary tumor and an isolated adrenal metastasis. The adrenal gland is a common site of metastasis from NSCLC: it is estimated that up to 4% of patients with an operable NSCLC present with a unilateral adrenal mass. About 40% of these masses may be malignant and the only metastatic site. Even if the best treatment that can be proposed to patients with a potentially operable or resected lung cancer and a single adrenal metastasis is debatable, several authors consider the surgical approach as the only "curative" strategy possible likely to improve survival, even if the exact role of surgery has yet to be defined. ASCO maintains that available data show that combined resection of lung primary along with an adrenalectomy is associated with long-term survival but that additional data are required before a more definitive recommendation can be made. The role of chemotherapy is not well defined in this setting but it is common to propose systemic therapy before and/or after the resection of malignant lesions.

16.3.3
Metastasis to the Lung

Differentiating primary lung cancer and synchronous or metachronous metastasis may be difficult, but the recent revised international system for staging lung cancer considers all separate metastatic tumor nodules in the ipsilateral nonprimary-tumor lobe as metastasis. The treatment of a single pulmonary metastasis is controversial. If the second neoplasm is synchronous, the surgical options can be different. In presence of a secondary lesion localized in the same lobe as the primary tumor, radical surgery (lobectomy or pneumonectomy) is indicated. If the metastasis is localized in the same lung, but in different lobes, treatment (surgery or systemic therapy) will be strongly influenced by the patient's general medical conditions (cardiological status, pulmonary function). When surgery is contraindicated, systemic treatments are often preferred. If the primary tumor and the second neoplasm are localized in different lungs, surgery is ill-advised for both lungs but the final decision will be dependent on each patient's general condition. If surgery is totally impossible, then systemic CT is administered. In all these cases, the size of the tumor (up to T2 maximum) and lymph node involvement are parameters that strongly influence the decision. After resection of NSCLC, the remaining portion of the lung or the contralateral lung may be the site of metachronous metastases.

16.3.4 Studies on Lung Metastasectomy

Numerous studies have been performed on surgery for pulmonary metastasis from different solid primary tumors, and have demonstrated enhanced survival when metastases are totally resected. Girard et al. (1994) conducted a retrospective review and analysis of survival of 186 adults who had surgery for lung metastases from various primaries and showed a 10-year survival rate of 23% for patients in whom a complete resection of all metastatic lesions was possible, while none of the patients whose resection was incomplete were alive. The types of resection performed are wedge resections, segmentectomies and lobectomies, with a mortality rate of 1.1%. This retrospective study confirms that complete resection of lung metastases can prolong survival in a significant number of patients. The International Registry of Lung Metastases (1997) has published its recent data. Having accrued 5206 cases of lung metastasectomies and demonstrated an actuarial survival of 36% after 5 years, 26% after 10 years, and 22% after 15 years, with a median of 35 months, the results of this study confirm that lung metastasectomy is a potentially curative procedure.

16.4 Conclusions

For a long time, the treatment of metastatic NSCLC has been controversial due to the absence of data strongly supporting the role of chemotherapy. Randomized trials and a meta-analysis recently performed show that systemic therapy is active in advanced NSCLC, modestly but significantly improving both median survival and the quality of life of patients. Platinum-based chemotherapy is considered the standard combination in advanced malignancies and several trials are ongoing to identify which drugs preferably must be combined with CDDP. Recent drugs such as vinorelbine, docetaxel, paclitaxel and gemcitabine in combination with CDDP, have all demonstrated clear activity and can be recommended as standard treatment for advanced NSCLC. Nevertheless, the drugs available are not curative and chemotherapy remains palliative for inoperable NSCLC. Curing stage IV NSCLC is exceptional but nonetheless possible in a very small subset of patients with a single metastasis. A wide experience of these patients must be acquired in clinical trials conducted by highly specialized anticancer centers where these patients should be referred.

References

Abratt RP, Bezwoda WR, Falkson G et al (1994) Efficacy and safety profile of gemcitabine in non-small cell lung cancer: a phase II study. J Clin Oncol 12:1535–1540

Anderson H, Lund B, Bach F et al (1994) Single-agent activity of weekly gemcitabine in advanced non-small cell lung cancer: a phase II study. J Clin Oncol 12: 1821–1826

Bonomi P, Kim K Chang A et al (1996) Phase III trial comparing etoposide (E) cisplatin (C) versus taxol (T) with cisplatin-G-CSF (G) versus taxol, cisplatin in advanced non-small cell lung cancer: an Eastern Cooperative Oncology Group (ECOG) trial. Proc ASCO 15:382 (abstract)

Bunn PA Jr (1986) The expanding role of cisplatin in the treatment of NSCLC. Semin Oncol 16[Suppl 6]:1–12

Burt ME, Hulan R, Coit D et al (1994) Prospective evaluation of unilateral adrenal metastasis in patients with operable non small cell lung cancer: impact of magnetic resonance imaging. J Thorac Cardiovasc Surg 107:584–589

Cairneross JG, Kim JH, Posner JB (1980) Radiation therapy for brain metastasis. Ann Neurol 7:529–541

Cartei G, Cartei F, Cantone A et al (1993) Cisplatin-cyclophosphamide-mitomycin combination chemotherapy withs upportive care versus supportive care alone for treatment of metastatic non-small-cell lung cancer. J Natl Cancer Inst 85:794–800

Cellerino R, Tummarello D, Guidi F et al (1991) A randomized trial of alternating chemotherapy versus best supportive care in advanced non-small-cell lung cancer. J Clin Oncol 9:1453–1461

Clinical practice guidelines for the treatment of unresectable non-small-cell lung cancer (1997) J Clin Oncol 15: 2996–3018

Cormier Y, Bergeron D, LaForge J et al (1982) Benefits of polichemotherapy in advanced non-small cell bronchogenic carcinoma. Cancer 50:845–849

Figlin RA, Piantadosi S, Feld R et al (1988) Intracranial recurrence of carcinoma after complete surgical resection of stage I, II and III non-small-cell lung cancer. N Engl J Med 318:1300–1305

Fossella FV, Lee JS, Murphy WK et al (1994) Phase II study of docetaxel for recurrent or metastatic non-small cell lung cancer. J Clin Oncol 12:1238–1244

Francis PA, Rigas JR, Kris MG et al (1994) Phase II trial of docetaxel in patient with stage III and IV non-small lung cancer. J Clin Oncol 12:1232–1237

Fukuoka M, Niitani H, Suzuki A et al (1992) A phase II study of CPT-11, a new derivative of camptothecin, for previously untreated non-small cell lung cancer. J Clin Oncol 10:16–20

Gandara DR, Crowley J, Livingston RB et al (1993) Evaluation of cisplatin intensity in metastatic non-small cell lung cancer: a phase II study of the Southwest Oncology Group. J Clin Oncol 11:873–878

Giaccone G, Postmus P, Debruyne C et al (1997) Final results of an EORTC phase III study of paclitaxel versus teniposide, in combination with cisplatin, in advanced NSCLC. Proc ASCO 16:1653 (abstract)

Girard P, Baldeyrou P, Le Chevalier T et al (1994) Surgery for pulmonary metastases: who are the 10 years survivors? Cancer 74:2791–2797

Grilli R, Oxman AD, Julian JM (1993) Chemotherapy for advanced non-small-cell lung cancer: how much benefit is enough? J Clin Oncol 11:1866–1872

Harpole D, Amos A, Alexander E et al (1996) Stage of the primary is important when treating isolated brain metastases from lung cancer. Proc ASCO 15:382 (abstract)

Ihde DC (1992) Chemotherapy of lung cancer. N Engl J Med 327:1434–1441

Jaakkimainen L, Goodwin PJ, Pater J et al (1990) Counting the costs of chemotherapy in a National Cancer Institute of Canada randomized trial in non small cell lung cancer. J Clin Oncol 8:1301–1309

Kaasa S, Lund E, Thorud E et al (1991) Symptomatic treatment versus combination chemotherapy for patients with extensive non-small-cell lung cancer. Cancer 67:2443–2447

Klastersky J, Sculier JP, Ravez P et al (1986) A randomized study comparing a high and a standard dose of cisplatin in combination with etoposide in the treatment of advanced non-small cell lung carcinoma. J Clin Oncol 4:1780–1786

Klastersky J, Sculier JP, Lacroix H et al (1990) A randomized study comparing cisplatin or carboplatin with etoposide in patients with advanced non-smallcell lung cancer: European Organization for Research and Treatment of Cancer Protocol 07861. J Clin Oncol 8:1556–1562

Le Chevalier T (1996) Single-agent activity of gemcitabine in advanced non-small cell lung cancer. Semin Oncol 23[5 Suppl 10]:36–42

Le Chevalier T, Brisgand D, Douillard JY et al (1994) Randomized study of vinorelbine and cisplatin versus vindesine and cisplatin versus vinorelbine alone in advanced non-small-cell lung cancer: results of a European multicenter trial including 612 patients. J Clin Oncol 12:360–367

Le Chevalier T, Pujol JL, Douillard JY et al (1997) Six year follow up of the European Multicentre Randomised Study comparing Navelbine (NVB) alone vs NVB + Cisplatin (CDDP) vs Vindesine (VDS) + CDDP in 612 patients (pts) with advanced non-small cell lung cancer(NSCLC). Lung Cancer 18[Suppl 1]:13(abstract)

Macchiarini P, Bonaguidi R, Hardin M et al (1991) Results and prognostic factors of surgery in the management of non-small cell lung cancer (NSCLC) with solitary brain metastasis (SBM). Proc Am Soc Clin Oncol 10:253 (abstract)

Marino P, Pampallona S, Prestoni A et al (1994) Chemotherapy versus supportive care in advanced non-small-cell lung cancer: results of a meta-analysis of the literature. Chest 106:861–865

Mountain C F (1997) Revision in the International System for Staging Lung Cancer. Chest 111:1710–1717

Mussi A, Janni A, Pistolesi M et al (1985) Surgical treatment of primary lung cancer and solitary brain metastasis. Thorax 40:191–193

Non-small cell Lung Cancer Collaborative Group (1995) Chemotherapy in non-small cell lung cancer: a meta-analysis using updated data on individual patients from 52 randomised clinical trials. BMJ 311:899–909

Noordijk EM, Vecht CJ, Haaxma-Reiche H et al (1994) The choice of treatment of single brain metastasis should be based on extracranial tumor activity and age. Int J Rad Oncol Biol Phys 29:711–717

Order SE, Hellman S, von Essen CF et al (1968) Improvement in quality of survival following whole-brain irradiation for brain metastasis. Radiology 91:149–153

Patchell RA, Tibbs PA, Walsh JW et al (1990) A randomized trial of surgery in the treatment of single metastases to the brain. N Engl J Med 322:494–500

Posner JB, Chernik NL (1978) Intracranial metastases from systemic cancer. Adv Neurol 19:579–592

Putnam JB, Suell DM, Natarajan G et al (1993) Extended resection of pulmonary metastases: is the risk justified? Ann Thorac Surg 55:1440–1446

Quoix E, Dietemann A, Charbonneau J et al (1991) La chimiothérapie comportant du cisplatine est-elle utile dans le cancer bronchique non microcellulaire au stade IV? Résultants d'une étude randomisée. Bull Cancer 78: 341–346

Rapp E, Pater J, William A et al (1988) Chemotherapy can prolong survival in patients with advanced non-small cell lung cancer: report of a Canadian multicenter randomized trial. J Clin Oncol 6:633–641

Shepard KV, Golomb HH, Bitran JD et al (1985) CAMP chemotherapy for metastatic non-oat cell bronchogenic carcinoma. Cancer 56:2385–2390

Shinkai T, Saijo N, Eguchi K et al (1986) Cisplatin and vindesine combination chemotherapy for non-small lung cancer: a randomized trial comparing two dosages of cisplatin. Jpn J Cancer Res 77:782–789

Souquet PJ, Chauvin F, Boissel JP et al (1993) Polichemotherapy in advanced non-small cell lung cancer: a meta-analisys. Lancet 342:19–21

The International Registry of Lung Metastases (1997) Long-term results of lung metastasectomy: prognostic analyses based on 5206 cases. J Thorac Cardiovasc Surg 113:37–49

Woods R, Williams C, Levi J et al (1990) A randomized trial of cisplatin and vindesine versus supportive care only in advanced non-small cell lung cancer. Br J Cancer 61: 608–611

Wronski N, Arbit E, Burt M et al (1995) Survival after surgical treatment of brain metastases from lung cancer: a follow-up study of 231 patients treated between 1976–1991. J Neurosurg 83:605–616

17 Intensive Therapy of Small Cell Lung Cancer: A Review of Recently Published Data

J. KLASTERSKY and D. DEVRIENDT

CONTENTS

17.1 Introduction

There are about 15 drugs with known activity in patients with small cell lung cancer (SCLC) and they are usually used in double or triple drug combinations. The cisplatin-etoposide combination proved to be one of the most active regimens but, as with other treatments, attempts to increase the delivered dose intensity of that combination did not improve the response rate or the survival but led to a significant augmentation of toxicity, namely myelosuppression (IHDE et al. 1994).

In spite of the earlier disappointing experience with high dose chemotherapy supported by autologous bone marrow transplantation (KLASTERSKY and SCULIER 1989), there is currently a renewed interest in high dose chemotherapy of SCLC, perhaps because of the relative simplicity of palliative therapy of myelosuppression through the use of hematopoietic colony stimulating factors (CSF) or the administration of peripheral blood progenitor cells (PBPC). As a consequence, in recent years several studies have aimed at escalating the dose intensity of chemotherapy again either with high dose chemotherapy or standard doses given at shorter intervals. So far, there is no evidence that an effect on survival has been achieved by these attempts. Moreover, the approach was often limited to a reduced number of courses, because of progressive anemia and thrombocytopenia (DEMETRI 1993). Nonetheless, many studies are still being undertaken to continue and explore this approach.

Thoracic radiotherapy in addition to chemotherapy for patients with limited-disease SCLC has been evaluated in a meta-analysis by PIGNON et al. (1992); it included 13 trials with 2140 patients. There was a 14% reduction in the mortality rate, corresponding to a 5% improvement in 3-year survival, in the combined treatment arm. The identification of the optimal combination of chemotherapy and radiotherapy, taking into account the potentiation of radiotherapy by chemotherapy, as well as the benefit of radiation for the bulky tumors, remain other areas requiring continuing research.

17.2 Concurrent Use of Radiotherapy and Chemotherapy

Patients with limited-stage SCLC were treated with concurrent twice daily chest radiotherapy and etoposide/cisplatin every 3 weeks, followed by cyclophosphamide, doxorubicin and vincristine, by JOHNSON et al. (1996). The 2-year survival rate was 43% but the principal cause of death in these patients was still relapse of the original cancer; moreover, brain metastases caused 30% of the deaths.

Weekly cisplatin and etoposide plus concurrent thoracic radiotherapy was used by TABATA et al. (1997); in 11 patients, 3 complete remissions (CR) and 8 partial remissions (PR) were observed; a phase II study with this feasible regimen is now underway. Along the same lines, FRYTAK et al. (1996) used infusion chemotherapy with cisplatin and hyper-

J. KLASTERSKY and D. DEVRIENDT, Service de Médecine et Service de Radiothérapie et Laboratoire de Recherche et d'Investigation Clinique, Institut Jules Bordet, Centre des Tumeurs de l'Université Libre de Bruxelles, 1 rue Héger-Bordet, 1000 Brussels, Belgium

fractionated thoracic radiotherapy. In patients with limited disease, the response rate was 100% (76% CR) and the 2-year survival was 90%. The regimen was felt to be safe and effective.

There are some indications that continuously administered cisplatin during radiotherapy of lung cancer leads to superior results to intermittent (weekly or monthly) therapy. The European Lung Cancer Working Party (ELCWP) is currently exploring this possibility. Patients with limited stage of SCLC are treated with radiation therapy, associated with concurrent standard (every 3 weeks) cisplatin/etoposide chemotherapy (cf. the Johnson approach) or continuous cisplatin as daily administrations (cf. the Frytak approach) with etoposide being given on 3 consecutive days, every 3 weeks. After completion of radiotherapy, four additionnal courses with cisplatin/etoposide are given.

Bunn et al. (1995) explored the possibility that granulocyte-macrophage (GM) CSF reduced the hematologic toxicity and morbidity induced by chemoradiotherapy in limited stage SCLC. In this multicenter prospective trial, 230 patients were randomized to receive chemotherapy and radiotherapy with or without GM-CSF. There was a statistically significant increase in the frequency and duration of life-threatening thrombocytopenia in GM-CSF treated patients who had significantly more toxic deaths and more frequent and severe morbidity. There was a non-significant lower response rate in the GM-CSF treated patients but no difference in survival. It was felt that simultaneous cisplatin/etoposide and radiotherapy produced severe neutropenia and thrombocytopenia in a small enough proportion of patients so that prophylactic hematopoietic growth factors are unnecessary.

Concomitant high dose chemotherapy (ifosfamide, epirubicin, carboplatin and etoposide) and radiotherapy, with G-CSF and PBSC support, was investigated by Weynants et al. (1997). The response rate consisted of 65% of CR and the median survival was 27 months. The local control was felt to be improved: 5/22 relapses in the chest but a high rate of relapse in the central nervous system was seen (12/22). Severe infections (WHO > 2) were observed in many patients but esophagitis and mucositis were rate.

A similar approach was used by De Marinis et al. (1997) for late intensification in limited stages of SCLC. Patients responding to induction chemotherapy (cyclophosphamide, epirubicine and vincristine) received radiotherapy and concurrent chemotherapy with carboplatin/etoposide plus G-CSF. All patients showed a major response to intensification with 75% CR. The median survival time was 19 months and relapses were due to local recurrence (11 patients), brain metastases (11 patients) and metastatic disease (13 patients). Neither sepsis or bleeding was recorded and no toxic deaths occurred.

These studies do not demonstrate that G-CSF is a necessary component of either initial or late high dose chemotherapy associated with concurrent radiotherapy. They do not prove either that high dose initial or late chemotherapy with concurrent radiotherapy is more beneficial than standard treatment for patients with limited stages of SCLC. The results reported by Weynants et al. (1997) look somewhat more encouraging than those reported by De Marinis et al. (1997), suggesting perhaps that an early aggressive therapy might be preferable.

17.3 Standard Versus High Dose Chemotherapy

One of the latest comparative trials between a high dose and a standard dose of etoposide and cisplatin, by Ihde et al. (1994), in patients with extensive SCLC, has already been mentionned. No therapeutic benefits resulted from increasing the planned dose by 67% for the first two cycles of etoposide and cisplatin in these patients; higher doses were associated with substantially worse toxicities.

Nonetheless, other comparative studies recently addressed the same question using different methodologies. Gatzmeier et al. (1994) compared etoposide/vincristine to etoposide/vincristine/carboplatin in extensive-stage SCLC. They found a significantly higher response rate with the triple drug regimen but no difference in median survival. A long term survival advantage was observed in patients with good performance status, less than 60 years, with no distant metastases and who achieved CR.

Standard versus high dose epirubicin (60 mg/m^2 and 120 mg/m^2) in combination with cisplatin and vincristine was investigated by Kolaric et al. (1994). The overall response rate was slightly but significantly superior in the patients treated with the higher dose of epirubicin and more CR were observed. However, no improvement of the progression free survival time was seen. Bleehen et al. (1996) conducted a randomized trial of four-drug versus less intensive two-drug chemotherapy in patients with poor prognosis SCLC. The regimens consisted of etoposide, cyclophosphamide, methotrexate and vincristine and of etoposide/vincristine. There was no difference overall in response or survival but the two-drug regimen was less toxic.

SANDLER et al. (1997) compared standard and intensive therapy within the frame of ECOG. Therapy consisted of cyclophosphamide, CCNU and methotrexate and the two arms differed only in the dosage of cyclosphamide (700 mg/m^2 and 1500 mg/m^2). Overall response rates were not different, but life threatening toxicity was significantly worse in the high-dose arm. However, in that study in which all the responders received the same maintenance therapy, time to progression and overall survival, although significantly better, was only marginally increased: 29 vs 23 and 41 vs 36 weeks, respectively; however, this slight advantage was seen only in patients with limited disease.

GONZALEZ-LARRIBA and the Spanish Lung Cancer Group (1997) compared high-dose epirubicin (100 mg/m^2) plus cisplatin to standard etoposide/cisplatin. The response rate and the duration of response were similar in both arms, as well as the toxicity.

MURRAY et al. (1997) compared the CODE regimen, designed to deliver a higher dose-intensity of vincristine, doxorubicin and etoposide in combination with cisplatin than the alternation of cyclophosphamide/adriamycin/vincristine with etoposide/cisplatin. Although CODE increased the response rate compared to the other regimen, progression free survival and overall survival were not improved. Moreover, the mortality during chemotherapy was higher with CODE (9% vs 1%). Despite supportive prednisone, cotrimoxazole and ketoconazole, febrile neutropenia occurred in 20% of the CODE treated patients. Another study by KUBOTA et al. (1997) used CODE plus G-CSF following concurrent etoposide/cisplatin plus radiotherapy; they reported grade 3–4 leukopenia in 50% of the patients but no treatment related deaths were observed.

These seven studies discussed above are summarized in Table 17.1.

Two of these studies (GATZEMEIER et al. 1994; BLEEHEN et al. 1996) used as a control regimen etoposide/vincristine, which might not be optimal; it is not surprising therefore that the addition of carboplatin resulted in a higher response and better survival at least in patients with limited disease; in patients with extensive disease no differences were seen in either study.

The study by GONZALEZ-LARRIBA et al. (1997) probably compares two regimens with adequate but similar dose-intensity; once again, it is a little surprising that no differences were found.

The other four studies, in which a higher dose-intensity was probably achieved in the study arm, report overall disappointing results. Two studies (KOLARIC et al. 1994; MURRAY et al. 1997) demonstrated a significant increase in the response rate that did not translate into a survival benefit; in one study, it was associated with a significantly increased toxicity and toxic deaths.

The other two studies (KLASTERSKY and SCULIER 1989; SANDLER et al. 1997) did not show an increased response rate or improved survival; both were associated with significantly increased toxicity.

Thus, overall high dose chemotherapy may increase the response rate in good prognosis patients without a significant prolongation of the survival; on

Table 17.1. Comparative studies of dose intensification with support of hematopoietic growth factors

Reference	Chemotherapy[a]	Results[b]		
		Response	Survival	Toxicity
IHDE et al. 1994	Standard vs high dose Cis/Eto	–	–	+
GATZEIMER et al. 1994	Eto/Vin ± Car	+	+	+
KOLARIC et al. 1994	Standard vs high dose Epi	+	–	–
BLEEHAN et al. 1996	Eto/Vin vs Eto/Vin/Cyc/Met	–	–	+
SANDLER et al. 1997	Standard vs high dose Cyc/Met/CCNU	–	(+)	+
GONZALEZ-LARRIBA et al. 1997	Epi/Cis vs Eto/Cis	–	–	–
MURPHY et al. 1997	Cis/Vin/Dox/Eto vs alternating Cyc/Dox/Vin and Eto/Cis	+	–	+

[a] Cis, cisplatin; Eto, etoposide; Vin, vincristine; Car, carboplatin; Epi, epirubicin; Cyc, cyclophosphamide; Met, methotrexate; Dox, doxorubicin.
[b] (+), experimental arm had more efficacy and/or toxicity; (–) no difference.

the other hand, it significantly increases the side-effects and morbidity.

17.4 High Dose Chemotherapy and the Use of Hematopoietic Growth Factors

A pivotal study by CRAWFORD et al. (1991) evaluated standard therapy (cyclophosphamide, doxorubicin, etoposide) in SCLC patients with or without G-CSF. A reduction of the duration of severe neutropenia could be demonstrated; the patients receiving G-CSF had fewer febrile episodes and documented infections; they also had shorter hospital stays and less antibiotic therapy.

PUJOL et al. (1997) investigated the dose-intensity of a four drug regimen with or without GM-CSF in extensive SCLC. In that multicenter randomized study, they were unable to achieve a 50% increase in dose intensity due to excessive toxicity. In spite of the use of GM-CSF, patients treated with the higher dosage of chemotherapy had more documented infections; actually, these patients had a shorter survival than those treated with standard therapy.

THATCHER et al. (1997) conducted a randomized trial of dose intensification with G-CSF; in the G-CSF treated patients, chemotherapy with doxorubicin, cyclophosphamide and etoposide was given every 2 weeks instead of 3 weeks in the other group. The G-CSF treated patients completed their treatment on average 1 month sooner and had an improved survival at 12 months: 48% vs 39%.

Phase I-II studies of dose intensified chemotherapy with support by G-CSF have been reported recently. JANSSEN et al. (1997) conducted a phase II study of dose intensified carboplatin/etoposide/vincristine with G-CSF. The use of G-CSF was felt to allow an increase in the dose intensity in comparison with previous studies. The median survival for patients with extensive disease was 10 months.

Goss et al. (1997) conducted a pilot study of high dose chemotherapy and irradiation with G-CSF. Patients received etoposide/cisplatin followed by high dose cyclophosphamide (1750 mg/m^2) etoposide/cisplatin, twice with concurrent radiotherapy and G-CSF support. Five patients out of 8 died (2 from definite treatment related toxicity) and the estimated median survival was 10 months.

ROBERT et al. (1997) investigated initial chemotherapy dose intensification with doxorubicin/etoposide/cisplatin/cyclosphosphamide with G-CSF support. One year survival was 77% and the median survival was 12.5 months. Two possible therapy related deaths were observed among 16 patients. It was felt that this approach produced an increased rate of infection and thrombocytopenia without producing a major improvement in survival. KATAKAMI et al. (1996) performed a dose escalation study of carboplatin with a fixed dose of etoposide plus G-CSF. The overall median survival was 9 months. It was concluded that no therapeutic benefit accrued from increasing the dose of carboplatin up to 700 mg/m^2.

The pharmaco-economic evaluation of the use of colony-stimulating factors with standard therapy has been performed by NICHOLS et al. (1994), who found that the incidence of neutropenic fever with standard therapy was actually only 18% and felt that it did not justify the routine use of the hematopoietic growth factors which are expensive and do not provide, under these circumstances and in those patients, an obvious therapeutic benefit or cost savings. The authors calculated the respective charge estimates for three models of the use of G-CSF in SCLC patients. The total charge for the prophylactic approach was calculated to be US $1 287 481; the use of G-CSF only in cycles following a febrile neutropenia episode cost US $276 154 and the policy of reducing by 25% the dose of chemotherapy was evaluated at US $192 820. In the three groups of patients, septic deaths, response rates and survivals were comparable.

MESSORI et al. (1996), in a meta-analysis and pharmaco-economic evaluation, concluded that G-CSF given prophylactically to patients with SCLC and receiving conventional chemotherapy did not affect mortality but significantly reduced the incidence of neutropenic fever from 68% to 39%. The cost-effectiveness ratio of prophylactic G-CSF, i.e., the average cost associated with the prevention of an episode of neutropenic fever, was US $41 088.

The use of G-CSF as a suppot for routine chemotherapy of patients with SCLC cannot be recommended on the basis of the presently available data. CRAWFORD's study (1991), using quite liberal definitions for neutropenia, has been rediscussed by NICHOLS et al. (1994), who pointed out the high cost of prophylactic G-CSF. Such a high cost was also found in Messori's study.

There is no doubt that the incidence of febrile neutropenia can be shortened by prophylactic administration of G-CSF. However, the overall incidence of severe neutropenia is relatively low and it is usually of short duration when conventionnal therapy is given. Episodes of febrile neutropenia are

Table 17.2. Studies of dose intensification with peripheral blood progenitor cell support

Reference	Regimen[a]	Median survival (months)	1-year survival (%)	Severe neutropenia during first course (%)
THATCHER et al. 1997	Accelerated Cyc/Dox/Eto	12	48	57
JANSSEN et al. 1997	Carb/Eto/Vin intensified	10	–	27
Goss et al. 1997	Cis/Eto then Cyc/Cis/Eto and radiotherapy	10	–	90
ROBERT et al. 1997	Dox/Cyc/Eto/Cis then Cis/Eto plus radiotherapy	12	77	60
KATAKAMI et al. 1996	Escalation Car	9	–	12

[a] Cis, cisplatin; Eto, etoposide; Vin, vincristine; Car, carboplatin; Cyc, cyclophosphamide; Dox, doxorubicin.

not very common and usually respon well to antibiotics, which can often be administered on an outpatient basis; the mortality due to sepsis is almost negligible under these circumstances. Therefore, it would appear wise to restrict the use of G-CSF to those patients at high risk of febrile neutropenia or those who had a severe episode of febrile neutropenia and in whom dose reduction of chemotherapy is not indicated.

The use of G-CSF with intensified chemotherapy of SCLC can probably have some favorable effects. As indicated in Table 17.2, two out of five studies did not find a therapeutic benefit but three did. Perhaps the most distressing observation is that all these studies report median survivals between 9 and 12 months, which does not look better than what can be obtained with standard therapy. Thus, G-CSF might allow dose escalation but neutropenia still remains a limiting factor. Most importantly, the course of the neoplastic disease is not improved. Further studies with dose escalation with neutropenia being controlled by G-CSF are probably not needed.

17.5 Dose Intensification with Peripheral Blood Progenitor Cell (PBPC) Support

The hematopoietic growth factors allow the collection of large amounts of peripheral blood progenitor cells in patients receiving chemotherapy. These cells can then be used for rapid reconstitution of the bone marrow function after intensive chemotherapy.

LEYVRAZ et al. (1997) treated 65 patients with SCLC, two-thirds of whom had extensive disease, with ifosfamide (10 g/m^2), carboplatin (1200 mg/m^2) and etoposide (1200 mg/m^2). Severe myelosuppression (20% of the patients), infection (21%) and mucositis (10%) were the major toxic effects. The study did not show a survival advantage. BRUGGER et al. (1997) conducted a similar study in patients with limited disease. Patients received etoposide (500 mg/m^2)/ifosfamide (12 g/m^2)/carboplatin (750 mg/m^2)/epirubicin (150 mg/m^2). Patients with I-IIA stage had a 3-year survival of 69% and those with IIIB, 33%. All the patients who had surgery after chemotherapy and PBPC were long term survivors. Unfortunately this is a very limited study; it is certainly encouraging but requires confirmation.

Other, even smaller studies have been reported but do not provide enough data to support or confirm these preliminary observations. Such a study in limited stage patients was reported by CHOU et al. (1997). After etoposide/cisplatin and concurrent radiotherapy, five patients received carboplatin (1600 mg/m^2), etoposide (1600 mg/m^2), ifosfamide (8 g/m^2) and prophylactic cranial irradiation. All these patients stayed in CR with a follow up period of 8–22 months. KITADA et al. (1997) have used carboplatin (1.2 g/m^2)/etoposide (1.2 g/m^2)/cyclophosphamide (120 mg/kg) after CR or PR was obtained with standard chemotherapy. The intensive regimen maintained CR or PR in these patients for 8–16 months.

WOLF et al. (1997) used cyclophosphamide (4 g/m^2)/etoposide (2100 mg/m^2)/carboplatin (1200 mg/m^2) in seven patients with limited stage disease; five patients were put into CR and two progressed. DUNLOP and FITZIMONS (1997) compared myelosuppression after ifosfamide (3 g/m^2)/carboplatin (400 mg/m^2)/etoposide (700 mg/m^2) supported with G-CSF, PBPC or unsupported. This small study suggested that G-CSF was superior to PBPC in supporting standard chemotherapy induced neutropenia. Once again, it is a preliminary observation which requires confirmation not only in SCLC patients treated with standard chemotherapy but mainly in those receiving more intensive regimens.

It is clearly too early to draw any conclusions about the use of PBPC after intensive chemotherapy in SCLC. The experience in patients, most of whom had extensive disease, is not very encouraging. The experience in patients with limited disease might be more positive if the very preliminary data so far available are confirmed. However, one should be aware that the same intensive regimens failed to alter the course of SCLC when used with autologous bone marrow transplantation. To avoid delays in our information and prevent the undertaking of many small trials – which may be seen as unethical – a major cooperative effort should be made to perform a large controlled study taking survival and treatment related morbidity as end points.

17.6 Weekly Chemotherapy

Administration of chemotherapy weekly can be seen as a way to obtain dose intensification. Souhami et al. (1994) studied 438 patients with either limited or extensive SCLC in a randomized investigation. The overall response was similar as was the median survival; the 2-year survival was 12% in both arms.

Similar conclusions were reached by the European Lung Cancer Working Party (Sculier et al. 1993); weekly multiple drug combination chemotherapy failed to improve survival. Actually, if the cumulative doses received by the patients in each arm were nearly equal to the scheduled cumulative doses, the total relative dose intensity was significantly higher in the standard treatment arm. More recently, Skarlos et al. (1997) found no differences between standard therapy and a weekly alternation of "non-cross resistant" drugs.

In patients with extensive disease, Joss et al. (1995) performed a randomized study comparing weekly carboplatin/etoposide designed as a regimen with low toxicity to cisplatin/adriamycin/etoposide alternating with cyclophosphamide/methotrexate/vincristine/lomustine. The alternating regimen produced a significantly prolonged median survival as well as a different 1-year survival (30% vs 4%). The weekly regimen was much less toxic, as expected.

Clearly, there is no justification for giving weekly chemotherapy to patients with SCLC. As an attempt for dose intensification, weekly chemotherapy is not superior to standard regimens; used at doses aimed at a reduction of the side effects, it is clearly inferior to standard therapy.

17.7 Maintenance Therapy

Maintenance therapy, after conventional treatment, can also be viewed as an intensification of therapy. Beith et al. (1996) used etoposide/cisplatin as an induction regimen followed by a randomization to vincristine/doxorubicin/cyclosphosphamide. Maintenance therapy was not associated with increased surival but led to a significant toxicity after induction therapy. On the other hand, the European Lung Cancer Working Party (Sculier et al. 1996) found that maintenance therapy was beneficial. After six courses of chemotherapy with ifosfamide/etoposide/epirubicin, patients were treated with etoposide/vindesine or no maintenance therapy. Progression-free survival was significantly improved by maintenance therapy with a median duration of 25 vs 12 weeks; however, the survival was not signicantly different (48 and 38 weeks, respectively).

In spite of these latter data, the overall benefit from maintenance therapy is small and probably not worth the alteration of quality of life that continued chemotherapy is likely to cause.

17.8 Conclusions

So far, there is no evidence that dose intensification, whatever the modality is, benefits patients with SCLC. Since attempts to intensify therapy often lead to increased toxicity, further attempts should require very strong justification and should be conducted only under strict investigational surveillance.

References

Beith JM, Clarke SJ, Woods RL et al (1996) Long-term follow-up of a randomised trial of combined chemoradiotherapy induction treatment, with and without maintenance chemotherapy in patients with small cell carcinoma of the lung. Eur J Cancer 32:438–443

Bleehen NM, Girling DJ, Hopwood P et al (1996) Randomised trial of four-drug vs less intensive two-drug chemotherapy in the palliative treatment of patients with small-cell lung cancer (SCLC) and poor prognosis. Br J Cancer 73:406–413

Brugger W, Fetscher S, Hasse J et al (1997) Early high-dose chemotherapy and peripheral blood progenitor cell transplantation in limited-disease small cell lung cancer. Proc ASCO 16:1665 (abstract)

Bunn PA Jr, Crowled J, Kelly K et al (1995) Chemoradiotherapy with or without granulocyte-macrophage colony-stimulating factor in the treatment of limited-stage small-cell lung cancer: a prospective phase III randomized study of the Southwest Oncology Group. J Clin Oncol 13:1632–1641

Chou T, Yokoyama A, Ishiguro T et al (1997) High-dose chemotherapy with peripheral blood stem cell transplantation (PBSCT) for limited-disease (LD) small cell lung cancer (SCLC). Proc ASCO 16:1668 (abstract)

Crawford J, Ozer H, Stoller R et al (1991) Reduction by granulocyte colony-stimulating factor of fever and neutropenia induced by chemotherapy in patients with small cell lung cancer. N Engl J Med 325:164–170

De Marinis F, Crino L, Corgna E et al (1997) Concurrent chemoradiotherapy as intensification in limited (LD) small cell lung cancer (SCLC). A phase II trial. Proc ASCO 16:1675 (abstract)

Demetri GD (1993) Impact of hematopoietic growth factors on the management of small cell lung cancer. Chest 103:427s–432s

Dunlop DJ, Fitzsimons EJ (1997) Peripheral blood stem cell (PBSC) support for ICE chemotherapy in small cell lung cancer (SCLC). Lung Cancer 18[Suppl 1]:30

Frytak S, Shaw EG, Jett JR et al (1996) Infusion cisplatin chemotherapy and hyperfractionated thoracic radiotherapy for small-cell lung cancer. Am J Clin Oncol Cancer Clin Trials 19:193–198

Gatzemeier U, Pawel JV, Laumen R et al (1994) Etoposide/vincristine-based chemotherapy with or without carboplatin in extensive-stage small cell lung cancer: a prospective randomized phase III trial. Semin Oncol 21:31–35

Gonzalez-Larriba JL, Artal A, Barneto I et al (1997) Prospective randomized trial of high-dose epirubicin-cisplatin (EP) vs etoposide-cisplatin (VP) in small cell lung cancer (SCLC). Lung Cancer 18[Suppl 1]:13

Goss G, Lochrin C, Gertler S et al (1997) A pilot study of high dose chemotherapy and irradiation with NEUPOGEN (G-CSF) in limited disease small cell lung cancer (SCLC). Lung Cancer 18[Suppl 1]:45

Ihed DC, Mulshine JL, Kramer BS et al (1994) Prospective randomized comparison of high-dose and standard-dose etoposide and cisplatin chemotherapy in patients with extensive-stage small-cell lung cancer. J Clin Oncol 12:2022–2034

Janssen B, Jagos U, Gatzemeier U et al (1997) Phase II study of dose intensified chemotherapy with carboplatin/etoposide/vincristine (CEV) with lenograstim support in small cell lung cancer (SCLC). Lung Cancer 18[Suppl 1]:31

Johnson BE, Bridges JD, Sobczeck M, et al. (1996) Patients with limited-stage small cell lung cancer treated with concurrent twice daily chest radiotherapy and etoposide/cisplatin followed by cyclophosphamide, doxorubicin and vincristine. J Clin Oncol 14:806–813

Joss RA, Alberto LP, Hurny C et al (1995) Quality versus quantity of life in the treatment of patients with advancd small-celll lung cancer? A randomized phase III comparison of weekly carboplatin and teniposide versus ciplatin, adriamycin, etoposide alternating with cyclophosphamide, methotrexate, vincristine and lomustine. Ann Oncol 6:41–48

Katakami N, Takada M, Negoro S et al (1996) Dose escalation study of carboplatin with fixed-dose etoposide plus granulocyte-colony stimulating factor in patients with small cell lung carcinoma: a study of the Lung Cancer Study Group of West Japan. Cancer 77:63–70

Kitada C, Yamanaka H, Tokumoto H et al (1997) High-dose chemotherapy with PBSCT for small cell lung cancer. Lung Cancer 18[Suppl 1]:40

Klastersky JA, Sculier JP (1989) Intensive chemotherapy of small cell lung cancer. Lung Cancer 5:196–206

Kolaric K, Oreskovic B, Vukas D et al (1994) Standard vs. high-dose epirubicin in combination chemotherapy of small cell lung cancer (SCLC) – results of a phase III randomized trial. Libri Oncol 23:177–185

Kubota K, Nishiwaki Y, Furuse K et al (1997) Feasibility study of concurrent cisplatin/etoposide (PE) and thoracic radiotherapy (TRT) followed by weekly dose intensive regimen (CODE) with human granulocyte colony-stimulating factor (G-CSF) for limited stage (LS) small cell lung cancer (SCLC): report of a Japan Clinical Oncology Group study (JCOG-9509). Proc ASCO 16:1701 (abstract)

Leyvraz S, Rosti G Lange A et al (1997) Early intensification chemotherapy for the treatment of small cell lung cancer (SCLC). Proc ASCO 16:1626 (abstract)

Messori A, Trippoli S, Tendi E (1996) G-CSF for the prophylaxis of neutropenic fever in patients with small cell lung cancer receiving myelosuppressive antineoplastic chemotherapy: meta-analysis and phamaco-economic evaluation. Clin Pharm Ther 21:5743

Murray N, Livingston R, Shepherd F et al (1997) A randomized study of CODE plus thoracic irradiation versus alternating CAV/EP for extensive stage small cell lung cancer (ESCLC): an intergroup study of the national cancer institute of Canada and the Southwest Oncology Group. Lung Cancer 18[Suppl 1]:6

Nichols CR, Fox EP, Roth BJ et al (1994) Incidence of neutropenia fever in patients treated with standard-dose combination chemotherapy for small-cell lung cancer and the cost impact of treatment with granulocyte colony-stimulating factor. J Clin Oncol 12:1245–1250

Pignon JP, Arriagada R Ihde, et al (1992) A meta-analysis of thoracic radiotherapy of small cell lung cancer. N Engl J Med 327:1618–1624

Pujol JL, Douillard JY, Rivière A et al (1997) Dose-intensity of a four-drug chemotherapy regimen with or without recombinant human granulocyte-macrophage colony-stimulating factor in extensive stage small-cell lung cancer: a multicenter randomized phase III study. J Clin Oncol 15:2082–2089

Robert F, Redden D, Jennelle RLS et al (1997) Initial chemotherapy dose intensification (DI) using granulocyte colony-stimulating factor (G-CSF) and prophylactic antibiotic therapy for patients with small cell lung cancer (SCLC). Proc ASCO 16:1725 (abstract)

Sandler A, Jiroutek M, Vogl S et al (1997) A comparison of standard with intensive combination chemotherapy in small cell lung cancer-mature results: an Eastern Cooperative Oncology Group Trial (ECOG). Proc ASCO 16:1730 (abstract)

Sculier JP, Paesmans M, Bureau G et al (1993) Multiple-drug weekly chemotherapy versus standard combination regimen in small-cell lung cancer: a phase III randomized study conducted by the European Lung Cancer Working Party. J Clin Oncol 11:1858–1865

Sculier JP, Paesmans M, Bureau G et al (1996) Randomized trial comparing induction chemotherapy versus induction chemotherapy followed by maintenance chemotherapy in small-cell lung cancer. J Clin Oncol 14: 2337–2344

Skarlos D, Samantas E, Pavlidis N et al (1997) Weekly chemotherapy with alternating non-cross resistant chemotherapy regimens in good-prognosis small cell lung cancer (SCLC) (Final results). Lung Cancer 18[Suppl 1]:42

Souhami RL, Rudd R, Ruiz de Elvira MC et al (1994) Randomized trial comparin weekly versus 3-week chemotherapy in small-cell lung cancer: a cancer research campaign trial. J Clin Oncol 12:1806–13

Tabata M, Ueoka H, Kiura K et al (1997) A phase I–II study of weekly cisplatin (CDDP) and etoposide (ETP) plus concurrent thoracic radiotherapy (TRT) for limited small cell lung cancer (LD-SCLC). Proc ASCO 16:1741 (abstract)

Thatcher N, Sambrook RJ, Stephens RJ et al (1997) First results of a randomised trial of dose intensification (DI) with G-CSF in small cell lung cancer (SCLC). Lung Cancer 18[Suppl 1]:7

Weynants P, Bosequée L, Canon JL et al (1997) Concomitant high-dose chemotherapy (HDCt) and radiotherapy (Rt) with G-CSF and peripheral blood stem cell (PBSC) rescue for limited (LD) small cell lung cancer (SCLC). Lung Cancer 18[Suppl 1]: 27

Wolf M, Hans K, Föller A et al (1997) Tandem high dose chemotherapy with peripheral blood stem cell support (PBSCS) in limited stage small cell lung cancer (SCLC). Lung Cancer 18[Suppl 1]:53

18 Best Supportive Care or Chemotherapy for Stage IV Non-Small Cell Lung Cancer

J.P. Sculier, T. Berghmans, C. Castaigne, Y. Lalami, S. Luce, C. Sotiriou, P. Vermylen, and M. Paesmans

CONTENTS

18.1 Introduction

Although cisplatin-based chemotherapy regimens were introduced in the late 1970s for the management of advanced non-small cell lung cancer, more than 15 years of randomized trials were required to produce convincing data showing survival improvement in comparison to best supportive care alone. The routine use of chemotherapy in this indication is still the object of considerable debate in Europe and North America as reflected by different recent editorials or reviews (Haskel 1991; Souhami 1996; Vokes 1995; White 1995; Souquet et al. 1995; Sorensen 1997).

In the present chapter, we will perform a systematic review on the randomized trials performed in patients with advanced non-small cell lung cancer and comparing systemic chemotherapy to best supportive care alone. It will not be possible to strictly limit the scope of our review to stage IV disease because the majority of the trials also deal with patients having advanced locoregional disease (stage III) and the reported results are rarely stratified according to disease extent. We will focus our analysis of the literature on survival because it was the primary endpoint of the trials and because other endpoints such as symptom control, quality of life and cost effectiveness have rarely been adequately investigated. However, a summary of the data available for these secondary endpoints will be presented. The published meta-analyses will be discussed and a qualitative assessment of the publications accompanied by an aggregation of the available data in the original articles that has been performed by the authors of the present chapter will be reported.

18.2 The Individual Randomized Trials

We identified the randomized trials comparing chemotherapy to best supportive care alone in advanced non-small cell lung cancer, on the basis of a prospective search of the published articles in the Current Contents since 1980. Nine studies have been so far reported in the English or French literature in a total of 11 articles (Cormier et al. 1982; Rapp et al. 1988; Gane et al. 1989; Woods et al. 1990; Williams et al. 1988; Kaasa et al. 1991; Quoix et al. 1991; Cellerino et al. 1988, 1991; Leung et al. 1992; Cartel et al. 1993). The chemotherapy regimens used in the experimental arm are described in Table 18.1, the number of patients that were registered, eligible or presenting with metastatic disease (stage IV) in Table 18.2 and the results in terms of response to chemotherapy, survival and statistical analysis in Table 18.3.

The first study was performed by Cormier et al. (1982) in Quebec. It was published in the early 1980s and is the only one not using a cisplatin-containing chemotherapy regimen. The survival was highly statistically significantly improved by the MACC combination. However, the trial was criticized because of the small number of patients included and the poor survival of the control group.

J.P. Sculier, T. Berghmans, C. Castaigne, Y. Lalami, S. Luce, C. Sotiriou, P. Vermylen and M. Paesmans, Service de Médecine Interne et Laboratoire d'Investigation Clinique H.J. Tagnon, Centre des Tumeurs de l'Université Libre de Bruxelles, B-1000 Brussels, Belgium
J.P. Sculier, Institut Jules Bordet, 1 rue Héger-Bordet, B-1000 Brussels, Belgium

Table 18.1. Chemotherapy regimens used in randomized trials

Reference	Chemotherapy regimen (mg/m²)		Number of courses
CORMIER et al. 1982	MACC:	MTX 40 i.v. d1 ADR 40 i.v. d1 CPA 400 i.v. d1 CCNU 30 p.o. d1	Q 3 weeks until progression or relapse
RAPP et al. 1988	I. CAP:	CPA 400 i.v. d1 ADR 40 i.v. d1 CDDP 40 i.v. d1	Q 4 weeks until progression or unacceptable toxicity
	II. VP:	VDS 3 i.v. weekly ×4 then every 2 weeks CDDP 120 i.v. dl, 29, then every 6 weeks	Q 6 weeks until progression or unacceptable toxicity
GANZ et al. 1989	CDDP: + VBL:	120 i.v. d1, 29 then every 6 weeks 6 i.v. weekly ×5 then every 2 weeks	Q 6 weeks
WOODS et al. 1990; WILLIAMS et al. 1988	VP:	VDS 3 i.v. weekly ×6 then every 2 weeks CDDP 120 i.v. d1, 29 then every 6 weeks	Maximum of 6 cycles
KAASA et al. 1991	CE:	CDDP 70 i.v. d1 VP16 100 i.v. d1 200 p.o. d2,3	Two to (responders) 4
QUOIX et al. 1991	VP:	VDS 3 i.v. weekly ×5 then every 2 weeks CDDP 120 i.v. d1	Q 4 weeks for a maximum of 8 cycles
CELLERINO et al. 1988, 1991	CE'P ~ MEC':	CPA: 500 i.v. d1 epirubicin 50 i.v. d1 CDDP 80 i.v. d1 MTX 30 i.v. d29 VP16 200 i.v. d29 CCNU 70 p.o. d29	Q 8 weeks until progression or relapse
LEUNG et al. 1992	CE:	CDDP 100 i.v. d1 VP16 125 i.v. d1 250 p.o. d2, 3	Q 3 weeks for 3 courses then chest irradiation (40 Gy in 20 fractions over 3 weeks)
CARTEI et al. 1993	CDDP 75 i.v. d1 MMC 10 i.v. d1 CPA 400 i.v. d1		Q 3 weeks for a maximum of 6 courses

MTX, methotrexate; ADR, doxorubicine; CPA, cyclophosphamide; CCNU, lomustine; CDDP, cisplatin; VBL, vinblastine; VP16, etoposide; MMC, mitomycin C.

Table 18.2. Number of patients registered in the randomized trials

Reference	Number of registered patients	BSC arm		Chemotherapy arm	
		No. eligible	% with stage IV	No. eligible	% with stage IV
CORMIER et al. 1982	39	17	53%	20	55%
RAPP et al. 1988	150	50	90%	I. 43	86%
				II. 44	82%
GANZ et al. 1989	63	26	100%	22	100%
WOODS et al. 1990; WILLIAMS et al. 1988	201	91	59%	97	73%
KAASA et al. 1991	87	43	100%	44	100%
QUOIX et al. 1991	49	22	100%	24	100%
CELLERINO et al. 1988, 1991	128	61	57%	62	60%
LEUNG et al. 1992	119	58	0%	42	0%
CARTEI et al. 1993	102	50	100%	52	100%

Table 18.3. Results of the randomized trials

Reference	BSC arm		Chemotherapy			P
	MST	1 yr S	OR	MST	1 yr S	
Cormier et al. 1982	8.5 wks	NR	35%	30.5 wks	NR	<0.0005
Rapp et al. 1988	17 wks	10%	I. 15%	24.7 wks	21%	<0.05
			II. 25%	32.6 wks	22%	<0.01
Ganz et al. 1989	14 wks	NR	22%	19 wks	NR	NS
Woods et al. 1990; Williams et al. 1988	17 wks	NR	28%	27 wks	NR	NS
Kaasa et al. 1991	3.8 mo	NR	11%	5.0 mo	NR	NS
Quoix et al. 1991	10 wks	NR	42%	28 wks	NR	<0.001
Cellerino et al. 1988, 1991	4.9 mo	23%	21%	8 mo	32%	NS
Leung et al. 1992	8.7 mo	30%	21%	12.4 mo	53%	<0.05
Cartei et al. 1993	4.0 mo	12%	25%	8.5 mo	38%	<0.0001

BSC, best supportive care; MST, median survival time; 1 yr S, 1 year survival rate; OR, objective response rate; wks, weeks; NR, not reported; NS, nonsignificant; mo, months.

The second Canadian study reported in 1988 by Rapp et al. had a three-aim design and compared two different chemotherapy regimens with best supportive care alone. The sample size was assessed prior to trial activation and both chemotherapy combinations resulted in significantly improved survival.

The UCLA study (Gane et al. 1989) had a particular design, using a double-consent prerandomization. After on-study registration and randomization of the patient, the physician explained the random assignment to the patient and requested consent. Once assigned to a treatment group, the patient remained a member of that group for survival analysis whether or not consent was obtained. Of 32 subjects randomized for support, 6 refused consent and of 31 randomized for chemotherapy, 9 refused. When all the patients were considered, median survival times were respectively 13.6 weeks in the supportive care arm and 20.4 weeks in the chemotherapy arm ($P = 0.09$). When only the patients who gave their consent were analysed, the respective times were 14.4 weeks and 18.6 weeks ($P = 0.26$).

The Australian trial (Woods et al. 1990; Williams et al. 1988) was the largest in terms of number of patients included. Results were similar for both arms but the statistical design has not been clearly reported with the publication or presentation of several probably unplanned interim analyses.

Four studies have been performed in Europe: one in Norway (Kaasa et al. 1991), one in France (Quoix et al. 1991) and two in Italy (Cellerino et al. 1988, 1991; Cartei et al. 1993). All but that by Cellerino et al. (1988, 1991) included patients with only metastatic disease. The Norwegian trial failed to show any significant survival improvement but a major problem in the interpretation of the results was the use of radiation therapy for the primary tumor and mediastinum that was administered with symptomatic intent for patients in both arms (18% in the chemotherapy arm and 42% in the supportive care arm). In the French study, chemotherapy significantly improved survival but the median survival time was unusually short in the control arm.

The Italian trial by Cellerino et al. (1988, 1991) failed to show any significant survival improvement although the final analysis reported (Cellerino et al. 1991) did not take into account prior published interim analyses (Cellerino et al. 1988), not mentioned in the statistical analyses of the final paper. The second Italian trial published in 1993 by Cartei et al. was significantly in favor of chemotherapy for patients with stage IV disease. No interim analysis was performed but the statistical analyses were not reported.

The last published trial (Leung et al. 1992) compared, in Hong Kong, chemotherapy followed by chest irradiation to best supportive care alone in patients with inoperable nonmetastatic non-small cell lung cancer. It showed a significant survival improvement in favor of the treatment arm. Although its design with stage III disease was quite different than that of the other trials, we have decided to keep it in our analysis because it has been included in the reviews and meta-analyses on this topic.

It should be noted that a large British trial has very recently been presented at the Eighth World Conference on Lung Cancer in Dublin in August 1997 (Cullen et al. 1997). A total of 351 eligible patients were randomized between palliative treatment only and 4 courses of chemotherapy (mitomycin C, ifosfamide, cisplatin). Results were significantly in favor of active treatment with respective median survival times of 4.8 and 6.7 months ($P = 0.03$).

18.3 The Meta-analyses

As summarized in Table 18.4, four meta-analyses have been published so far: three were based on the results reported in the articles (Souquet et al. 1993; Grilli et al. 1993; Marind et al. 1994) and one was performed with the individual patient data (Non-Small Cell Lung Cancer Collaborative Group 1995). We will briefly review and comment on these publications before presenting our own meta-analysis of the literature.

Souquet et al. (1993) used seven trials. They excluded three studies, because they investigated monochemotherapy (etoposide and nitrogen mustard) or because the supportive care group was in fact a "wait and see" group with treatment by chemotherapy or radiotherapy only when symptoms appeared. The authors used the mortality rates at 3, 6, 9, 12 and 18 months as endpoints. The way they obtained these numbers is not clearly explained. With chemotherapy they obtained a significant reduction in the mortality rate at 3, 6, 9 and 12 months but not at 18 months, with relative risks of 0.65 (reported in Table 18.4), 0.73, 0.86, 0.91 and 0.96 (of observing an event in the chemotherapy arm compared to the control arm).

Grilli et al. (1993) performed a similar literature selection but without the trial by Quoix et al. (1991) because it was published in French and not in English. They estimated the numbers of deaths at 3, 6, 9 and 12 months from survival curves by simple multiplications, ignoring therefore the censoring mechanism. Their meta-analysis showed a 24% reduction in the likelihood of death (relative risk = 0.76; 95% confidence interval or CI: 0.66–0.87). The effect of chemotherapy varied with time, with a 37% risk reduction at 3 months that increased later. The mean potential gain in survival 1 year after initiation of chemotherapy was estimated to be approximatively 6 weeks (95% CI: 1–10 weeks).

Marino et al. (1994) selected the same studies as Souquet but also included the trial by Buccheri et al. (1990), which is in fact not a true randomized trial. As described by the authors themselves (p. 89 of the article), a "non-conventional randomized procedure was adopted: all eligible patients, seen during the first years of study, were treated with chemotherapy (the MACC regimen as reported by Cormier); in contrast, all the eligible ones, treated during the subsequent years, received no specific antitumor therapy." The authors have considered

Table 18.4. Meta-analyses results

Meta-analysis Trials included	Souquet et al. 1993	Grilli et al. 1993	Marino et al. 1994	Non-Small Cell Lung Cancer Collaborative Group 1995
Laing et al. 1975	–	–	–	NS
Cormier et al. 1982	S	S	S	NS
Anderson and Payne 1985	–	–	–	NS
Rapp et al. 1988	NS	S	S	NS
Ganz et al. 1989	NS	NS	NS	NS
Woods et al. 1990; Williams et al. 1988	S	NS	NS	
– England				NS
– Australia				NS
Buccheri et al. 1990	–	–	NS	–
Kaasa et al. 1991	NS	NS	NS	NS
Quoix et al. 1991	S	–	S	S
Cellerino et al. 1988, 1991	NS	NS	NS	NS
Leung et al. 1992	–	–	–	–
Cartei et al. 1993	–	–	–	S
OR or HR (95% CI)	0.65	0.76	0.44	0.73[a]
	–	0.66–0.87	0.32–0.59	–
	S	S	S	S

Comment: an OR or HR equal to 1 indicates no effect of chemotherapy, and an OR or HR less or greater than 1 indicates that chemotherapy is beneficial or harmful, respectively.
S, significant; NS, nonsignificant; –, not included; OR, odds ratio; HR, hazard rate; CI, confidence interval.
[a] Cisplatin-containing chemotherapy regimens only.

survival at 6 months as the endpoint and have extrapolated the numbers of events from the survival curves, with the assumption of no censoring before 6 months. The pooled odds ratio at 6 months was 0.44 (95% CI: 0.32–0.59). In terms of median survival time, the gain obtained with chemotherapy has been estimated to be about 3 months.

Stewart and Pignon have reported, for the NON-SMALL CELL LUNG CANCER COLLABORATIVE GROUP (1995), a meta-analysis using updated data on individual patients. Trials were eligible if they started recruitment after 1 January 1965 and completed recruitment by 31 December 1991. To avoid publication bias, both published and unpublished studies were included. Updated information on survival status and date of last follow-up were requested together with treatment allocated, date of randomization, age, sex, histological cell type, stage and performance status. Survival analyses (comparisons by log-rank tests) were stratified by trial and the expected and observed numbers of deaths were used to calculate individual and overall pooled hazard ratios (HR), representing the instantaneous risk of dying when receiving treatment compared with best supportive care. Data were available from 11 trials (1190 patients and 1144 deaths), including two using alkylating agents (CORMIER et al. 1982; LAING et al. 1975) and one with etoposide as single agent (ANDERSON and PAYNE 1985). An estimate of the global hazard ratio, on the basis of patient's individual data, is presented in Table 18.4. There was considerable overall statistical heterogeneity, the trials using the alkylating agents suggesting a detrimental effect of chemotherapy (HR: 1.26; 95% CI: 0.96–1.66; $P = 0.095$) and the cisplatin based trials showing a benefit (HR: 0.73; $P < 0.0001$) with an absolute improvement in survival of 10% at 1 year or an increased median survival of 1.5 months. Subgroup analysis failed to reveal any particular advantage of chemotherapy according to sex, histology, type, performance status or stage.

We performed a meta-analysis based on the published literature including papers in both English and French, based on crude numbers of patients dead at the time of publication as reported by the authors in their article, in order to avoid the extrapolation from the survival curves as performed in the prior reported studies and the assumption that no censoring was done before the endpoint time. We did not include the LAING et al. (1975) and ANDERSON and PAYNE (1985) trials using inactive drugs and the BUCCHERI et al. (1990) one for the reason previously given. The meta-analysis was performed according to the method of YUSUF et al. (1985). This method is based on the estimation of the odds ratio describing the relative risk of surviving in the experimental arm in comparison to the control arm, by combining the data of the studies where the information was available In the present analysis, by definition, an OR above 1 is in favor of the experimental arm, the results being statistically significant if the 95% CI of the OR is above 1.

The results are shown in Table 18.5. Crude data on the number of patients dead or alive were available for six of the nine trials selected (Table 18.1). Although the difference was never significant in the individual trials, due, perhaps, to a lack of statistical power, the overall OR was significantly ($P < 0.05$) in favor of chemotherapy, with a relative risk of 2.07 (95% CI: 1.06–4.04). When only cisplatin-based trials were considered (without the study by Cormier), the difference has a lower significance probability

Table 18.5. Authors' own meta-analysis of the results published in the literature

Trial	No. of events/ No. of patients eligible		OR	95% CI
	BSC	CT		
CORMIER et al. 1982	17/17	17/20	7.1	0.70–73.35
RAPP et al. 1988	48/50	92/97	1.3	0.26–6.36
GANZ et al. 1989	25/26	19/22	3.5	0.46–26.73
CELLERINO et al. 1988, 1991	60/61	58/62	3.4	0.57–20.22
LEUNG et al. 1992	45/58	27/42	1.9	0.80–4.63
CARTEI et al. 1993	50/50	52/52	1	–
Pooled results				
– Total			2.07	1.06–4.04
– Cisplatin based trials (without CORMIER)			2.27	1.20–4.32

OR, odds ratio; CI, confidence interval; BSC, best supportive care; CT, chemotherapy.

($P < 0.02$), with an OR of 2.27 (95% IC: 1.20–4.32) in favor of active treatment. There was no statistically significant difference between the negative and positive trials in terms of cisplatin dosage planned by the protocol and in terms of rate of patients with stage IV disease.

In conclusion, the five meta-analyses are all in favor of chemotherapy in comparison to best supportive care alone in patients with advanced non-small cell lung cancer, especially when a cisplatin-containing regimen is used.

18.4 The Qualitative Assessment of the Randomized Trials

A meta-analysis, as we performed, consists of a quantitative aggregation of the results of randomized trials, not taking into account the individual quality of each study. In order to analyse this important aspect of clinical research, we used two different methods. The first was the quality scale developed by Chalmers et al. (1981), which has two components, the internal validity (scientific) and the external validity (allowing the generalization of the results to the entire cancer patient population concerned). Respective maximal scores are 63 and 25 points, the total being 88. The second method (Appendix) has been developed by our group, the European Lung Cancer Working Party (ELCWP), and is called the ELCWP scale. It assesses the following qualitative aspects: the study protocol (as usually described in the "Patients and methods" section of the article) and the performed analysis (as reported in the "Results" section). Respective maximal scores are 42 and 60 points, the total being 102. When an item does not apply to a trial, the theoretically concerned points are omitted from the theoretical total (denominator). The final scores are expressed in percentages, a higher rate meaning a higher methodological quality as reported in the publication.

Table 18.6 summarizes the scores obtained for each trial by the two methods. The mean Chalmers and ELCWP scores were respectively 42.5% (SD: 13.2%; median: 47.5%) and 66.2% (SD: 8.7%; median 64.1%). The numbers were low, as already reported by Marino et al. in their meta-analysis. They reported a median Chalmers score of 41% (range: 34%–73%). The scores obtained by the ELCWP method were higher and the correlation of the results obtained by the two methods was not significant (Bravais-Pearson coefficient $r = 0.45$).

The studies obtaining in the publication a statistically significant advantage of survival in favor of chemotherapy had no better quality score as evaluated by the Mann-Whitney nonparametric test. The mean rates of the negative and positive trials were respectively 38.8% and 45.4% on the Chalmers scale ($P = 0.62$) and 64.9% and 67.3% on the ELCWP scale ($P = 0.62$). When the analysis was restricted to studies using the cisplatin-containing regimen by excluding the Cormier trial, the results were similar.

The studies reporting crude data on dead patients to allow the meta-analysis were compared to those not giving these data. Their quality was not significantly improved with mean rates respectively of

Table 18.6. Quality scores of the published randomized trials comparing chemotherapy to best supportive care alone for advanced non-small cell lung cancer

Trial	Scoring system			
	Chalmers (%) Total	ELCWP (%)		
		Protocol	Analysis	Total
Cormier et al. 1982	34.2	42.9	63.0	53.4
Rapp et al. 1988	49.3	78.6	85.2	82.3
Ganz et al. 1989	52.9	54.8	62.5	58.9
Woods et al. 1990; Williams et al. 1988	22.9	64.3	64.0	64.1
Kaasa et al. 1991	24.7	54.8	66.7	61.1
Quoix et al. 1991	47.5	59.5	67.4	63.6
Cellerino et al. 1988, 1991	59.7	78.6	73.1	75.5
Leung et al. 1992	37.3	69.0	66.7	67.8
Cartei et al. 1993	58.9	76.2	63.0	69.3

Table 18.7. Reporting of some important items in quality scoring for the individual randomized trials

Trial	Items							
	A	B	C	D	E	F	G	H
Cormier et al. 1982	1	0	0	2	0	0	2	NA
Rapp et al. 1988	2	0	2	2	0	2	2	NA
Ganz et al. 1989	0	2	0	2	2	2	2	0
Woods et al. 1990; Williams et al. 1988	0	0	0	2	0	2	0	0
Kaasa et al. 1991	2	0	0	2	2	2	0	1
Quoix et al. 1991	0	0	0	2	0	2	0	NA
Cellerino et al. 1988, 1991	2	2	1	2	2	2	2	0
Leung et al. 1992	2	0	0	2	0	0	2	NA
Cartei et al. 1993	2	1	0	2	0	2	2	NA

A, primary objective definition; B, technique of randomization used; C, a priori estimate of the sample size; D, survival statistical analysis; E, confidence interval on the estimated parameters; F, intent to treat analysis; G, crude number of deaths observed per arm; H, a posteriori estimate of study power (for negative trial): 2 = adequate; 1 = inadequate; 0 = not reported; NA = not applicable.

47.9% vs 31.7% on the Chalmers scale ($P = 0.07$) and 67.9% vs 62.9% on the ELCWP scale ($P = 0.44$).

Table 18.7 reports some important items of the quality scoring scales and shows that very important items like the description of method of randomization used, the a priori estimate of the sample size and, for negative trials, the a posteriori estimate of the study power or confidence intervals on the evaluated parameters were rarely reported in the publication.

In conclusion, the analyzed trials lacked good methodological quality. A possible explanation might be the ethical difficulties of obtaining patients who agreed to participate in this type of investigation or the biases due to poor reports of adequately performed and analyzed studies. Whatever the reason, the poor quality of a trial can provide arguments against chemotherapy, even if the results are reported as significantly positive.

18.5 Other Endpoints than Survival

Important secondary endpoints are the subjective effect of chemotherapy sensed by the patient and the cost of the treatment procedure.

Subjective effect can be evaluated by symptom control and quality of life evaluation. Published data are rare so far in this field. Toxicity has been assessed in the conventional way but that approach does not necessarily reflect the feeling of the patient. Ganz et al. (1989) measured the evolution of Karnofsky performance status in the two groups and did not detect any difference in the average score over the first 24 weeks between the patients receiving chemotherapy and those treated by supportive care only. Billingham et al. (1997) presented for the previously discussed trial (Cullen et al. 1997) quality of life data obtained for patients included in the study. These data mainly assessed symptoms and toxicity with a significant improvement after 6 weeks when chemotherapy was administered. In the same congress, another English group reported on a trial (Anderson et al. 1997) comparing in advanced non-small cell lung cancer single agent chemotherapy with gemcitabine to best supportive care. Their study, including 300 patients, had as primary endpoint quality of life measured by symptom scales and the EORTC questionnaire. A significant improvement was reported with gemcitabine but without better survival.

Costs of chemotherapy have been analyzed for the three-arm Canadian trial performed by Rapp et al. In the Canadian health care system, the investigators have shown (Jaakkimainen et al. 1990) that chemotherapy, especially the CAP regimen, was cost-effective, mainly because of a reduction of the number of days of hospitalization.

18.6 Conclusions

The systematic literature review that we have performed on randomized trials on the role of systemic chemotherapy in advanced non-small cell lung cancer has identified multiple positive points in favor of active treatment of these patients: modest but significant survival improvement as shown in some randomized trials and in all the meta-analyses when cisplatin is present in the regimen, better symptom control and cost-effectiveness. However, the trials are not of excellent methodological quality, probably because they are difficult to conduct from an ethical point of view. These methodological problems might be the source of further discussion on the true impact of chemotherapy in this indication. Nevertheless the large effort put into this type of investigation over more than 15 years and the convergence of all the data available, whether the observed differences are statistically significant or not, should encourage us to improve the available regimens and no longer try to reproduce trials that are becoming more and more ethically questionable.

Appendix: The Quality Scoring Method for Publication Proposed by the European Lung Cancer Working Party (ELCWP)

Item identification or category	Maximal category	Definition
		I. Study protocol description
A	2	*Definition of the number of participating centers*
B		*Selection criteria for the study*
B1	2	– Performance status
B2	2	– Age
B3	2	– Histological type
B4	2	– Disease extent
B5	2	– Prior therapy
B6	2	– Comorbidity
C	2	*Randomization method*
D		*Treatment description*
D1	2	– Radiotherapy: energy, dose, fractionation, fild, duration – Chemotherapy: drugs, dose, route – Course number
D2	2	– Dose adaptation plan
E		*Work-ups*
E1	2	– Initial
E2	2	– At response assessment
E3	2	– During follow-up after therapy
F		*Evaluation criteria*
F1	2	– Response
F2	2	– Response or disease-free duration
F3	2	– Survival
F4	2	– Toxicity
G		*Statistical methods and trial objectives*
G1	2	– Primary objective definition
G2	2	– Secondary objective definition
G3	2	– Statistical methods and tests used
G4	2	– A priori estimate of sample size
		II. Study analysis report
A		*Analysis timing*
A1	2	– Dates of first and last patient registration
A2	2	– Type of analysis (definitive or planned interim)
B		*Patient characteristics*
B1	2	– Ineligibility rate (per arm)
B2	2	– Causes of ineligibility
B3		– *Eligible patient characteristics*
B31	2	– Age
B32	2	– Performance status
B33	2	– Sex
B34	2	– Histological type
B35	2	– Disease extent or stage
B4	2	– Arms balancing according to stratification
C		*Survival*
C1	2	– Rates
C2	2	– Crude numbers of deaths
C3	2	– Statistical test results
C4	2	– Confidence intervals on rates
C5	2	– Intent to treat analysis
D		*Antitumoral response*
D1	2	– Unassessable rate (per arm)
D2	2	– Cause for nonassessability
D3	2	– Response rates
D4	2	– Confidence intervals on rates
D5	2	– Statistical test results
D6	2	– Inclusion of toxic deaths and early deaths by cancer in the rate calculation
E		*Local control*
E1	2	– Actuarial rate
E2	2	– Statistical test results
F		*Toxicity*
F1	2	– Description per arm
F2	2	– Statistical test results
F3	2	– Confidence intervals on rates
G		*Prognostic factors for survival*
G1	2	– Univariate analysis
G2	2	– Multivariate analysis
H		*Discussion*
H1	2	– Author's conclusions in accordance with results
H2	2	– For negative trials: a posteriori estimate of study power
Quotation:	2 points:	description adequate and complete
	1 point:	partially described or not optimal
	0 point:	not performed or not mentioned

References

Anderson G, Payne H (1985) Response rate and toxicity of etoposide (VP-16) in squamous carcinoma of the lung: report from the Lung Cancer Treatment Study Group. Semin Oncol 12:21–22

Anderson H, Cottier B, Nicoloson M, Milroy R, Maughan T, Bond M, Falk S, Burt P, Carmichael J, Thatcher N (1997) Phase III study of gemcitabine (Gemzar©) versus best supportive care (BSC) in advanced non-small cell lung cancer (NSCLC). Lung Cancer 18 [Suppl 1]:9

Billingham LJ, Cullen MH, Woods J, Chetiyawardana AD, Joshi RC, Cook J, Woodroffe CM (1997) Mitomycin, ifosfamide and cisplatin (MIC) in non-small cell lung cancer (NSCLC): 3. Results of a randomized trial evaluating palliation and quality of life. Lung Cancer 18 [Suppl 1]:9

Buccheri G, Ferrigno D, Rosso A, Vola F (1990) Further evidence in favour of chemotherapy for inoperable non-small cell lung cancer. Lung Cancer 6:87–98

Cartei G, Cartei F, Cantone A, Causarano D, Genco G, Tobaldin A, Interlandi G, Giraldi T (1993) Cisplatin-cyclophosphamide-mitomycin combination chemotherapy with supportive care versus supportive care alone for treatment of metastatic non-small cell lung cancer. J Natl Cancer Inst 85:794–800

Cellerino R, Tummarello D, Porfiri E, Guidi F, Isidori P, Raspugli M, Biscottini B, Fatati G (1988) Non-small cell lung cancer (NSCLC) – a prospective randomized trial with alternating chemotherapy CEP/MEC' versus no treatment. Eur J Cancer Clin Oncol 24:1839–1843

Cellerino R, Tummarello D, Guidi F, Isidori P, Raspugli M, Biscottini B, Fatati G (1991) A randomized trial of alternating chemotherapy versus best supportive care in advanced non-small cell lung cancer. J Clin Oncol 9: 1453–1461

Chalmers TC, Smith HJ, Blackburn B, Silverman B, Schroeder B, Reitman D, Ambroz A (1981) A method for assessing the quality of a randomized clinical trial. Contr Clin Trials 2:31–49

Cormier Y, Bergeron D, La Forge J, Lavandier M, Fournier M, Chenard J, Desmeules M (1982) Benefits of polychemotherapy in advanced non-small cell bronchogenic carcinoma. Cancer 50:845–849

Cullen MH, Woodroffe CM, Billingham LJ, Chetiyawardana AD, Joshi R, Ferry D, Connolly CK, Bessell E (1997) Mitomycin, ifosfamide and cisplatin (MIC) in non-small cell lung cancer (NSCLC): 2. Results of a randomized trial in patients with extensive disease. Lung Cancer 18 [Suppl 1]:5

Ganz PA, Figlin RA, Haskell CM, La Soto N, Siau J (1989) Supportive care versus supportive care and combination chemotherapy in metastatic non-small cell lung cancer. Cancer 63:1271–1278

Grilli R, Oxman AD, Julian JA (1993) Chemotherapy for advanced non-small cell lung cancer: how much benefit is enough? J Clin Oncol 11:1866–1872

Haskell CM (1991) Chemotherapy and survival of patients with non-small cell lung cancer: a contrary view. Chest 99:1325

Jaakkimainen L, Goodwin PJ, Pater J, Warde P, Murray N, Rapp E (1990) Counting the costs of chemotherapy in a National Cancer Institute of Canada randomized trial in non-small cell lung cancer. J Clin Oncol 8:1301–1309

Kaasa S, Lund E, Thorud E, Hatlevoll R, Host H (1991) Symptomatic treatment versus combination chemotherapy for patients with extensive non-small cell lung cancer. Cancer 67:2443–2447

Laing AH, Berry RJ, Newman CR, Peto J (1975) Treatment of inoperable carcinoma of bronchus. Lancet i:1161–1164

Leung WT, Shiu WCT, Pang JCK, Lau J, Tao M, Leung SF, Teo F (1992) Combined chemotherapy and radiotherapy versus best supportive care in the treatment of inoperable non-small cell lung cancer. Oncology 49:321–326

Marino P, Pampallano S, Preatoni A, Cantoni A, Invernizzi F (1994) Chemotherapy vs supportive care in advanced non-small cell lung cancer. Chest 106:861–865

Non-small Cell Lung Cancer Collaborative Group (1995) Chemotherapy in non-small cell lung cancer: a meta-analysis using updated data on individual patients from 52 randomised clinical trials. BMJ 311:899–909

Quoix E, Dietemann A, Charbonneau J, Boutin C, Meurice JC, Orlando JP, Ducolone A, Pauli G, Roegel E (1991) La chimiothérapie comportant du cisplatine est-elle utile dans le cancer bronchique non microcellulaire au stade IV? Résultats d'une étude randomisée. Bull Cancer 78:341–346

Rapp E, Pater JL, Willan A, Cormier Y, Murray N, Evans WK, Hodson DI, Clark DA, Feld R, Arnold AM, Ayoub JI, Wilson KS, Latreille J, Wierzbicki RF, Hill DP (1988) Chemotherapy can prolong survival in patients with advanced non-small cell lung cancer – report of a Canadian multicenter randomized trial. J Clin Oncol 6:633–641

Sorensen JB (1997) The increased armament in the battle against non-small cell lung cancer. Ann Oncol 8:513–514

Souhami RL (1996) Chemotherapy in non-small cell lung cancer: time to re-examine our attitudes. Thorax 51:231–232

Souquet PJ, Chauvin F, Boissel JP, Cellerino R, Cormier Y, Ganz PA, Kaasa S, Pater JL, Quoix E, Rapp E, Tumarello D, Williams J, Woods BL, Bernard JP (1993) Polychemotherapy in advanced non-small cell lung cancer: a meta-analysis. Lancet 342:19–21

Souquet PJ, Lombard-Bohas CH, Bernard JP (1995) Est-il encore licite en 1994 de préconiser l'abstention thérapeutique pour les cancers bronchiques non à petites cellules de stade IIIB et IV? Rev Mal Respir 12:71–72

Vokes EE (1995) Should non-small cell carcinoma of the lung be treated with chemotherapy? Pro: chemotherapy is for non-small cell lung cancer. Am J Respir Crit Care Med 151:1285–1287

White SR (1995) Should non-small cell carcinoma of the lung be treated with chemotherapy? Con: therapeutic empiricism – the case against chemotherapy in non-small cell lung cancer. Am J Respir Crit Care Med 151:1288–1291

Williams CJ, Woods R, Levi J, Page J (1988) Chemotherapy for non-small cell lung cancer: a randomized trial of cisplatin/vindesine vs no chemotherapy. Semin Oncol 15 [Suppl 7]:58–61

Woods RL, Williams CJ, Levi J, Page J, Bell D, Byrne M, Kerestes ZL (1990) A randomized trial of cisplatin and vindesine versus supportive care only in advanced non-small cell lung cancer. Br J Cancer 61:608–611

Yusuf S, Peto R, Lewis J (1985) Beta-blocked during and after myocardial infarction: an overview of randomized trials. Prog Cardiovasc Dis 27:335–371

19 Do We Have the Real Tools to Evaluate Lung Radiotoxicity?

F. Mornex[1] and L.J. Boersma[2]

CONTENTS

19.1 Introduction

Lung cancer remains a devastating disease. In many situations, radiation therapy represents a chance of cure. However, due to the high radiosensitivity of the lung, it is often not possible to achieve a tumoricidal dose of radiation in lung cancer patients. In addition, in patients who are cured by radiotherapy, the quality of life may be compromised by an impaired respiratory function. Radiation-induced pulmonary symptoms occur in up to approximately 20% of patients irradiated for lung, breast cancer, lymphoma and thymoma (Marks 1997b). Subclinical changes in whole-lung function, manifested by asymptomatic reductions in quantitative pulmonary function tests, are seen in a larger fraction of patients. For an individual patient, there are presently no good means of predicting the probability of developing symptoms, nor of predicting the severity of the lung injury induced by radiation therapy, alone or combined with chemotherapy, which is becoming the standard treatment in some situations (Peckham and Collis 1981; Schaake-Koning et al. 1992). This problem may become even more critical with the radiation dose escalation, which is necessary to improve local control and survival in lung cancer, and which is now realistic, with the recent advent of three-dimensional conformal therapy, allowing the radiation dose to be increased in a limited volume (Armstrong et al. 1993; Hazuka et al. 1993; Lichter et al. 1992; Perez et al. 1986, 1987). However, to design the optimal treatment technique, it should be possible to predict the risk of lung injury more precisely. Thus, the limited tolerance of the lung to radiation is of great importance in the radiotherapeutic management of malignant chest tumors, and the recent improvements in radiation therapy equipment make the need for prediction more crucial.

The purpose of this chapter is to identify the different tools available which can help evaluating (and potentially predicting) the lung parenchyma radiotoxicity, and to present the SOMA/LENT scale (Pavy et al. 1995a).

1 F. Mornex, Radiation Oncology Department, EA 643, Centre Hospitalier Lyon-Sud, 69310 Pierre-Bénite, France

2 L.J. Boersma, Radiotherapy Department, The Netherlands Cancer Institute/Antoni van Leeuwenhoek Huis, Plesmanlaan 121, 1066 CX Amsterdam, The Netherlands

19.2 Characteristics of Radiation-Induced Lung Injury

19.2.1 Introduction

The earliest reports of radiation-induced lung injury were presented at the beginning of this century, with description of clinical and radiological changes in the lung and pleura, which were attributed to previous irradiation (Groover et al. 1921; Phillips and Margolis 1972; Rubin and Casarett 1968; Tyler and Blackman 1992). This description was then confirmed by several publications.

Radiation-induced lung injury occurs in two phases: an early phase, radiation pneumonitis, developing 1–8 months after irradiation, which can be followed by a late phase, radiation fibrosis (Gross 1977). The severity of the injury can vary from slight dyspnea and cough, to severe impairment of respiratory function, which may eventually lead to death.

The histopathologic changes and the resultant physiological abnormalities of cancer therapy are relatively similar for radiation and chemotherapy. Although cytotoxic drugs affect the entire lung, radiation injury is generally limited to the irradiated volume.

A great number of histologic changes have been documented in animals (Down 1986; Law 1985; Law and Ahier 1989); however, data for humans are incomplete. The effects of doses of radiation on the lung parenchyma, with resulting congestion and intra-alveolar edema, become evident within weeks to months after exposure to radiation (Travis 1980).

The most important factors which influence the severity and the probability of developing radiation damage include treatment-related factors such as total radiation dose, fractionation schedule, and irradiated volume (Boersma 1995a,b; Bornstein et al. 1990; Choi et al. 1985; Hermann et al. 1997; Marks et al. 1997a,b; Moldofsky et al. 1988; Van Dyk et al. 1981, 1989; Van Dyk and Keane 1989). Other factors are concomitant or previous chemotherapy, previous irradiation, steroid withdrawal, and pre-existing pulmonary disease (Choi et al. 1985; Gross 1977). Only little evidence has been found for the influence of age, presence of atherosclerosis and previous surgery. There are additional unknown factors contributing to the development of radiation damage. It may occur "at random," but it is also possible that individual sensitivity partially determines the reaction (Mah et al. 1987). This could correlate with the hypothesis that autoimmunity or a delayed hypersensitivity reaction are pathogenic mechanisms in developing radiation pneumonitis, particularly in cases where damage occurs outside the treatment fields (Gross 1977).

To reduce or even prevent radiation-induced lung damage, the pathogenesis of this type of injury should be known, as well as the quantitative influence of the above-mentioned factors on the severity and probability of developing radiation-induced injury (e.g., radiation dose, irradiated volume, additional treatment with chemotherapy).

19.2.2 Pathogenesis

19.2.3 Early Phase

The changes due to radiation affect several types of cells: capillary endothelial cells, and epithelial cells such as pneumocytes I and II (Katzenstein and Askin 1990; Phillips 1981; Stone et al. 1956).

Endothelial cell damage results in an increased capillary permeability, in occlusion of the microvasculature by platelets, fibrin, collagen and debris, and in metabolic activity changes, affecting vasodilation and constriction. This injury results in interstitial inflammation, thickening of alveolar walls, and alveolar collapse, leading to impairment of gas exchange.

Type I pneumocytes are desquamated into the alveolar lumen, and this injury is followed by proliferation of type II pneumocytes, which produce surfactant and maintain patent alveoli. An increased level of alveolar surfactant is one of the earliest detectable changes following lung irradiation starting within hours of irradiation and persisting a maximum of 2–6 weeks (Travis et al. 1987). Subsequently, surfactant levels return to and remain at normal levels during the pneumonic phase (MacDonald et al. 1995). Although abnormalities are found in most elements and no specific lesion is entirely characteristic of pneumonitis, current evidence suggests that damage to the type II pneumocyte and the endothelial cell is closely linked to the pneumonic process. Changes in bronchiolar epithelium have also been reported: focal bronchial necrosis, squamous metaplasia and bronchiectasis. In addition, slight pleural thickening may be seen. Mild radiation-induced pneumonitis may reverse to normal, but the inflammatory response may lead to distorsion of the lung architecture and result in the late and irreversible phase of fibrosis (Roswit and White 1977).

19.2.4 Late Phase

The principal characteristic lesions of pulmonary radiation fibrosis are progressive vascular sclerosis and interstitial fibrosis, which includes a pathological organization of collagen fibers and fibrosis of the alveolar walls, peribronchial and perivascular regions, subpleural zone and interlobular septa. This process results in a marked thickening of the septa and pleura (Ward et al. 1979). An imbalance between collagen production and degradation seems to be one of the major factors underlying late radiation damage. Recently, it has been suggested that cytokines (especially transforming growth factor β) released immediately after irradiation may play a major role in the development of radiation fibrosis (Anscher et al. 1993, 1998; Border and Noble 1994; Finkelstein et al. 1994). The fibrotic collapse of lung tissue finally leads to dilatation of bronchi (bronchiectasis) with accumulation of intraluminal secretions and secondary infections.

19.3 Tools to Evaluate Radiation-Induced Lung Toxicity

There are several "tools" available to evaluate the radiation-induced injury: these include clinical examination, radiological findings, functional tests and blood tests. This chapter will review all these aspects, as well as the potential new tools to predict radiation-induced injury.

19.3.1 Clinical Evaluation

Symptomatic pneumonitis occurs in approximately 5%–20% of patients irradiated for mediastinal lymphoma, lung, or breast cancer (Davis et al. 1992; Morgan et al. 1985; Shapiro et al. 1990). The symptoms of radiation damage of the lung vary from very mild signs of dyspnea and cough, to lethal respiratory failure. The clinical syndrome of the early phase, acute radiation pneumonitis, usually occurs 1–3 months after completion of radiation, and is characterized by a hacking cough, dyspnea on exertion, fever and, rarely, chest pain. The cough is initially nonproductive, but rather accompanied by the production of thick white sputum. The fever may be subfebrile, but can also be high and spiking. The physical signs are scant; sometimes there is evidence of consolidation, dry and moist rales may be heard and occasionally a pleural friction rub is heard. Sometimes signs of pleural effusion can be found.

The early phase 1–8 months after irradiation may be followed by a late fibrotic phase, which is usually asymptomatic, but sometimes chronic respiratory failure develops. The clinical signs are dyspnea, reduced exercise tolerance, orthopnea, cyanosis and finger clubbing. Sometimes even a cor pulmonale develops. These symptoms may persist for the life of the patient (Gross 1977). In addition the lung becomes very susceptible to invasion by microorganisms due to the diminished tissue resistance. Bronchiectasis is accompanied by chronic respiratory infections, which are often resistant to therapy.

In terms of treatment, steroids may help to decrease the severity of clinical symptoms (Cosgriff and Kligerman 1951; Moss et al. 1960; Roswit and White 1977). Abrupt withdrawal of corticosteroids may provoke radiation pneumonitis and therefore withdrawal has to be gradual. The beneficial effect of the prophylactic use of corticosteroids has not been established. Steroids are not of benefit in the late fibrotic phase (Moss et al. 1960). Because in this late phase the lungs become more susceptible to infections, antibiotics are often needed. In addition, conventional asthma medicines as bronchodilatators may be helpful in cases of severe dyspnea. The use of anticoagulants (e.g., heparin) has been studied, as well as many other agents (Moss et al. 1960; McDonald et al. 1995). However, none of these agents has yet been shown to be of beneficial effect in clinical studies.

19.3.2 Radiological Evaluation

The radiographic changes in the lung occurring 7–10 days after radiotherapy can be described as a diffuse haze and a ground glass opacification, having the appearance of either pleuritis or pneumonitis (Bate and Guttmann 1957; Bell et al. 1988; Davis et al. 1992; Libshitz and Southard 1974). Usually air bronchograms are visible as well. These changes have a sharp edge and are confined to the margin of the treatment field.

When fibrosis occurs, the changes gradually alter to linear fibrotic densities (PRATO et al. 1977). These densities are centered upon the irradiated region, but may extend outside it. Other radiographic features of the late phase are mediastinal shift with loss of volume, lung contraction, shrinkage of the pulmonary vessels, pleural thickening, bronchiectasis and bronchial stenosis. Sometimes pleural effusion is seen. Even if pneumonitis has not occurred, fibrosis may develop. Cases of radiographic changes outside treatment portals have been described, but this phenomenon is rare and has been attributed to opportunistic infections or other causes.

Chest radiographs are generally less sensitive for detecting radiation damage than CT-scan images of the thorax (MAH et al. 1988; VAN DYK and HILL 1983; VAN DYK and KEANE 1989; VAN DYK et al. 1989). Abnormalities are generally apparent on CT within 16 weeks after radiotherapy, and can be described in a few cases even if no abnormalities are seen on chest radiographs. Further characteristic findings are extension of the injury over anatomical tissue margins (50%), air bronchograms (25%), loss of volume (15%), and pleural thickening (55%) (MAH et al. 1986, 1987; VAN DYK and HILL 1983). Computerized tomographic findings demonstrate a well-defined dose-response relationship. Four patterns of radiation-induced changes in lung on CT have been identified (LIBSHITZ and SOUTHARD 1974): homogeneous, slight increase in radiodensity; patchy consolidation; discrete consolidation; and solid consolidation. In the past few years high resolution CT (HRCT) has been used to study radiation-induced lung damage in more detail. It is claimed that with HRCT a differentiation can be made between fibrosis (e.g., reticular densities, honeycombing) and reversible alveolitis, which cannot be distinguished by density measurements on conventional CT (SCHRATTERER-SEHN et al. 1993).

19.3.3 Overall Pulmonary Function Tests

The clinical toxicity of irradiation of the lungs is not only determined by the incidence of radiation pneumonitis or CT density changes, but also by the functional changes associated with irradiation of the lung.

Patients with lung carcinoma frequently have compromised lung function because of coexistent chronic obstructive airways disease. Surgery or radiotherapy for lung carcinoma can only be undertaken if it is estimated that patients will tolerate the loss of normal lung tissue.

Patients are normally not considered candidates for surgery if their estimated postoperative forced expiratory volume in 1 s (FEV_1) is less than 800–1000 ml, as this is associated with carbon dioxide retention and decreased exercise tolerance (GROSS 1977). This postoperative FEV_1 may be predicted with the help of regional lung perfusion scans using the formula: postoperative FEV_1 = preoperative FEV_1 × percent perfusion of remaining lung (ABRATT and WILCOX 1995). This method results in a statistically significant correlation between predicted and measured results.

Radiation-induced lung injury is usually accompanied by a decrease in lung volumes in all compartments (total lung capacity, vital capacity, residual volume, inspiratory capacity, tidal volume and FEV_1) (CIONINI et al. 1984; GROSS 1977). These decreases are first seen at 4–8 weeks after treatment, and are maximal after 6–9 months (BOERSMA 1995a; MORNEX et al. 1997). After 1–2 years most studies report some recovery, with respect to the early phase, but there is no agreement as to whether this recovery reaches pre-treatment levels or whether a significant reduction of lung volumes remains present (COSSET et al. 1991; CURRAN et al. 1992; RUBENSTEIN 1988). Long-term follow-up studies after treatment for Hodgkin's disease show a minor but significant reduction of lung volumes (3–11% of predicted from a normal healthy population) at 2–18 years after irradiation (GROTH et al. 1989; LINGOS et al. 1991; MORGAN et al. 1985; SHAPIRO et al. 1990).

Other pulmonary function tests with respect to the physiological aspects of total lung function are transfer factor for carbon monoxide (T_{LCO}), compliance and breathing work (JENSEN et al. 1990). T_{LCO} decreases as well during the early phase, but most authors did not find a subsequent recovery. Due to the progressive scarring of lung tissue, compliance of the lung decreases after irradiation, which results in an increase of the work of breathing. ABRATT showed the superiority of T_{LCO} on FEV_1, with respect to clinical symptoms: a worsening of the dyspnea score occurred only in patients with a >10% decrease in transfer factor (T_{LCO}) irrespective of the change in FEV_1 (ABRATT et al. 1990; ABRATT and WILLCOX 1995). In addition, they found a relation between pulmonary functional tests and perfusion scans, with a statistically significant correlation between the amount of perfusion in the zones at risk and a decreased transfer factor (T_{LCO}) at follow-up. They suggest a potential predictive value of pretreatment

T_{LCO} assessment to radiation clinical tolerance (ABRATT et al. 1990; ABRATT and WILLCOX 1995).

19.3.4 Local Lung Function

Scintigraphic techniques offer the opportunity to investigate functional changes (perfusion and ventilation) regionally. Nuclear medicine ventilation/perfusion scans are very frequently abnormal following thoracic irradiation (CHOI et al. 1985; MCDONALD et al. 1995). Perfusion defects are seen more commonly than ventilation defects and approximately correspond to the irradiated volume (SHAPIRO et al. 1990). This supports the concept that abnormal shunts occur following irradiation, with some irradiated areas remaining ventilated but not adequately perfused. The perfusion deficit seems to precede the ventilation decrease, which correlates with the histologic findings that the earliest damage occurs to the capillary endothelium. The first decrease in blood flow (Q) has been reported to occur 3 weeks after the start of radiotherapy, while the maximal decrease has been seen at approximately 150 days after the treatment (COSSET et al. 1991). Hereafter a slight improvement has been reported (BOERSMA 1995a). The decrease in ventilation (V) starts about 45 days after radiotherapy. Beyond 300 days after radiation, more or less similar values for perfusion and ventilation are found (BOERSMA et al. 1996).

With more sophisticated techniques, such as single photon emission computed tomography (SPECT), ventilation/perfusion scans provide a 3D display of the V/Q data and may be even more sensitive in detecting regional lung injury. Quantification of local functional changes has become possible (BELL et al. 1988). ZWIJNENBURG performed pre- and postradiotherapy SPECT V and Q scans and found a decrease of perfused lung volume, which was maximal at 5–7 months after irradiation (ZWIJNENBURG et al. 1988).

By combining CT-thorax scans and SPECT ventilation and perfusion scans, BOERSMA has shown that it is possible to quantify local functional injury, in relation with the 3D dose distribution (BOERSMA 1995; BOERSMA et al. 1994, 1995, 1996). Before quantifying V and Q from the measured number of counts, a correction was applied to account for attenuation of the photons due to interactions with the different body tissues. CT-thorax scans were performed to calculate the 3D dose distribution. Subsequently SPECT and CT were spatially correlated, and quantification of V and Q was carried out per dose-interval of 4 Gy. The locally delivered radiation dose could be calculated with a maximal uncertainty of 11%, while the uncertainty of the image correlation was 0.5 cm. This method was illustrated using data from five patients: in all patients a dose-dependent decrease in perfusion was seen, and in four patients a dose-dependent decrease in ventilation was seen. In the low-dose regions an increase in local perfusion and ventilation was found. This increase was suggested to represent a redistribution phenomenon, and has been shown to be dependent on the dose distribution in the rest of the lung. It was concluded that the combined use of SPECT and CT data is an effective method for determining the dose-effect relations for regional lung function in each individual patient. Using this method, the average dose-effect relations for local V and Q were derived over 25 lymphoma patients (BOERSMA 1995).

19.3.5 Laboratory Tests of Serum or Blood

The usefulness of laboratory tests is still undefined, there being a need for early biochemical markers of normal tissue damage that would predict late injury and would allow the radiation oncologist and medical oncologist to determine if their treatment is exceeding normal tissue tolerance (MCDONALD et al. 1995; ROTSTEIN et al. 1990). If biochemical markers of tissue damage could be detected in the subclinical phase, prior to the accumulation of significant injury, one could terminate therapy or institute treatment to prevent or attenuate later lesion. There are a large number of substances whose release potentially may reflect or predict the degree of radiation and/or chemotherapy injury to the lung. Besides the surfactant apoprotein, procollagen type 3 can be measured in the blood. It is possible that angiotensin converting enzyme, blood plasminogen activating factor, and prostacyclin could be measured as well. These various substances have been correlated with either acute or delayed radiation pneumopathy. Significant additional work is required to evaluate the usefulness of such blood level measurements but they should be considered in any prospective evaluation of toxicity grading. Finally, although the preliminary data suggested that plasma TGF-β may be a predictor for the later development of complications, recent results published by the group at Duke University no longer support this hypothesis (CANNEY and DEAN 1990, MARKS et al. 1997b).

19.4 How to Quantify and Potentially Predict the Effect of Radiation

There is, so far, no ideal parameter allowing the quantification of the potential radiation damage on an individual basis. Studies following radiation are difficult as there is a delay in the onset of radiation fibrosis and the mechanism of lung damage is complex, occurring mainly at the capillary-alveolar level. Several models have been developed to estimate the probability of developing normal tissue injury from an inhomogeneous (3D) dose distribution. These models can be divided into two categories: phenomenological models and more biological models.

The most widely used model of the first category uses a sigmoidal relation between dose and NTCP, for homogeneous irradiation of a partial volume of an organ at risk (LYMAN 1985; LYMAN and WOLBARST 1987, 1989). For homogeneous irradiation of partial lung volumes, EMAMI proposed an estimation of TD_5 and TD_{50} for radiation pneumonitis, which occurs during the early phase of radiation-induced lung injury, i.e., 1–8 months after irradiation (EMAMI 1991; GROSS 1977). The diagnosis of radiation pneumonitis is made as the severity of symptoms and radiographic changes cross a certain threshold. The TD_5 and TD_{50} for whole lung irradiation were estimated to be 17.5 Gy and 24.5 Gy, for irradiation of two-thirds of the lung 30 Gy and 40 Gy, and for one-third of the lung 40 Gy and 65 Gy, respectively. Subsequently, BURMAN applied the model of Lyman (1985) to these estimations, resulting in $TD_{50} = 24.5$ Gy, $m = 0.18$, and $n = 0.87$ (BURMAN et al. 1991; LYMAN 1985). For an inhomogeneous dose distribution, the dose volume histogram (DVH) first has to be reduced into a single step (HAMILTON et al. 1992; TEN HAKEN et al. 1993). This is usually done using a power-law relationship between tolerance dose and irradiated volume (KUTCHER and BURMAN 1989), with a power equal to $n = 0.87$.

Models of the second category are based on the concept of functional subunits (FSUs) (WITHERS et al. 1988). This model (NIEMIERKO and GOITEIN 1992; JACKSON et al. 1993; YORKE et al. 1993) is a full probabilistic model, which uses a local dose-effect relation to determine the probability of destruction of an FSU (for instance using the linear quadratic model of cell survival and an assumed number of cells per FSU), and calculates the NTCP as a cumulative binomial probability of destroying a certain minimum fraction of FSUs. Therefore it is assumed that in organs with parallel organized FSUs such as the lung, a complication occurs if a certain fraction of these FSUs is destroyed, and for organs with a serial organization, such as the spinal cord, if any FSU is destroyed.

Apart from knowledge of the probability of developing a complication secondary to a certain irradiation plan, one should like to know the severity of the symptoms of the normal tissue damage. Several attempts have been made to develop a reliable and reproducible scoring system (see below). One clinically relevant way to quantify the graded response of lung damage is to measure lung function. Based on the FSU model, the fraction of nonfunctioning FSUs (i.e., the integral response parameter) can be calculated by combining the dose-effect relation for FSUs with the 3D dose distribution. Since this integral response parameter thus directly represents the fraction of an organ that is considered to be nonfunctioning due to irradiation, the FSU model seems a suitable tool to estimate the reduction in pulmonary function for a certain dose distribution. The next step now is to investigate whether the predicted amount of injury using these theoretical models correlates with the observed amount of injury.

19.4.1 Prediction of the Incidence of Radiation Pneumonitis

Observed Incidence of Pneumonitis Vs Predicted by the Kutcher and Lyman Model. The group at Michigan (MARTEL et al. 1994) discussed that the TD_{50} value should be corrected to 28 Gy, to account for tissue heterogeneity. Using this value, they observed a good correlation between the calculated normal tissue complication probability (NTCP) and the observed incidence of radiation pneumonitis in lymphoma patients treated with mantle field irradiation. However, for lung cancer patients, the correlation was weak (MARTEL et al. 1994). In the 60 lung cancer patients studied by GRAHAM et al. (1994) also a weak correlation between the calculated NTCP (using a TD_{50} of 26 Gy) and the observed incidence of radiation pneumonitis was observed. The group of OETZEL et al. (1995) did find a good correlation in a patient group irradiated for lung and esophageal cancer, using the original value for TD_{50} of 24.5 Gy. Recently, MARKS et al. (1997b) reported findings similar to MARTEL et al. (1994): a reasonable correlation was observed between the observed incidence of pneumonitis and the NTCP (calculated with a TD_{50} of 29.5 Gy) in a study of 100 patients (67 patients with lung cancer, 17 with breast cancer, 12 with lymphoma, and 4 with other malignant diseases in the thorax). However, in the subgroup of the 67 lung cancer patients the correlation was weak, but when patients with a poor pulmonary function prior to radiotherapy were excluded (15 patients), the correlation improved considerably. Therefore, the same group (Marks et al. 1993, 1995, 1997b) proposed to take into account not only the 3D dose distribution, but also the pre-treatment lung function, by calculating functional dose volume histograms (*f*). These *fs* were based on pre-treatment SPECT perfusion data, and were used to take into account the local lung function in the design of the optimal treatment plan. This resulted in beam set-ups, which minimized the incidental irradiation of functioning tissue. Although this approach certainly may have theoretical advantages, it is based on the assumption that nonfunctioning areas do not *and will not* contribute to the overall lung function. However, Marks et al. (1995) have shown in a study of 50 lung cancer patients that reperfusion occurs adjacent to the tumor, which probably explains why in a recent paper of Marks et al. (1997b) the prediction of radiation pneumonitis was not improved using the *fs* compared to the conventional *s*. In The Netherlands Cancer Institute, SPECT lung perfusion scans of 23 lung cancer patients have been evaluated (data not yet published), with regard to homogeneity of lung perfusion prior to radiotherapy. In all patients, less or no perfusion was found at the tumor site relative to the average perfusion in the lung. Adjacent to the tumor, 20 patients (87%) showed a relative reduced perfusion. Twelve patients (52%) had spots or regions of hypoperfusion at areas separate from the tumor. These data are in agreement with the data reported by Marks et al. (1995), as mentioned above. To evaluate potential reperfusion due to tumor shrinkage after radiotherapy, the group at The Netherlands Cancer Institute quantitatively compared post-RT scans with pre-RT scans of 12 patients. To visualize local reperfusion in the lung, the ratio of the relative number of SPECT counts post-RT and pre-RT (normalized on the low-dose well-perfused region) was calculated. At low dose regions separate from the tumor, four patients showed strong reperfusion effects, in three patients no trace of reperfusion could be observed, while in five cases the amount of reperfusion was dubious. Considering that about 33% of these patients showed reperfusion after irradiation separate from the tumor, care should be taken to differentiate between permanent and reversible hypoperfusion, when one considers using functional *s* (based on the perfusion) for dose optimization.

In conclusion, most authors found a rather good correlation in the case of patients without intrapulmonary tumor, whereas in lung cancer patients, or patients with a poor lung function, the correlation was worse. It should be mentioned, however, that there were several differences between the studies mentioned in this section. First of all, different values for TD_{50} were used. In addition, in the study of Martel et al. the best correlation was observed when the lungs were considered to be a paired organ, whereas Oetzel et al. found the best results when the lungs were considered as independent separate organs (Martel et al. 1994; Oetzel et al. 1995). Another difference is that Martel and Oetzel scored any grade of radiation pneumonitis as a complication, whereas Graham only considered severe complications (≥ grade 3) as a complication (Martel et al. 1994; Oetzel et al. 1995).

19.4.2 Observed Incidence of Pneumonitis vs Predicted by the Functional-Subunit (FSU) Model

Boersma applied the FSU model to clinical data of 25 patients treated for malignant lymphoma (Boersma et al. 1993, 1994; Boersma 1995; Niemierko and Goitein 1992; Jackson et al. 1993; Yorke et al. 1993). Dose-effect relations were determined for local changes in perfusion and ventilation (Boersma et al. 1993, 1994). The same dose-effect relation for perfusion was found by Marks et al. (1993, 1997a). An "overall response parameter" (ORP) was calculated (Boersma 1995; Boersma et al. 1995), which represents the average reduction of local perfusion over the whole lung (analogue to the integral response parameter, if the dose-effect relation for perfusion represents the dose-effect relation for the function of FSUs). A strong correlation was observed between the ORP and the incidence of radiation pneumonitis. However, the limited number of patients and the low incidence of pneumonitis did not allow a reliable comparison with the other NTCP models (Damen et al. 1994).

19.4.3 Observed Incidence of Pneumonitis vs Predicted by Simple Parameters

Apart from fitting the data to the theoretical models, GRAHAM et al. (1995) investigated whether a straightforward parameter as the percentage of the total lung volume that received more than 20 Gy ($V_{>20Gy}$) was related to the incidence of radiation pneumonitis, in patients irradiated for lung cancer. They found a reasonable correlation ($r = 0.45$) between the $V_{>20Gy}$ and the incidence of pneumonitis (by grade). Similar findings were reported by MARKS et al. (1997b) for the lung volume receiving ≥30 Gy. Another rather straightforward parameter as the mean dose seems to be correlated with the incidence of pneumonitis as well. In the study by MARTEL, the mean lung dose in the 5 lymphoma patients with complications was 26.1 Gy, whereas the mean dose in the 16 lymphoma patients without complications was 21 Gy (MARTEL et al. 1994). For the 9 lung cancer patients with complications and the 33 patients without complications these figures were 24 Gy and 18 Gy, respectively. These differences were even larger when the lungs were considered to be independent separate organs (30 Gy vs 21.3 Gy, and 34.2 Gy vs 18.2 Gy, respectively). In the study by OETZEL these differences were somewhat smaller: the mean physical lung dose in the 37 lung cancer patients without complications was 20.1 Gy, whereas this figure was 23.8 Gy for the 9 patients with pneumonitis (OETZEL et al. 1995). Graham showed that out of the 50 lung cancer patients without complications, only 18% had a mean lung dose >26 Gy, whereas in 75% of the 10 patients with a complication the mean dose exceeded this level (GRAHAM et al. 1994).

These results have been elaborated recently in a large multicenter[1] study of 540 patients (KWA 1998). The results show that the mean lung dose, which is relatively easy to calculate, can be used to predict the risk of radiation pneumonitis, grade ≥2. However, for lung cancer patients this prediction still has an uncertainty of about 11%, which may be explained by differences in patient and treatment related factors.

19.4.4 Prediction of the Reduction in Overall Lung Function

Since the ORP represents the average reduction in local perfusion over the complete lung, Boersma (BOERSMA 1995; BOERSMA et al. 1995) and THEUWS et al. (1998) investigated whether this parameter could be used to predict the reduction in overall lung function. In addition, the predictive value of the mean lung dose with respect to the reduction in overall lung function was investigated. For 81 patients (41 lymphoma patients and 40 breast cancer patients) the correlation coefficients were calculated between these dose volume parameters (ORP and mean lung dose) and the change in overall lung function parameters, measured prior to radiotherapy and 3–4 months after therapy. All different dose volume parameters showed a similar positive correlation with the reduction of the alveolar volume, vital capacity, FEV_1 and T_{LCO}, with correlation coefficients of 0.73, 0.70, 0.69 and 0.58 respectively, when the mean lung dose was used. The relation between the mean lung dose and the reduction in overall lung function parameters could be described with one regression line through the origin and a slope of 1% reduction in overall lung function for each increase of 1 Gy in mean lung dose. For patients treated with MOPP/ABV chemotherapy prior to radiotherapy, the overall lung function was 7%–12% lower prior to the start of radiotherapy than for patients without irradiation. CMF chemotherapy given after radiotherapy caused an additional decrease in T_{LCO} of 6%, which should be added to the estimated radiation-induced reduction of T_{LCO}.

In a recent paper from the group at Duke University (MARKS et al. 1997b), it was investigated whether the reduction in FEV_1 and T_{LCO} was correlated with the lung volume irradiated to ≥30 Gy. In a study of 100 patients only a poor correlation was found between these parameters. However, when patients with a poor pulmonary function prior to therapy were excluded, the correlation improved. Considering these results, it may be useful to take the pretreatment pulmonary function into account. In the first attempts to estimate the radiation-induced

---

1 KWA SLS, LEBESQUE JV, THEUWS JCM, Department of Radiation Oncology, The Netherlands Cancer Institute, Amsterdam, The Netherlands; MARKS LB, MUNLEY MT, BENTEL G, Department of Radiation Oncology, Duke University Medical Center, NC, USA; OETZEL D, SPAHN U, Department of Clinical Radiology, University of Heidelberg, Heidelberg, Germany; GRAHAM MV, DRZYMALA RE, PURDY JA, Radiation Oncology Center, Mallinckrodt Institute of Radiology, Washington University School of Medicine, St. LOUIS, MO, USA; LICHTER AS, MARTEL MK, TEN HAKEN RK, Department of Radiation Oncology, University of Michigan, Ann Arbor, MI, USA.

reduction in lung function (FEV_1) after treatment (CHOI et al. 1990; MOLDOFSKY et al. 1988), the pre-treatment FEV_1 was multiplied by the percentage of the perfused lung volume (determined from planar perfusion scans) outside the radiation portal, thereby assuming that tissue irradiated to doses higher than 40 Gy would no longer contribute to the FEV_1. Using this method, the reduction of lung function was usually overestimated, probably due to the fact that radiation-induced pulmonary injury occurs later and less definitively than after surgery and, in addition, due to the fact that the full 3D dose distribution was not taken into account. Although the prediction of radiation pneumonitis did not improve using *fs*, a slight adaptation of this approach (MARKS et al. 1993, 1995, 1997b) may improve the prediction of the reduction in lung function. This may be reached by discriminating between reversible and irreversible hypoperfusion, with the help of CT data.

In conclusion, it should be noted that several investigators have tried to develop a reliable parameter which is predictive for the functional outcome. Until now the complicated theoretical models have not given a better estimation of the risk than more simple parameters such as the mean lung dose and the percentage lung volume irradiated to more than 20 Gy. However, so far only physical parameters such as radiation dose and irradiated volume have been taken into account. Possibly, the estimation of the functional outcome can be improved by incorporation of biological factors in the models, for example, the distribution of the local lung function prior to radiotherapy. Therefore, more clinical data are needed optimize the models, and thereby the prediction in overall outcome. A better estimation of the functional outcome may lead to a better quality of life by preventing or reducing side effects, and may eventually also lead to better local control and survival in a selected group of patients, by increasing the total dose to the tumor.

19.5 Late Effects of Radiation on Normal Tissues Scoring System: The SOMA Scale

19.5.1 Joint Statement of Mission by the EORTC/RTOG Working Groups

Over the years, various systems for recording morbidity have been developed, such as the WHO Handbook for Reporting Results of Cancer Treatment (World Health Organization, Geneva, 1979), which is widely used, but is particularly concerned with acute morbidity, devoting only one paragraph to late effects (WHO 1979); the well-designed system developed by Stanley Dische, based on a dictionary made up of elements of morbidity in all anatomical sites (DISCHE et al. 1989); and the EORTC/RTOG late effects classification (Late Radiation Morbidity Scoring Criteria, LRMSC), used in the past by both groups in several trials, and which covers nearly all systems dealing with delayed reactions (COX et al. 1995; RUBIN 1995). This last system recognized the difficulty of comparing one study with another because of the absence of common language with regard to late effects morbidity: There was no indication that this system was strictly tested for reliability and validity. In this context, the SOMA/LENT system (see description below) is the result of an international collaboration (DISCHE et al. 1989, 1997; PAVY et al. 1995a,b; RUBIN 1995; RUBIN et al. 1988, 1995a–d). The two large organizations that initiate and coordinate multicenter clinical trials in Europe and in North America, the EORTC and the RTOG, have formed specific subcommittees or working groups to update their systems for assessing the late injury to normal tissues. This was regarded as necessary to standardize and improve the recording, so that there can be uniform reporting of toxicity, at agreed and regular intervals in different clinical studies. The RTOG and EORTC have been in active collaboration to produce the new scoring system, which is a logical extension of the previous scales, focusing on the data agreed to be of most use. A concerted effort has been made to harmonize the two proposals so that there will be uniformity in reporting, not only within each organization, but also on both sides of the Atlantic.

19.5.2 The Late Effects Scoring System: The SOMA/LENT Scale

Late effects to normal tissues (LENT) and organs are currently defined as those toxicities that occur or are persistent 90 days or more from the start of therapy. Ideally, the scoring criteria can be either applied prospectively (based on patient examination) or retrospectively (based on the patient's clinical chart). The LENT scores/scales should be simple, reproducible, widely applicable, accurate and designed to provide an ascending order of severity of the complication from radiation treatment or chemotherapy. The format devised by the RTOG working group has been adopted (SOMA scales), and the degree of injury represented by the allocated grades has been extensively discussed. The common features of injury in a range of tissues, for example, bleeding, ulceration, or pain, have been made uniform across the score scales. The SOMA scales have been designed to allow the acquisition of data by several different methods, which it is hoped are not inevitably dependent one upon the other:

Two acronyms introduce the new scoring system for late effects toxicity:

LENT: Late Effects Normal Tissues
SOMA: Subjective, Objective, Management, Analytic

19.5.2.1 The SOMA Scoring System (Table 19.1)

LENT encompasses the four domains: Subjective, Objective, Management and Analytic evaluation of injury.

Subjective. The injury, if any, will be recorded from the subject's point of view, that is, as perceived by the patient. This can be either derived from interviews,

Table 19.1. Lung SOMA Scale (from LENT SOMA Tables 1995b)

	Grade 1	Grade 2	Grade 3	Grade 4
Subjective				
Cough	Occasional	Intermittent	Persistent	Refractory
Dyspnea	Breathless on intense exertion	Breathless on mild exertion	Breathless at rest, limits all activities	Prevents any physical activity
Chest pain/discomfort	Occasional and minimal	Intermittent and tolerable	Persistent and intense	Refractory and excruciating
Objective				
Pulmonary fibrosis	Radiological abnormality	Patchy dense abnormalities on radiograph	Dense confluent radiographic changes limited to radiation field	Dense fibrosis, severe scarring and major retraction of normal lung
Lung function	10%–25% reduction of respiration volume and/or diffusion capacity	25%–50% reduction of respiration volume and/or diffusion capacity	>50%–75% reduction of respiration volume and/or diffusion capacity	>75% reduction of respiration volume and/or diffusion capacity
Management				
Pain	Occasional non-narcotic	Regular non-narcotic	Regular narcotic	Surgical intervention
Cough		Non-narcotic	Narcotic, intermittent corticosteroids	Respiratory, continuous corticosteroids
Dyspnea		Occasional O_2	Continuous O_2	
Analytic				
PFT	Decrease to >75%–90% of pretx value	Decrease to >50%–75% of pretx value	Decrease to >25%–50% of pretx value	Decrease to <25% of pretx value
DLCO	Decrease to >75%–90% of pretx value	Decrease to >50%–75% of pretx value	Decrease to >25%–50% of pretx value	Decrease to <25% of pretx value
% O_2/CO_2 saturation	>70% O_2 <50% CO_2	>60% O_2 <60% CO_2	>50% O_2 <70% CO_2	<50% O_2 >70% CO_2
CT/MRI	Assessment of lung volume and zones of fibrosis			
Perfusion scan	Assessment of pulmonary blood flow and alveolar filling			
Lung lavage	Assessment of cells and cytokines			

or perhaps more effectively by involving the patient directly in the completion of carefully designed questionnaires or by filling out a diary.

Objective. The morbidity is assessed as objectively as possible by the clinician during a clinical examination. The clinician may be able to detect signs of tissue dysfunction which are still below the threshold that will give the patient symptoms, but are an indication of how close to tissue tolerance the treatment is, or they may be indicators of more serious problems that are developing and will be expressed later.

Management. This indicates the active steps that have been taken in an attempt to ameliorate the symptoms.

Analytic. This involves tools by which tissue function can be assessed even more objectively or with more biological insight than by simple clinical examination. It is recognized that the tools available for such an analysis may differ widely from one center to another, and may evolve as the clinical trials progress. The invasiveness and cost of any tool used to quantify the late effects must be reasonable and proportional to the severity of the symptoms and the possible therapeutic consequences. The scale lists the techniques that could yield valuable data, but it is not envisaged that all such tests would be feasible or even desirable in all studies.

For each of these domains a score will be given and together comprise the SOMA score (LENT SOMA 1995a,b). This will allow a comparison within each set of data of the clinical perception of injury, the patient's view of treatment efficacy, the medical measures that are available and implementable to correct the idiopathic injuries and the underlying pathobiology.

It has not yet been determined which scoring system should be used. It was originally recommended that the scores should be summed and divided by the number of elements scored. This is no longer advocated: it is possible to imagine a situation where the patient scores would be 0 or 1 for most of the elements in the SOMA scale, but there could be a grade 4 for just one of two components on injury. These high scores would be diluted out by the low scores for the other elements and would clearly give a misleading average. A mean score of 1 obtained in that way could give false optimism and could even lead to more patients being put into a continuation of a toxic regimen and suffering unacceptable late complications. It has not yet been agreed how an overall score can be derived from the elements of these scales, but it is agreed that a simple average is not advisable. It remains to be decided how these four individual scores will be summarized for each organ or tissue assessed within the LENT scale.

19.5.2.2 The Grading System

There is a general agreement that LENT toxicity should include four grades. Neither grade 0 nor 5 is included since grade 0 indicates no toxicities and grade 5 indicates fatality or loss of an organ or structure.

Grade 1 represents the most minor symptoms that require no treatment.
Grade 2 represents moderate symptoms, requiring only conservative treatment.
Grade 3 represents severe symptoms, which have a significant negative impact on daily activities, and which require more aggressive treatment.
Grade 4 represents irreversible functional damage, necessitating major therapeutic intervention.

The severity of symptoms is classified as occasional (monthly), intermittent (weekly), persistent (daily), or refractory (constant). Intensity of pain is evaluated according to the strength of the analgesic used, that is, non-narcotic versus narcotic.

Whenever possible, exact values are recorded. It is also important to obtain a "baseline score" for each patient before treatment, because organ function may already show mild to moderate deviations from normal, especially in ageing patients, even before any intervention. A good example is the pretreatment damaged lung parenchyma in emphysema patients. For any treatment site a combination of different organ-specific scales would be selected. For example, a lung cancer treatment protocol may include some or all the following scales: lung/heart and vessels/esophagus/cervical-thoracic spinal cord/mucosa-pharyngeal/skin-subcutaneous tissue/bone marrow/peripheral nerves/muscle-soft tissue/thyroid/mature bone.

The SOMA scale for lung includes the four cited categories of parameters, and will probably be improved in the future, according to the current evaluation step, as well as the different tools which are currently being evaluated and are the subject of this chapter: pulmonary functional tests are included, as well as TLCO, CT/MRI, perfusion scan, and lung lavage, but the models have not yet been proposed as effective tools.

19.5.3 Validation: The Next Step

It is essential that this system should be validated before being adopted as a substitute for the existing scales. The intention in the validation process is to see which analysis of information collected in this way gives the best discrimination of the evolution and severity of injury. Validation protocols are being undertaken in EORTC and RTOG to determine the best parameter for scoring a summary grade in addition to the maximum grade of toxicity. A statistical method needs to be agreed upon in reporting late effects as a function of time.

Case report forms will be used to compare analyses of injury using the new and old scales on a defined group of patients for each tumor localization. The validation exercise will include translation of the scales and of questionnaires into several languages. In addition, comparison with the abbreviated EORTC/RTOG scales currently in use, the late radiation morbidity scoring criteria (LRMSC), is critical to determine if these will improve the accuracy of reporting. Pilot studies are being developed to prospectively compare the results of the two systems in a uniform fashion.

19.5.4 Future Objectives

Objectives for the future are as follows:

1. Develop a uniform toxicity scoring system to assess late effects in vital organs as a result of multimodal cancer treatment, which includes radiation therapy, chemotherapy and surgery.
2. Clearly define endpoints in terms of somatic, genetic and second malignant tumors with appropriate time scales set, as an evolutionary process with and from existing toxicity scoring systems.
3. Develop protocols for longitudinal studies of key dose-limiting normal tissues and organs, and statistical methods to validate the new scoring systems.
4. Develop methods of actuarial risk reporting and recall of long-term survivors, namely survivors beyond 2 years.
5. Ensure that publications routinely present therapeutic ratios and use standard toxicity and late effects scoring along with tumor response rates and survival.

References

Abratt RP, Willcox PA (1995) The effect of irradiation on lung function and perfusion in patients with lung cancer. Int J Radiat Oncol Biol Phys 31:915–919

Abratt RP, Willcox PA, Smith JA (1990) Lung cancer in patients with borderline lung functions-zonal lung perfusion scans at presentation and lung function after high dose irradiation. Radiother Oncol 19:317–322

Anscher MS, Peters WP, Reisenbichier H et al (1993) Transforming growth factor b as a predictor of liver and lung fibrosis after autologous bone marrow transplantation for advanced breast cancer. N Engl J Med 328:1592–1598

Anscher MS, Peters WP, Reisenbichier H et al (1998) Transforming growth factor b as a predictor of liver and lung fibrosis after autologous bone marrow transplantation for advanced breast cancer. N Engl J Med 328:1592–1598

Armstrong JG, Burman C, Leibel S et al (1993) Three-dimensional conformal radiation therapy may improve the therapeutic ratio of high dose radiation therapy for lung cancer. Int J Radiat Oncol Biol Phys 26:685–689

Bate D, Guttmann RJ (1957) Changes in lung and pleura following two-million-volt therapy for carcinoma of the breast. Radiology 69:372–383

Bell J, McGivern D, Bullimore J et al (1988) Diagnostic imaging of post-irradiation changes in the chest. Clinical Radiol 39:109–119

Boersma LJ (1995) Lung function and radiotherapy: an analysis of local and overall radiation effects. Thesis, University of Amsterdam, The Netherlands

Boersma LJ, Damen, EMF, de Boer RW et al (1993) A new method to determine dose-effect relations for local lung-function changes using correlated SPECT and CT data. Radiother Oncol 29:110–116

Boersma LJ, Damen EMF, de Boer RW et al (1994) Dose-effect relations for local functional and structural changes of the lung after irradiation for malignant lymphoma. Radiother Oncol 32:201–209

Boersma LJ, Damen EMF, de Boer RW et al (1995) Estimation of overall pulmonary function after irradiation using dose-effect relations for local functional injury. Radiother Oncol 36:15–23

Boersma LJ, Damen EMF, de Boer RW et al (1996) Recovery of overall and local lung function loss 18 months after irradiation for malignant lymphoma. J Clin Oncol 14:1431–1441

Border WA, Noble NA (1994) Transforming growth factor b in tissue fibrosis. N Engl J Med 19:1286–1292

Bornstein BA, Cheng CW, Rhodes LM et al (1990) Can simulation measurements be used to predict the irradiated lung volume in the tangential fields in patients treated for breast cancer? Int J Radiat Oncol Biol Phys 18:181–187

Burman C, Kutcher GJ, Emami B, Goitein M (1991) Fitting of normal tissue tolerance data to an analytic function. Int J Radiat Oncol Biol Phys 21:123–135

Byhardt RW (1995) The evolution of Radiation Therapy Oncology Group (RTOG) protocols for nonsmall cell lung cancer. Int J Radiat Oncol Biol Phys 32:1513–1525

Canney PA, Dean S (1990) Transforming growth factor beta: a promoter of late connective tissue injury following radiotherapy? Br J Radiol 63:620–623
Choi NC, Kanarek DJ, Kazemi H (1985) Physiologic changes in pulmonary function after radiotherapy for patients with lung cancer and role of regional pulmonary function studies in predicting post-radiotherapy pulmonary function before radiotherapy. Cancer Treatment Symposia 2:119–130
Choi NC, Kanarek DJ, Grillo HC (1990) Effect of postoperative radiotherapy on changes in pulmonary function in patients with stage Il and IIIA lung carcinoma. Int J Radiat Oncol Biol Phys 18:95–99
Cionini L, Pacini P, De Paola E et al (1984) Respiratory function tests after mantle irradiation in patients with Hodgkin's disease. Acta Radiologica 23:401–409
Cosgriff SW, Kligerman MA (1951) Use of ACTH and cortisone in treatment of postirradiation pulmonary reaction. Radiology 57:536
Cosset JM, Henry-Amar M, Meerwaldt JH (1991) Long-term toxicity of early stages of Hodgkin's disease therapy: the EORTC experience. Ann Oncol 2:77–82
Cox JD, Stetz J, Pajak TF (1995) Toxicity criteria of the Radiation Therapy Oncology Group (RTOG) and the European Organization for Research and Treatment of Cancer (EORTC). Int J Radiat Oncol Biol Phys 31:1341–1346
Curran WJ, Moldofsky PJ, Solin LJ (1992) Observations on the predictive value of perfusion lung scans on post-irradiation pulmonary function among 210 patients with bronchogenic carcinoma. Int J Radiat Oncol Biol Phys 24:31–36
Damen EMF, Boersma LJ, de Boer RW, Muller SH, Lebesque JV (1994) Predicting overall lung function loss based on clinically determined dose-effect relations and the full 3-dimensional dose distribution. In: Housell AR, Wilkinson JM, Williams PC (eds) Proceedings of XIth ICCR, Manchester, 204–205
Davis SD, Yankelevitz DF, Henschke C (1992) Radiation effects on the lung: clinical features, pathology, and imaging findings. Am J Roentgenol 159:1157–1164
Denekamp J, Bartelink H, Rubin P. On behalf of the American and European LENT Working Committees (1996) Radiother Oncol 39:191
Dische S, Vaeth JM, Meyer JL (1989) Conference summary. Radiation tolerance of normal tissues. Front Radiat Ther Oncol 23:419–427
Dische S, Warburton MF, Jones D, Lartigau E (1997) The recording of morbidity related to radiotherapy. Radiother Oncol 16:103–108
Down JD (1986) The nature and relevance of late lung pathology following localized irradiation of the thorax in mice and rats. Br J Cancer 53:330–332
Emami B, Lyman J, Brown A et al (1991) Tolerance of normal tissue to therapeutic irradiation. Int J Radiat Oncol Biol Phys 21:109–122
Finkelstein JN, Johnston CJ, Saggs R (1994) Early alterations extracellular matrix and transforming growth factor b, gene expression in mouse lung indicative of late radiation fibrosis. Int J Radiat Oncol Biol Phys 28:621–631
Graham MV (1989) Predicting radiation response. Int J Radiat Oncol Biol Phys 39:561–562
Graham MV, Matthews JW, Harms WB et al (1994) Three-dimensional radiation treatment planning study for patients with carcinoma of the lung. Int J Radiat Oncol Biol Phys 29:1105–1117
Graham MV, Purdy JA, Emami B, Matthews JW, Harms B (1995) Preliminary results of a prospective trial using three-dimensional radiotherapy for lung cancer. Int J Radiat Oncol Biol Phys 33:993–1000
Groover TA, Christie AC, Merritt EA (1921) Intrathoracic changes following roentgen treatment of breast carcinoma. Am J Roentgenol 10:471–476
Gross NJ (1977) Pulmonary effect of radiation therapy. Ann Int Med 86:81–92
Groth S, Johansen H, Sorensen PB, Rossing et al (1989) The effect of thoracic irradiation for cancer of the breast on ventilation, perfusion and pulmonary permeability. A one year follow-up. Acta Oncol 28:671
Hamilton CS, Chan LY, McElwain DLS, Denham JW (1992) A practical evaluation of five dose volume histogram reduction algorithms. Radiother Oncol 24:251–260
Hazuka MB, Turrisi AT, Lutz ST et al (1993) Results of high-dose thoracic irradiation incorporating beam's eye view display in non-small-cell lung cancer: a retrospective multivariate analysis. Int J Radiat Oncol Biol Phys 27:273–284
Hermann T, Baumann M, Voigtman L, Knorr A (1997) Effect of irradiated volume on lung damage in pigs. Radiother Oncol 44:35–40
Jackson A, Kutcher GJ, Yorke ED (1993) Probability of radiation-induced complications for normal tissues with parallel architecture subject to non-uniform irradiation. Med Phys 20:613–625
Jensen BV, Carlsen NLT, Groth S (1990) Late effects on pulmonary function of mantle field irradiation, chemotherapy or combined modality therapy for Hodgkin's disease. Eur J Haematol 44:165–171
Katzenstein AA, Askin FB (1990) Acute lung injury patterns: diffuse alveolar damage: acute interstitial pneumonia. In: Surgical pathology of non-neoplastic disease, bronchiolitis obliterans organizing pneumonia, 2nd edn, WB Saunders, Philadelphia, pp 9–57
Kutcher GJ, Burman C (1989) Calculation of complication probability factors for non uniform normal tissue irradiation: the effective volume method. Int J Radiat Oncol Biol Phys 16:1623–1630
Kwa SLS, Lebesque JV, Theuws JCM et al (1998) Radiation pneumonitis as a function of mean lung dose: an analysis of pooled data of 540 patients. Int J Radiat Oncol Biol Phys (in press)
Law MP (1985) Vascular permeability and late radiation fibrosis in mouse lung. Rad Res 103:60–76
Law MP, Ahier RG (1989) Vascular and epithelial damage in the lung of the mouse after X rays or neutrons. Rad Res 117:128–144
LENT SOMA Scales for All Anatomic Sites (1995a) Int J Radiat Oncol Biol Phys 31:1049–1092
LENT SOMA Tables (1995b) Table of contents. Radiother Oncol 35:17–60
Libshitz HI, Southard ME (1974) Complications of radiation therapy: the thorax. Sem Roentgenol 9:41–49
Lichter AS, Sandler HM, Robertson JM et al (1992) Clinical experience with three-dimensional treatment planning. Sem Radiat Oncol 2:257–266
Lingos TI, Recht A, Vicini F et al (1991) Radiation pneumonitis in breast cancer patients treated with conservative surgery and radiation therapy. Int J Radiat Oncol Biol Phys 21:355–360
Lyman JT (1985) Complication probability as assessed from dose volume histograms. Rad Res 104:S13–Sl9
Lyman JT, Wolbarst AB (1987) Optimization of radiation therapy, Ill: a method of assessing complication probabilities from dose volume histograms. Int J Radiat Oncol Biol Phys 13:103–109

Lyman JT, Wolbarst AB (1989) Optimization of radiation therapy, IV: a dose-volume histogram reduction algorithm. Int J Radiat Oncol Biol Phys 13:103–109

Mah K, Van Dyk J (1988) Quantitative measurement of changes in human lung density following irradiation. Radiother Oncol 11:169–179

Mah K, Poon PY et al (1986) Assessment of acute radiation-induced pulmonary damage using computed tomography. J Comp Assist Tomogr 10:736–743

Mah K, Van Dyk J, Keane T (1987) Acute radiation-induced pulmonary damage: a clinical study on the response to fractionated radiation therapy. Int J Radiat Oncoi Biol Phys 12:179–188

Marks LB, Spencer DP, Bentel GC et al (1993) The utility of SPECT lung perfusion scans in minimizing and assessing the physiologic consequences of thoracic irradiation. Int J Radiat Oncol Biol Phys 23:659–668

Marks LB, Spencer DP, Sherouse GW et al (1995) The role of three dimensional functional lung imaging in radiation treatment planning: the functional dose-volume histogram. Int J Radiat Oncol Biol Phys 33:65–75

Marks LB, Munley MT, Spencer DP et al (1997a) Quantification of radiation-induced regional lung injury with perfusion imaging. Int J Radiat Oncol Biol Phys 38:399–409

Marks LB, Munley MT, Bentel G et al (1997b) Physical and biological predictors of changes in whole-lung function following thoracic irradiation. Int J Radiat Oncol Biol Phys 39:563–570

Martel MK, Ten Haken RK, Hazuka MB et al (1994) Dose-volume histogram and 3-D treatment planning evaluation of patients with pneumonitis. Int J Radiat Oncol Biol Phys 28:575–581

McDonald S, Rubin P, Phillips TL, Marks LB (1995) Injury to the lung from cancer therapy: clinical syndromes, measurable endpoints, and potential scoring systems. Int J Radiat Oncol Biol Phys 31:1187–1203

Moldofsky P, Rubinstein JH, Richter MP, Solin LJ, Gatenby RA, Broder GJ (1988) Quantitative lung scans for prediction of postradiotherapy pulmonary function. Clin Nucl Med 13:644–646

Morgan GW, Freedman AP, McLean RG, Jarvie BH, Giles RW (1985) Late cardiac, thyroid, and pulmonary sequelae of mantle radiotherapy for Hodgkin's disease. Int J Radiat Oncol Biol Phys 11:1925–1931

Mornex F, Méré P, Pélisson H, Ginestet C, Wiesendanger, Pérol M (1997) Tolérance à l'irradiation des patients ayant eu une pneumonectomie pour cancer bronchique: place de l'exploration fonctionnelle respiratoire. Cancer / Radiother 1:181–185

Moss WT, Haddy FJ, Sweany SK (1960) Some factors altering the severity of acute radiation pneumonitis: variation with cortisone, heparin and antibiotics. Radiology 75:50–54

Niemierko A, Goitein M (1992) Modelling of normal tissue response to radiation: the critical volume model. Int J Radiat Oncol Biol Phys 25:135–145

Oetzel D, Schraube P, Hensley F et al (1995) Estimation of pneumonitis risk in three-dimensional treatment planning using dose-volume histogram analysis. Int J Radiat Oncol Biol Phys 33:455–460

Pavy JJ, Denekamp J, Letschert J et al (1995a) EORTC late effects working group. Late effects toxicity scoring: the SOMA scale. Radiother Oncol 35:11–15

Pavy JJ, Denekamp J, Letschert J et al (1995b) EORTC late effects working group. Late effects toxicity scoring: the SOMA scale. Int J Radiat Oncol Biol Phys 31:1043–1047

Peckham MJ, Collis CH (1981) Clinical objectives and normal tissue responses in combined chemotherapy and radiotherapy. Bull Cancer 68:132–141

Perez CA, Bauer M, Edelstein S et al (1986) Impact of tumor control on survival in carcinoma of the lung treated with irradiation. Int J Radiat Oncol Biol Phys 12:539–547

Perez CA, Pajak TF, Rubin P et al (1987) Long-term observations of the patterns of failure in patients with unresectable non-oat cell carcinoma of the lung treated with definitive radiotherapy. Cancer 59:1874–1881

Phillips TL (1981) Pulmonary section-cardiorespiratory workshop. Cancer Clin Trials 4:45–52

Phillips TL, Margolis L (1972) Radiation pathology and the clinical response of lung and esophagus. Front Radiat Ther Oncol 6:254–273

Prato FS, Kurdyak R, Saibil AE et al (1977) Physiological and radiographic assessment during development of pulmonary radiation fibrosis. Radiology 122:389–397

Roswit P, White DC (1977) Severe radiation injuries of the lung. Am J Roentgenol 129:127–137

Rotstein S, Lax I, Svane G (1990) Influence of radiation therapy on the lung-tissue in breast cancer patients: CT-assessed density changes and associated symptoms. Int J Radiat Oncol Biol Phys 18:173–180

Rubenstein JH, Richter MP, Moldofsky PJ, Solin LJ (1988) Prospective prediction of post-radiation therapy lung function using quantitative lung scans and pulmonary function tests. Int J Radiat Oncol Biol Phys 15:83–87

Rubin P (1995) Editors note. Int J Radiat Oncol Biol Phys 31:1035–1036

Rubin P, Casarett G (1968) Chapter 12: clinical radiation pathology, WB Saunders, Philadelphia, pp 423–327

Rubin P, Constine LS, Van Ess J (1988) Late effects of toxicity scoring. Natl Cancer Instit Monogr 6:9–18

Rubin P, Constine S, Fajardo LF et al (1995a) Introduction: joint statement of mission by RTOG/EORTC Working Groups. Int J Radiat Oncol Biol Phys 31:1037–1039

Rubin P, Constine S, Fajardo LF, Phillips TL, Wasserman TH (1995b) RTOG late effects working group. Overview: late effects of normal tissues (LENT) scoring system. Int J Radiat Oncol Biol Phys 31:1041–1042

Rubin P, Constine S, Fajardo LF et al (1995c) Introduction: late effects consensus conference: RTOG/EORTC. Radiother Oncol 35:5–7

Rubin P, Constine S, Fajardo LF, Phillips TL, Wasserman TH (1995d) RTOG late effects working group. Overview of late effects normal tissues (LENT) scoring system. Radiother Oncol 35:9–10

Schaake-Koning C, Van den Bogaert W, Dalesio O et al (1992) Effects of concomitant cisplatin and radiotherapy in inoperable non small-cell lung cancer. A randomised phase III study of the EORTC Radiotherapy and Lung Cancer Cooperative Group. N Eng J Med 326:524–530

Schratterer-Sehn AU, Schurawitzki H, Zach M, Schratterer M (1993) High resolution computed tomography of the lungs in irradiated breast cancer patients. Radiother Oncol 27:198–202

Shapiro SJ, Shapiro SD, Mill WB, Campbell EJ (1990) Prospective study of longterm pulmonary manifestations of mantle irradiation. Int J Radiat Oncol Biol Phys 19:707–714

Stone DJ, Schwartz MJ, Green RA (1956) Fatal pulmonary insufficiency due to radiation effect upon the lung. Am J Med 21:211–225

Ten Haken RK, Martel MK, Kessler ML et al (1993) Use of Veff and iso-NTCP in the implementation of dose escalation protocols. Int J Radiat Oncol Biol Phys 27:689–695

Theuws JCM, Kwa SLS, Wagenaar AC et al (1998) Prediction of overall pulmonary function loss in relation to the 3-D dose distribution, for patients with breast cancer and malignant lymphoma. Radiother Oncol (submitted)

Travis EL (1980) Early indicators of radiation injury in the lung: are they useful predictors for late changes? Int J Radiat Oncol Biol Phys 6:1267–1269
Travis EL, Newman RA, Helbing SJ (1987) WR 2721 modification of type II cell and endothelial cell function in mouse lung after single doses of radiation. Int J Radiat Oncol Biol Phys 13:1355–1359
Tyler AF, Blackman JR (1992) Effect of heavy radiation on the pleurae and the lungs. J Radiol 3:469–475
Van Dyk J, Hill RP (1983) Post-irradiation lung density changes measured by computerized tomography. Int J Radiat Oncol Biol Phys 9:847–852
Van Dyk J, Keane TJ (1989) Determination of parameters for the linear quadratic model for radiation induced lung damage. Int J Radiat Oncol Biol Phys 17:695–698
Van Dyk J, Keane TJ, Kan S, Rider WD, Fryer CJH (1981) Radiation pneumonitis following large single dose irradiation: a reevaluation based on absolute dose to lung. Int J Radiat Oncol Biol Phys 7:461–467
Van Dyk J, Mah K, Keane TJ (1989) Radiation-induced lung damage: dose-time fractionation considerations. Radiother Oncol 14:55–69
Ward WF, Shih-Hoeilwarth A, Port CD, Kim YT (1979) Modification of radiation-induced pulmonary fibrosis in rats. Radiology 131:751–758
WHO Handbook for reporting results of cancer treatment (1979) Geneva: World Health Organization
Withers HR, Taylor JMG, Maciejewski B (1988) Treatment volume and tissue tolerance. Int J Radiat Oncol Biol Phys 14:751–759
Yorke ED, Kutcher GJ, Jackson A, Ling CC (1993) Probability of radiation-induced complications in normal tissues with parallel architecture under conditions of uniform whole or partial organ irradiation. Radiother Oncol 26:226–237
Zwijnenburg A, Klumper A, Roos CM et al (1988) Lung volume calculations from ^{81m}Kr SPECT for the quantification of regional ventilation. Clin Phys Physiol MEAS 9:147–154

20 Treatment Indications and Clinical Target Volume

P. Van Houtte, D. Ball, S. Danhier, and P. Scalliet

CONTENTS

20.1 Introduction

In the modern management of lung cancer, radiation continues to play an important role not only in terms of palliation but also as a means of prolonging survival used either alone or as part of a multimodality approach. In addition to patient and disease characteristics, some technical factors of radiotherapy delivery have been shown to be of prognostic significance. As well as TNM stage, performance status and weight loss, several radiation treatment parameters have been shown to have an impact not only on local control but also on survival: these include total dose, fractionation, duration of treatment and quality of radiation procedure. Several audit procedures performed within or outside the scope of randomised trials have clearly demonstrated the negative impact of major protocol variation on local control and survival. In the classical Radiation Therapy Oncology Group Trial 73-01, the median survival dropped from 50 weeks in patients treated according to the protocol to 23 weeks for patients in whom the target volume was not adequately covered (Perez et al. 1982). In another classical trial demonstrating the benefit of induction chemotherapy with cisplatin and vinblastine published by Dillman et al., a review of the radiation protocol showed that the tumour was not adequately incorporated in the treated volume in 22% of the patients (Dillman et al. 1990).

Furthermore, a number of national or international surveys of radiation practice have shown a wide range of treatment approaches and indications for radiotherapy as well as differences in the radiotherapy prescription. New developments in radiotherapy planning and delivery, including three-dimensional treatment planning and conformal radiotherapy, will certainly require greater precision in definition of the intended target volume and the highest standards of treatment delivery.

20.2 Patterns of Practice Study

20.2.1 Treatment Indications

Defining the clinical target volume may be directly influenced by our treatment approach depending on whether the aim is cure or palliation, and whether treatment involves radiotherapy alone or is to be combined with chemotherapy or surgery. Before the IASLC (International Association for the Study of Lung Cancer) workshop held in June 1996 in Bruges, a questionnaire was sent to the participants; all had a major interest in the management of lung cancer and were considered to be international experts: we received 58 responses. The same questionnaire was sent in November 1996 to 959 Australian physicians involved in the management of lung cancer; these were predominantly thoracic physicians (55%) with a smaller number of radiation oncologists (9%),

P. Van Houtte, S. Danhier, Service de Radiothérapie, Institut Jules Bordet, Brussels, Belgium
D. Ball, Division of Radiation Oncology, Peter MacCallum Cancer Institute, Melbourne, Australia
P. Scalliet, Service de radiothérapie oncologique, Cliniques Universitaires Saint-Luc, Brussels, Belgium

Table 20.1. Preferred management strategy for a T2N0 adenocarcinoma of the left lower lobe not a candidate for surgical resection

Treatment options	IASLC survey	Australian survey
Curative radiotherapy	75.8%	49.8%
Radiotherapy and chemotherapy	17.2%	7.0%
Palliative radiotherapy		4.9%
Wait and see	5.2%	24.7%
Supportive treatment	1.7%	7%

Table 20.2. Preferred management strategy for a T2N2MO of the left main bronchus with positive subcarinal lymph node and left lower lobe atelectasia

Treatment options	IASLC survey	Australian survey
Induction chemotherapy, surgery and radiotherapy	10.3%	18.8%
Surgery	6.9%	17.8%
Induction chemotherapy and surgery	36.2%	17.1%
Preoperative radiotherapy and chemotherapy	17.2%	3.5%
Curative radiotherapy	10.3%	13.2%
Induction chemotherapy and radiotherapy	6.9%	4.5%
Concurrent radiotherapy and chemotherapy	10.3%	9.4%
Palliative radiotherapy	1.7%	13.2%
Supportive treatment	1.7%	1%
Chemotherapy plays a role in	80.9%	53.3%
Radiotherapy plays a role in	56.7%	62.6%

medical oncologists (1%) and surgeons (5%). The remainder were trainee physicians. Here are the results:

The first case was that of a 77-year-old man with a 4-cm tumour mass located in the left lower lobe. The complete work-up was negative including chest CT except for the primary tumour and mediastinoscopy. The pathological report revealed an adenocarcinoma. The patient might have tolerated a lobectomy. In both surveys, there was a clear consensus in favour of surgery: less than 5% of the physicians recommended a course of curative radiotherapy or a wait-and-see policy. In contrast, if the patient was not a candidate for surgery for medical reasons, a majority favoured a course of curative radiotherapy either alone or with chemotherapy (Table 20.1). Interestingly, only four respondents (6%) in the IASLC survey chose a non-curative approach compared to a rate of 36% for the Australian respondents.

The second case was that of a 55-year-old man who had a squamous cell carcinoma of the left main bronchus located at 2 cm from the carina with a complete left lower lobe collapse. There were positive subcarinal lymph nodes. The patient had a Karnofsky index of 80% and might have tolerated a pneumonectomy. In both surveys, there was a wide variety of treatment approaches but respondents favoured a multimodality approach including chemotherapy (81% for the IASLC and 53% for the Australian survey) and surgery (81% and 57%, respectively) (Table 20.2). A single treatment modality such as surgery or radiotherapy was only recommended by 17% and 31%, respectively, but chemotherapy alone was not recommended. The Australian physicians tended to recommend a palliative approach more often (13%).

The last example was a 55-year-old man with a squamous cell carcinoma of the right upper lobe with four pathologically positive ipsilateral-paratracheal nodes established at mediastinoscopy. The clinical staging was T2N2M0 and the patient's lung function was sufficient for a pneumonectomy. Again, surgery was favoured by most physicians either alone or in combination with chemotherapy and radiotherapy, but opinion as to a preferred approach was still not clearly defined (Table 20.3).

Both surveys showed: a strong preference for surgery whenever possible, despite a low number of surgeons among the respondents; a wide variety of treatment approaches for stage III disease, but mostly favouring a multidisciplinary approach; and, finally, the greatest consensus was seen in recommendations for the treatment of early stage disease.

Table 20.3. Preferred management strategy for a T2N2MO of the right upper lobe with four positive lymph nodes

Treatment options	IASLC survey	Australian survey
Induction chemotherapy surgery and radiotherapy	8.6%	20.9%
Surgery	5.2%	16.7%
Induction chemotherapy and surgery	34.4%	7.3%
Preoperative radiotherapy and chemotherapy	20.6%	3.8%
Curative radiotherapy	8.6%	14.6%
Induction chemotherapy and radiotherapy	12.0%	16.0%
Concurrent radiotherapy and chemotherapy	10.3%	0.3%
Palliative radiotherapy	1.7%	5.6%
Supportive treatment	1.7%	2.4%
Chemotherapy plays a role in	85.9%	48.3%
Radiotherapy plays a role in	61.8%	61.2%

Furthermore, there was a general trend for the experts of the IASLC to recommend a more aggressive approach, reflecting, possibly, the larger proportion of oncologists compared with the Australian physicians who tended to favour a more palliative or observation only policy, reflecting the larger proportion of chest physicians. Even so, a palliative approach was only chosen by a minority of the respondents in both surveys. Chemotherapy alone was not considered to be a treatment option for localised lung cancer and some form of locoregional treatment was usually part of the strategy. Still, chemotherapy is more often advocated than radiotherapy in these complex but not infrequent situations by IASLC experts and much less by the Australian physicians.

20.2.2 Surveys of Radiation Practice

In a survey of radiation practice in Australia and New Zealand, 14 radiation oncologists were asked to draw the gross tumour and clinical target volumes on 12 sample cases of non-small cell lung cancer using orthogonal radiographic views from a simulator and selected computed tomography slices (Denham et al. 1993). There were large variations in definition of the volumes, including failure to define macroscopic tumour extensions (34.5%), mistaken definition of normal structure as tumour (25.5%) and incorporation of microscopic extension in the gross tumour volume (47%). There was frequent misinterpretation by the clinician of normal structures such as the superior vena cava or the pulmonary artery; however, the oncologists had not been supplied with a full set of CT images and the amount of vascular contrast used was variable. Once the physicians had chosen their gross tumour volume, there was still surprising variation in the margins added for the target volume, both in radically and palliatively treated patients. The average margin size was 1.27 cm with a range of 0.35–4.25 cm. It was also noted that when the clinical target volume was defined on the basis of CT images, it was smaller than when the same volume was based on the simulator films.

In the study by Valley and Mirimanoff (1993), the ten participating centers in Switzerland were asked to apply their standard technique to a case of inoperable non-small cell lung cancer (T3N2M0). The authors observed wide variations in prescription method (seven centers used a point prescription and three used isodose prescription), in fractionation, in technique and also in tumour and target volume definitions: in the central plane, the tumour surface area ranged from 7 cm^2 to 65 cm^2 and for the target volume from 22 cm^2 to 110 cm^2.

During the workshop held in Bruges, a number of radiation oncologists were asked to draw, on a CT-based treatment planning system, their clinical target volume (CTV) according to the ICRU definition using two different cases of stage III non-small cell lung cancer. In each case, CT images taken in the treatment position were provided in addition to a summary of the patient record. The first patient was a 54-year-old female with a 5-cm squamous cell carcinoma in the right upper lobe with positive hilar and right paratracheal nodes. The second case was a 65-year-old male presenting with weight loss and dyspnea. The workup revealed an adenocarcinoma with positive hilar and subcarinal lymph nodes. Both patients had good performance status and normal lung functions. There was a wide range of CTVs cho-

the boost field 242 cm^3. The margins added to the CTV and the GTV ranged from 7 and 10 mm.

Defining the precise limits of a lung tumour may be a very complex task; this is especially so in the presence of additional inflammatory disease, collapse or consolidation of adjacent lung or pleural effusion. One method of overcoming this problem is to include the whole area of solid lung within the CTV but, according to the IASLC survey, this was only done by 45% of radiation oncologists (Van Houtte et al. 1994). This approach necessarily leads to the treatment of a very large area as illustrated in Fig. 20.3. Alternatively it may be possible to reduce the target volume by administering endobronchial treatment either with laser or endoluminal brachytherapy before or during the course of external radiation and repeated simulation during the treatment so the field can be reduced if lung re-expansion has occurred (Cotter et al. 1993). PET scan images may also be helpful in the future but will require a precise co-registration with the CT image to define the gross tumour volume, as demonstrated in Fig. 20.4.

Treatment of tumours of the superior sulcus requires prophylactic irradiation of the spinal cord since the tumour may spread through the intervertebral foramen directly into the spinal canal. In a previous report, when the treatment field just en-

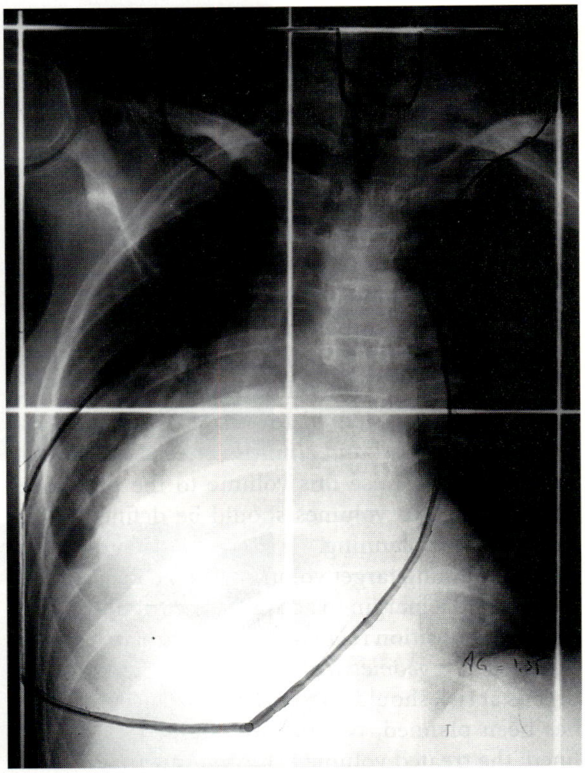

Fig. 20.3. Patient with a partial right lower lobe atelectasia. *Black line* represents the limits of the individualized blocks. Note the mediastinal displacement

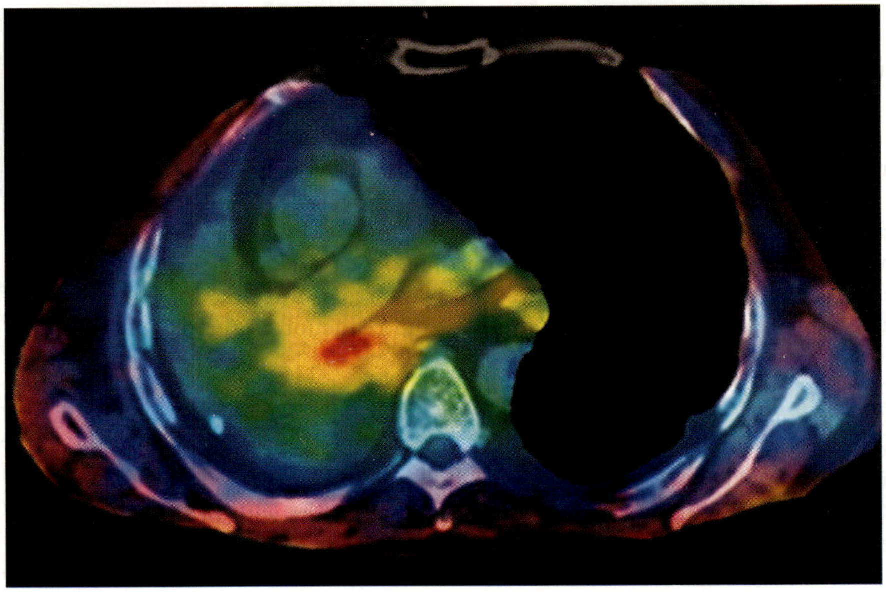

Fig. 20.4. Manually co-registered CT scan and PET image in a patient with complete right lung collapse showing centrally located tumour *in red*. (Image courtesy of Peter MacCallum, Cancer Institute PET Centre)

compassed the lung tumour and was limited by the vertebral body medially, it was not uncommon for tumour progression to result in spinal cord compression.

20.5 Normal Tissue Tolerance

The dose limiting factor in clinical radiotherapy is the risk of severe normal tissue injury. If with increasing radiation doses more and more neoplastic cells are killed to ultimately achieve the complete destruction of all clonogenic cells, the same principle also applies to normal tissues. The normal tissues can be classified according to their proliferative activities, i.e., rapid or slow. The former group is characterized by an active proliferation as well as by maintenance of a steady-state number: they are directly involved in the acute side effects and they include the bone marrow, the intestinal epithelium, the skin and the mucosa. Slowly proliferating tissues include the liver, the lung, the kidney, the central nervous system and the connective tissues. Acute effects are related to the balance between loss of stem cells and the regeneration potential of the tissue and occur within days to weeks of treatment delivery. On the other hand, in a slow renewal system or nonrenewal system, late damage may occur months or years after the treatment and may be irreversible.

Another factor influencing radiation injury and recovery relates to organisation and function of the tissue or an organ i.e., whether functional subunits are arranged in series or in parallel. For example, in the thorax localised lung damage (fibrosis) may be functionally compensated by the remaining normal lung through hypertrophy of adjacent alveoli (functional subunits in parallel) but in the esophagus severe late damage in the form of a stricture cannot be compensated and the function of the whole system is impaired (functional subunits in series).

The concept of tolerance dose has been introduced as an aid for the radiation oncologist but it should never replace clinical judgement, by which the balance between benefit and risk is weighed. RUBIN and CASARETT (1972) have proposed the concept of TD5/5 or TD50/5: they are the doses which will result in no more than 5% or 50% severe complications respectively within a period of 5 years. Table 20.4 presents the tolerance doses for several thoracic organs according to risk and volume treated but the figures are only valid for conventional treatments (2 Gy/fraction, 5 fractions a week) (EMAMI et al. 1991). The recent progress in computerised treatment planning and the use of dose volume histograms should further refine the importance of volume in determining tolerance.

20.6 Nodal Irradiation

The rationale for elective nodal irradiation is that it may, by eradicating subclinical disease, improve either symptom-free or overall survival but, because of competing risks, any benefit of improved nodal control can only occur with a high rate of control at the primary site and provided treatment of the mediastinum does not result in excessive toxicity. In the RTOG's landmark study 73-01, the guidelines for irradiation portals of non-small cell lung cancer included all areas of lung involvement as well as the ipsilateral hilar and mediastinal lymph nodes, with at least 2-cm margins, and as well as the contralateral mediastinum and hilum with a 1-cm margin (PEREZ et al. 1982, 1987). The supraclavicular lymph nodes were included in the irradiated volume only with primary tumours located in the upper lobes or when

Table 20.4. Normal tissue tolerance to thoracic irradiation. Doses are in grays (for 2 Gy/fraction) (adapted from EMAMI et al. 1991)

Organ	TD 5/5 volume			TD 50/5 volume			Endpoint
	1/3	2/3	3/3	1/3	2/3	3/3	
Rib cage	50			65			Pathologic fracture
Spinal cord	5 cm	10 cm	20 cm	5 cm	10 cm	20 cm	Myelitis necrosis
	50	50	47	70	70	–	
Brachial plexus	62	61	60	77	76	75	Nerve damage
Lung	45	30	17.5	65	40	24.5	Pneumonitis
Heart	60	45	40	70	55	50	Pericarditis
Oesophagus	60	58	55	72	70	68	Stricture/perforation

there was evidence of superior mediastinum or supraclavicular lymph node involvement. In a review of protocol compliance, the survival of patients with normal contralateral hilar lymph nodes was improved when the hilar nodal regions were treated with full compliance or minor variations from the protocol: median survival dropped from 49.9 months after irradiation of both hila to 22.6 months after inadequate coverage of the contralateral hilum (Perez et al. 1982). Furthermore, none of the 17 patients with major protocol violations survived more than 1 year.

In a survey of radiation practice carried out in 1993, one of the most striking observations was the difference in opinion regarding the coverage of the contralateral hilum and the supraclavicular fossae (Van Houtte et al. 1994). In the five examples used, the contralateral hilum was included in the irradiation portal by fewer than 40% of the radiation oncologists even when the nodes of the ipsilateral hilum or mediastinum were positive. One example was a T3N2 tumour of the right upper lobe with extension in the right main bronchus and two ipsilateral paratracheal lymph nodes. The contralateral hilum was included in the initial radiation volume by 38.8% of the 111 radiation oncologists surveyed. In a second example of a 4-cm tumour located in the left lower lobe with positive ipsilateral lymph nodes (T2N1), only 28.8% of oncologists included the contralateral hilum. Prophylactic irradiation of the supraclavicular fossae was only advocated in the presence of upper mediastinal lymph node involvement.

The main limiting factor of thoracic irradiation, especially when escalating the total dose, is often the volume of normal lung irradiated and not the spinal cord. Any extension of the margins will be at the expense of normal tissue and increases the risk of radiation pneumonitis or fibrosis (Emami 1994). Dose volume histogram (DVH) analysis has indicated a relationship between volume of lung receiving doses in excess of 25 Gy and subsequent risk of radiation pneumonitis: Graham et al. (1997) reported no case of grade 3 pneumonitis when less than 25% of the lung received more than 20 Gy, but if the volume of lung receiving more than 20 Gy was greater than 37% then the incidence of pneumonitis was 19%. By avoiding elective nodal irradiation, the amount of normal lung spared allows a dose escalation of about 30% without an increase in the probability of radiation pneumonitis (Belderbos et al. 1997). Modern nuclear medicine techniques may prove useful due to their ability to detect non-functioning lung, the irradiation of which is unlikely to have a significant future effect on a patient's vital capacity (Robertson et al. 1997). Matching PET or SPECT imaging with CT is probably one road to be explored in the near future.

Acute oesophagitis has more recently proven to be a dose-limiting factor, especially when accelerating the radiation procedure or when combining drugs concurrently with radiation. Grade 3 oesophageal toxicity implies severe dysphagia with a weight loss of more than 15% requiring artificial alimentation. In the trial conducted in Australia by Ball et al., patients were randomised to receive 60 Gy in 30 fractions over 6 weeks or the same dose in the same number of fractions over 3 weeks with or without concomitant carboplatin (Ball et al. 1995). In an interim analysis of the first 100 randomised patients, the estimated median duration of oesophagitis was 1.4 months for the conventional treatment and 3.2 months for the accelerated treatment. The rates of grade 3 and 4 oesophagitis were significantly higher in patients having accelerated treatment (respectively 9% and 0% for the conventional treatment and 31% and 4% for the accelerated schedule); furthermore, six patients required dilatation for an oesophageal stricture and one patient died as a result of a laryngoesophageal fistula without evidence of tumour at autopsy. The most extreme example of an accelerated program is CHART (continuous, hyperfractionated, accelerated, radiation therapy), a radiation schedule introduced by the Mount Vernon team. The main concept was first not to leave any gap during the treatment by treating every day including the weekend and to complete the treatment before the onset of repopulation or acute effects such as acute oesophagitis: the schedule consisted of three fractions of 1.5 Gy/day separated by 6-h intervals for 12 consecutive days. Initially 37.5 Gy was delivered to a large volume including the whole mediastinum and the remaining dose was given to the gross tumour volume. It was hypothesised that the reduction of total radiation dose (54 Gy for the CHART vs 60 Gy for conventional therapy) was more than compensated for by a reduction in tumour repopulation. In patients treated with the CHART, the incidence of severe dysphagia was 49% compared to 19% in patients treated with conventional fractionation (Saunders et al. 1996). Seven percent of the CHART patients developed oesophageal stricture compared with 4% of the conventionally treated patients. Grade 3 oesophagitis may require the interruption of the radiation treatment even if this does not necessarily always translate into permanent late damage such a stenosis requiring repeated dilatation procedures. In addition to accelerated fractionation, the length of the oesophagus irradiated may also be a risk factor for oesophagitis: this was the case with the concomitant boost technique as proposed by the Amsterdam team (SCHUSTER-UITTERHOEVE et al. 1993).

So, given that mediastinal irradiation increases the risk of lung and oesophageal toxicity, can we reduce these risks by omitting elective nodal irradiation without increasing the probability of the geographic miss. Table 20.5 summarises the results of different studies using conformal radiotherapy for non-small cell lung cancers and limiting the treated volume to the GTV (HAZUKA et al. 1993; GRAHAM et al. 1997; MARTEL et al. 1997; ARMSTRONG et al. 1997; SIBLEY et al. 1995). Although there is little available information on the precise pattern of failure, the main problem continues to be failure to control disease at the primary site. In the experience of SIBLEY et al. (1995), local progression was always within the GTV and no isolated regional failure outside the treated area was observed in his 37 patients with stage III NSCL cancers. The study of HAZUKA et al. (1993) examined the effect of volume on survival and progression free survival after patients had been planned according to the modern beam's eye view technique. Some patients had only the primary site, ipsilateral hilum and mediastinal nodes irradiated whereas others had additional supraclavicular and contralateral hilar nodes irradiated according to the classical RTOG recommendations. This was a retrospective study and the choice of treatment volume was left to the physician's preference. Eighty-eight consecutive patients were treated with doses of 60 Gy or more. No differences in progression-free survival or overall survival were observed between the small volume and extended volume groups. These observations were independent of tumour stage. Furthermore, all local failures occurred within the high dose region except in three patients: two failed in the supraclavicular nodes and concomitantly with primary site failure; both had irradiation of the supraclavicular regions with doses of 36 and 45 Gy. Only one patient failed at a single regional node site which had received 54 Gy.

Last but not least, in a more recent analysis 1705 patients, derived from 4 different RTOG protocols, were studied to assess the impact of regional nodal irradiation on survival. Three groups of patients experienced significant differences in outcome when the radiation was not performed according to protocol. These included patients in whom the margins on the ipsilateral hilum were inadequate or those in whom the doses to the ipsilateral hilar nodes or to the mediastinal lymph nodes were below those specified. This study did not reveal a beneficial effect of irradiation of the contralateral hilum (EMAMI et al. 1996). It should be remembered, however, that these RTOG studies were conducted over a long period of time in which there had been major developments in imaging techniques and accuracy.

The last issue is whether or not to treat clinically normal supraclavicular nodes. Even if relapse rates in the supraclavicular region are low in an unirradiated patient, the addition of a supraclavicular field or fields is considered to add little toxicity. In the RTOG 73-01 study, the failure rate in the supraclavicular area was 8% in the absence of irradiation, 14% for doses between 8 and 35 Gy, 5% for 35–45 Gy and 2% for doses in excess of 45 Gy (PEREZ et al. 1987). In another series of 76 patients with locally advanced non-small cell lung cancer staged by CT and treated with radical radiotherapy, without a neck field, none relapsed in the supraclavicular fossa (PIGGOT and SAUNDERS 1993). In a pattern of failure study of 159 patients treated at the Peter MacCallum Cancer Institute, within a randomised trial, only 3% relapsed in the neck as their first and only site of failure. One way of resolving this issue is

Table 20.5. Conformal radiotherapy for NSC lung cancer

Authors	No. patients	Stage I/II(%)	Doses (Gy)	Local failure rate (%)	Two-year survival rate (%)
Hazuka	88	22	60–74	29	37
Graham	99	23	60–74	Stage I–II 33% III 11%	45
Martel	76	21	64–82	29	Stage I/II 56 IIIa 26 IIIb 9
Armstrong	45	13	52–72	46	32
Sibley	37	0	60–70	49	Stage IIIa 49 IIIb 26

to better define patients at high risk of failure in the supraclavicular fossa, e.g. patients with high mediastinal involvement and patients whose disease is located in the upper part of the upper lobe such as superior sulcus tumour (in whom the lower neck is usually incorporated in the clinical targeted volume anyway). Another clinical situation may be a positive mediastinoscopy: in the practice of some, the mediastinoscopy scar is always included in the initial field.

Another approach may be to plan our clinical target volume (CTV) according to the probability of lymph node involvement. The position of the lymph nodes within the mediastinum is described according to the American Thoracic Society (ATS map), which defines nodal station in relation to fixed anatomical structures allowing a correlation between imaging procedures, CT, MRI and surgical findings. In essence, lymph from the right upper lobe drains to the right tracheobronchial lymph nodes and lymph from the right middle and lower lobes drains to the lobar, interlobar and finally to the hilar nodes and subcarinal, ipsilateral and mediastinal nodes. On the left hand side, lymph from the upper lobe drains not only to the angle of the confluence of the subclavian and internal jugular veins on the same site but also crosses over to the right lower and upper mediastinum. Lymph drainage from both lower lobes can also go to the pulmonary ligament and paraoesophageal nodes (Nohl-Oser 1981). In the case of chest wall involvement there is a risk of spread along the intercostal spaces or to the axillary region. At present, the only sign of nodal involvement on CT is nodal enlargement. This criterion for involvement has major limitations: the normal lymph node size varies within the mediastinum and enlargement may be due to another cause of metastasis, e.g. distal infection and incidental granulomatous lung disease. In the study by MacLoud, the rate of positive mediastinal lymph node involvement rose from 13% when the node measured less than 1 cm to 62% for nodes of 2–2.9 cm (MacLoud et al. 1992). In the presence of obstructive pneumonitis, the rate of false positive lymph node increased to 45%. One way to improve the accuracy of CT is to take into account natural lymphatic drainage: if nodes in the draining territory of the tumour are enlarged (more than 10 mm in short axis) and are at least 5 mm larger than nodes in non-draining territories, the CT specificity improves with a positive predictive value of 95% (Buy 1988). Indeed, taking into account the natural pattern of drainage may be helpful in drawing the CTV. Minet et al. (1993) have proposed a table of probability of lymph node invasion according to the primary tumour location (Table 20.6). The data are mainly based on surgical series and may represent an underestimate of the probability of involvement for more advanced primary tumours. These data have been used by Derycke et al. (1997), who calculated the GTV and the GTV plus the regional lymph nodes with a probability greater than 10% of involvement according to the tumour loca-

Table 20.6. Average probability (%) of lymph node involvement according to tumour location (adapted from Minet et al. 1993)

	Station	Tumour location				
		RUL	RML	RLL	LUL	LLL
Supraclavicular: left	1	4	2	2	21	6
Right	1	25	9	7	4	4
Upper paratracheal: left	2	2	5	3	17	11
Right	2	30	19	18	6	9
Lower paratracheal: left	4	2	5	3	19	12
Right	4	25	14	17	5	8
Aortopulmonary	5	0	0	0	10	7
Anterior	6	0	0	0	5	5
Subcarinal	7	14	15	33	19	41
Paraesophageal: left	8	0	0	0	1	3
Right	8	1	1	2	0	0
Pulmonary ligament: left	9	0	0	0	1	1
Right	9	1	1	2	0	0
Peribronchial: left	10	0	0	0	12	7
Tracheobronchial: right	10	13	11	9	1	1
Intrapulmonary: left	11	0	0	0	5	6
Right	11	41	46	55	0	0

tion in a series of ten patients with stage III non-small cell lung cancer: five stage IIIa and five stage IIIb (excluding N3 disease) (DERYCKE et al. 1997). The volume of GTV alone varied from 66 to 244 ml with an average of 147 ml compared with the GTV plus the possible lymph node extension, which ranged from 192 to 542 ml with an average of 319 ml.

KIRICUTA et al. (1994) carried out a retrospective study on the pretherapy CT scans of 512 patients who were candidates for radiation. On the basis of pure CT criteria (lymph node larger than 10 mm along the short axis or 15 mm along the long axis), 266 were considered to be node positive. They correlated their observations with the tumour location using a modified mapping scheme of the ATS. The incidence of positive nodes in the supraclavicular area or in the contralateral hilum was less than 10% (Table 20.7). In their experience using a volume of irradiation modified according to the nodal extent based on the CT observations, none of the patients with positive supraclavicular or contralateral hilar nodes survived over 2 years.

In our general practice with stage III disease nodal irradiation is limited to the mediastinum. When the primary lies in the apex of the upper lobe close to the clavicle, the ipsilateral supraclavicular fossa is usually included in the clinical target volume by default. In patients who have had a positive mediastinoscopy, it is not unreasonable to include the surgical scar, in which case the medial parts of the supraclavicula fossa will also be irradiated. We do not attempt to irradiate the clinically normal contralateral hilum, but the aortopulmonary window and the subcarinal regions are always included in the clinical target volume. The lower mediastinum containing the paraoesophageal nodes is rarely included even for lower lobe lung tumours because of the risk of excessive toxicity.

Table 20.7. Incidence of positive lymph node for NSCL cancer based on CT information (adapted from KIRICUTA et al. 1994)

	Tumour location	
	Right	Left
Number of cases	161	105
Supraclavicular: right	8.6	9.5
Left	1.8	3.8
Upper mediastinal	0.6	0
Paratracheal: right	19.9	5.7
Left	2.5	6.7
Lower tracheobronchial: right	77	43.8
Left	30.4	76.2
Hilar: right	34.2	4.8
Left	3.7	41.9
Anterior tracheal	27.3	25.7
Subcarinal	50.9	44.8

20.7 Elective Nodal Irradiation for Early Stage NSCLC

Although surgery remains the standard treatment for stage I lung cancer, some patients refuse surgery or are considered inoperable because of co-morbidities, but they can be treated with radiotherapy with curative intent. The issue in these patients is whether the clinical target volume should be limited to the primary tumour in the absence of CT evidence of nodal involvement or whether the hilar and mediastinal nodes should be treated prophylactycally. In our survey carried out in 1993, we asked specifically for a definition of the area to be irradiated in the case of a 4-cm tumour mass located in the left lower lobe without nodal invasion (T2N0) (VAN HOUTTE et al. 1994). Of the 111 respondents, 98% included the ipsilateral hilum in the initial clinical target volume, 88% included the subcarinal lymph nodes, 70.2% the lower mediastinal lymph node and 70.2% and 69.4% the right and left paratracheal lymph nodes respectively. The contralateral hilum and the supraclavicular fossae were only irradiated by one radiation oncologist in five. This survey suggested that conventional practice favoured elective nodal irradiation.

However, the data available from the literature do not allow us to draw any definitive conclusions. In fact, the 3- and 5-year survival rates are not dissimilar regardless of whether the regional nodes were electively irradiated or not (Table 20.8). In two series in which patterns of failure analysis were performed after the irradiation was restricted to the primary tumour, the incidence of relapse in the regional nodes as the first and only site of failure was low: in the series of SLOTMAN et al. (1996) including 31 patients, three locoregional recurrences were observed; in the study of KROL et al. (1996), of 50 patients achieving a complete remission at the primary site, 4 developed locoregional failure including two nodal relapses (SLOTMAN et al. 1996; KROL et al. 1996). In contrast, MORITA et al. (1997) reported better results after elective hilar/mediastinal irradiation: 5-year survival rate reached 31.3% with elective irradiation vs 14.9% after a limited irradiation (MORITA et al. 1997). However, patients in whom the nodes were not treated were more likely to have adenocar-

Table 20.8. Definitive radiation for early NSC lung cancer

Authors	No. of pts.	Radiation scheme		Elective nodal irradiation	Survival rate (%)	
		(Gy)	(weeks)		3 years	5 years
Coy and Kennelly (1980)	141	50–57	4	Yes	18	10
Dosoretz et al. (1992)	152	50–70	5–7	Yes		10
Gauden et al. (1995)	347	50	4	Yes		27
Graham et al. (1995)	150	60	6	Yes		14
Krol et al. (1996)	108	60/65	6–7 S	No	31	15
Noordijk et al. (1988)	50	60	6–7 S	No		16
Sandler et al. (1990)	77	60	6	Yes	21	17
Talton et al. (1990)	77	60	6	Yes	21	17
Zhang et al. (1989)	44	55–70	6–7	Yes		16
Slotman et al. (1996)	31	48	2.5	No	42	8
Morita et al. (1997)	66	55–74	6–7	Yes		31
	83			No		15
Burt et al. (1989)	133	50–55	3	No		20

cinoma and tumours located in the lower lobe (here the treatment was often limited to the primary to avoid an excessively large field).

Additional information is obtainable on patterns of failure data after surgical resection. Loco-regional relapse has been reported in 6%–14% for T1 and T2N0 tumours (Table 20.9) (Pairolero et al. 1984; Feld et al. 1984; Laffitte et al. 1996; Immerman et al. 1981). In surgically treated patients loco-regional relapse includes all recurrences within the same lobe, ipsilateral hilum and mediastinum. In our randomised trial on the role of postoperative radiotherapy, pattern of failure analysis was carried out taking into account the theoretical radiation field: after complete resection for a T1, T2 or T3N0 tumour of the main bronchi, the rate of "in-field" loco-regional relapse was 13.4%. Furthermore, the Lung Cancer Study Group conducted a randomised trial in T1N0 tumours to compare lobectomy to more limited resection (segmentectomy or wedge resection): 247 patients were included. The study demonstrated a clear benefit in terms of locoregional recurrence and survival in favour of patients randomised to lobectomy. The locoregional recurrence rate dropped from 17% after a limited resection to 5% after lobectomy (Ginsberg and Rubinstein 1995).

Current available radiotherapy techniques allow us to achieve local cure in only a limited number of patients, and relapse at the primary site remains the major cause of failure. Increasing the total radiation dose is a promising strategy but will require a reduction in the amount in the volume of normal lung irradiated, especially in patients whose lung function is already compromised. Individualisation of treatment is probably the only way to determine if elective nodal irradiation is possible without reducing the dose to the primary and without increasing the volume of lung tissue irradiated above patient tolerance. This is well illustrated by the following two cases. Both patients had non-small cell lung cancer with poor lung function. As a result of tumour location, it was possible in one case to treat the first nodal station because the tumour was close to the mediastinum, whereas in the second case the peripheral location of the tumour necessitated limiting the irradiated volume of the primary tumour alone (Figs. 20.5, 20.6). In both cases, PET scanning did not reveal any uptake in the mediastinum. Both patients are alive at 3 years without any evidence of disease.

Table 20.9. Pattern of failure after curative surgery

Authors	Stage	No. of patients	Pattern of failure (%)	
			Local	Distant
Pairolero	T1NO	170	6	15
	T2NO	158	6	23
Feld	T1NO	162	9	17
	T2NO	196	11	30
Laffite	T2NO	70	14	26
Immermam	T1-2, NO	77	12	27

20.8 Conclusions

Radiation remains an important component in the treatment of localised non-small cell lung cancer. Nevertheless, current radiation programs are only

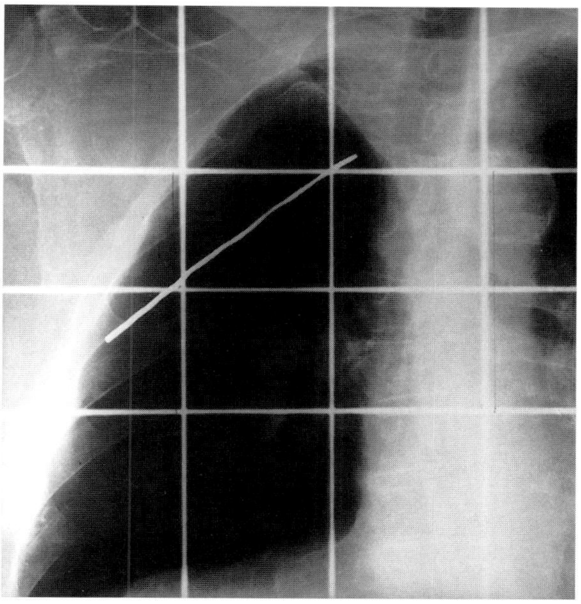

Fig. 20.5. Patient with a squamous cell carcinoma of the right lung not candidate for surgery due to poor lung function. The first nodal station was irradiated due to its proximity with the tumour. The PET scan did not show any uptake in the mediastinum

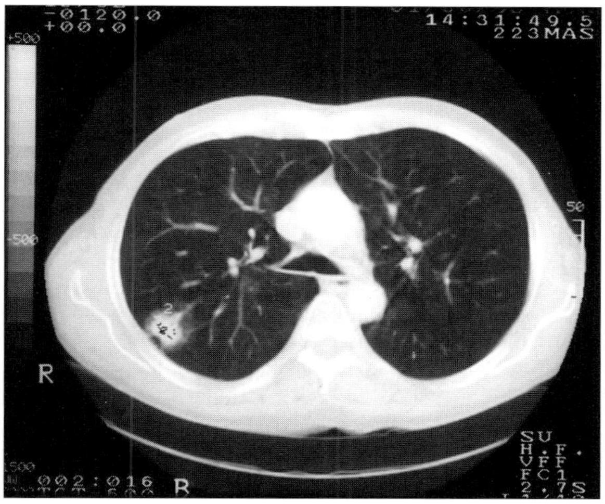

Fig. 20.6. Patient with a peripheral lung tumour and poor lung function. Only the tumour was irradiated with three tangential fields to spare as much as possible of the normal lung

able to control a limited number of tumours, and we have to improve our treatment strategies. Several avenues of investigation are currently being explored including modification of the fractionation, increasing the total dose with endoluminal brachytherapy, three-dimensional conformal radiotherapy and multimodality treatment. There is still some controversy regarding the precise definition of clinical target volume. Additional studies are necessary to define a common language and to specify the volume to be treated both in relation to the primary tumour and elective nodal stations. Furthermore, the quality of the radiation procedure remains a major determinant for success even in a multimodality approach.

Acknowledgements. The authors would like to acknowledge the assistance of Eli Lilly (Australia) in making possible the survey of Australian patterns of practice.

References

Armstrong J, Raben A, Zelefsky M, Burt M, Leibel S, Burman C, Kutcher G, Harrison L, Hahn C, Ginsberg R, Rusch V, Kris M, Fuks Z (1997) Promising survival with three-dimensional conformal radiation therapy for non-small cell lung cancer. Radiother Oncol 44:17–22

Ball D, Bishop J, Smith J, Crennan E, O'Brien P, Davis S, Ryan G, Joseph D, Walker Q (1995) A phase III study of accelerated radiotherapy with and without carboplatin in nonsmall cell lung cancer: an interim toxicity analysis of the first 100 patients. Int J Radiat Oncol Biol Phys 31:267–272

Belderbos JSA, Lebesque JV, Barillot I (1997) Normal tissue complication probabilities for irradiation of NSCLC patients with and without elective nodal irradiation. Lung Cancer 18:126

Burt PA, Hancock BM, Stout R (1989) Radical radiotherapy for carcinoma of the bronchus: an equal alternative to radical surgery? Clin Oncol 1:86–90

Buy JN, Ghossain MA, Poirson F (1988) Computed tomography of mediastinal lymph nodes in non-small cell lung cancer: a new approach based on the lymphatic pathway of tumor spread. J Comput Assist Tomogr 12:545–552

Cotter GW, Lariscy C, Ellingwood KL, Herbert D (1993) Inoperable endobronchial obstructing lung cancer treated with combined endobronchial and external beam irradiation: a dosimetric analysis. Int J Radiat Oncol Biol Phys 27:531–536

Cox P, Kennelly GM (1980) The role of curative radiotherapy in the treatment of lung cancer. Cancer 45:698–702

De Neve W, De Gersem W, Fortan L, Van Den Heuvel F (1996) Clinical implementation of electronic portal imaging: correction strategies and set-up errors. Bull Cancer/Radiother 83:401–405

Denham JW, Hamilton CS, Joseph DJ, Lamb DS, Spry NA, Gray AJ, Atkinson CH, Wynne CJ, Abdelaal A, Bydder PV, Chapman PJ, Matthews JHL, Stevens G, Ball DL, Kearsley J, Ashcroft JB, Janke P, Gutmann A (1993) The use of simulator and CT information in the planning of radiotherapy for non-small cell lung cancer: an Australian pattern of practice study. Lung Cancer 8:275–284

Derycke S, Van Duyse B, De Gersem W, De Wagter C, De Neve W (1997) Non-coplanar beam intensity modulation allows large dose escalation in stage III lung cancer. Radioth Oncol 45:253–261

Dillman RO, Seagren SL, Propert KJ, Guerra J, Eaton WL, Perry MC, Carey RW, Frei EF, Green MR (1990) A randomized trial of induction chemotherapy plus high-dose versus radiation alone in stage III non-small cell lung cancer. N Engl J Med 323:940–945

Dosoretz DE, Katin MJ, Blitzer PH, Rubenstein JH, Salenius S, Rashid M, Dosani RA, Mestas G, Siegel AD, Chadha TT, Chandrahasa T, Hannan SE, Bhat SB, Metke M (1992) Radiation therapy in the management of medically inoperable carcinoma of the lung: results and implications for future treatment strategies. Int J Radiat Oncol Biol Phys 24:3–9

Emami B, Lyman J, Brown A, Coia L, Goitein M, Munzenrider JE, Shank B, Solin LJ, Wesson M (1991) Tolerance of normal tissue to therapeutic irradiation. Int J Radiat Oncol Biol Phys 21:109–122

Emami B, Graham MV, Purdy JA (1994) Three-dimensional conformal radiotherapy in bronchogenic carcinoma considerations for implementation. Lung Cancer 11 [Suppl 3]:117–128

Emami B, Scitt C, Byhardt R, Graham MV, Andras EJ, John M, Herskovic A, Urtasun RC, Asbell SO, Perez CA, Cox J (1996) The value of regional nodal radiotherapy (dose/volume) in the treatment of unresectable non-small cell lung cancer: an RTOG analysis. Int J Radiat Oncol Biol Phys 36[Suppl 1]:209

Feld R, Rubinstein LV, Weisenberger TH and the Lung Cancer Study Group (1984) Sites of recurrence in resected stage I non small cell lung cancer: a guide for future studies. J Clin Oncol 2:1352–1358

Gauden S, Ramsay J, Tripciony L (1995) The curative treatment by radiotherapy alone of stage I non-small cell lung cancer. Chest 108:1278–1282

Ginsberg RJ, Rubinstein LV (1995) Lung Cancer Study Group Randomized trial of lobectomy versus limited resection for T1N0 non-small cell lung cancer. Ann Thorac Surg 60:615–622

Graham MV, Matthews JW, Harms WB, Emami B, Glaze HS, Purdy JA (1994) Three-dimensional radiation treatment planning study for patients with carcinoma of the lung. Int J Radiat Oncol Biol Phys 29:1105–1117

Graham PH, Gebski VJ, Langlands AO (1995) Radical radiotherapy for early nonsmall cell lung cancer. Int J Radiat Oncol Biol Phys 31:261–266

Graham MV, Purdy JA, Harms W, Emami B, Drzymala R (1997) Clinical results of three-dimensional radiation therapy for non-small cell lung cancer. Lung Cancer 18:124–125

Harris KM, Adams H, Lloyd DC, Harvey DJ (1993) The effect on apparent size of simulated pulmonary nodules of using three standard CT window settings. Clin Radiol 47:241–244

Hazuka MB, Turrisi AT, Lutz ST, Martel MK, Ten Haken RK, Strawderman M, Borema PL, Lichter AS (1993) Results of high-dose thoracic irradiation incorporating beam's eye view display in non-small cell lung cancer: a retrospective multivariate analysis. Int J Radiat Oncol Biol Phys 27:273–284.

Hobday P, Hodson NJ, Husband J, Parker RP, Macdonald JS (1979) Computed tomography applied to radiotherapy treatment planning: techniques and results. Radiology 133:477–482

Huang DT, Tercilla O, Lutz S, Silverman L, Schmidt-Ullrich R (1996) A patient self-gated technique for radiotherapy to lung cancers. Int J Radiat Oncol Biol Phys 36[Suppl 1]:349

ICRU (1993) International Commission on Radiation Units and Measurements: prescribing, recording and reporting photon beam therapy. ICRU Report 50, Bethesda, USA

Immerman SC, Vanecko RM, Fry WA, Shields TW (1981) Site of recurrence in patients with stages I and II carcinoma of the lung resected for cure. Ann Thorac Surg 32:23–26

Jacobs I, Vanregemorter J, Scalliet P (1996) Influence of respiration on calculation and delivery of the prescribed dose in external radiotherapy. Radiother Oncol 36:123–128

Kiricuta IC, Mueller G, Stiess J, Bohndorf W (1994) The lymphatic pathways of non-small cell lung cancer and their implication in curative irradiation treatment. Lung Cancer 11:71–82

Krol ADG, Aussems P, Noordijk EM, Hermans J, Leer JWH (1996) Local irradiation alone for peripheral stage I lung cancer: could we omit the elective regional nodal irradiation? Int J Radiat Oncol Biol Phys 34:297–302

Lafitte J, Ribert ME, Prévost BM, Gosselin BH, Copin MC, Brichet AH (1996) Postresection irradiation for T2NOMO non-small cell carcinoma: a prospective, randomized study. Ann Thorac Surg 62:830–834

MacLoud TC, Bourgouin PM, Greenberg RW, Kosiuk JP, Templeton PA, Shepard JA, Moore EH, Wain JC, Mathisen DJ, Grillo HC (1992) Bronchogenic carcinoma: analysis of staging in the mediastinum with CT by correlative lymph node mapping and sampling. Radiology 182:319–323

Martel MK, Strawderman M, Hazuka MB, Turrisi AT, Fraass BA, Lichter AS (1997) Volume and dose parameters for survival of non-small cell lung cancer patients. Radiother Oncol 44:23–30

Minet P, Constant ML, Biquet JF, Lemaire M (1993) Probability of lymph node invasion in lung cancer: a tool to delineate the target volume. In: Minet P (ed) Three dimensional treatment planning. WHO Headquarters, Geneva, pp 57–68

Morita K, Fuwa N, Suzuki Y, Nishio M, Sakai K, Tamaki Y, Niibe H, Chujo M, Wada S, Sugawara T, Kita M (1997) Radical radiotherapy for medically inoperable non-small cell lung cancer in clinical stage I: a retrospective analysis of 149 patients. Radiother Oncol 42:31–36

Nohl-Oser HC (1981) Surgery of the lung. In: Nohl-Oser HC, Nissen R, Schreiber HW (eds) Surgery of the lung. Thieme, Stuttgart, pp 37–184

Noordijk EM, Van Poest Clement E, Hermans J, Wever AMJ, Leer JWH (1988) Radiotherapy as an alternative to surgery in elderly patients with resectable lung cancer. Radioth Oncol 13:83–89

Paiorolero PC, Williams, DE, Bergstrahl MS, Piehlen JM, Bernartz PE, Payne WJ (1984) Post-surgical stage I bronchogenic carcinoma: morbid implications of recurrent disease. Ann Thorac Surg 38:331–338

Perez CA, Stanley K, Grundy G, Hanson W, Rubin P, Kramer S, Brady L, Marks JE, Perez-Tamayo R, Brown GS, Concannon JP, Rotman M (1982) Impact of irradiation technique and tumor extent in tumor control and survival of patients with unresectable non-oat cell carcinoma of the lung. Report by the Radiation Therapy Oncology Group. Cancer 50:1091–1099.

Perez CA, Pajak TF, Rubin P, Simpson JR, Mohiuddin M, Brady LW, Perez-Tamayo R, Rotman M (1987) Long-term observations of the patterns of failure in patients with unresectable non oat-cell carcinoma of the lung treated with definitive radiotherapy. Cancer 59:1874–1881.

Pigott KH, Saunders MI (1993) The long term outcome after radical radiotherapy for advanced localized non-small cell carcinoma of the lung. Clin Oncol 5:360–354

Rabinowitz I, Broomberg J, Goitien M, McCarthy K, Leong J (1985) Accuracy of radiation field alignment in clinical practice. Int J Radiat Oncol Biol Phys 11:1857–1867

Roberston JM, Ten Haken RK, Hazuka MB, Turrisi AT, Martel MK, Pu AT, Litlles JF, Martinez FJ, Francis IR, Quint LE, Lichter AS (1997) Dose escalation for non-small cell lung cancer using conformal radiation therapy. Int J Radiat Oncol Biol Phys 37:1079–1085

Rubin P, Casarett G (1972) A direction for clinical radiation pathology. Front Radiat Ther Oncol 6:1–16

Sandler HM, Curran WJ, Turrisi AT (1990) The influence of tumor size and pre-treatment staging on outcome following radiation therapy alone for stage I non small cell lung cancer. Int J Radiat Oncol Biol Phys 19:9–13

Saunders MI, Dische S, Barrett A, Parmar MKB, Harvey A, Gibson D on behalf of the CHART Steering Committee (1996) Randomised multicentre trials of CHART vs conventional radiotherapy in head and neck and non-small-cell lung cancer: an interim report. Br J Cancer 73:1455–1462

Sause W, Scott C, Taylor S, Johnson D, Livingston R, Komaki R, Emami B, Curran WJ, Byhardt RW, Turrisi AT, Dar AR, Cox JD (1994) Radiation Therapy Oncology Group (RTOG) 88-08 and Eastern Cooperative Oncology Group (ECOG) 4588 Preliminary analysis of a phase III trial in regionally advanced unresectable non-small cell lung cancer. J Natl Cancer Inst 87:198–205

Schaake-Koning C, van den Bogaert W, Dalesio O, Festen NJ, Hoogenhout J, Van Houtte P, Kirkpatrick A, Koolen M, Maat B, Nijs A, Renaud A, Rodrigus P, Schuster-Uitterhoeve L, Sculier JP, Van Zandwijk N, Bartelink H (1992) Effects of concomitant cisplatin and radiotherapy on inoperable non-small cell lung cancer. N Engl J Med 326:524–530

Schuster-Uitterhoeve ALF, Hulshof MCC, Gonzalez DG, Koolen M, Sminia P (1993) Feasibility of curative radiotherapy with a concomitant boost technique in 33 patients with nonsmall cell lung cancer. Radiother Oncol 28:247–251

Sibley GS, Munct AJ, Shapiro C, Jacobs R, Chen G, Weichselbaum R, Vijayakumar S (1995) The treatment of stage III nonsmall cell lung cancer using high dose conformal radiotherapy. Int J Radiat Oncol Biol Phys 33:1001–1007

Slotman BJ, Njo KH, Karim ABMF (1994) Curative radiotherapy for technically operable stage I nonsmall cell lung cancer. Int J Radiat Oncol Biol Phys 29:33–37

Slotman BJ, Antonisse IE, Njo KH (1996) Limited field irradiation in early stage (T1-2,N0) non-small cell lung cancer. Radiother Oncol 41:41–44

Talton BM, Constable WC, Kersh CR (1990) Curative radiotherapy in non-small cell carcinoma of the lung. Int J Radiat Oncol Biol Phys 19:15–21

Valley JF, Mirimanoff RO (1993) Comparison of treatment techniques for lung cancer. Radiother Oncol 28:168–173

Van Houtte P, Gregor A, Philips P (1994) An international survey of radiotherapy practice for radical treatment of non-small cell lung cancer. Lung Cancer 11:S129–138

Zhang HX, Yin WB, Yang ZY, Zang ZX, Wang M, Chen DF, Gu XZ (1989) Curative radiotherapy of early operable non small cell lung cancer. Radioth Oncol 14:89–94

21 Radiotherapy and the Challenge of Palliation

F. MACBETH

CONTENTS

21.1 Introduction

Despite the best intentions of doctors and the advances in treatment, more than 90% of patients diagnosed with lung cancer will still eventually die of their disease. The majority of these will at some stage have significant symptoms, either from the primary tumour or from metastatic disease. The successful palliation of symptoms is therefore a major management problem and a challenge.

Evidence-based medicine has been defined as the "conscientious and judicious use of research evidence in the management of individual patients" (SACKETT et al. 1996). It is about the skilled synthesis of evidence, clinical expertise and patient preference in making clinical decisions. The application of radical, potentially curative treatment for lung cancer requires skill and experience, but the initial decisions to treat are often straightforward. With palliative treatment the decision-making is sometimes more difficult with trade-offs to make between the inconvenience and toxicity of treatment and its possible benefits.

Radiotherapy has been used for many years to relieve the symptoms of advanced lung cancer and policies for its use and suitable dose regimens have evolved in a pragmatic way from collective clinical experience. Comparative studies of clinical practice (PRIESTMAN et al. 1989; MAHER et al. 1992) have shown that different clinical policies about the use of radiotherapy and what regimens are most appropriate have evolved in different health care systems. It is interesting to note that in a recent survey of radiotherapy practice from one American radiotherapy centre (LUTZ et al. 1997) only 12% of lung cancer patients received low dose, palliative radiotherapy, whereas a typical British centre would probably treat 85% of patients palliatively (MACBETH, unpublished observations). In this paper I will discuss the use of radiotherapy in less than radical doses given with the intention of controlling symptoms rather than prolonging survival. It is only in recent years that the use of radiotherapy in this context has been subjected to the same critical research and evaluation as chemotherapy or radical radiotherapy. How good is the research evidence which we can use to support our decisions about when and how to use palliative radiotherapy?

The studies referred to in this review were identified from a search of Medline in March 1998, from a check of the references in the papers found and in other previous reviews, and from a personal collection.

21.2 Palliative Radiotherapy to the Chest

21.2.1 How Effective Is It?

Although radiotherapy has been used for many years for palliating the local symptoms of lung cancer, evidence of its effectiveness is limited. There have been

F. MACBETH Clinical Effectiveness Support Unit (Wales), Llandough Hospital, Cardiff, CF642XX, UK

Table 21.1. Published results of the effect of palliative thoracic radiotherapy

First author	Year	No. of patients	Symptoms assessed by	Cough	Haemoptysis	Chest pain	Dyspnoea	Anorexia
Simpson	1985	409	Clinician	99/180 (55)	71/75 (95)	67/134 (50)	63/171 (37)	NR
Papavasiliou	1987	18	Clinician	8/10 (80)	5/7 (71)	3/4 (75)	3/3 (100)	NR
Collins	1988	96	Clinician	58/86 (67)	42/48 (87)	28/39 (72)	45/85 (53)	24/59 (41)
Teo	1988	255	Clinician	Overall symptom control 146/255 (57)				
MRC LCWP	1991	369	Clinician	206/341 (60)	144/172 (84)	162/208 (78)	156/255 (61)	141/213 (66)
MRC LCWP	1992	235	Clinician	114/220 (52)	80/109 (73)	90/137 (66)	84/198 (42)	77/148 (52)
Muers	1993	289	Clinician	(72)	(98)	(82)	(82)	NR
Stevens and Begbie	1995	38	Clinician	(91)	(92)	(78)	(40)	NR
MCRC LCWP	1996a	509	Patient questionnaire	210/404 (52)	NR	188/289 (65)	146/255 (57)	NR
Rees et al.	1997	216	Patient questionnaire	107/168 (64)	78/81 (95)	78/89 (88)	128/78 (72)	NR
Lutz et al.	1997	54	Retrospective	9/27 (33)	11/17 (65)	6/17 (35)	19/41 (46)	9/29 (31)

Number of patients with palliation/number with symptoms (%); NR, not recorded. Note: Different definitions of palliation are used in different studies.

no randomised clinical trials (RCTs) comparing radiotherapy with other means of palliation, and in trials comparing chemotherapy with "best supportive care" the use of radiotherapy has been variable. The best evidence comes for the RCTs that compare different doses of radiotherapy that are discussed in detail below, and from a few other published series. These are summarised in Table 21.1.

Symptom palliation is a difficult endpoint to measure and there are no well validated, universally applicable ways of doing it; and the studies in Table 21.1 used a variety of techniques and measures. Some symptoms, especially haemoptysis, may be intermittent or self-limiting making the effect of treatment difficult to estimate. All symptoms are by definition subjective and how they are rated may vary between patients and between patients and clinicians, and it unusual for them to be assessed by an impartial observer. Data from the Medical Research Council Lung Cancer Working Party (MRC LCWP) suggest that clinicians tend to underestimate the severity of physical symptoms compared to the patients (Stephens 1994). It is also usual for patients to be on medication, such as pain killers or anti-tussives, the dose of which may be changed at the same time as treatment, and unless carefully recorded, this fact may affect the evaluation of effectiveness. For all these reasons comparison or summation of the numerical results in Table 21.1 would be misleading.

However, it can be seen that palliative radiotherapy to the chest does result in more than 50% of patients getting symptom improvement. Haemoptysis and chest pain seem to be better palliated than cough. The palliation of dyspnoea is more variable between the studies with recorded rated ranging from 37% to 100%, probably reflecting the difficulty of assessing this symptom and the varied causes in patients with lung cancer.

Five studies reported the duration of palliation. In two of the MRC LCWP trials (MRC LCWP 1991, 1992), it was reported that the median length of palliation was more than 50% of the survival time. In the third study (MRC LCWP 1996a), including fitter patients, around 50% of patients had palliation of their symptoms at 3 months. Stevens and Begbie (1995) reported that 70% of patients had "a complete symptomatic response" until death or last review. On the other hand the study from Bristol (Rees et al. 1997) showed more disappointing results with haemoptysis being the only symptom that disappeared in more than 50% of patients at 8 weeks.

21.2.2 What Are the Most Effective Dose Regimens?

Radiotherapy regimens have evolved in a pragmatic way over the years from collective clinical experience. It is only in recent years that the use of radiotherapy in this context has been subjected to the same critical research and evaluation as chemotherapy or radical radiotherapy.

There are now five published RCTs that have investigated the most appropriate dose regimen for the palliation of lung cancer (Table 21.2). This shows that, in general, short regimens of radiotherapy with one or two fractions are as effective as longer

Table 21.2. Randomised trials of palliative radiotherapy

First author	Year	No. of patients	Patients	Doses	Palliation	Survival	Side-effects
Simpson	1985	409	Good PS (Karnofsky >70)	30 Gy/10 f/2 w vs 40 Gy/20 f/4 w vs 40 Gy/10 f/4 w "split" course	No difference	No difference	Worse radiation pneumonitis with 40-Gy split course
Teo	1987	291	Any PS	45 Gy/18 f/4.5 w vs 31.2 Gy/4 f/4 w	Better with 45 Gy	Not reported	No difference
MRC LCWP	1991	369	Any PS	30 Gy/10 f vs 17 Gy/2 f	No difference	No difference	No difference; myelopathy: 1 case after 17 Gy
MRC LCWP	1992	235	Poor PS (WHO 2–4)	17 Gy/2 f vs 10 Gy/1 f	No difference	No difference	Fewer immediate with 10 Gy; myelopathy: 1 case after 17 Gy
MRC LCWP	1996	509	Good PS (WHO 1)	39 Gy/13 f or 36 Gy/12 f vs 17 Gy/2 f	Quicker with 17 Gy	Longer with 39/36 Gy (3% at 2 years)	Fewer immediate with 17 Gy; myelopathy: 2 cases after 39 Gy, 1 after 17 Gy
Rees et al.	1997	216	Any PS	22.5 Gy/5 f vs 17 Gy/2 f	No difference	No difference	Not reported

PS, performance status.

ones in palliating the major intrathoracic symptoms of lung cancer. In four trials the effect on survival was investigated, and in three there was no significant difference between the regimens, with median survivals ranging from 4 to 6 months depending on the performance status (PS) of the patients included.

The one exception was the third MRC LCWP trial (MRC LCWP 1996a), which compared 17Gy/2f/8d with 39Gy/13f/18d (or 36Gy/12f/17d) in patients with good PS (WHO 0 or 1). This showed that there was a significant difference in survival (2-month increase in median and 3% difference in 2-year survival) in favour of the higher dose regimen. Interestingly there was also a significant difference in the incidence in metastases (64% vs 77% at 12 months). This is consistent with a similar finding in a trial investigating the use of post-operative radiotherapy in node-positive patients (MRC LCWP 1996b) when a dose of 40Gy/15f/23d was used. It is therefore reasonable to conclude that radiotherapy to the mediastinum can delay systemic metastatic spread even with non-radical doses.

21.2.3 What Are the Risks of Toxicity?

It has long been recognised that palliative radiotherapy to the chest can produce significant toxicity both in the short and long term. Transient nausea and anorexia are common, as is radiation oesophagitis. These symptoms were investigated in detail in the MRC LCWP trials (MRC LCWP 1991, 1992, 1996a) by the use of a daily diary card which the patients completed and on which they rated important symptoms on a five point scale. This demonstrated very clearly the time course and severity of radiation oesophagitis. With regimens of 30Gy/10f/12d and 17Gy/2f/8d it was very similar, starting on day 7, peaking around days 15–20, when 50% of patients recorded dysphagia, and subsiding by day 28. The regimen of 10Gy/1f/1d caused significantly less oesophagitis and, as would be expected, with the higher dose regimens of 36 and 39 Gy dysphagia was more frequent (around 70% of patients recording some dysphagia) and prolonged.

What has been, until recently, less well recognised is that palliative radiotherapy to the chest is associated with other acute symptoms. Stevens and Begbie (1995) noted acute chest pain in 5 of 38 patients receiving 17Gy/2f/8d. Devereux et al. (1997) also found, in a study of 118 patients who completed a questionnaire 24 h after RT, that almost 50% recorded acute chest pain, and over 30% experienced systemic symptoms, such as sweating, fever and rigors. Only 49 patients recorded no symptoms. The majority of the patients were being treated with 8.5- or 10-Gy fractions. The symptoms were usually transient but could cause distress and anxiety, and in some patients the chest pain required opiates. The temporal relationship to the radiotherapy suggests that it is the cause but the mechanism is obscure. Stevens (Stevens and Begbie 1995) observed that chest pain occurred despite prophylactic corticosteroids.

There has always been concern that radiotherapy might make the symptoms of patients with stridor acutely worse and standard practice is to treat such patients with corticosteroids and use more prolonged fractionated regimens. A recent study (Hatton et al. 1997) of 56 patients in whom peak expiratory flow (PEFR) was recorded for 72 h after radiotherapy, with a variety of dose regimens, reported that 49 patients (87%) showed a decrease in PEFR, with a mean fall of 20.3%, and maximal around 6 h. There was no clear correlation with fraction size, and the phenomenon was observed in patients receiving 2-Gy fractions, but the sample sizes were small.

The most serious late toxicities of thoracic irradiation are pneumonitis and myelopathy. Provided that the radiation portals are not too large, pneumonitis is not usually a problem in this context, because the dose is not very high and most patients usually do not survive long enough. Radiation myelopathy (RM) is a rare but potentially disastrous late effect.

Clinical experience over the years has demonstrated that regimens such as 30Gy/10f/12d and 20Gy/5f/5d are within the tolerance of the spinal cord, but that higher dose regimens, particularly with larger fractions, are associated with an unacceptable risk of RM. The first MRC LCWP study reported one possible case of RM after 17Gy/2f/8d and two other cases following the use of this regimen were subsequently reported (Stevens and Begbie 1995). The cumulative experience from all three MRC LCWP studies was reported by Macbeth et al. (1996). Five cases of probable RM were identified in 1048 patients; 3 of these were from the 524 patients treated with the 17Gy/2f/8d regimen and 2 from the 153 patients treated with 39Gy/13f/18d. The time of onset ranged from 8 to 42 months from treatment and the cumulative risk was estimated as being 2%–3% at 2 years.

21.2.4 What Are the Most *Appropriate* Regimens?

The art of good palliative medicine is in making therapeutic decisions for individual patients which balance the possibilities of benefit, of making the patient feel better, against the risks of toxicity and discomfort. For a variety of social and psychological reasons lung cancer sufferers may be less vocal and demanding of health care professionals than other groups of patients, and the quality of the care they receive may be correspondingly less good. The challenge, then, is to ensure that appropriate and humane clinical decisions are made.

Palliative radiotherapy to the chest does seem to be effective in controlling the local symptoms of lung cancer. The evidence summarised above suggests that for the majority of patients short courses of palliative radiotherapy, using one or two fractions, are as effective as more prolonged ones. They also have the advantage of requiring the patients who are often ill and frail to travel less often to the radiotherapy centre. For poor performance status patients the evidence from the MRC LCWP trial (MRC LCWP 1992) is quite clear that a regimen of 10 Gy is effective and causes less radiation oesophagitis. Although nausea and rarely vomiting can occur with this regimen, it does not seem from the evidence available to be more frequent than with other regimens. It can be simply managed with anti-emetics, which may be appropriate to give prophylactically. There does seem to be a risk of systemic symptoms such as chest pain and rigors, but again it is not clear whether this risk is higher in patients having large fraction treatment. Warning the patient and carers, and the prophylactic use of analgesics and anti-pyretics are probably necessary and sufficient. There seems to be no significant risk of myelopathy with this regimen.

It is more difficult to make a clear recommendation for the management of patients with better performance status. The MRC LCWP trial (MRC LCWP 1996a) showed a modest survival benefit but no better palliation from a higher dose and more prolonged regimen, but at the expense of greater toxicity. In this situation it is probably best to discuss the options openly with the patient in order to make a fully informed decision. The regimen of 17Gy/2f/8d is now widely used in the United Kingdom (Maher et al. 1993), and for the majority of patients it appears to be a safe and effective regimen. However, the increasing evidence of a small but significant risk of spinal cord damage means that it should be used with care. There are techniques by which the cord dose can be reduced (Macbeth et al. 1996; Slotman et al. 1993) and so the clear advantages in terms of convenience and resource use should not be forfeited because of anxiety about this complication.

21.2.5 When Should Palliative Radiotherapy Be Given?

This may seem to be a pointless question because any patient referred for palliative radiotherapy should have symptoms and so should be treated as soon as possible. There are, however, some patients who are diagnosed at a stage when they are asymptomatic or their presenting symptom has resolved and is no longer troubling them. What should be done with these patients? Should they be treated immediately or not until their symptoms become more troublesome?

There has been one study that has looked at what happens to a group of patients who were assigned to a "watch" policy and only treated when they became symptomatic (Carroll et al. 1986). Of 48 patients, 26 (54%) developed symptoms requiring thoracic radiotherapy, while the remainder died without needing treatment. Reinfuss et al. (1993) identified a group of 332 patients who were asymptomatic or had "minimal" symptoms, of whom 170 were treated (40Gy/10f/56d, "split" course) and 162 were not because of refusal or "logistic problems". Significantly improved survival was observed but only in patients with stage IIIA disease and good performance status. Symptom control was not reported.

It therefore not clear what the best policy is for this group of patients and the MRC LCWP is currently investigating the question in a prospective RCT.

21.3 What Is the Role of Endobronchial Brachytherapy?

Endobronchial brachytherapy (EBT) is a technique that has been used for many years but has increased in popularity since the introduction of remote afterloading machinery. It has the advantage of delivering treatment to the site of the tumour while minimising the dose of radiation to adjacent normal structures, but the disadvantage of only being effective if there is visible endobronchial tumour rather than adjacent nodal disease causing symptoms. It also means the patient has to have a bronchoscopy for placement of the delivery catheter.

The use of EBT has been widely reported (Baas and van Zandwijk 1995) but the reports are largely of treated series rather than prospective trials. There has, however, been one published randomised trial comparing two different dose schedules (Huber et al. 1995) and two others, reported in abstract only (Burt 1997), comparing EBT with external beam radiotherapy.

As with the studies of external beam palliative radiotherapy there is no consistency in the methods of assessment or reporting. The patient groups are different; some only include patients who had recurrent disease previous to radiotherapy, others those who had had no previous treatment and others mixed groups. Also some reports include patients who had undergone laser or cryotherapy immediately before EBT.

However, it is reasonable to conclude that EBT:

- Is effective in controlling symptoms of cough, haemoptysis and breathlessness, caused by endobronchial tumour and/or external compression by tumour in 75% of patients
- Results in radiological improvement of atelectasis due to tumour obstruction
- Can produce measurable changes in lung function
- Is associated with significant improvement in airway obstruction seen at bronchoscopy.

There are similar problems with the estimates of side-effects. In general the procedure seems to be well tolerated acutely, with very few reports of acute morbidity. Occasional patients seem to develop bronchospasm during and after the procedure.

Of more concern is the incidence of late morbidity, especially massive fatal haemoptysis, airway stenosis and broncho-oesophageal fistula. The last two appear to be rare (probably <5%), but massive fatal haemoptysis is commoner. The average rate is 18% in nine studies, with a range from 3% to 50%. In one detailed long term follow up study of 406 (Collins et al. 1996), it occurred in only 32 (8%) and only 6 of these appeared to be tumour free at the time of death.

Massive fatal haemoptysis can result from tumour growth into one of the major pulmonary blood vessels in any patient with lung cancer, but it appears to be more common in patients who have had EBT. The variable incidence may be due to a number of factors, such as previous laser therapy, dose of radiation, the site of the tumour, the presence of local recurrence and the length of survival. The series reporting a high incidence of fatal haemoptysis tend to be those in which the patients have had combined treatment or have been treated with a high radiation dose. When used in patients with symptomatic recurrent disease with a dose of less than 20 Gy, the overall rate appears to be <10%. But ORNADEL et al. (1997) calculate the actuarial risk in their series to be 20% at 2 years.

There is only one report of a randomised trial comparing EBT with external beam palliative radiotherapy (BURT 1997) in a dose of 36Gy/8f (maximum subcutaneous dose). This is reported in abstract form and suggests that EBT is no more effective in palliating symptoms. A further trial is being conducted with a different dose regimen of external beam radiotherapy, which may eventually give more information.

On the present evidence it would therefore seem that, although EBT is effective, because of the additional complexity of treatment and the long term risks of fatal haemoptysis, its use should be restricted to those patients who have a symptomatic local recurrence in whom more external beam radiotherapy would be inappropriate.

21.4 How Should Radiotherapy Be Used in the Palliation of Metastatic Disease?

There are two main sites of metastasis for which radiotherapy is used frequently, bone and brain. As with thoracic radiotherapy, regimens evolved from experience that appeared to be safe and effective and only recently have they been subjected to critical review in RCTs.

For both sites RCTs (GAZE et al. 1997; NIEWALD et al. 1996; PRIESTMAN et al. 1997) have shown that there is no substantial difference in the palliative effect of short regimens of radiotherapy compared to longer ones, especially for patients with poor performance status or limited prognosis. Since most patients with metastatic lung cancer will fall into one of these categories, it seems inappropriate for the majority of them to be treated with regimens longer than one or two fractions.

21.5 What Is the Role of Radiotherapy in the Palliation of SCLC?

There is much less research information about the role of palliative radiotherapy in the management of small cell lung cancer (SCLC) than for NSCLC. It is well known that SCLC is a radio-responsive tumour and radiotherapy has an established place as consolidation and prophylaxis against brain metastases. Previous authors (BLEEHEN 1986; PAYNE 1994) have implied that its role in palliation is "unquestioned" and "useful".

There are only two studies that have tried to look critically at the role of radiotherapy in patients who have failed treatment with first line chemotherapy. In the first study (IHDE et al. 1979), which was retrospective, the outcome of 23 patients who were treated with radiotherapy with a variety of schedules (median dose 32 Gy) after progressing on chemotherapy was evaluated. All patients relapsed and the time to progression was, curiously, shorter in those who responded to radiotherapy than in those who did not. The sample size was small and it is difficult to draw conclusions from this study.

Another retrospective study (SALAZAR et al. 1991) reported 36 patients (27 with limited disease) treated solely with radiotherapy following relapse after induction chemotherapy. A range of doses from 38 to 60 Gy (in 2-Gy fractions) was used. There was a 77% response rate (25% complete) and more than 60% of patients who had not responded to induction chemotherapy did respond to radiotherapy. The median survival in a subgroup with limited disease and a good response was 40 weeks.

There are two reports of the role of radiotherapy in the primary management of patients presenting with superior venal cava obstruction (SVCO). EGELMEERS et al. (1996) reported that 94% of 17 patients with SCLC presenting with SVCO responded and remained symptom free for an average of 90% of their remaining life. CHAN et al. (1997) described 76 patients with SCLC and SVCO, either at presentation or first relapse, who were treated with radiotherapy in a variety of regimens. A very high response rate was again seen and more than 70% were free of SVCO symptoms to death. Because both of these are retrospective series of patients collected over 7- and 10-year time periods, in whom a variety of chemotherapy and radiotherapy regimens were used, it is difficult to draw firm conclusions beyond saying that radiotherapy is effective in this situation and should be considered as part of a combined approach with chemotherapy, especially in patients with limited disease and in patients considered unfit for chemotherapy.

It therefore seems that there may be a role for high dose radiotherapy in managing patients with limited disease and incomplete response or localised relapse in the thorax. But it is not clear exactly what place low dose, palliative radiotherapy has in the less fit, symptomatic patient at the time of relapse, nor what dose of radiotherapy is the most appropriate. In the absence of good evidence it is probably appropriate to treat these patients with short hypofractionated regimens in the same way as patients with NSCLC. The same also applies to the management of metastatic disease.

21.6 Conclusion

Despite the recent developments in chemotherapy and the increasing efficacy of individual drugs and regimens, radiotherapy still has a very important role in the palliation of patients with advanced and metastatic lung cancer. Research over the past 10 years has given us more insights into the most appropriate regimens to use, what the risks of toxicity are and how to minimise them. Some important questions are, however, still not answered. The challenge for all of us treating these unfortunate patients is not only to integrate the available knowledge into our daily practice but also to continue to ask the right questions from our patients and through research to make the experience of terminal lung cancer as symptom-free as possible.

References

Baas P, van Zandwijk N (1995) Endobronchial treatment modalities in thoracic oncology. Ann Oncol 6:523–531

Bleehen NM (1986) Radiotherapy for small cell lung cancer. Chest 89:268S–276S

Burt P (1997) High dose rate brachytherapy in endobronchial tumours. Lung Cancer 18(S2):35

Carroll M, Morgan SA, Yarnold JR, Hill JM, Wright NM (1986) Prospective evaluation of a watch policy in patients with inoperable non-small cell lung cancer. Eur J Cancer Clin Oncol 22:1353–1356

Chan RH, Dar A, Yu E et al (1997) Superior vena cava obstruction in small cell lung cancer. Int J Radiat Oncol Biol Phys 38:513–520

Collins TM, Ash DU, Close HJ, Thorogood J (1988) An evaluation of the palliative role of radiotherapy in inoperable carcinoma of the bronchus. Clin Radiol 39:284–286

Devereux S, Hatton MQ, Macbeth FR (1997) Immediate side effects of large fraction radiotherapy. Clin Oncol 9:96–99

Egelmeers A, Goor C, van Meerbeeck J, van den Weyngaert D, Scalliet P (1996) Palliative effectiveness of radiation therapy in the treatment of superior vena cava syndrome. Bull Cancer Radiother 83:153–157

Gaze MN, Kelly CG, Kerr GR et al (1997) Pain relief and quality of life following radiotherapy for bone metastases: a randomised trial of two fractionation schedules. Radiother Oncol 45:109–116

Gollins SW, Ryder W, Burt P, Barber P, Stout R (1996) Massive haemoptysis death and other morbidity associated with high dose rate intraluminal radiotherapy for carcinoma of the bronchus. Radiother Oncol 39:105–116

Hatton MQ, Nixon DL, Macbeth FR, Symonds RP (1997) Acute changes in peak expiratory flow rate following palliative radiotherapy for bronchial carcinoma. Radiother Oncol 44:31–34

Huber RM, Fischer R, Hautmann H et al (1995) Palliative endobronchial brachytherapy for central lung tumors. A prospective, randomized comparison of two fractionation schedules. Chest 107:463–470

Ihde DC, Bilek F, Cohen M, Bunn PA, Eddy J, Minna JD (1979) Response to thoracic radiotherapy in patients with small cell carcinoma of the lung after failure of combination chemotherapy. Radiology 132:443–446

Lutz ST, Huang DT, Ferguson CL, Kavanagh BD, Tercilla OF, Lu J (1997) A retrospective quality of life analysis using the Lung Cancer Symptom Scale in patients treated with palliative radiotherapy for advanced nonsmall cell lung cancer. Int J Radiat Oncol Bio Phys 37:117–122

Macbeth FR, Wheldon TE, Girling DJ et al (1996) Radiation myelopathy: estimates of risk in 1048 patients in three randomized trials of palliative radiotherapy for non-small cell lung cancer. The Medical Research Council Lung Cancer Working Party. Clin Oncol 8:176–181

Maher EJ, Coia L, Duncan G, Lawton PA (1992) Treatment strategies in advanced and metastatic lung cancer: differences in attitude between the USA, Canada and Europe. Int J Radiat Oncol Biol Phys 23:239–244

Maher EJ, Timothy A, Squire CJ et al (1993) Audit: the use of radiotherapy for NSCLC in the UK. Clin Oncol 5:72–79

Medical Research Council Lung Cancer Working Party (1991) Inoperable non-small-cell lung cancer (NSCLC): a Medical Research Council randomised trial of palliative radiotherapy with two fractions or ten fractions. Report to the Medical Research Council by its Lung Cancer Working Party. Br J Cancer 63:265–270

Medical Research Council Lung Cancer Working Party (1992) A Medical Research Council (MRC) randomised trial of palliative radiotherapy with two fractions or a single fraction in patients with inoperable non-small-cell lung cancer (NSCLC) and poor performance status. Br J Cancer 65: 934–941

Medical Research Council Lung Cancer Working Party (1996a) Randomized trial of palliative two-fraction versus more intensive 13-fraction radiotherapy for patients with inoperable non-small cell lung cancer and good performance status. Clin Oncol 8:167–175

Medical Research Council Lung Cancer Working Party (1996b) The role of post-operative radiotherapy in non-small cell lung cancer; a multicentre randomised trial. Br J Cancer 74:632–639

Muers MF, Round CE (1993) Palliation of symptoms in non-small cell lung cancer: a study by the Yorkshire Regional Cancer Organisation Thoracic Group. Thorax 48:339–343

Niewald M, Tkocz HJ, Abel U et al (1996) Rapid course radiation therapy vs. more standard treatment: a randomized trial for bone metastases Int J Radiat Oncol Biol Phys 36:1085–1089

Ornadel D, Duchesne G, Wall P, Hetzel M (1997) Defining the roles of high dose rate endobronchial brachytherapy and laser resection for recurrent bronchial malignancy. Lung Cancer 16:203–213

Papavasiliou C, Kouvaris J, Vasilopoulos P, Ioannou R, Riris C (1987) Effective palliation of advanced lung cancer by short duration irradiation. Radiother Oncol 9:269–272

Payne D (1994) The role of radiation in small cell lung cancer. Crit Rev Oncol Haematol 16:113–127

Priestman TJ, Bullimore JA, Godden TP, Deutsch GP (1989) The Royal College of Radiologists' Fractionation Survey. Clin Oncol 1:39–46

Priestman TJ, Dunn J, Brada M, Rampling R, Baker PG (1997) Final results of the Royal College of Radiologists' trial comparing two different radiotherapy scedules in the treatment of cerebral metastases. Clin Oncol 8:308–315

Rees GJ, Devrell CE, Barley VL, Newman HF (1997) Palliative radiotherapy for lung cancer: two versus five fractions. Clin Oncol 9:90–95

Reinfuss M, Skolyszewski J, Kowalska T, Rzepecki W, Kociolek D (1993) Palliative radiotherapy in asymptomatic patients with locally advanced, unresec-table, non-small cell lung cancer. Strahlenther Onkol 169:709–715

Sackett DL, Rosenberg WC, Muir Gray JA, Haynes RB, Richardson WS (1996) Evidence based medicine:what it is and what it isn't. Br Med J 312:71–72

Salazar OM, Yee GJ, Slawson RG (1991) Radiation therapy for chest recurrences following induction chemotherapy in small cell lung cancer. Int J Radiat Oncol Bio Phys 21:645–650

Simpson JR, Francis ME, Perez-Tamayo R, Marks RO, Rao DV (1985) Palliative radiotherapy for inoperable carcinoma of the lung: final report of a PTOG multi-institutional trial. Int J Radiat Oncol Biol Phys 11:751–758

Slotman BJ, Njo KH, de Jonge A, Meijer OW, Karim ABMF (1993) Palliative radiotherapy in advanced metastatic and non-metastatic non-small cell lung cancer. Lung Cancer 8:285–292

Stephens RJ (1994) Quality of life (QL) in randomised clinical trials: are doctors' assessments as valid as the patients'? Lung Cancer 11 [Suppl 1]:81

Stevens MJ, Begbie SD (1995) Hypofractionated irradiation for inoperable non-small cell lung cancer. Austr Radiol 39:265–270

Teo P, Tai TH, Choy D, Tsui KH (1988) A randomised study on palliative radiation therapy for inoperable non-small cell carcinoma of the lung. Int J Radiat Oncol Biol Phys 14:867–871

22 New Drugs in Lung Cancer

J.E. Dancey and F.A. Shepherd

CONTENTS

22.1 Introduction

Lung cancer is the most common cause of death due to cancer in the western world (Boring et al. 1994). Approximately 75%–80% of all lung cancer patients are diagnosed with non-small cell lung cancer (NSCLC), which comprises several histological subtypes: squamous cell, adenocarcinoma, large cell and bronchoalveolar. Most patients with NSCLC present with unresectable disease or relapse following resection. The survival rate as a whole is poor with only about 10%–15% of all patients surviving 5 years from diagnosis (Ginsberg et al. 1994). Previously, the list of drugs with activity against NSCLC has been brief: in addition to cisplatin, only ifosfamide, the vinca alkaloids, and mitomycin C have had consistent response rates greater than 15% (Green 1993). Combinations of active drugs have demonstrated increased response rates over single agents.

However, objective responses are seen in less than 50% of patients and complete responses are rare. Despite treatment, median survival of patients with advanced disease is 20–25 weeks and less than 25% survive 1 year (Finkelstein et al. 1986).

Small cell lung cancer (SCLC) is found in 20%–25% of patients. Without treatment, it is a rapidly progressive tumor associated with a median survival of less than 3 months. Fortunately, SCLC is highly sensitive to both radiotherapy and chemotherapy, with 80%–90% of patients responding initially to treatment. The list of drugs with activity against SCLC includes alkylating agents, anthracyclines, vinca alkaloids, platinum complexes, and antimetabolites. To improve efficacy, different strategies have been tried such as combining non-cross resistant agents and increasing dose intensity by using hematopoietic growth factors or stem cell transplantation to overcome dose-limiting myelosuppression. Unfortunately, these efforts to increase doses or recombine existing agents have not led to major advances in the treatment of SCLC. With combination chemotherapy, the median survival for patients with extensive disease is approximately 10 months. The median survival for patients with limited stage remains less than 18 months and only 10%–20% survive more than 2 years (Klastersky 1995).

Despite over 30 years of clinical research, most patients with lung cancer still die of their disease. Improved treatment requires the identification of new drugs and drug combinations that will enhance not only response rates but also survival duration. Recently, several new drugs with novel mechanisms of action have been identified. These drugs include the taxoids, paclitaxel, docetaxel, topoisomerase I inhibitors, irinotecan, topotecan, the antimetabolite gemcitabine, and the vinca alkaloid vinorelbine.

J.E. Dancey, MLW 2-031, Princess Margaret Hospital, 610 University Avenue, 5-109, Toronto, Ontario, Canada, M5G 2M9

F.A. Shepherd, Princess Margaret Hospital, 610 University Avenue, 5-109, Toronto, Ontario, Canada, M5G 2M9

22.2 The Taxoids

22.2.1 Mechanism of Action

The taxoids, represented by the prototypic agent paclitaxel and the semisynthetic analog docetaxel, are spindle poisons which function by stabilizing microtubules. Paclitaxel, a novel dipterpene plant product isolated from the western yew *Taxus breviofolia* (Wani et al. 1971), consists of a 14-member taxoid ring linked to a rare oxetan ring at positions 3 and 4 and an ester side chain at position 13. All the taxoid compounds with significant antitumor activity possess this chain. Docetaxel is a semisynthetic taxoid prepared from a precursor compound, 10-deacetylbaccatin III, extracted from the needles of the European yew *Taxus baccata*. Paclitaxel and docetaxel share the taxoid skeleton but have differing substituents at C-10 and on the C-13 side chain. Both taxoids induce the formation of very stable microtubule bundles by promoting microtubule assembly and subsequent inhibiting normal depolymeratization. Hence, cell replication is blocked in G2 and M phases of the cell cycle (Gelmon 1994). Paclitaxel is insoluble in aqueous solutions and is formulated in Cremophor EL and alcohol. Docetaxel, being more water soluble, is formulated in polysorbate 80 (Tween 80) and in in vitro models is more potent at promoting tubulin polymerization compared with paclitaxel.

Both paclitaxel and docetaxel exhibit triphasic patterns of elimination with prolonged terminal half lives. Both components are highly protein bound with hepatic metabolism and biliary excretion being important for elimination. Toxicities common to both compounds include neutropenia, infusion-related hypersensitivity reactions, alopecia, peripheral neurotoxicity, mucositis, diarrhea, mylagias and fatigue (Francis et al. 1995).

22.2.2 Paclitaxel

22.2.2.1 Phase I Trials

Paclitaxel is a potent agent against both NSCLC and SCLC. Initial phase I trials of paclitaxel utilized a number of schedules ranging from infusions of 3–24 h every 3 weeks to a daily for 5 days. Recently, even shorter 1-h administrations and longer infusions of 72–96 h have been evaluated (Donehower and Rowinsky 1993). If a short infusion is used, the recommended dose of paclitaxel is 175–225 mg/m^2. Since myelosuppression is greater with longer administration time, the recommended dose is lower, in the range of 135–175 mg/m^2 when administered without granulocyte-colony stimulating factor (G-CSF). With G-CSF support, maximally tolerated doses range from 200 to 250 mg/m^2. The toxicity profile of paclitaxel changes depending on its schedule of administration. Shorter infusion times more frequently cause neurotoxicity and myalgias.

Regardless of the schedule, the dose-limiting toxicity is non-cumulative neutropenia. Acute hypersensitivity reactions are also seen, but prophylactic premedication with corticosterioids as well as H_1 and H_2 histamine antagonists reduces the incidence of severe reactions from as high as 30% to less than 5%. Neuromuscular toxicity has been marked by peripheral neuropathy affecting sensory, motor, and autonomic pathways, myopathy and rare episodes of central nervous system effects. Dose, co-morbid diseases such as diabetes mellitus or alcoholism, and prior or concurrent neurotoxic chemotherapy are risk factors for the development of neurotoxicity. Transient myalgias and arthralgias are generally mild but occasionally patients require narcotic analgesics for relief. Other reported toxicities include mucositis, diarrhea, alopecia and, rarely, cardiac arrhythmias (Donehower and Rowinsky 1993).

22.2.2.2 Non-Small Cell Lung Cancer

22.2.2.2.1

SINGLE AGENT PHASE II TRIALS

Initial phase II trials of paclitaxel in untreated patients with NSCLC given 200–250 mg/m^2 over 24 h with G-CSF every 3 weeks showed response rates of 21%–24% (Murphy et al. 1993; Chang et al. 1993). Recent trials have employed more convenient administration times of 1–3 h without an obvious loss of efficacy. Response rates of 22%–38% have been reported with paclitaxel doses of 200–250 mg/m^2 administered over 3 h every 3 weeks (Gatzemeier et al. 1995; Sekine et al. 1996; Tester et al. 1997; Alberola et al. 1995; Hainsworth et al. 1995). Interestingly, Millward and colleagues administered paclitaxel at a lower dose of 175 mg/m^2 over 3 h to 51 chemotherapy naive patients and observed a rather unimpressive 10% response rate (Millward et al.

1996). These results suggest that there may be a dose-response relationship; however, the confidence intervals for response rates overlap, making it impossible to reach a definitive conclusion.

Despite these rather impressive results in untreated NSCLC patients, paclitaxel does not appear to be active in platinum-pretreated patients. Two trials have attempted to assess paclitaxel non-cross resistance to platinum compounds by evaluating drugs in second-line treatment of NSCLC (Murphy et al. 1994; Ruckdeschel et al. 1994). The combined response rate was a mere 6% in a total of 46 patients.

22.2.2.2.2 Combination Chemotherapy Trials with Paclitaxel

Paclitaxel in combination with platinum compounds has been tested extensively. The combination of paclitaxel and cisplatin is particularly attractive since these agents demonstrate additive or synergistic cytotoxicity in preclinical studies and because the drugs possess slightly different toxicity profiles (Jekunen et al. 1994). Paclitaxel 135 mg/m^2 over 24 h can be given with cisplatin 75 mg/m^2 without hematopoietic growth factors (Rowinsky et al. 1991). With the addition of G-CSF, the dose of paclitaxel can be escalated to 250 mg/m^2 with neurotoxicity being dose-limiting (Rowinsky et al. 1993).

Two phase III trials comparing paclitaxel and cisplatin regimens to standard cisplatin combinations in patients with advanced NSCLC have reported conflicting results. In the Eastern Cooperative Oncology Group (ECOG) phase III trial (E5592), cisplatin 75 mg/m^2 with etoposide was tested against cisplatin and paclitaxel infused over 24 h at dose levels of either 135 mg/m^2 or 250 mg/m^2 with G-CSF (Bonomi et al. 1996). Among 574 randomized patients, response rates and survival were higher for those receiving the high dose and standard dose paclitaxel combinations compared to the etoposide combination (32% vs 27% vs 12%; median survival 10.1 vs 9.6 vs 7.4 months; P = 0.053). Of note, response rates and survival were not significantly different between the paclitaxel regimens. Hematological toxicity was comparable amongst the regimens; however, neurotoxicity was more frequent with the high dose paclitaxel regimen. Paclitaxel with cisplatin has become the reference arm for future ECOG phase III studies. European investigators compared cisplatin 80 mg/m^2 and paclitaxel 175 mg/m^2 by 3 h infusion to cisplatin and teniposide. Preliminary results indicate a higher response rate (47% vs 29%) and less toxicity with the paclitaxel combination without a corresponding improvement in median survival (9.3 vs 9.1 months) (Giaccone et al. 1996). These preliminary results are at odds with those reported in the ECOG trial and may reflect the use of the lower dose or the shorter schedule of administration. Longer follow-up is needed to fully assess the significance of the EORTC trial.

Paclitaxel has been combined with other active drugs including carboplatin, ifosfamide, gemcitabine and vinorelbine. Phase II results with paclitaxel plus carboplatin are particularly interesting, with response rates as high as 40%–60% and median survival approaching 1 year in selected studies (Langer et al. 1995; Johnson et al. 1996; Rowinsky et al. 1995). Most trials used paclitaxel doses of 225 mg/m^2 and carboplatin at area under the curve (AUC) 6.0. Not surprisingly, myelosuppresion is common although hospitalization for febrile neutropenia is unusual. Although G-CSF was not routinely administered during the first cycle, the majority of patients required growth factor support with subsequent therapy. Cumulative peripheral neuropathy was relatively common with grade 3 toxicity occurring in up to 15% of patients.

The ECOG and EORTC randomized trials indicate that cisplatin with paclitaxel is a useful combination with an acceptable toxicity profile. The ease of administrating a 3 h infusion of paclitaxel makes such a regimen appealing; however, the lack of survival benefit in the EORTC randomized trial suggests continued study of optimal infusion time and dose is warranted. Data from phase II studies of carboplatin and paclitaxel suggest that substituting carboplatin for cisplatin may reduce the incidence of nausea, vomiting and peripheral neuropathy. The question of which platinum-paclitaxel combination is most beneficial to patients in terms of survival, toxicity and quality of life will need to be answered by a randomized trial.

22.2.3 Docetaxel

22.2.3.1 Phase I Trials

In phase I trials of docetaxel, the highest recommended dose and dose intensity was reached with a 1 h infusion of 100 mg/m^2 every 3 weeks. Dose-limiting toxicity of docetaxel is neutropenia, but the incidence of docetaxel-induced hypersensitivity reactions is lower than for paclitaxel. The incidence of hypersensitivity reactions among patients on the phase I studies who were not routinely premedicated was 18%, with all but 4% described as mild to moderate (GELMON 1994). Two unique side effects of docetaxel are cutaneous reactions and fluid retention. Although these are usually mild, severe skin reactions causing onycholysis and desquamation over the extremities and edema presenting with pleural effusions, ascites, leg edema and anasarca have been dose-limiting in some patients. Other toxicities include alopecia, neuropathy, mucositis, diarrhea and myalgias. The appearance of cutaneous toxcities, edema as well as hypersensitivity reactions has led to the routine use of premedication with corticosteroids to avoid these side-effects.

22.2.3.2 *Non-Small Cell Lung Cancer*

22.2.3.2.1 SINGLE AGENT PHASE II TRIALS

Most phase II trials of single agent docetaxel in chemotherapy-naive patients with NSCLC evaluated the dose and schedule of 100 mg/m^2 every 3 weeks (CORTES and PAZDUR 1995; FOSSELLA et al. 1994; FRANCIS et al. 1994). Response rates ranged from 18% to 38%. Up to 89% of patients developed grade 3/4 neutropenia and 24% of patients developed febrile neutropenia. Two phase II studies suggested that a lower dose of doxetaxel might be equally efficacious with significantly less toxicity. In a small trial of 20 untreated patients treated with 75 mg/m^2, a response rate of 25% and a 1 year survival of 71% were seen (MILLER et al. 1995). A larger study of 75 patients treated at 60 mg/m^2 reported a response rate of 19% and median survival of 42 weeks (KUNITOH et al. 1996). Fluid retention occurred in 66% of patients but was severe in only 8%. This was cumulative, typically occurring after a median total dose of 400 mg/m^2. Subsequent studies have shown that dexamethasone decreases the severity of fluid retention.

Unlike paclitaxel, docetaxel appears to be active in platinum pretreated NSCLC patients. Phase II studies of doxetaxel 100 mg/m^2 every 3 weeks in patients with cisplatin-refractory disease have reported response rates of 16%–22% and median survivals of 30–39 weeks (FOSSELLA et al. 1995; CERNY et al. 1994). The incidence of febrile neutropenia and neurotoxicity appeared to be higher in this group of pretreated patients.

22.2.3.2.2 COMBINATION CHEMOTHERAPY TRIALS WITH DOCETAXEL

Docetaxel in combination with cisplatin has been tested extensively (MILLWARD et al. 1997; COLE et al. 1995; LE CHEVALIER et al. 1995). Phase II studies have evaluated doxetaxel 75–100 mg/m^2 with cisplatin 75–100 mg/m^2 every 21 days. Response rates from 21%–41% were reported. Grade 4 neutropenia was seen in up to 66% of patients and febrile neutropenia ranged from 6% to 27%. Other grade 3 and 4 toxicities reported were diarrhea, nausea and vomiting, and fatigue. Severe and dose-limiting fluid retention has been rare with corticosteroid premedication. Both vinorelbine and ifosfamide are being evaluated in combination with docetaxel. Although preclinical studies in murine xenografts suggest that docetaxel is synergistic with vinorelbine when the drugs are administered simultaneously (BISSERY et al. 1995), preliminary results from phase I/II trials of this combination indicate that hematologic toxicity limits the delivery of full doses of either drug, which potentially may compromise the efficacy of this non-platinum regimen (KOUROUSIS et al. 1996).

Results to date suggest that docetaxel has promising activity in untreated and previously treated NSCLC patients with acceptable toxicity. Concerns about hypersensitivity reactions, cutaneous side effects and fluid retention have been alleviated with the demonstration that routine premedication with corticosteroids can reduce their incidence and severity. The evidence of antitumor effect in pretreated patients is particularly encouraging. Ongoing multicenter phase III studies comparing doxetaxel 100 mg/m^2 every 3 weeks to supportive care in chemotherapy-naive and in platinum-pretreated NSCLC patients will better define the impact of doxetaxel on survival and quality of life.

22.2.4 Small Cell Lung Cancer

There have been fewer trials of taxoids in SCLC than NSCLC. Paclitaxel 250 mg/m^2 intravenously over 24 h with G-CSF every 3 weeks has been evaluated in two phase II studies of untreated patients with extensive SCLC (ETTINGER et al. 1995; KIRSCHLING et al. 1994). Twenty-six of 69 evaluable patients had confirmed responses for a combined response rate of 38%. Similar activity has been reported in previously treated patients. In a small study of paclitaxel

175 mg/m² over 3 h, 5 of 14 patients (36%) had partial responses (SMIT et al. 1996).

The results with docetaxel in SCLC have been less impressive. The European Organization for Research and Treatment of Cancer (EORTC) conducted a phase II study of docetaxel 100 mg/m² every 3 weeks in 34 previously treated patients with extensive disease SCLC and reported only seven partial responses among 28 evaluable patients (SMYTHE et al. 1994). In contrast, a Canadian multicenter phase II study of docetaxel 75 mg/m² intravenously every 3 weeks showed only an 8% response in 12 previously untreated patients (LATREILLE et al. 1996). These two studies suggest that the activity of docetaxel in SCLC is modest and that paclitaxel is the preferred taxoid for this disease. Studies of paclitaxel with platinum compounds and/or etoposide, doxorubicin and vinca alkaloids are underway to further define its role in the treatment of SCLC.

22.2.5 Combination Trials with Radiation

Both paclitaxel and docetaxel are radiosensitizing agents in vitro (CHOY et al. 1992). This effect may be due to their ability to block the cells in the G2/M phase, which is the radiation sensitive phase of the cycle. Although strategies to combine both taxoids with radiation are underway, to date only studies using paclitaxel have been published. In the phase I study of this regimen, esophagitis is the principle dose-limiting toxicity of weekly paclitaxel and thoracic radiation (CHOY et al. 1994). A phase II trial using concurrent radiation to a total dose of 60 Gy in 6 weeks and weekly paclitaxel 60 mg/m² over 3 h is underway. In a phase II trial of weekly paclitaxel and split course radiotherapy in NSCLC patients, an unexpectedly high incidence of interstitial pneumonitis was observed. In this study, patients with inoperable stage IIIA/B NSCLC were treated with paclitaxel at dose levels between 50 mg/m² and 86 mg/m² over 3 h on day 1 in weeks 1–3 and 6–8 with simultaneous radiotherapy in daily doses of 2 Gy, 5 days/week, in weeks 1–3 and 6–8 up to a total dose of 56 Gy (RECKZEH et al. 1996). Although the 78% response rate was impressive among 14 evaluable patients, 7 patients developed moderate to severe interstitial pneumonia while an 8th patient had a cytomegalovirus infection. The major myelotoxic effect observed was moderate to severe lymphocytopenia. During treatment and a 3-month follow-up period, all lymphocyte subsets were reduced with the most pronounced toxicity seen in CD4+ T and B cells. These results suggest that patients receiving this regimen may require long-term antibiotic and antimycotic prophylaxis.

Phase I and II studies are exploring the feasibility of combining paclitaxel with platinum compounds and radiation. In one study, paclitaxel 50 mg/m²/week as a 1-h infusion and carboplatin AUC of 2/week for 7 weeks was given with a total radiation dose of 66 Gy (CHOY et al. 1996). In addition, patients received two additional cycles of paclitaxel 200 mg/m² and carboplatin (AUC of 6) 3 weeks apart. Twenty-three patients entered the study and their overall response rate was 82%. Nine patients (45%) experienced grades 3 or 4 esophagitis but only one patient (4%) had grade 4 pneumonitis. A phase II trial designed to determine the feasibility of giving paclitaxel plus cisplatin concurrently with thoracic radiation entered nine patients with stage IIIB NSCLC (ANTONIA et al. 1995). Paclitaxel was given as a 24-h infusion (135 mg/m²) followed by cisplatin (75 mg/m²) every 4 weeks, for a total of four cycles. Thoracic radiation was given concurrently with the first two cycles of chemotherapy, to a total dose of 64.8 Gy over 6 weeks. Sixty-six percent of patients experienced grade 3 or 4 neutropenia, 55% experienced grade 3 or 4 esophagitis, and grade 3 pulmonary toxicity developed in 33% of patients. All patients were able to receive the full dose of radiation, although half required some modification of the chemotherapy regimen. There was one complete response and four partial responses. These studies demonstrate that it is feasible to treat patients with locally advanced lung cancer with paclitaxel and either carboplatin or cisplatin plus concurrent thoracic radiation with a degree of toxicity comparable to that associated with other concurrent combined-modality regimens for this disease.

22.3 The Camptothecins

22.3.1 Mechanism of Action

Over 30 years ago, camptothecin, the active compound extracted from the Chinese tree *Camptotheca acuminata*, was found to have antitumor activity in experimental systems (WALL et al. 1966). Despite promising antitumor activity in phase I studies, results in phase II trials indicated the drug was ineffective and highly toxic (MOERTEL et al. 1972;

Gottlieb and Luce 1972). Interest in camptothecins was renewed with the identification of topoisomerase I as the cellular target of the drug (Hsiang and Liu 1988) and the development of the water soluble synthetic and semisynthetic analogs topotecan and irinotecan.

Topoisomerases are nuclear enzymes that modulate the three-dimensional structure of DNA by inducing transient breaks that allow unwinding of supercoiled DNA (Pommier 1993). Topoisomerase I binds to DNA and allows the formation of a break in a single DNA strand. Camptothecin binds to and stabilizes the topoisomerase I enzyme-DNA complex after DNA cleavage, preventing re-sealing of DNA (Hsiang et al. 1989; Hsiang and Liu 1988). The subsequent interaction between the advancing replication fork of drug-stabilized DNA-enzyme complex results in an arrest of DNA replication and formation of double-strand breaks. These in turn activate endonucleases, triggering further DNA fragmentation and cell death (Zhang et al. 1990).

22.3.2 Irinotecan (CPT-11)

22.3.2.1 Phase I Trials

Irinotecan, a pro-drug with limited activity, is converted in plasma by de-esterification to SN-38, which has 1000 times the potency of the parent compound (Kawato et al. 1991a). Phase I trials evaluated various schedules: 30 min infusion every week and every 3 weeks; 30–90 min infusion daily for 3 days every 3 weeks; 90 min infusion every week and every 3 weeks; and 120 h continuous intravenous infusion every 3–4 weeks. Dose-limiting toxicities were somewhat dependent on the treatment schedule. Dose-limiting leukopenia, neutropenia and diarrhea were prominent in single-dose regimens, while gastrointestinal toxicities prevailed with continuous intravenous infusion schedules.

Diarrhea is the most significant gastrointestinal toxicity and may occur early or late following treatment. The early syndrome starts during or shortly after the infusion of irinotecan and is often associated with flushing, sweating, nausea, vomiting and abdominal cramps. It can be managed by the administration of diphenhydramine or atropine with a serotonin antagonist. Late diarrhea occurs 1–3 weeks after treatment and may last 5–7 days. It is refractory to most antidiarrheal agents but early aggressive treatment with loperamide 2 mg every 2 h (24 mg/24 h) reduces the incidence of severe diarrhea to 6% (Abigerges et al. 1994). Other toxic effects of irinotecan include thrombocytopenia, eosinophilia, anemia, alopecia, fatigue, transient elevation of liver function tests, rash and mucositis. Rarely, cases of interstitial pneumonitis have occurred in patients with previously treated lung cancer.

The pharmacokinetics of irinotecan are complex. In plasma, carboxylesterases rapidly convert the pro-drug into SN-38. Both irinotecan and SN-38 are converted by pH dependent hydrolysis from the active lactone to inactive carboxylate forms. Biliary and urinary excretion are both important routes of elimination. Both irinotecan and SN-38 undergo glucuronic acid conjugation and are eliminated in bile (Narita et al. 1993; Gupta et al. 1994). Indirect estimates of biliary concentration of SN-38 and its glucuronide have shown good correlation between the concentration of SN-38 and the occurrence of late diarrhea (Araki et al. 1993).

22.3.2.2 Non-Small Cell Lung Cancer

22.3.2.2.1 PHASE II SINGLE AGENT TRIALS

Based on the results of phase I studies, the recommended doses and schedules of 100–125 mg/m^2/week and 350 mg/m^2 every 3 weeks have been evaluated in phase II lung cancer trials. In single agent phase II trials testing schedules of 100 mg/m^2 weekly and 350 mg/m^2 every 3 weeks, irinotecan response rates of 34% and 36% respectively were observed in untreated patients with NSCLC (Douillard et al. 1995; Negoro et al. 1991b). In contrast, there were no responses seen in 26 previously treated NSCLC patients (Masuda et al. 1992).

22.3.2.2.2 COMBINATION CHEMOTHERAPY TRIALS WITH IRINOTECAN

Preclinical studies showed that the efficacy of camptothecins is synergistic or additive when combined sequentially with alkylating agents such as cisplatin (Kano et al. 1992), and topoisomerase II inhibitors like etoposide (Del Bino et al. 1992). In these in vitro studies, the efficacy of drug combinations depended not only on choice of drug but also on schedule as the concurrent administration of camptothecins with some chemotherapeutic agents leads to antagonistic rather than synergistic effects

(BERTRAND et al. 1992; KAUFMANN 1991). Initial combination studies focused on the use of irinotecan with cisplatin or etoposide. Two phase I studies evaluated irinotecan with differing schedules of cisplatin. In the first, cisplatin was administered by 5-day continuous intravenous infusion at 20 mg/m^2 per day and irinotecan was administered by bolus on day 1 (MORI et al. 1997a). The optimum dose appeared to be cisplatin 20 mg/m^2 per day and irinotecan 80 mg/m^2. Granulocytopenia was dose-limiting. This regimen resulted in a partial response in 9 out of 19 assessable patients. With G-CSF, irinotecan dose was escalated to 160 mg/m^2 with the same schedule of cisplatin. Dose-limiting toxicities were granulocytopenia and diarrhea. However, the response rate was similar (11 of 20 patients) with the more intensive regimen (MORI et al. 1997b). In the second study, 14 previously untreated NSCLC patients were treated with irinotecan (90 min intravenous infusion on days 1, 8, and 15) plus cisplatin (60 mg/m^2, intravenously on day 1). The recommended dose was 80 mg/m^2 of irinotecan, and 60 mg/m^2 of cisplatin and diarrhea was the dose-limiting toxicity. There were one complete and five partial responses among the 14 patients for an overall response rate of 43% (MASUDA et al. 1993). With the use of G-CSF, the irinotecan dose could be increased by 33% to 90 mg/m^2, and diarrhea remained dose-limiting (MASUDA et al. 1994b).

In a phase II study of irinotecan 80 mg/m^2 days 1, 8, and 15 and etoposide 80 mg/m^2 days 1 to 3, 13 of 59 evaluable patients achieved a partial response. The median survival time was 10.0 months and the 1-year survival rate was 36.1%. Twenty-four (39%) patients experienced grade 3 or 4 neutropenia. The results were equivalent to those expected with other cisplatin-based chemotherapy or with irinotecan alone, suggesting that this regimen of etoposide and irinotecan is not advantageous despite preclinical evidence favoring the combination of topoisomerase I and II inhibitors (OSHITA et al. 1997).

22.3.2.3
Small Cell Lung Cancer

Irinotecan given at a dose of 100 mg/m^2 weekly is also active in SCLC, with response rates of 50% and 33% seen in untreated and previously treated patients respectively (MASUDA et al. 1992). The major toxicities were myelosuppression (83% grade 3 and 4), diarrhea (7% grade 3) and pulmonary toxicity (13% grade 3 and 4). Toxic effects are usually manageable but late diarrhea can be severe despite maximal medical therapy.

Irinotecan in combination with etoposide or cisplatin appears to be active in patients with SCLC. In a phase I trial of 25 advanced lung cancer patients, escalating doses of irinotecan were given as a 90-min intravenous infusion on days 1, 8, and 15 with a fixed dose of etoposide 80 mg/m^2 intravenously on days 1 to 3 with G-CSF every 4 weeks. The recommended dose for phase II studies in previously untreated patients is 80 mg/m^2 of irinotecan and 80 mg/m^2 of etoposide with diarrhea and leukopenia being dose-limiting (MASUDA et al. 1994a). The response rates for patients with SCLC was 58% (seven of 12 patients). In a phase II study of untreated SCLC patients, irinotecan 60 mg/m^2 day 1, 8, and 15 and cisplatin 60 mg/m^2 response rates were 79% and 78% in patients with limited and extensive disease respectively (FUJIWARA et al. 1994). The major toxicities were leukopenia (6% grade 4) and diarrhea (21% grade 3 and 4). These results are comparable to standard therapies and suggest the combination of irinotecan with either cisplatin or etoposide is effective in SCLC.

Future study of irinotecan will likely fall into three major areas: the pursuit of effective (preferably mechanism based) methods of overcoming the late diarrhea, the development of rational, safe combination regimens and the randomized comparison of irinotecan-based regimens with standard therapy.

22.3.3
Topotecan

22.3.3.1
Phase I Studies

Topotecan (9-(demethylamino)methyl-10-hydroxycamptothecin) is a camptothecin derivative with aqueous solubility conferred by the charged amino group on the 9-substituent. Preclinical testing indicated that, in topotecan-sensitive tumors, longer exposure to the drug increased the magnitude of response (BURRIS et al. 1992; FRIEDMAN et al. 1994). Phase I studies of short, intermediate and prolonged infusion schedules have been reported including: single intravenous injection every 21 days; 30 min infusion on 5 consecutive days every 21–28 days; 24, 72, 96, and 120 h continuous intravenous infusions every 21–28 days, and a 21-day continuous intravenous infusion every 28 days. Since several antitumor responses were seen in the daily times 5 phase I trial, this schedule was selected for phase II evaluation. In all studies, myelosuppression was dose-limiting, although the pattern of myelosuppression varied with the method of administration. Intermittent bolus and short infusion schedules resulted in noncumulative neutropenia as the predominant toxicity while prolonged continuous infusions were followed by neutropenia, thrombocytopenia and anemia. Attempts to improve dose intensity on the daily times 5 schedule by using hematopoietic growth factors have been unsuccessful (Murphy et al. 1992; Rowinsky et al. 1992; Janik et al. 1993). Non-hematologic toxic effects were generally mild and included alopecia, nausea, vomiting, diarrhea, elevations in hepatic enzymes, mucositis, skin rash and fatigue.

Pharmacokinetic studies of topotecan show that the drug is rapidly hydrolyzed in plasma to the open-ring carboxylate form following intravenous administration (Rowinsky et al. 1992). Patients with reduced creatinine clearance require dose adjustment as they are at increased risk of toxicity from topotecan. However, hyperbilirubinemia does not alter topotecan disposition or toxicity and no dose adjustment is required in patients with serum bilirubin as high as 170 µmol/l (Grochow et al. 1994).

22.3.3.2 Non-Small Cell Lung Cancer

22.3.3.2.1 Phase II Single Agent Trials

Studies of topotecan in untreated patients with NSCLC have reported response rates of only 0%–18%, with the highest response rate seen with a 72-h continuous intravenous infusion schedule (Weitz et al. 1995; Perez-Soler et al. 1996a; Lynch et al. 1994). These results compare unfavorably to those reported for existing agents; thus it is unlikely that topotecan will become an important drug in the treatment of NSCLC.

22.3.3.3 Small Cell Lung Cancer

22.3.3.3.1 Phase II Single Agent Trials

The results of phase II studies of topotecan in SCLC have been more impressive. Forty-eight patients with previously untreated, extensive-stage SCLC received 2.0 mg/m^2 topotecan daily for 5 days every 3 weeks (Schiller et al. 1996). The first 13 patients were treated without G-CSF; the next 35 patients received 5 µg/kg G-CSF for 10–14 days starting on day 6. Patients who had a partial response to topotecan after four cycles, stable disease after two cycles, or progressive disease at any time received salvage chemotherapy with cisplatin and etoposide. In this trial, 19 patients had a partial response for an objective response rate of 39%. The overall median survival time was 10.0 months, and the 1-year survival rate was 39%. Ninety-two percent of patients treated without G-CSF developed grade 3 or 4 neutropenia, compared with 29% who received G-CSF. However, the incidence of neutropenic fevers was similar between the two groups (8% and 11% respectively), and there were no differences in objective tumor response, duration of response, time to treatment failure, or survival.

Intriguing results have been obtained from studies assessing the efficacy of topotecan in previously treated SCLC. Attempts have been made to assess the activity of topotecan in both chemotherapy "sensitive" disease and "refractory" disease. Refractoriness to chemotherapy has been defined as lack of response to frontline therapy or progression during or within 3 months of the last dose. Pooled analysis of data from three multicenter, international phase II studies in patients with "sensitive" disease treated with second-line topotecan has shown a response rate of 18% in 168 patients and a median survival of 30 weeks (Eckardt et al. 1997). Grade 4 neutropenia occurred in 38% of courses and was associated with infection or fever in 4% of courses. Grade 4 thrombocytopenia and grades 3–4 anemia occurred in 11% of courses. Non-hematologic toxicity was mild, with alopecia, asthenia, nausea, and vomiting reported most frequently.

The EORTC studied patients with chemotherapy "refractory" disease, i.e., failed first-line treatment less than 3 months from chemotherapy discontinuation and those with "sensitive" disease, i.e., failed after 3 months (Ardizzoni et al. 1997). Topotecan was administered as a 30-min daily infusion at a dose of 1.5 mg/m^2 for 5 consecutive days every 3 weeks. Ninety-two patients (47 refractory and 45 sensitive) were eligible and assessable for response. Among refractory patients, there were two partial responses and one complete response for an overall response rate of only 6.4%. However, in the sensitive group, there were 11 partial responses and 6 complete responses for an overall response rate of 37.8%. Grade 3 and 4 neutropenia occurred in 46.8% of cycles. Non-hematological toxicity was mild with fatigue or malaise reported in 39% and transient elevation of liver enzymes in 17% of cycles.

To address the issue of cross-sensitivity between topoisomerase I and II agents, a phase II study was designed to assess the anti-tumor activity of topotecan in patients with SCLC refractory to etoposide (Perez-Soler et al. 1996b). Topotecan was administered at a dose of 1.25 mg/m^2/day for 5 days over 30 min every 21 days. Three of 28 assessable patients (11%) achieved a partial remission. Grade 3 to 4 granulocytopenia and thrombocytopenia occurred after 70% and 31% of courses administered, respectively. No grade 3 to 4 non-hematological toxicities were observed. The modest response rate observed in this trial indicates that instead of conferring cross-sensitivity to topotecan, clinical resistance to the topoisomerase II poison etoposide actually is associated with near complete cross-resistance topotecan.

These favorable results have been reproduced in a multicentred phase III trial of topotecan versus cyclophosphamide, doxorubicin, and vincristine as second-line therapy in patients off first-line treatment greater than 60 days before relapse (Clarke et al. 1997). Among the 125 evaluable patients, partial responses were seen in 16/64 (25%) of topotecan treated patients and 9/61 (15%) of CAV patients. Median survival was 21.7 vs 23.1 weeks. Incidences of hematological and non-hematological toxicity were similar between the two arms. These results suggest that single-agent topotecan has efficacy similar to CAV with manageable toxicity in patients with SCLC who responded to first-line therapy. Further follow-up is required to determine whether quality of life and survival are affected.

22.3.3.3.2 Combination Chemotherapy Trials with Topotecan

Phase I studies with topotecan in combination with cisplatin and paclitaxel have been reported. There have been two phase I studies of topotecan administered as a 30-min infusion daily for 5 days with cisplatin. In both trials, neutropenia and thrombocytopenia were dose-limiting. In the first trial, the recommended phase II doses were topotecan 1.0 mg/m^2/day for 5 days in combination with cisplatin 50 mg/m^2 on day 1 without G-CSF or cisplatin 75 mg/m^2 on day 1 with G-CSF support (Miller et al. 1994). In the second trial, each patient was given cisplatin either before topotecan on day 1 or after topotecan on day 5 on an alternating basis every 3 weeks (Rowinsky et al. 1996). The sequence of cisplatin before topotecan induced significantly worse neutropenia and thrombocytopenia than the alternate sequence. Pharmacokinetic studies suggested that the differences in toxicity were due, in part, to lower topotecan clearance and exposure when cisplatin preceded topotecan. The sequence of cisplatin before topotecan at doses of 50 and 0.75 mg/m^2, respectively, was recommended for subsequent clinical trials. Clearly, the combination of topotecan and cisplatin causes more myelotoxicity than either drug given alone at the same dosage. Whether the significant attenuation of cisplatin and topotecan doses required for their concurrent administration compromises the clinical efficacy of this combination will require further study. Myelosuppression has also limited dose escalations of topotecan and paclitaxel in combination. The recommended doses of topotecan on a daily times-five schedule combined with paclitaxel given as a 24 h infusion were merely 0.75 mg/m^2/day and 135 mg/m^2, respectively, despite G-CSF support (O'Reilly et al. 1997). Greater success has been achieved by giving paclitaxel over 3 h. Paclitaxel 80 mg/m^2 on day 1 in combination with topotecan 1.0 mg/m^2/day for 5 days could be given safely without G-CSF. With G-CSF, the dose of paclitaxel would be escalated to 230 mg/m^2 with the same dose of topotecan without dose-limiting effects (Lilenbaum et al. 1995). The dose of topotecan is much lower than the topotecan dose at which single-agent activity has been observed. Due to the inability to administer close to the maximum single-agent doses of both drugs in combination as well as the requirement for G-CSF support, further evaluations of this regimen are necessary before it can be recommended.

22.3.3.3.3 Combination Topotecan with Radiation

Attempts have been made to combine topotecan with thoracic radiation. In vitro data suggests that the scheduling of the modalities will be important. In tissue culture cell lines, synergy was seen only when the drugs were administered shortly after irradiation, suggesting low dose radiation triggers cells to enter S-phase rendering them sensitive to the cytotoxic effects of camptothecins (Tamura et al. 1997; Mattern et al. 1991; Kim et al. 1992). In a phase I study of NSCLC, patients received thoracic irradiation to a total tumor dose of 60 Gy in 30 fractions. Topotecan was delivered by bolus injection days 1 through 5, and days 22 through 26 beginning on the same day as the radiation therapy. The combination of topotecan and thoracic radiotherapy could be given safely at a dose level of only 0.5 mg/m² days 1 to 5 and 22 to 26 with 60 Gy of external beam radiotherapy. Higher doses of topotecan were associated with dose limiting neutropenia and esophagitis. (Graham et al. 1996).

Topotecan has a much more favorable toxicity profile than irinotecan and clearly further studies of topotecan in combination with other effective cytotoxic agents and radiation are warranted in SCLC. Topotecan with either cisplatin, etoposide or paclitaxel are potentially interesting combinations; however, determining optimal dosages and schedules of these agents clearly requires further evaluation. In SCLC, the role of topotecan as first-line treatment should be explored and a study addressing this question is currently ongoing in the United States.

22.4 Gemcitabine

22.4.1 Mechanism of Action

Gemcitabine (2′, 2′-difluoro-2′-dioxycytidine) is a new nucleoside analog of deoxycytidine in which two fluorine atoms have been substituted in the geminal configuration. It is a pro-drug which is phosphorylated intracellularly to its active form by deoxycytidine kinase (Plunkett et al. 1995). The diphosphate form is then converted to gemcitabine triphosphate by nucleoside diphosphate kinase. Gemcitabine is deactivated by cytidine deaminase to the biologically inert 2′, 2′-diflourodeoxyuridine. Gemcitabine differs from other nucleoside analogs by its substrate efficiency for deoxycytidine kinase, which is fivefold greater than that of cytosine arabinoside, and by the exceedingly long terminal half-life of its triphosphate.

The major cytotoxic effect of gemcitabine is directed at DNA synthesis with lesser effects on RNA production. DNA polymerases incorporate gemcitabine triphosphate into extending primer strands of DNA. After gemcitabine is incorporated, one more deoxynucleotide is added and thereafter, DNA polymerases cannot proceed with further strand elongation. DNA proofreading enzymes are unable to remove gemcitabine from this penultimate position, resulting in "masked chain termination" which inhibits both DNA replication and repair (Plunkett et al. 1995). In addition, gemcitabine diphosphate is a substrate for ribonucleotide reductase, the enzyme that produces the deoxynucleotides required for both DNA replication and repair. Inhibiting the production of these normal deoxynucleotides potentiates the incorporation of gemcitabine nucleotides into DNA.

22.4.2 Phase I Trials

Phase I studies of gemicitabine have reported different dose intensities and dose-limiting toxicities depending on the schedule of administration. In one of the first schedules examined, gemcitabine was given once daily for five consecutive days, every 3 weeks (O'Rourke et al. 1994). The maximum tolerated dose was 12 mg/m² per day, and further dose escalation was limited by flu-like symptoms and hypotension. When gemcitabine was administered twice weekly for 3 weeks with a 1 week rest, a maximum tolerated dose of 65 mg/m² was observed, and the dose-limiting toxicity was neutropenia (Poplin et al. 1992). Administration of gemcitabine every other week resulted in a maximum tolerated dose of 4560 mg/m² with dose-limiting toxicities of fatigue, myelosuppression and transient increases in liver enzymes (Clavel et al. 1989). Several trials evaluated a schedule of weekly gemcitabine given 3 out of every 4 weeks (Storniolo et al. 1997). In heavily pretreated patients, the maximum tolerated dose was 800 mg/m². Dose-limiting toxicities included neutropenia, thrombocytopenia, fever and rash.

In most of the phase I studies, gemcitabine was administered over 30 min. However, preclinical studies have suggested that the administration of higher gemcitabine doses over a short infusion time is unlikely to result in higher response rates. It has been postulated that prolonged infusion times may maximize gemcitabine triphosphate accumulation in tumor cells, and may lead to higher response rates. A phase I study of gemcitabine administered over 24 h showed that the maximum tolerated dose was 180 mg/m² weekly for 3 weeks. Neutropenia was the dose-limiting toxicity (Anderson et al. 1994).

22.4.3 Non-Small Cell Lung Cancer

22.4.3.1 Single-Agent Phase II Trials

Since the schedule with the most favorable toxicity profile was weekly administration of gemcitabine over 30 min for 3 weeks with a 1 week break, phase II trials were initiated in chemotherapy-naive patients with advanced NSCLC at a starting dose of 800 mg/m^2 per week. In a small American trial, the response rate was only 3% (Eli Lilly and Company data on file). However, in two larger studies, the starting doses for gemcitabine were increased to 1000 and 1250 mg/m^2, and encouraging response rates of 22.5% and 20% were achieved (Burkes and Shepherd 1995). In a large international confirmatory trial of 161 patients, the starting dose for all patients was 1250 mg/m^2, and one dose escalation was allowed in the absence of toxicity (Gatzemeier and Shepherd 1996). A response rate of 22% was achieved, with 2% of patients having a complete clinical response. Toxicity was modest with grade 4 neutropenia in only 5.7% of patients. Mild elevations of hepatic enzymes were seen, but these were usually not dose-limiting.

The issue of a dose-response effect for gemcitabine remains as yet unresolved. In a trial limited to patients with NSCLC, doses ranged from 1000 to 2800 mg/m^2 per week times three with a 1 week break. Partial responses were seen in 8 of 32 assessable patients, a rate which appears comparable to that achieved with lower doses (Fosella et al. 1997).

The favorable toxicity profile of gemcitabine suggests that it might be an alternative treatment for elderly patients with NSCLC. A review of more than 300 patients treated on phase II trials showed that gemcitabine was equally active in elderly patients (≥65 years of age), and that older age was not associated with increased toxicity or lower dose delivery (Shepherd et al. 1997a).

22.4.3.2 Combination Chemotherapy Studies with Gemcitabine

The combination of gemcitabine and cisplatin has been shown to be synergistic in vitro, and at least additive in vivo (Peters et al. 1995). There have been several trials of gemcitabine and cisplatin in patients with NSCLC. In most of these studies, gemcitabine, at a dose of 1000 mg/m^2 weekly for 3 weeks followed by a 1 week break, was combined with a single dose of cisplatin 100 mg/m^2 given either on day 1 (Einhorn 1997) or day 2 (Crino et al. 1997), or day 15 (Steward et al. 1996; Abratt et al. 1997; Anton et al. 1997). All investigators reported high overall response rates ranging from 37% to 54%. Medial survival times ranged from 8.4 to 14.2 months and 1 year survival rates ranged from 35% to 61%. These very favorable results should be viewed with some caution as most studies, with the exception of that reported by Einhorn, had a high proportion of patients with stage IIIA and IIIB tumors. Overall, the combination of cisplatin and gemcitabine was relatively well-tolerated. Grade 3 and 4 thrombocytopenia and neutropenia were seen in approximately 50% of patients but non-hematologic toxicity rates, with the exception of nausea and vomiting, were similar to those seen with gemcitabine alone.

In a Canadian phase II trial, gemcitabine 1500 mg/m^2 and cisplatin 30 mg/m^2 were administered weekly for 3 weeks (Shepherd et al. 1997b). The weekly administration of both drugs at these doses resulted in more severe myelosuppression and a lower overall response rate (29%) compared to the other five gemcitabine-cisplatin studies.

Gemcitabine has also been combined successfully with ifosphamide 1500 mg/m^2 daily from day 8 to 12 (Gatzemeir et al. 1997). An overall response rate of 22% was reported with a 1 year survival rate of only 11%.

Gemcitabine has also been assessed in several prospectively randomized phase II and III trials. In two studies (Perng et al. 1997; Manegold et al. 1997), gemcitabine alone was compared to the combination of cisplatin and etoposide. In both studies, the overall response rate achieved with single-agent gemcitabine was similar to that with the combination of cisplatin and etoposide. Survival also was similar but toxicity was considerably lower for the patients treated with gemcitabine monotherapy.

In a third randomized phase II trial (Cardenal et al. 1997), a gemcitabine and cisplatin combination was compared to single-agent etoposide. The response rate in the gemcitabine arm was 48% compared to only 22% in the etoposide arm. Survival rates for this study are not yet available.

Three large, randomized, phase III trials are currently ongoing in Europe and North America. In the European trial, gemcitabine and cisplatin are being compared to a combination of mitomycin C, ifosphamide and cisplatin. In a Hoosier Oncology Group study in North America, gemcitabine and cisplatin are being compared to cisplatin alone and in the large, Eastern Cooperative Oncology Group trial, gemcitabine and cisplatin are being compared to three other regimens including paclitaxel and cisplatin, docetaxel and cisplatin, and paclitaxel and carboplatin. The results of these trials will help define the role of gemicitabine as a single agent and in combination with cisplatin in NSCLC.

Gemcitabine has demonstrated potent radiosensitizing activity in a variety of human tumor cell lines

(LAWRENCE 1995). In a phase II clinical trial of full-dose gemcitabine (1000 mg/m^2 weekly for six consecutive weeks) administered with thoracic radiotherapy, 60 Gy over 6 weeks to patients with locally advanced NSCLC, severe esophagitis and pneumonitis were observed (GOOR et al. 1996). Phase I and II trials are now ongoing with lower doses of gemcitabine to assess the ability to deliver this agent safely with thoracic irradiation.

22.4.4 Small Cell Lung Cancer

There has been only one small trial of single-agent gemcitabine in patients with small cell lung cancer (CORMIER et al. 1994). In this National Cancer Institute of Canada study, the starting dose of gemcitabine was 1000 mg/m^2 but was increased to 1250 mg/m^2 when significant hematologic toxicity was not encountered in the first 17 patients. Twenty patients entered the trial, and the overall response rate was 27%. The median response duration was 12.5 weeks and the median survival was 12 months.

Despite the promising activity seen in this trial, there have been few combination chemotherapy studies of gemcitabine in small cell lung cancer. A phase I study undertaken in patients with both SCLC and NSCLC showed that gemcitabine 1000 mg/m^2 weekly for 3 weeks could be administered safely with etoposide 80 mg/m^2 daily on days 8, 9, and 10 (RASSMANN et al. 1997). A phase II trial limited to patients with SCLC is currently ongoing. In a phase I Canadian trial, gemcitabine was combined with both etoposide and cisplatin. At all dose levels, cisplatin 75 mg/m^2 was administered on day 1. Gemcitabine was administered on days 1 and 8 and etoposide on days 1–5. Severe myelotoxicity was encountered at gemcitabine and etoposide doses of 800 mg/m^2 and 100 mg/m^2 respectively. Both drugs were lowered at subsequent dose levels, and to date, acceptable toxicity has been seen with gemcitabine 1000 mg/m^2 days 1 and 8 and etoposide 50 mg/m^2 days 1–5 with cisplatin 75 mg/m^2 on day 1. This study is ongoing and response and survival rates are not yet available.

It is clear that gemcitabine is active in both SCLC and NSCLC. As a single agent, it is extremely well-tolerated, and when combined with cisplatin favorable response and survival rates have been observed in many studies. The true role of gemcitabine awaits the results of future randomized trials.

22.5 Vinorelbine

22.5.1 Mechanism of Action

Vinorelbine (Navelbine) is a novel semisynthetic vinca alkaloid that differs from others in this class by the presence of an 8-member rather than a 9-member catharanthine ring. Its antitumor effect is exerted by binding to tubulin during polymerization, inhibiting microtubule assembly and preventing mitotic spindle formation required for cell division (SORENSON 1995). Vinorelbine differs functionally from other vinca alkoids by being relatively selective for mitotic microtubules compared to axonal microtubules, suggesting that vinorelbine should be associated with less neurotoxicity and an improved therapeutic ratio (BINET et al. 1989).

22.5.2 Phase I Trials

On the basis of broad antitumor activity shown in preclinical studies compared to other vincas, phase I clinical studies were initiated. The recommended phase II dose was 25–30 mg/m^2/week, with neutropenia being the dose limiting toxicity (LEVEQUE et al. 1992). Severe non-hematologic toxicity is uncommon; however, alopecia, asthenia, neuropathy, pain and respiratory reactions characterized by dyspnea, bronchopasm, or cough occurring within 1 h of infusion have been reported. Like other vinca alkaloids, vinorelbine is a vesicant. Phlebitis occurs in 6% of patients; however, shortening infusion times to 6–10 min may reduce the incidence (HOHNEKER 1994). Vinorelbine exhibits a triexponential pattern of elimination with a prolonged terminal phase half-life ranging from 27.7 to 43.6 h. The primary pathways for elimination are hepatic metabolism and biliary excretion (WARGIN and SOLLUCAS 1994).

22.5.3 Non-Small Cell Lung Cancer

22.5.3.1 Phase II Single Agent Trials

There have been four phase II studies of single agent vinorelbine in chemotherapy-naive patients with advanced NSCLC. When vinorelbine was administered at a dose of 20–30 mg/m^2 weekly, response rates ranged from 29% to 37% (Depierre et al. 1991; Crivellari et al. 1992; Lonardi et al. 1992; Yokoyama et al. 1992). Vinorelbine does not have substantial activity in pretreated patients (Pronzato et al. 1994).

22.5.3.2 Combination Chemotherapy Trials with Vinorelbine

Four randomized trials comparing vinorelbine to other agents in patients with stage III or IV NSCLC have been reported. Le Chevalier and colleagues randomly assigned 612 patients with stage III or IV NSCLC to receive one of three treatments: vinorelbine alone, vinorelbine and cisplatin, or vindesine and cisplatin. Response rates were 14%, 30% and 19% and median durations of survival for the 3 treatment arms were 31 weeks, 40 weeks, and 32 weeks respectively. The differences in response rates and overall survival were statistically significant in favor of the vinorelbine-cisplatin combination compared to the other treatment arms. Toxic effects were noted most frequently in the cisplatin arms. Neutropenia occurred more frequently in the vinorelbine plus cisplatin group than in the vindesine plus cisplatin group (78% vs 47.6%, $P < 0.001$) and neurotoxic effects occurred more frequently in the vindesine plus cisplatin group (17% vs 7%, $P < 0.04$) (Le Chevalier et al. 1994).

In contrast, Depierre and colleagues randomly assigned 240 patients with stage III or IV NSCLC to receive either vinorelbine alone or vinorelbine and cisplatin. Although the response rates were significantly different and favored the combination (16% vs 43%, $P = 0.0001$), the median durations of survival were strikingly similar (32 weeks and 33 weeks). Nausea and vomiting, neurologic effects, renal impairement and myelosuppression were noted more frequently in the combination chemotherapy group (Depierre et al. 1994).

Crawford and colleagues used a 2:1 randomization schedule to assign 216 patients with stage IV NSCLC to receive either vinorelbine or leucovorin and 5-fluorouracil. This latter chemotherapy regimen is considered to be virtually inactive in NSCLC. While response rates did not differ significantly between groups: 12% in the vinorelbine group vs 3% in the 5-FU leucovorin group, the median duration of survival was significantly better among patients receiving vinorelbine (30 weeks vs 22 weeks, $P = 0.03$) (Crawford et al. 1996).

These three studies have shown consistently that treatment with vinorelbine as a single agent or in combination with cisplatin results in superior survival. The important question of whether vinorelbine adds to the activity of cisplatin was addressed in a recently completed study which compared single-agent cisplatin to cisplatin and vinorelbine in 432 patients with stage IV disease. Response rates, median and 1 year survival were 10% and 25%, 6 and 7 months, and 12% and 33% respectively in favor of the combination (Wozniak et al. 1996).

Although this two-drug regimen appears to be superior to other vinca-cisplatin combinations, substituting one vinca for another in a three-drug combination has not been shown to produce better results. In a randomized phase III study which compared vindesine to vinorelbine in a cisplatin, mitomycin and vinca alkaloid chemotherapeutic regimen, substitution with vinorelbine did not lead to a significant improvement in objective response rate or survival among 227 stage III and IV NSCLC patients. There was a reduction in neurotoxicity (23% vs 6% grade 2–4) but an increase in hematologic toxicity (61% vs 87% grade 3 to 4 neutropenia) with the vinorelbine containing combination (Perol et al. 1996).

Collectively, these studies suggest that cisplatin and vinorelbine should be considered a standard regimen for treating NSCLC and a standard arm in future randomized trials evaluating newer combinations. They also suggest that vinorelbine as a single agent is an effective, well tolerated agent for patients unable to receive cisplatin. Studies of vinorelbine and cisplatin are now underway to determine the efficacy of this regimen in earlier stage disease.

22.5.4 Small Cell Lung Cancer

22.5.4.1 Single Agent Phase II Trials

Vinorelbine is active against SCLC. In a phase II trial of vinorelbine 30 mg/m^2 weekly, 11 of 30 (26.7%) chemotherapy-naive patients responded (Depierre et al. 1997). Three phase II trials have assessed vinorelbine 25–30 mg/m^2 weekly in previously treated patients. Collectively, the response rate was 25% (range 12.5%–46%) among 75 evaluable patients (Depierre et al. 1997; Furuse et al. 1996;

Jassem et al. 1993). Grade 3 and 4 leukopenia occurred in 32%–66.7% and grade 3 anemia occurred in up to 20.8% of patients. Peripheral neuropathy has occurred in cisplatin pretreated patients.

22.5.5 Combined Modality Therapy with Radiation

Radiation sensitizing effects have been observed with vinorelbine in cell culture. The greatest potentiation was seen when irradiated cells were exposed to vinorelbine after they had plateaued in the G2/M phase of the cycle (Edelstein et al. 1996). There is clinical evidence to support these in vitro effects. In a phase I study of vinorelbine administered once weekly with cisplatin 100 mg/m^2 every 21 days and concomitant thoracic radiation therapy (2 Gy/day times 30 fractions for 60 Gy) (Vokes et al. 1996), dose-limiting myelosuppression was seen at a vinorelbine dose of 25 mg/m^2/week. Grade 4 neutropenia occurred in two of three patients and one patient died from neutropenic sepsis. At vinorelbine 20 mg/m^2/week, grade 3 or 4 esophagitis developed in three of six patients near the end or after completion of radiation therapy. The significant dose reduction of vinorelbine that is necessary with concomitant radiation therapy provides the first in vivo evidence of a strong radiosensitizing effect of vinorelbine. The schedule is currently being modified to reduce the incidence of esophagitis.

22.6 Conclusion

In the coming decades, lung cancer will remain a major health problem worldwide. Thus, treatment strategies must focus on improvements in early detection and on the development of innovative therapies. The last few years have seen a doubling of the number of active agents for this classically chemoresistant tumor. There is no doubt that the clinical data has confirmed that the taxoids, camptothecins, gemicitabine and vinorelbine all represent exciting new chemotherapeutic agents. Already, phase III studies have demonstrated that two of these new agents, paclitaxel and vinorelbine in combination with cisplatin, are superior to older regimens. However, the role each drug will play in improving survival or palliating symptoms of lung cancer patients is still evolving with the present generation of randomized trials. Optimization of combination chemotherapy, radiotherapy regimens, and timing of the modalities are areas requiring further development. Hopefully, these regimens will produce clinically meaningful survival benefits and decrease therapy-related toxicities to ensure that the added quantity of life translates into improved quality of life.

References

Abigerges D, Armand JP, Chabot GG et al (1994) Irinotecan (CPT-11) high-dose escalation using intensive high-dose loperamide to control diarrhea. J Natl Cancer Inst 86: 446–449

Abratt RP, Bezwoda WR, Goedhals L et al (1997) Weekly gemcitabine with monthly cisplatin: effective chemotherapy for advanced, non-small cell lung cancer. J Clin Oncol 15:744–749

Alberola V, Rosell R, Gonzalez-Larriba JL et al (1995) Single agent Taxol, 3-hour infusion, in untreated advanced non-small cell lung cancer. Ann Oncol 6[Suppl 3]:S49–S51

Anderson H, Thatcher N, Walling J et al (1994) A phase I study of 24 hour infusion of gemcitabine in patients with previously untreated, locally advanced non-small cell lung cancer. Proc Am Soc Clin Oncol 13:348 (abstract)

Anton A, Artal A, Carrato A et al (1997) Gemcitabine plus cisplatin in advanced NSCLC: final phase II results. Proc Am Soc Clin Oncol 16:461 (abstract)

Antonia SJ, Wagner H, Williams C et al (1995) Concurrent paclitaxel/cisplatin with thoracic radiation in patients with stage IIIA/B non-small cell carcinoma of the lung. Semin Oncol 22[4 Suppl 9]:34–7

Araki E, Ishikawa M, Iigo M, Koide T, Itabashi M, Hoshi A (1993) Relationship between development of diarrhea and the concentration of SN-38, an active metabolite of CPT-11, in the intestine and the blood plasma of athymic mice following intraperitoneal administration of CPT-11. Jpn J Cancer Res 84:697–702

Ardizzoni A, Hansen H, Dombernowsky P et al (1997) Topotecan, a new active drug in the second-line treatment of small-cell lung cancer: a phase II study in patients with refractory and sensitive disease. J Clin Oncol 15: 2090–2096

Bertrand R, O'Connor PM, Kerrigan D, Pommier Y (1992) Sequential administration of camptothecin and etoposide circumvents the antagonistic cytotoxicity of simultaneous drug administration in slowly growing human colon carcinoma HT-29 cells. Eur J Cancer 28A:743–748

Binet S, Fellous A, Meininger V (1989) In situ analysis of the action of Navelbine on various types of microtubules using immunofluorescence. Semin Oncol 16[Suppl 4]:5–8

Bissery MC, Vrignaud P, Bayssas M et al (1995) Preclinical in vivo activity of docetaxel-containing combinations. Proc Am Soc Clin Oncol 14:489

Bonomi P, Kim K, Chang A et al (1996) Phase II trial comparing etoposide, cisplatin versus Taxol with cisplatin-G-CSF versus Taxol-cisplatin in advanced non-small cell lung cancer. An Eastern Cooperative Group (ECOG) trial. Proc Am Soc Clin Oncol 15:382 (abstract)

Boring CC, Squires TS, Tong TT et al (1994) Cancer statistics. CA 44:7–26

Burkes RL, Shepherd FA (1995) Gemcitabine in the treatment of non-small-cell lung cancer. Ann Oncol 6:S57–60

Burris HA, Hanauske AR, Johnson RK, Marshall MH, Kuhn JG, Hilsenbeck SG, Von Hoff DD (1992) Activity of topotecan, a new topoisomerase I inhibitor, against human tumor colony-forming units in vitro. J Natl Cancer Inst 84:1816–1820

Cardenal F, Rosell R, Anton A et al (1997) Gemcitabine plus cisplatin versus etoposide in advanced non-small cell lung cancer patients: preliminary randomized phase III results. Proc Am Soc Clin Oncol 16:458 (abstract)

Cerny T, Kaplan S, Pavlidis N et al (1994) Docetaxel (Taxotere) is active in non small cell lung cancer: a phase II trial of the EORTC Early Clinical Trials Group (ECTG). Br J Cancer 70:384–387

Chang AY, Kim K, Glick J et al (1993) Phase II study of taxol, merbarone, and piroxantrone in stage IV non-small cell lung cancer: the ECOG results. J Natl Cancer Inst 85: 388–393

Choy H, Rodriguez F, Koester S et al (1992) Synergistic effects of Taxol/Taxotere on radiation sensitivity on human tumor cells. Int J Radiat Oncol Biol Phys 24:274–275 (abstract)

Choy H, Akerley W, Safran H et al (1994) Phase I trial of outpatient weekly paclitaxel and concurrent radiation therapy for advanced non-small-cell lung cancer. J Clin Oncol 12:2682–2686

Choy H, Akerley W, Safran H, Graziano S, Chung C (1996) Paclitaxel plus carboplatin and concurrent radiation therapy for patients with locally advanced non-small cell lung cancer. Seminars in Oncology 23[6 Suppl 16]: 117–119

Clarke P, Schiller JH, Von Pawel J et al (1997) Preliminary results of a randomized comparative phase III trial of topotecan versus CAV as second-line therapy of small cell lung cancer. Eur J Cancer 33[Suppl 8]:S228 (abstract)

Clavel M, Guastella J, Peters G (1989) Phase I study of LY188011, 2′ 2′-difluorodeoxycytadine. Invest New Drugs 7:379

Cole JT, Gralla RJ, Marques CB et al (1995) Phase I-II study of cisplatin + docetaxel (Taxotere) in non-small cell lung cancer (NSCLC). Proc Am Soc Clin Oncol 14:357 (abstract)

Cormier Y, Eisenhauer E, Muldal A et al (1994) Gemcitabine is an active new agent in previously untreated extensive small cell lung cancer (SCLC). A study of the National Cancer Institute of Canada Clinical Trials Group. Ann Oncol 5:283–285

Cortes JE, Pazdur R (1995) Docetaxel. J Clin Oncol 13:2643–2655

Crawford J, O'Rourke M, Schiller JH et al (1996) Randomized trial of vinorelbine compared with fluorouracil plus leucovorin in patients with Stage IV non-small cell lung cancer. J Clin Oncol 14:2774–2784

Crino L, Scagliotti G, Marangolo M et al (1997) Cisplatin-gemcitabine combination in advanced non-small cell lung cancer: a phase II study. J Clin Oncol 15:297–303

Crivellari D, Veronesi A, Sacco C et al (1992) Phase II study of vinorelbine (V) in 50 patients with non-small cell lung cancer (NSCLC). Proc Am Soc Clin Oncol 11:1192 (abstract)

Del Bino G, Lassota P, Darzynkiewicz Z (1991) The S-phase cytotoxicity of camptothecin. Exp Cell Res 193:27–35

Del Bino G, Bruno S, Yi PN, Darzynkiewicz Z (1992) Apoptotic cell death triggered by camptothecin or teniposide. The cell cycle specificity and effects of ionizing radiation. Cell Proliferation 25:537–548

Depierre A, Lemarie E, Dabouis G et al (1991) A phase II study of Navelbine (vinorelbine) in the treatment of non-small cell lung cancer. Am J Clin Oncol 14:115–119

Depierre A, Chastang CI, Quoix E et al (1994) Vinorelbine versus vinorelbine plus cisplatin in advanced non-small cell lung cancer: a randomized trial. Ann Oncol 5:37–42

Depierre A, Le Chavalier T, Quoix E et al (1997) Phase II trial of navelbine (NVB) in small cell lung cancer (SCLC). Lung Cancer 18[Suppl 1]:3 (abstract)

Donehower RC, Rowinksy EK (1993) An overview of experience with Taxol (paclitaxel) in the U.S.A. Cancer Treat Rev 19[Suppl C]:63–78

Douillard JY, Ibrahim N, Riviere A, Spaeth D, Chomy P, Soussan K, Mathieu-Boue A (1995) Phase II study of CPT-11 in non small cell lung cancer (NSCLC). Proc Am Soc Clin Oncol 14:365 (abstract)

Eckardt J, Depierre A, Ardizzoni A et al (1997) Pooled analysis of topotecan (T) in the second-line treatment of patients (pts) with sensitive small-cell lung cancer (SCLC). Proc Am Soc Clin Ocol 16:1624 (abstract)

Edelstein MP, Wolfe LA 3rd, Duch DS (1996) Potentiation of radiation therapy by vinorelbine (Navelbine) in non-small cell lung cancer. Sem Oncol 23[2 Suppl 5]:41–47

Einhorn L (1997) Phase II trial of gemcitabine plus cisplatin in non-small cell lung cancer: a Hoosier Oncology Group study. Semin Oncol 24:S8-24–S8-26

Ettinger DS, Finkelstein DM, Sarma RP, Johnson DH (1995) Phase II study of paclitaxel in patients with extensive-disease small-cell lung cancer: an Eastern Coo perative Oncology Group study. J Clin Oncol 13:1430–1435

Finkelstein DM, Ettinger DS, Ruckdeschel JC (1986) Long-term survivors in metastatic non-small cell lung cancer: an Eastern Cooperative Oncology Group study. J Clin Oncol 4:702–709

Fosella FK, Lippman SM, Shin DM et al (1997) Maximum-tolerated dose defined for single-agent gemcitabine: a phase I dose-escalation study in chemotherapy-naive patients with advanced non-small-cell lung cancer. J Clin Oncol 15:310–316

Fossella FV, Lee JS, Murphy WK et al (1994) Phase II study of docetaxel for recurrent or metastatic non-small cell lung cancer. J Clin Oncol 12:1232–1244

Fossella FV, Lee JS, Shin DM et al (1995) Phase II study of docetaxel for advanced or metastatic platinum-refractory non-small cell lung cancer. J Clin Oncol 13:645–651

Francis P, Rigas JF, Kris MG et al (1994) Phase II trial of docetaxel patients with stage III and IV non-small-cell lung cancer. J Clin Oncol 12:1232–1237

Francis PA, Dris MG, Rigas JR, Grant SC, Miller VA (1995) Paclitaxel (Taxol) and Docetaxel (Taxotere): active chemotherapeutic agents in lung cancer. Lung Cancer 12[Suppl 1]:S163–S172

Friedman HS, Houghton PJ, Schold SC, Keir S, Bigner DD (1994) Activity of 9-dimethylaminomethyl-10-hydroxycamptothecin against pediatric and adult central nervous system tumor xenografts. Cancer Chemother Pharmacol 34:171–174

Fujiwara Y, Yamakido M, Fukuoka M et al for the West Japan Lung Cancer Study Group (1994) Phase II study of irinotecan (CPT-11) and cisplatin (CDDP) in patients with small cell lung cancer (SCLC). Proc Am Soc Clin Oncol 13:335 (abstract)

Fukuoka M, Niitani H, Suzuki A et al (1992) A phase II study of CPT-11, a new derivative of camptothecin, for previously untreated non-small-cell lung cancer. J Clin Oncol 10:16–20

Furuse K, Kubota K, Kawahara M et al (1996) Phase II study of vinorelbine in heavily previously treated small cell lung cancer. Oncology 53:169–172

Gandia D, Abigerges D, Armand JP et al (1993) CPT-11-induced cholinergic effects in cancer patients. J Clin Oncol 11:196–197

Gatzemeier U, Shepherd FA (1996) Activity of gemcitabine in patients with non-small cell lung cancer: a multicentre, extended phase II study. Eur J Cancer 32(2):243–248

Gatzemeier U, Heckmayr M, Neuhauss R et al (1995) Phase II study with paclitaxel for the treatment of advanced inoperable non-small cell lung cancer. Lung Cancer 12[Suppl 2]:S101–S106

Gatzemeier U, Manegold CH, Eberhard W et al (1997) A phase II trial of gemcitabine and ifosphamide in non-small cell lung cancer. Semin Oncol 24:S8-36–S8-38

Gelmon K (1994) The taxoids: paclitaxel and docetaxel. Lancet 344:1267–1272

Giaccone G, Splinter T, Postmus P et al (1996) Paclitaxel-cisplatin versus teniposide-cisplatin in advanced non-small cell lung cancer (NSCLC). Proc Am Soc Clin Oncol 15:1109 (abstract)

Ginsberg RJ, Kris MG, Armstrong JG (1994) Non-small cell lung cancer. In: DeVita VT Jr, Hellman S, Rosenberg SA (eds) Cancer principles and practice of oncology, 4th edn. Lippincott, Philadelphia, p 673

Goor C, Scalliet P, Vanmeerbeek J et al (1996) A phase II study combining gemcitabine and radiotherapy in stage III NSCLC. Ann Oncol 7[Suppl 5]:101

Goto K, Nishiwaki Y, Saijo N et al (1995) A phase II study of irinotecan (CPT-11) and etoposide (VP-16) for metastatic non-small cell lung cancer (NSCLC): Japanese Clinical Oncology Group (JCOG) trial. Proc Am Soc Clin Oncol 14:362 (abstract)

Gottlieb JA, Luce JK (1972) Treatment of malignant melanoma with camptothecin (NSC-100880). Cancer Chemother Rep 56:103–105

Graham MV, Jahanzeb M, Dresler CM et al (1996) Results of a trial with topotecan dose escalation and concurrent thoracic radiation therapy for locally advanced, inoperable non-small cell lung cancer. Int J Rad Oncol Biol Phys 36:1215–1220

Green MR (1993) New directions for chemotherapy in non-small cell lung cancer. Chest 103:370s-372s

Grochow LB, Slichenmeyer W, Rowinsky E, Donehower R, Forastiere A, Chen TL (1994) Phase I clinical and pharmacologic study of topotecan (top) in patients with hepatic or renal dysfunction. Ann Oncol 5[Suppl 5]:191 (abstract)

Gupta E, Lestingi TM, Mick R, Ramirez J, Vokes EE, Ratain MJ (1994) Metabolic fate of irinotecan in humans: correlation of glucuronidation with diarrhea. Cancer Res 54: 3723–3725

Hainsworth JD, Thompson DS, Greco FA (1995) Paclitaxel by 1-hour infusion: an active drug in metastatic non-small cell lung cancer. J Clin Oncol 13:1609–1614

Hohneker JA (1994) A summary of vinorelbine (Navelbine) safety data from North American Clinical Trials. Semin Oncol 21[Suppl 10]:42–47

Hsiang YH, Liu LF (1988) Identification of mammalian DNA topoisomerase I as an intracellular target of the anticancer drug camptothecin. Cancer Res 48:1722–1726

Hsiang YH, Liu LF, Wall ME et al (1989) DNA topoisomerase I-mediated DNA cleavage and cytotoxicity of camptothecin analogues. Cancer Res 49:4385–4389

Janik J, Miller L, Smith J, Kopp W, Alvord G, Gause B, Curit B, Urba WJ, Longo DL (1993) Prechemotherapy granulocyte-macrophage colony stimulating factor (GM-CSF) prevents topotecan-induced neutropenia. Proc Am Soc Clin Oncol 12:437 (abstract)

Jassem J, Karnicka-Mlodkowska H, van Pottelsberghe C et al (1993) Phase II study of vinorelbine (Navelbine) in previously treated small cell lung cancer patients. Eur J Cancer 29A:1720–1722

Jekunen AP, Cristen RD, Shalinsky DR, Howell SB (1994) Synergistic interaction between cisplatin and taxol in human ovarian carcinoma cells in vitro. Br J Cancer 69: 299–306

Johnson DH, Paul DM, Hande KR et al (1996) Paclitaxel plus carboplatin in advanced non-small cell lung cancer – a phase II trial. J Clin Oncol 14:2054–2060

Kano Y, Suzuki K, Akutsu M, Suda K, Inoue Y, Yoshida M, Sakamoto S, Miura Y (1992) Effects of CPT-11 in combination with other anti-cancer agents in culture. Int J Cancer 50:604–610

Kaufmann SH (1991) Antagonism between camptothecin and topoisomerase II-directed chemotherapeutic agents in a human leukemia cell line. Cancer Res 51:1129–1136

Kawato Y, Aonuma M, Hirota Y, Kuga H, Sato K (1991a) Intracellular roles of SN-38, a metabolite of the camptothecin derivative CPT-11, in the antitumor effect of CPT-11. Cancer Res 51:4187–4191

Kim JH, Kion SH, Kolozsvary A Khil MS (1992) Potentiation of radiation response in human carcinoma cells in vitro and murine fibrosarcoma in vivo by topotecan, an inhibitor of DNA to poisomerase I. Int J Rad Oncol Biol Phys 22: 515–518

Kirshlong RJ, Jung SH, Jett JR (1994) A phase II study of Taxol and G-CSF in previously untreated patients with extensive stage small cell lung cancer (SCC). Proc Am Soc Clin Oncol [abstract] 13:326

Kawato Y, Furuta T, Aonuma M, Yasuoka M, Yokokura T, Matsumoto K (1991b) Antitumor activity of a camptothecin derivative, CPT-11, against human tumor xenografts in nude mice. Cancer Chemother Pharmacol 28:192–198

Klastersky J (1995) Small cell lung cancer: can treatment results be improved? Semin Oncol 22[Suppl 2]:1–2

Kourousis C, Kakoyris S, Androullakis N et al (1996) First-line treatment of non-small cell lung carcinoma with docetaxel and vinorelbine: a phase II study. Proc Am Soc Clin Oncol 15:374 (abstract)

Kunitoh H, Watanabe K, Onoshi T et al (1996) Phase II trial of docetaxel in previously untreated advanced non-small-cell lung cancer: a Japanese cooperative group study. J Clin Oncol 14:1649–1655

Langer CJ, Leighton JC, Comis RL et al (1995) Paclitaxel and carboplatin in combination in the treatment of advanced non-small cell lung cancer (NSCLC): a phase II toxicity, response and survival analysis (FCCC 93-024). J Clin Oncol 13:1860–1870

Latreille J, Cormier Y, Martins H, Goss G, Fisher B, Eisenhauer EA (1996) Phase II study of docetaxel (taxotere) in patients with previously untreated extensive small cell lung cancer. Investigational New Drugs 13:343–345

Lawrence TS, Eisbruch A, Shewach DS (1997) Gemcitabine mediated radiosensitization. Sem Oncol 24[2 Suppl 7]: S7-24–S7-28

Le Chevalier T, Brisgand D, Douillard JY et al (1994) Randomized study of vinorelbine and cisplatin versus vindesine and cispltin versus vinorelbine alone in advanced non-small cell lung cancer: results of a European multicenter trial including 612 patients. J Clin Oncol 12:360–367

Le Chevalier T, Belli L, Monnier A et al (1995) Phase II study of docetaxel (Taxotere) and cisplatin in advanced non-small cell lung cancer (NSCLC), an interim analysis. Proc Am Soc Clin Oncol 14:350 (abstract)

Leveque D, Jehl F, Quoix E et al (1992) Clinical pharmacokinetics of vinorelbine alone and combined with cisplatin. J Clin Pharmacol 32:1096–1098

Lilenbaum RC, Ratain MJ, Miller AA et al (1995) Phase I study of paclitaxel and topotecan in patients with advanced tumors: a cancer and leukemia group B study. J Clin Oncol 13:2230–2237

Lonardi F, Pavanoto G, Jirillo A et al (1992) Vinorelbine (VNB) as single agent chemotherapy (CT) in advanced non-small cell lung cancer (NSCLC) patients (pts). Proc Am Soc Clin Oncol 11:A1123

Lynch TJ Jr, Kalish L, Strauss G et al (1994) Phase II study of topotecan in metastatic non-small-cell lung cancer. J Clin Oncol 12:347–352

Manegold C, Bergman B, Chemaissani A et al (1997) Single-agent gemcitabine versus cisplatin-etoposide: early results of a randomized phase II study in locally-advanced or metastatic non-small cell lung cancer. Ann Oncol 8: 525–529

Masuda N, Fukuoka M, Kusunoki Y et al (1992) CPT-11: a new derivative of camptothecin for the treatment of refractory or relapsed small-cell lung cancer. J Clin Oncol 10: 1225–1229

Masuda N, Fukuoka M, Kudoh S et al (1993) Phase I and pharmacologic study of irinotecan in combination with cisplatin for advanced lung cancer. Br J Cancer 68:777–782

Masuda N, Fukuoka M, Kudoh S et al (1994a) Phase I and pharmacologic study of irinotecan and etoposide with recombinant human granulocyte colony-stimulating factor support for advanced lung cancer. J Clin Oncol 12:1833–1841

Masuda N, Fukuoka M, Kudoh S et al (1994b) Phase I study of irinotecan and cisplatin with granulocyte colony-stimulating factor support for advanced non-small-cell lung cancer. J Clin Oncol 12:90–96

Mattern MR, Hofmann GA, McCabe FL, Johnson RK (1991) Synergistic cell killing by ionizing/radiation and topoisomerase I inhibitor topotecan (SkbF104864) Cancer Res 51:5813–5816

Miller AA, Hargis JB, Lilenbaum RC, Fields SZ, Rosner GL, Schilsky RL (1994) Phase I study of topotecan and cisplatin in patients with advanced solid tumors: a cancer and leukemia group B study. J Clin Oncol 12:2743–2750

Miller VA, Rigas JR, Francis PA et al (1995) Phase II trial of 75 mg/m^2 dose of docetaxel with prednisone premedication for patients with advanced non-small cell lung cancer. Cancer 75:968–972

Millward MJ, Bishop JF, Friedlander M et al (1996) Phase II trial of a 3-hour infusion of paclitaxel in previously untreated patients with non-small-cell lung cancer. J Clin Oncol 14:142–148

Millward MJ, Zalcberg J, Bishop JF et al (1997) Phase I trial of docetaxel and cisplatin in previously untreated patents with advanced non-small cell lung cancer. J Clin Oncol 15:750–758

Moertel CG, Schutt AJ, Reitemeier RJ, Hahn RG (1972) Phase II study of camptothecin (NSC-100880) in the treatment of advanced gastrointestinal cancer. Cancer Chemother Rep 56:95–101

Mori K, Ohnishi T, Yokoyama K, Tominaga K (1997a) A phase I study of irinotecan and infusional cisplatin for advanced non-small-cell lung cancer. Cancer Chemother Pharmacol 39:327–332

Mori K, Hirose T, Machida S, Yokoyama K, Tominaga K (1997b) A phase I study of irinotecan and infusional cisplatin with recombinant human granulocyte colony-stimulating factor support in the treatment of advanced non-small cell lung cancer. Eur J Cancer 33:503–505

Muggia FM, Creaven PJ, Hansen HH, Cohen MH, Selawry OS (1972) Phase I clinical trial of weekly and daily treatment with camptothecin (NSC-100880): correlation with preclinical studies. Cancer Chemother Rep 56: 515–521

Murphy B, Saltz L, Sirott M et al (1992) Granulocyte-colony stimulating factor (G-CSF) does not increase the maximum tolerated dose (MTD) in a phase I study of topotecan. Proc Am Soc Clin Oncol 11:139 (abstract)

Murphy WK, Fossella FV, Winn RJ et al (1993) Phase II study of taxol in untreated advanced non-small cell lung cancer. J Natl Cancer Inst 85:384–387

Murphy WK, Win RJ, Humber M et al (1994) Phase II study of Taxol in patients with non-small lung cancer who have failed platinum containing chemotherapy. Proc Am Soc Clin Oncol 13:357 (abstract)

Narita M, Nagai E, Hagiwara H, Aburada M, Yokoi T, Kamataki T (1993) Inhibition of beta-glucuronidase by natural glucuronides of kampo medicines using glucuronide of SN-38 (7-ethyl-10-hydroxycamptothecin) as a substrate. Xenobiotica 23:5–10

Negoro S, Fukuoka M, Masuda N et al (1991a) Phase I study of weekly intravenous infusions of CPT-11, a new derivative of camptothecin, in the treatment of advanced non-small-cell lung cancer. J Natl Cancer Inst 83:1164–1168

Negoro S, Fukuoka M, Niitani H et al (1991b) A phase II study of CPT-11, a camptothecin derivative, in patients with primary lung cancer. CPT-11 Cooperative Study Group. Gan To Kagaku Ryoho 18:1013–1019

O'Rourke TJ, Brown TD, Havlin K et al (1994) Phase I clinical trials of gemcitabine given as an intravenous bolus on five consecutive days. Eur J Cancer 30A:417–418

O'Reilly S, Fleming GF, Barker SD et al (1997) Phase I trial and pharmacologic trial of sequences of paclitaxel and topotecan in previously treated ovarian epithelial malignancies: a Gynecologic Oncology Group study. J Clin Oncol 15:177–186

Oshita F, Noda K, Nishiwaki Y et al (1997) Phase II study of irinotecan and etoposide in patients with metastatic non-small-cell lung cancer. J Clin Oncol 15:304–309

Perez-Soler R, Fossella FV, Glisson BS et al (1996a) Phase II study of topotecan in patients with advanced non-small-cell lung cancer previously untreated with chemotherapy. J Clin Oncol 14:503–513

Perez-Soler R, Glisson BS, Lee JS et al (1996b) Treatment of patients with small-cell lung cancer refractory to etoposide and cisplatin with the topoisomerase I poison topotecan. J Clin Oncol 14:2785–2790

Perng RP, Chen YM, Liu JM et al (1997) Gemcitabine versus the combination of cisplatin and etoposide in patients with inoperable non-small-cell lung cancer in a phase II randomized study. J Clin Oncol 15:2097–2102

Perol M, Guerin JC, Thomas P et al (1996) Multicenter randomized trial comparing cisplatin-mitomycin-vinorelbine versus cisplatin-mitomycin-vindesine in advanced non-small cell lung cancer. Lung Cancer 14: 119–134

Peters GJ, Bergman AM, Ruiz van Haperen V, Veerman G, Kuiper C, Braakhuis B (1995) Interaction between cisplatin and gemcitabine in vitro and in vivo. Semin Oncol 22[Suppl 11]:72–29

Plunkett W, Huang P, Xu YZ, Heinemann V, Grunewald R, Gandhi V (1995) Gemcitabine: metabolism, mechanisms of action and self-potentiation. Semin Oncol 22[Suppl 11]: 3–10

Pommier Y (1993) DNA topoisomerase I and II in cancer chemotherapy: update and perspectives. Cancer Chemother Pharmacol 32:103–108

Poplin EAD, Corbett T, Flaherty L et al (1992) Difluorodeoxycytadine (dFdC gemcitabine): a phase I study. Invest New Drugs 10:165–170

Pronzato P, Landucci M, Vaira F, Vigani A, Bertelli G. (1994) Failure of vinorelbine to produce responses in pretreated non-small cell lung cancer patients. Anticancer Res 14:1413–1416

Rassmann I, Thodtmann R, Depenbrock H et al (1997) Gemcitabine and etoposide in small cell lung cancer: phase I and II trial. Semin Oncol 24:S775–S778

Reckzeh B, Merte H, Pfluger KH et al (1996) Severe lymphocytopenia and interstitial pneumonia in patients treated with paclitaxel and simultaneous radiotherapy for non-small-cell lung cancer. J Clin Oncol 14:1071–1076

Rowinsky EK, Gilbert M, McGuire WP et al (1991) Sequences of taxol and cisplatin: a phase I and pharmacologic study. J Clin Oncol 9:1692–1703

Rowinsky EK, Grochow LB, Hendricks CB et al (1992) Phase I and pharmacologic study of topotecan: a novel topoisomerase I inhibitor. J Clin Oncol 10:647–656

Rowinsky EK, Chaudhry V, Forastiere AA et al (1993) Phase I and pharmacologic study of paclitaxel and cisplatin with granulocyte colony-stimulating factor: neuromuscular toxicity is dose-limiting. J Clin Oncol 11:2010–2020

Rowinsky EK, Grochow LB, Ettinger DS et al (1994) Phase I and pharmacological study of the novel topoisomerase I inhibitor 7-ethyl-10-[4-(1-piperidino)-1-piperidino] carbonyloxycamptothecin (CPT-11) administered as a ninety-minute infusion every 3 weeks. Cancer Res 54:427–436

Rowinsky EK, Flood WA, Sartorius SE et al (1995) Phase I study of paclitaxel as a 3-hour infusion followed by carboplatin in untreated patients with stage IV non-small cell lung cancer. Semin Oncol 22[4 Suppl 9]:48–54

Rowinsky EK, Kaufmann SH, Baker SD et al (1996) Sequences of topotecan and cisplatin: phase I, pharmacologic, and in vitro studies to examine sequence dependence. J Clin Oncol 14:3074–3084

Ruckdeschel J, Wagner H Jr, Williams C et al (1994) Second-line chemotherapy for resistant, metastatic non-small cell lung cancer (NSCLC): the role of Taxol. Proc Am Soc Clin Oncol 13:357 (abstract)

Schewach D, Lawrence T (1995) Radiosensitization of human tumor cells by gemcitibine in vitro. Sem Oncol 22:68–71

Schiller JH, Kim K, Hutson P et al (1996) Phase II study of topotecan in patients with extensive-stage small-cell carcinoma of the lung: an Eastern Cooperative Oncology Group Trial. J Clin Oncol 14:2345–2352

Sekine I, Nishiwaki Y, Watanabe K et al for the East Japan Paclitaxel Study Group (1996) Phase II study of 3 hour infusion of paclitaxel in previously untreated non-small cell lung cancer. Clin Cancer Res 2:941–945

Shepherd FA, Abratt RP, Anderson H, Gatzemeier U, Anglin G, Iglesias J (1997a) Gemcitabine in the treatment of elderly patients with advanced non-small cell lung cancer. Semin Oncol 24[Suppl 7]:50–55

Shepherd FA, Cormier Y, Burkes R et al (1997b) Phase II trial of gemcitabine and weekly cisplatin for advanced non-small cell lung cancer. Semin Oncol 24[Suppl 8]:27–30

Smit EF, Kloosterziel C, Groen HJM et al (1996) A phase II study of paclitaxel (P) in heavily pretreated patients with extensive stage small cell lung cancer (SCLC). Proc Am Soc Clin Oncol 15:394 (abstract)

Smyth JF, Smith IE, Sessa C, Schoffski P, Wanders J, Franklin H, Kaye SB (1994) Activity of docetaxel (Taxotere) in small cell lung cancer. The Early Clinical Trials Group of the EORTC. Eur J Cancer 30A:1058–1060

Sorensen JB (1995) Current position of vinorelbine in cancer chemotherapy. Ann Oncol 6:105–106

Steward WP, Dunlop DJ, Dabouis G et al (1996) A phase I/II study of gemcitabine and cisplatin in the treatment of advanced non-small cell lung cancer: preliminary results. Semin Oncol 23:43–47

Storniolo A, Allerheiligen SRB, Pearce HL (1997) Preclinical, pharmacologic and phase I studies of gemcitabine. Semin Oncol 24[Suppl 7]:S2–S7

Tamura K, Takada M, Kawase I et al (1997) Enhancement of tumor radio-response by irinotecan in human lung tumor xenografts. Jpn Cancer Res 88:218–223

Tester WJ, Jin PY, Reardon DH et al (1997) Phase II study of patients with metastatic non-small cell carcinoma of the lung treated with paclitaxel by 3-hour infusion. Cancer 79:724–729

Vokes EE, Haraf DJ, Masters GA et al (1996) Vinorelbine (Navelbine), cisplatin, and concomitant radiation therapy for advanced malignancies of the chest: a phase I study. Semin Oncol 23[2 Suppl 5]:48–52

Wall ME, Wani MC, Nicholas AW et al (1993) Plant antitumor agents. 30. Synthesis and structure activity of novel camptothecin analogues. J Med Chem 36:2689–2700

Wall ME, Wani MC, Cook CE, Palmer KH, Mcphail AT, Sim GA (1966) A. Plant antitumor agents. I. The isolation and structure of camptothecin, a novel alkaloidal leukemia and tumor inhibitor from Camptotheca acuminata. J Am Chem Soc 88:3888–3889

Wani MC, Taylor HL, Wall ME et al (1971) Plant antimor agents, VI: the isolation and structure of TAXOL, a novel antileukemic and antimor agent from *Taxus brevifolia*. Am Chem Soc 93:2325–2327

Wargin WA, Sol Lucas V (1994) The clinical pharmacokinetics of vinorelbine (Navelbine). Semin Oncol 21[suppl 10]: 21–27

Weitz JJ, Jung SH, Marschke RF Jr, Fitch TR, Jett JR (1995) Randomized phase II trial of two schedules of topotecan for the treatment of advanced stage non-small cell lung carcinoma (NSCLC): a North Central Cancer Treatment Group (NCCTG) trial. Proc Am Soc Clin Oncol 14:348 (abstract)

Wozniak AJ, Crowley JJ, Balcerzak SP et al (1996) Randomized phase III trial of cisplatin (CDDP) vs. CDDP plus Navelbine (NVB) in the treatment of advanced non-small cell lung cancer (NSCLC): report of a Southwest Oncology Group Study (SWOG-9308). Proc Am Soc Clin Oncol 15:374 (abstract)

Yokoyama A, Furuse K, Niitani H (1992) Multi-institutional phase II study of Navelbine (vinorelbine) in non-small cell cancer. Proc Am Soc Clin Oncol 11:287 (abstract)

Zhang H, D'arpa P, Liu LF (1990) A model for tumor cell killing by topoisomerase poisons. Cancer Cells 2: 23–27

23 Supportive Treatment in the Management of Lung Cancer

L. Crino

CONTENTS

23.1 Introduction

Lung cancer is the leading cause of cancer-related death in the Western world as well as in most Eastern and developing countries. Despite recent advances in diagnosis and treatment, mortality rates remain very similar to incidence rates: in Europe in the period 1978–1985, the 5-year relative survival was 8% for males and 10% for females (Berrino et al. 1995) and in North America it was 14% in a more recent survey (Parker et al. 1997). Approximately 70% of patients with non-small cell lung cancer (NSCLC) present with locally advanced (stage IIIB) or metastatic (stage IV) disease, and their 5-year survival is a dismal 2%, whereas in small cell lung cancer the overall survival rate at 5 years is less than 2% (Souhami and Law 1990). According to these data, cure must be considered unlikely for the great majority of lung cancer patients, and supportive treatment and the symptoms' palliation become the prime therapeutic objective.

L. Crino, Divisione di Oncologica Medica, Policlinico Monteluce, I-06122 Perugia, Italy

In recent years a number of randomized trials have compared best supportive care with combination chemotherapy plus best supportive care in patients with advanced NSCLC, and a meta-analysis of most of these studies shows a significant improvement for the patients treated with chemotherapy (Non-Small Cell Lung Cancer Collaborative Group 1995). Best supportive care includes palliative radiotherapy as required for superior vena caval obstruction, hemoptysis, painful bone metastases, brain metastases or bronchial obstruction. Antibiotics were used to control infections, corticosteroids to treat hypercalcemia or increased intracranial pressure. Analgesics and cough suppressants were given to all patients without restriction. Best supportive care measures produce median survivals of 16–17 weeks, and only 10–15% of patients were anticipated to be alive at 1 year, compared with a survival of approximately 26 weeks and a 1-year survival of 25% for patients receiving cisplatin-based chemotherapy.

Recently, a large randomized trial from the United Kingdom confirmed these results in 350 patients with extensive NSCLC randomized to receive mitomycin, ifosfamide, cisplatin (MIC) chemotherapy with supportive care versus supportive care alone. In this study a survival benefit was reported for patients receiving MIC compared with patients receiving supportive care (median survival 7 months and 1-year survival rate of 28% versus 4.8 months and 1-year survival rate of 18% (Cullen et al. 1997).

In all these studies combination chemotherapy induced subjective symptom improvement, enhanced performance status and increased length of remission and prolongation of life. On the basis of these considerations, the American Society of Clinical Oncology's NSCLC Guidelines include the recommendation that cisplatin-based combination chemotherapy should be offered to good PS, advanced NSCLC patients (American Society of Clinical Oncology 1997).

However, it is clear that not all advanced NSCLC patients should be treated with chemotherapy and, at the same time, that supportive treatment should be maximized and incorporated into treatment protocols of advanced NSCLC and SCLC in order to get the best results in terms of both survival and quality of life improvement.

23.2 Symptoms in Advanced Lung Cancer

In most clinical trials the efficacy of different palliation regimens has been evaluated by response to treatment, survival time, toxicity and variation in PS. A few studies specifically addressed the key question of symptom improvement. In 1992, Kreeck et al. (Curtis et al. 1991) described the most frequent symptoms in 100 patients with lung cancer referred to a palliation care service: moderate or severe pain, dyspnea, weight loss, anorexia, constipation, easy fatigue, weakness, early satiety, sleep problems and lack of energy.

More recently, in two lung cancer randomized trials conducted by the Medical Research Council, symptoms at presentation were evaluated in over 650 patients, with a patient self-reported measure of quality of life (the Rotterdam Symptom Check list), which consisted of a patient-completed questionnaire containing a core of 30 symptoms covering a number of domains (physical, psychological, sexual) plus four symptoms specific to lung cancer (cough, hemoptysis, chest pain and hoarseness) and one further item (restlessness) (Frith 1992).

The more frequently reported pretreatment symptoms included general symptoms (tiredness, lack of appetite) and psychological distress (worry, anxiety) in addition to disease-related chest symptoms (chest pain, cough, dyspnea) and were equally distributed both in small and non-small lung cancer (Hopwood et al. 1995).

Thus to fully evaluate the impact of supportive treatment in lung cancer patients, it is necessary to take into account the physical dimension including the most relevant symptoms for lung cancer (anorexia, fatigue, cough, dyspnea, hemoptysis and pain) (Hollen et al. 1994) and the functional dimension, a variable related to those activities associated with cognitive and social functioning which may be affected in the cancer experience.

23.3 Supportive Treatment of Physical Symptoms

In advanced lung cancer, fatigue, anorexia-cachexia, dyspnea and pain represent the most distressing and common symptoms of disease. Recently, Hollen et al. (1994) tested, in 144 NSCLC patients enrolled in a chemotherapy trial, a conceptual model for quality of life for lung cancer patients, the Lung Symptoms Scale, to develop a subjective measure for clinical trials. Fatigue was the greatest significant predictor of symptomatic distress across all three assessments throughout therapy and it is particularly relevant because fatigue is related to both treatment and malignancy.

Fatigue should be viewed as a multidimensional experience involving not only biochemical or pathophysiological causes, but also psychological and behavioral aspects (Glaus 1993), which remains very difficult both to assess and to evaluate in its outcome despite the recent emergence of measurement tools in quality of life studies.

Fatigue is often found as a single item in self-report evaluation of symptoms and psychological status, reflecting the possible interaction with other symptoms related to quality of life.

Recent research suggests that some correlation does exist between fatigue and depression, especially in the context of advanced disease (Visser and Smets 1998), indicating the opportunity for specific psychological support beside the traditional physical treatments.

Anorexia and cachexia are very common symptoms in cancer patients involving more than 80% of patients, and cachexia is the main cause of death in more than 20% of patients (Dunlops 1996). Their causes are related to severe metabolic abnormalities such as profound lipolysis, wasting in muscle protein, increased metabolic rate and production of cytokines and tumor by-products such as tumor necrosis factor (TNF) and interleukin-1 (Billingsly and Alexander 1996). Anorexia and cachexia worsen with tumor progression and disappear in patients responsive to cancer treatment.

The great majority of cachectic cancer patients, all of them with lung cancer, have incurable disease and the main therapeutic goal should be to improve symptoms and performance status.

Therapeutic intervention should be multidirected because anorexia-cachexia is a multi-casual syndrome, depending on gastrointestinal dismotility, depression, nausea, pain and side effects of pain drugs and chemotherapy.

Progestational drugs (megestrol acetate), corticosteroids and prokinetic agents (metoclopramide) have an established role in the treatment of anorexia-cachexia (BRUERA 1998).

Megestrol acetate seems to act by mechanisms other than weight gain, causing increasing appetite and decreasing fatigue, suggesting common features between cachexia and fatigue (BRUERA 1998).

Of the newly emerging drugs, thalidomide, melatonin, clenbuterol, pentoxifylline, and the cannabinoids have provided preliminary suggestions of activity in animal models and in some clinical trials, justifying further investigations (BRUERA 1998).

Dyspnea is a very common and troublesome symptom for patients with lung cancer. It can result directly from the obstruction of the central airways due to neoplastic growth in the trachea, bifurcation or main stem bronchi.

Laser disobliteration is the safest and quickest way to treat patients with severe obstruction, with good palliation being obtained in most situations.

Other methods have been developed to obtain median and long-term relief of central airways stenosis, such as photodynamic laser treatment, brachytherapy and endoscopic implantation of devices for disobliteration and internal stabilization, i.e., stenting of airways. However, dyspnea is also a prevalent symptom in the terminal stages, as 50–70% of all cancer patients will experience dyspnea during the last 6 weeks of life.

The etiology of dyspnea in terminal patients is often multifactorial, including progression of primary lung cancer or pulmonary metastases, development of pleural effusions, anemia, pulmonary emboli, infections, lymphangitic spread or multiple combinations of these variables. Dyspnea can also be worsened because of ascites or weakness of respiratory muscles as in cachexia or lung fibrosis secondary to chemotherapy or radiotherapy.

Management of dyspnea in cancer patients relies mainly on the possibility of removing its cause, correcting anemia, tapping pleural fluid, and treating infections or tumor growth by chemotherapy.

General measures in palliative treatment of dyspnea in terminal patients include oxygen therapy and steroids to reduce edema and inflammation of obstruction lesions or to treat lymphangitic cancer dissemination. Scopolamine or hyoscine given by subcutaneous injection can be very useful in reducing upper airway secretions, whereas bronchodilatators are controversial, causing tachycardia, tachypnea and increasing anxiety (FARCOMBE 1997).

Oral or subcutaneous opioids decrease the perception of breathlessness and improve dyspnea in the majority of patients without inducing respiratory depression (BRUERA et al. 1993). Evaluation of small doses of nebulized opioids acting peripherally on lung receptors is still ongoing (FARCOMBE et al. 1994). The management of anxiety associated with dyspnea through relaxation, breathing techniques and psychological support is very important for the improvement of the comfort level of the patient and family in the terminal stage of the disease.

Pain is a common and distressing symptom of lung cancer. It results from neoplastic infiltration of the thoracic wall, mediastinum or superior sulcus with consequent tissue nervous termination injury: the biochemicals released by tissue injury excite nociceptors or increase their sensitivity in the mechanism of primary hyperalgesia.

Secondary hyperalgesia depends on the peripheral sensitization of nociceptors induced by the release of neuropeptides such as neuropeptide substance P from an axon reflex after stimulation of fine afferent fibers.

Pain from large infiltration tumor should be managed with palliative radiotherapy and it can improve after active chemotherapy, but in all patients a specific supportive analgesic treatment is mandatory. Non-narcotic analgesics, including acetaminophen and non-steroidal anti-inflammatory drugs alone or in combination with opioids such as codeine, should be used in starting treatment for mild or moderate pain. Morphine, hydromorphone, oxycodone, levorphanol, methadone, and fentanyl are commonly used for severe cancer pain. Agonist-antagonist opioids such as pentazocine are not indicated for cancer pain management. Opioid analgesic drugs should be given by oral administration whenever possible, or by subcutaneous, epidural or intrathecal administration at effective doses and appropriate intervals.

23.4 Infective Complications in Lung Cancer Patients

Pulmonary hemorrhage, emboli, edema of cardiac and non-cardiac origin, chemo-radiotherapy side effects, neoplastic lymphangiosis, and superinfection of a necrotic poorly oxygenated tumor mass can produce febrile pneumonitis with or without infectious varieties of pneumonia.

Diagnosis of the specific disease requires a histological or bacterial culture documentation. Often, diffuse interstitial infiltrates on X-ray or CT scan constitute a difficult diagnostic problem and require bronchoalveolar lavage to define a possible opportunistic infection, more frequently due to *Pneumocystis carinii*, cytomegalovirus and mycobacteria (STOVEN et al. 1984).

Necrotic tumors are often complicated by the development of abscess mainly caused by anaerobic bacteria, such as *Bacteroides* and anaerobic cocci. Poor blood supply with resulting low oxygen tension may favor the growth of anaerobes in necrotic tumors (BROOK 1990).

Febrile neutropenia is a common complication of cancer chemotherapy mainly in high-dose chemotherapy regimens. In lung cancer, treatment-related neutropenia occurs more frequently in poor performance status patients, with serious underlying medical conditions. In small cell lung cancer, febrile neutropenia is statistically more frequent in doxorubicin-containing chemotherapy, such as CAV (cyclophosphamide, Adriamycin, vincristine) or CAE (cyclophosphamide, Adriamycin, etoposide) (DEVORE and JOHNSON 1996). The most common microorganisms causing infections during neutropenia include gram-negative (Enterobacteriaceae, *Pseudomonas aeruginosa*, *Salmonella*), gram-positive (*Staphylococcus*, *Streptococcus pneumoniae*), anaerobic cocci and bacilli, and opportunistic agents (*Candida*, *Aspergillus*, *Pneumocystis carinii* and *Nocardia*).

In any case, when possible, antimicrobical therapy should be based on the isolation of specific organisms, both aerobes and anaerobes. Antimicrobial agents that generally provide coverage for *S. auerus* in addition to anaerobic bacteria include cefoxitin, clindamycin, imipenem and a combination of a β-lactamase inhibitor (i.e., clavulanic acid) and a penicillin (i.e., ticarcillin) and the combination of metronidazole plus a β-lactamase-resistant penicillin.

Gram-negative aerobic bacilli are also covered by cefoxitin, imipenem and penicillin plus a β-lactamase inhibitor, but are more effectively treated with aminoglycosides and quinolones. G-CSF or GM-CSF hematological growth factors should be used in the treatment of febrile neutropenia according to American Society Clinical Oncology Guidelines, i.e., in the case of febrile neutropenia with less than 500 granulocytes/mm^3 or in the case of anamnestic chemotherapy-induced febrile neutropenia (American Society of Clinical Oncology).

An empiric therapeutic approach of febrile episodes in neutropenic patients includes combination antibiotic therapy with cephalosporin ± aminoglicoside ± vancomycin, modified after 48–72 h evaluation in the absence of identified pathogens by the eventual addition of amphotericin B and colony-stimulating growth factors (KLASTERSKY 1994).

However, an overview of randomized studies proved no superiority of empiric antibiotic combinations versus monotherapy with ceftazidime or meropenem in the empirical treatment of neutropenic cancer patients. Thus, monotherapy with either ceftazidime or meropenem is a reasonable approach in patients with uncomplicated febrile neutropenia (SANDERS et al. 1991).

Sulfamethoxazole/trimetroprim has been largely employed for prophylaxis of infective complications during chemotherapy in both small and non-small cell lung cancer and has been reported to prevent *Pneumocystis carinii* (HUGHES et al. 1977).

Recently, quinolones have been widely employed as prophylaxis or treatment because of their activity in gram-negative bacilli and the frequent appearance of drug-resistant microorganisms (WINSTON et al. 1987).

Severe acute radiation febrile pneumonitis is a treatment-related complication occurring in less than 5% of patients receiving high-dose lung irradiation, and requires aggressive supportive care with hydration and i.v. steroid administration (1 mg prednisone per kg i.v.) to be tapered slowly once symptoms improve, to avoid pneumonitis relapse.

In most patients with mild symptoms of radiation pneumonitis only a brief course of oral steroids (50 mg prednisone for 10 days) is usually recommended. The resolution time of acute radiation pneumonitis is quite variable, ranging from a few days to many weeks (EVANS et al. 1992).

23.5 Supportive Treatment of Specific Problems in Lung Cancer

23.5.1 Management of Recurrent Malignant Pleural Effusions

Malignant pleural effusion is a rather frequent complication of lung cancer, occurring in approximately

10% of patients. Systemic chemotherapy can be considered the initial treatment and it is usually effective in SCLC and also in most patients with NSCLC. On the other hand, recurrent pleural effusion no longer responsive to chemotherapy needs different palliation.

The treatment of choice is based on obtaining effective pleurodesis by the introduction of a sclerosing agent through a tube thoracostomy inserted to achieve complete drainage of pleural space and apposition of the visceral and parietal pleura. Talc insufflation is safe and effective (Feutiman 1987); each failed attempt may, however, determine loculated fluid collection, preventing lung expansion and leading to "trapped lung" (Lynch 1993).

Doxycycline, bleomycin, and quinacrine have been used as sclerosing agents with a response rate ranging from 50% to 87%. When pleurodesis fails, the only alternative palliation of malignant pleural effusion is pleuroperitoneal shunts.

A new attempt to treat pleural effusion consists of the intrapleural continuous infusion of cytokines, mainly interleukin-2, over 5 days, with a response of 22–50% (Viallat et al. 1993).

23.5.2 Central Airway Obstruction

Obstruction of the trachea, bifurcation or main stem bronchi from lung cancer is a life-threatening situation which is only occasionally suitable for curative treatment with resection of the trachea or sleeve resection of the bronchus, or by pulmonary resection, whereas for the majority of cases only palliation is possible. Intraluminal tumor can be cored out and resected by diathermy, laser, cryotherapy, or argon beamer.

Airways disobliteration can be produced by thermic destruction of neoplastic tissues with heat transformation of the energy of a high-frequency current passing through the tissue (Hooper and Jackson 1985). The major disadvantage of this technique, which should not be applied in patients wearing metallic devices (metallic stents or pacemaker), is the ensuing risk of bleeding. The insufflation of argon gas as a vehicle for the current can enhance the diathermy effects: the coagulation effect of the electric gas cloud makes the argon beamer superior to all other methods of coagulation, especially laser in the cases of profuse bleeding from superficial lesions (Grund et al. 1994).

Cryotherapy as a disobliterative technique is not as rapid as other methods and it has been widely replaced. The energy transfer of the Nd:Yag laser light occurs with tranformation into heat of energy absorbed and dispersed inside the tumor. The energy absorption depends largely on the tissue colors, red or dark absorbing a lot of energy whereas white-colored tissue needs more energy for destruction. There is a general consensus about applying the Nd:Yag laser at lower energies of 20–30 w for coagulation of tumor tissue and tumor vessels, and up to 40–50 w for thermal destruction (Cavaliere et al. 1994).

In recent years, new bronchoscopic methods have been developed for long-term treatment of persistent tumor inside or close to airways, i.e., photodynamic laser, brachytherapy, and the endoscopic implantation of devices for disobliteration and internal stabilization, the so-called stents, such as silicone plastic tubes, metallic meshworks and composite materials (Becher et al. 1995).

Goldstraw recently presented a retrospective review of 51 patients treated with endoluminal stents for distal obstruction. All but two patients gained immediate dyspnea relief with, in some cases, a 53% improvement in FEV1 (Abratt 1994).

23.5.3 Supportive Treatment of Painful Osteolytic Bone Metastasis

Painful bone metastases commonly occur in advanced lung cancer patients and represent a difficult management problem because of pain and reduction in mobility and performance status. Palliative radiotherapy is indicated in the treatment of unique painful bone lesion or multiple close lesions as in metastatic involvement of the spine. Recently, pamidronate has been recognized as useful in the management of painful osteolytic bone disease: biphosphonates are specific inhibitors of the osteoclast-mediated bone reabsorption and have an established role in the treatment of tumor-induced hypercalcemia. Intravenous pamidronate and daily oral clodronate or pamidronate have shown an analgesic effect in patients with osteolytic bone metastasis, mainly in prostate and breast cancer patients.

Recently two different papers showed a dose-effect correlation for pamidronate in i.v. infusion (Thurlimann et al. 1994; Cascinu et al. 1998). In both trials a statistically significant change in pain and mobility was noted for a dose intensity of 45 mg/weeks vs. 15–30 mg/weeks and for 90 mg/m^2 vs. 60 and 45 mg/ml every 3 weeks. The majority of patients in both studies were breast cancer patients, but it seems likely that biphosphonates should be indicated in all patients with bone metastases.

23.5.4 Management of Hypercalcemia in Lung Cancer

About 10% of lung cancer patients develop hypercalcemia, mainly caused by osteoclast-mediated bone resorption; however, in 10–15% of cases, mainly in squamous cell carcinoma hypercalcemia, there is a paraneoplastic syndrome due to ectopic production of a parathyroid analogue, and several cytokines secreted by tumors (Broadus et al. 1988). The osteoclast plays a central role as the final target of peptide hormone and cytokine action.

General treatment measures for hypercalcemia include vigorous rehydration with normal saline to establish good diuresis and to correct hypovolemia since hypercalcemia induces osmotic diuresis. Biphosphonates are the most important agents by intravenous administration because of their specific counteraction on osteoclastic-mediated bone reabsorption, although they appear to be less active in treating the hypercalcemia associated with high levels of parathyroid hormone-related peptide. Salmon calcitonin is probably less effective than biphosphates but it is useful in rapidly lowering elevated serum calcium levels.

Corticosteroids are still used but they no longer play a major role in the management of hypercalcemia, with the exception of steroid-responsive malignancies such as myeloma and lymphomas.

Diuretics such as furosemide may be employed, but careful attention should be given to the electrolyte depletion (Harvey 1995).

23.6 Conclusions

At present, more than 50% of cancer patients cannot be cured of their disease and this is true for more than 80% of lung cancer patients. These data alone explain why supportive care aimed at symptom palliation and at the preservation of an optimal quality of life plays a central role in the management strategies of all lung cancer patients.

References

Abratt R (1994) IASLC Workshop in improving quality of life and the supportive management of patients with lung cancer. Lung Cancer 10:375–380

American Society of Clinical Oncology (1996) Update of recommendations for the use of hematopoietic colony-stimulating factors: evidence based clinical practice guidelines. J Clin Oncol 14:1957–1960

American Society of Clinical Oncology (1997) Special article: clinical practice guidelines for treatment of unresectable non-small cell lung cancer. J Clin Oncol 15:2996–3018

Becher HD, Wagner B, Lierman D et al (1995) Stenting of the central airways. In: Lieramn (ed) Stents. State of art and future developments. Polyscience Publications, pp 249–255

Berrino F, Sant M, Verdecchia A et al (1995) Survival of cancer patients in Europe. IARC Scientific Publications No. 132, Lyon

Billingsly KG, Alexander HR (1996) The pathophysiology of cachexia in advanced cancer and AIDS. In: Bruera E, Higginson I (eds) Cachexia-anorexia in cancer patients, vol 1. Oxford University Press, Oxford, pp 1–22

Broadus AE, Maugin M, Ikeda K et al (1988) Humoral hypercalcemia of malignancy. N Engl J Med 319:556–563

Brook I (1990) Bacteria from solid tumours. J Med Microbiol 32:207–210

Bruera E, McEachern T, Ripamonti C et al (1993) Subcutaneous morphine for dyspnea in cancer patients. Ann Inter Med 119:906–907

Bruera E (1998) Pharmacological treatment of cachexia: any progress? Support Care Cancer 6:109–113

Cascinu S, Graziano F, Alessandroni P (1998) Different dose of pamidronate in prostate with painful osteolytic bone metastasis 6:139–143

Cavaliere S, Foccoli P, Toninelli C et al (1994) Laser therapy in lung cancer: an 11-year experience with 2253 applications in 1528 patients. J Bronchol 1:105–111

Cullen MH, Woodroffe CM, Billingham LJ et al (1997) Mitomycin, ifosfamide and cisplatin (MIC) in non-small cell lung cancer (NSCLC): results of a randomized trial in patients with extensive disease. Lung Cancer 18:5 (Suppl 1) Abstract 10

Curtis EB, Kreech RL, Walsh TD (1991) Common symptoms in patients with advanced cancer. J Palliative Care 7:25–29

De Vore R, Johnson D (1996) Chemotherapy of small cell lung cancer. In: Pass H, Mistchell J, Johnson D, Turrisi A (eds) Lung cancer: principles and practice. Lippincott Raven Press, pp 825–838

Dunlops R (1996) Clinical epidemiology of cancer cachexia. In: Bruera E, Higginson I (eds) Cachexia-anorexia in cancer patients, vol 5. Oxford University Press, Oxford, pp 76–82

Evans ML, Grahan MM, Mahler PA (1992) Use of steroids to suppress vascular response to radiation. Int J Radiat Oncol Biol Phys 13:563–567

Farcombe M (1997) Dyspnea: assessment and treatment. Support Care Cancer 5:94–99

Farcombe M, Chater S, Gillin A et al (1994) The use of nebulized opioids for breathlessness: a chart survey. palliat Med 8:306–312

Feutiman IS (1987) Effective treatment of malignant pleural effusions. Br J Hosp Med 37:423

Frith LI (1992) Quality of life as assessed by the Rotterdam Symptoms checklist in patients with lung cancer. MSc Thesis, University of Southampton

Glaus A (1993) Assessment of fatigue in cancer and non cancer patients and in healthy individuals. Support Care Cancer 1:305–315

Grund KE, Storek D, Farin G (1994) Endoscopic argon plasma coagulation. First clinical experiences in flexible endoscopy. End Surg 2:42–46

Harvey H (1995) The management of hypercalcemia of malignancy 3:123–129

Hollen PJ, Gralla R, Kris M et al (1993) Quality of life assessment in individuals with lung cancer: testing the Lung Cancer Symptom Scale (LCSC). Eur J Cancer 29A:S51–S52

Hollen PJ, Gralla R, Kris M et al (1994) Quality of life during clinical trials: conceptual model for the Lung Cancer Symptom Scale (LCSS). Support Care Cancer 2:213–223

Hooper RG, Jackson FN (1985) Endobronchial electrocautery. Chest 87:712–714

Hopwood P, Stephens RJ and half of the Medical Research Council (MRC) (1995) Lung cancer Working Party. Symptoms at presentation for treatment in patients with lung cancer: implications for the evaluation of palliative treatment. Br J Cancer 71:633–636

Hughes WT, Kubn S, Chandhary S et al (1977) Successful chemoprophylaxis for Pneumocystis carinii pneumonitis. N Engl J Med 297:1419–1426

Klastersky J (1994) Empirical therapy for bacterial infections in neutropenic patients. Support Care Cancer 2:347–354

Lynch TY (1993) Management of malignant pleural effusions. Chest 103:3855

Non-Small Cell Lung Cancer Collaborative Group (1995) Chemotherapy in non-small cell lung cancer: a meta-analysis using updated data on individual patients from 52 randomized clinical trials. Br Med J 311:899–909

Parker L, Touy T, Bolden S, Wingo PA (1997) Cancer statistics, CA. Cancer J Clin 47:5–27

Sanders JW, Powe NR, Moore RD (1991) Ceftazidime monotherapy for empiric treatment of febrile neutropenic patients. A meta-analysis. J Infect Dis 164:907–916

Souhami RL, Law K (1990) Longevity in small cell lung cancer. Br J Cancer 61:584–589

Stoven DE, Zaman MB, Hayden SI (1984) Bronchoalveolar lavage in the diagnosis of diffuse pulmonary infiltrates in the immunosuppressed host. Ann Intern Med 101:1–7

Thurlimann B, Morant R, Jungu WF (1994) Pamidronate for pain control in patients with malignant osteolytic bone disease: a prospective dose-effect study. Support Care Cancer 2:61–66

Viallat JR, Boutin C, Ray F et al (1993) Intrapleural immunotherapy with escalating doses of interleukin-2 in metastatic pleural effusions. Cancer 71:4067

Visser M, Smets E (1998) Fatigue depression and quality of life in cancer patients: how are they related? Support Care Cancer 6:101–108

Winston DJ, Ho WG, Chaplin RE et al (1987) Norfloxacin for prevention of bacterial infections in granulocytopenic patients. Am J Med 82:40–46

Subject Index

List of Contributors

KATHY S. ALBAIN, MD
Professor of Medicine
Division of Hematology/Oncology
Loyola University Medical Center
Cardinal Bernadin Cancer Center, Room 109
2160 South First Avenue
Maywood, IL 60153
USA

J. JAVIER ARISTU, MD
Department of Oncology
Clínica Universitaria de Navarra
E-31080 Pamplona
Spain

PETER ARMSTRONG, MD
Department of Academic Radiology
The Royals Hospitals NHS Trust
St. Bartholomew's Hospital
West Smithfield
London ECIA 7BE
UK

PIERRE BALDEYROU, MD
Departments of Radiotherapy and Medicine
Institut Gustave Roussy
39, rue Camille Desmoulins
F-94805 Villejuif Cédex
France

DAVID BALL, MD
Division of Radiation Oncology
Peter MacCallum Cancer Institute
Rocked Bays A'Beckett Street
Melbourne, Vic. 300
Australia

THIARY BERGHMANS, MD
Institut Jules Bordet
Service de Médecine Interne
et Laboratoire d'Investigation Clinique H.J. Tagnon
Centre des Tumeurs de L'Université Libre de Bruxelles
1 rue Héger-Bordet
B-1000 Brussels
Belgium

LIESBETH J. BOERSMA, MD
Radiotherapy Department
The Netherlands Cancer Institute
Antoni van Leeuwenhoek Huis
Plesmanlaan 121
1066 CX Amsterdam
The Netherlands

H. BUENEMANN, MD
Hermann-Holthusen-Institut für Strahlentherapie
Allgemeines Krankenhaus St. Georg
Lohmühlenstrasse 5
D-20099 Hamburg
Germany

FELIPE A. CALVO, MD
Professor
Department of Oncology
Hospital General Universitario Gregorio Marañon
Doctor Esquerdo, 46
E-28007 Madrid
Spain

MATTEO CAPPELLO, MD
Department of Thoracic Surgery
Hôpital Erasme
Université Libre de Bruxelles
808 Route de Lennik
B-1070 Brussels
Belgium

FEDERICO CAPPUZZO, MD
Department of Medicine
Institut Gustave Roussy
39, rue Camille Desmoulins
F-94805 Villejuif
France

CATHERINE CASTAIGNE, MD
Institut Jules Bordet
Service de Médecine Interne
et Laboratoire d'Investigation Clinique H.J. Tagnon
Centre des Tumeurs de l'Université Libre de Bruxelles
1 rue Héger-Bordet
B-1000 Brussels
Belgium

James D. Cox, MD, FACR
Professor and Chairman
Department of Radiation Oncology
The University of Texas M.D.
Anderson Cancer Center
1515 Holcombe Blvd., Box 97
Houston, TX 77030
USA

Lucio Crino, MD
Medical Oncology Department
Ospedale Bellaria
Via Altura, 3
I-40100 Bologna
Italy

Ann Cull, MD
Imperial Cancer Research Fund Psychology
Research Group
University of Edinburgh
Western General Hospital NHS Trust
Crewe Road
Edinburgh EH4 2XU
UK

Janet E. Dancey, MD, FRCPC
Princess Margareth Hospital
610 University Avenue
Toronto, Ontario M5G 2M9
Canada

Serge Danhier, MD
Institut Jules Bordet
Service de Radiothérapie
1, rue Héger-Bordet
B-1000 Brussels
Belgium

David Devriendt
Service de Radiotherapie
Recherche et d'Investigation Clinique
Institut Jules Bordet
1, rue Héger-Bordet
B-1000 Brussels
Belgium

Bahmam Emami, MD
Professor and Chairman
Department of Radiation Oncology
Loyola University Medical Center
2160 South First Avenue
Maywood, IL 60153
USA

Scot A. Fisher, MD
Department of Radiation Oncology
Allegheny University Hospitals Graduate
1800 Lombard St.
Philadelphia, PA 19146
USA

Philippe De Francquen, MD
Department of Thoracic Surgery
Hôpital Erasme
Université Libre de Bruxelles
808 Route de Lennik
B-1070 Brussels
Belgium

Mark R. Green, MD
Professor of Oncology
Hollings Cancer Center
Medical University of South Carolina
171 Ashley Avenue
Charleston, SC 29425-2225
USA

Anna Gregor, MD
Department of Clinical Oncology
University of Edinburgh
Western General Hospital NHS Trust
Crewe Road
Edinburgh EH4 2XU
UK

Julian A. Hanson, MD
Department of Diagnostic Imaging
The Royals Hospitals NHS Trust
St. Bartholomew's Hospital
West Smithfield
London ECIA 7BE
UK

Hans-Peter Heilmann, MD
Professor
Hermann-Holthusen-Institut für Strahlentherapie
Allgemeines Krankenhaus St. Georg
Lohmühlenstrasse 5
D-20099 Hamburg
Germany

Jean Klastersky, MD
Professor d'Investigation Clinique
Institut Jules Bordet
Centre des Tumeurs de l'Université Libre
de Bruxelles
1, rue Héger-Bordet
B-1000 Brussels
Belgium

Ritsuko Komaki, MD, FACR
Professor Radiation Oncology
The University of Texas M.D.
Anderson Cancer Center
1515 Holcombe Blvd., Box 97
Houston, TX 77030
USA

Yassine Lalami, MD
Institut Jules Bordet
Service de Médecine Interne
et Laboratoire d'Investigation Clinique H.J. Tagnon
Centre des Tumeurs de l'Université Libre de Bruxelles
1, rue Héger-Bordet
B-1000 Brussels
Belgium

Eric Lartigau, MD, PhD
Departments of Radiotherapy and Medicine
Institut Gustave Roussy
39, rue Camille Desmoulins
F-94805 Villejuif Cédex
France

Thierry Le Chevalier, MD
Department of Medicine
Institut Gustave Roussy
39, rue Camille Desmoulins
F-94805 Villejuif Cédex
France

Swan S. Leong, MD
Hollings Cancer Center
Medical University of South Carolina
171 Ashley Avenue
Charleston, SC 29425-2225
USA

Sylvie Luce, MD
Institut Jules Bordet
Service de Médecine Interne
et Laboratoire d'Investigation Clinique H.J. Tagnon
Centre des Tumeurs de l'Université Libre de Bruxelles
1, rue Héger-Bordet
B-1000 Brussels
Belgium

Fergus Macbeth, MD
Director, Clinical Effectiveness Support Unit (Wales)
Llandough Hospital and NHS Trust
Roseway
Penarth, South Wales CF6 42XX
UK

Hugo Marsiglia, MD
Divisione di Radioterapia
Istituto Europeo di Oncologia
Via Ripamonti, 435
I-20141 Milano
Italy

René O. Mirimanoff, MD
Professor
Department of Radiation Oncology
Centre Hospitalier Universitaire Vaudois, CHUV
CH-1011 Lausanne
Switzerland

Marta Moreno, MD
Department of Oncology
Clínica Universitaria de Navarra
E-31080 Pamplona
Spain

Françoise Mornex, MD
Professor
Radiation Oncology Department, EA 643
Centre Hospitalier Lyon-Sud
Chemin du Grand Revoyer
F-69310 Pierre-Bénite
France

Kell Østerlind, MD
Department of Internal Medicine F
Hillerød County Hospital
DK-3400 Hillerød
Denmark

Marianne Paesmans, MD
Institut Jules Bordet
Service de Médecine Interne
et Laboratoire d'Investigation Clinique H.J. Tagnon
Centre des Tumeurs de l'Université Libre de Bruxelles
1 rue Héger-Bordet
B-1000 Brussels
Belgium

Caio Max S. Rocha Lima, MD
Hollings Cancer Center
Medical University of South Carolina
171 Ashley Avenue
Charleston, SC 29425-2225
USA

Pierre Rocmans, MD
Professor of Surgery
Department of Thoracic Surgery
Hôpital Erasme
Université Libre de Bruxelles
808 Route de Lennik
B-1070 Brussels
Belgium

Manuel Santos, MD
Instituto Madrileño de Oncología
Emilio Vargas 16
E-28043 Madrid
Spain

Michele I. Saunders, MD
Professor
Marie Curie Research Wing
Mount Vernon Hospital
Rickmansworth Road
Northwood, Middlesex HA6 2RN
UK

Pierre Scalliet, MD
Professor
Service de Radiothérapie Oncologique
Cliniques Universitaires Saint-Luc
Avenue Hippocrate
B-1200 Brussels
Belgium

Christiaan Schiepers, MD, PhD
UCLA School of Medicine
Nuclear Medicine, CHS-AR144
10833 LeConte Avenue
Los Angeles, CA 90095-6942
USA

Jean-Paul Sculier, MD
Institut Jules Bordet
Service de Médecine Interne
et Laboratoire d'Investigation Clinique H.J. Tagnon
Centre des Tumeurs de L'Université Libre de Bruxelles
1, rue Héger-Bordet
B-1000 Brussels
Belgium

Frances A. Shepherd, MD, FRCPC
Princess Margareth Hospital
610 University Avenue
Toronto, Ontario M5G 2M9
Canada

Jens Benn Sørensen, MD
Chief Physician
The Finsen Center
Department of Oncology
Copenhagen University Hospital
9 Blegdamsvej
DK-2100 Copenhagen Ø
Denmark

Christophe Sotiriou, MD
Institut Jules Bordet
Service de Médecine Interne
et Laboratoire d'Investigation Clinique H.J. Tagnon
Centre des Tumeurs de l'Université Libre de Bruxelles
1, rue Héger-Bordet
B-1000 Brussels
Belgium

Paul Van Houtte, MD
Professor, Department of Radiation Oncology
Institut Jules Bordet
Service de Radiothérapie
1, rue Héger-Bordet
B-1000 Brussels
Belgium

Pierre Vermylen, MD
Institut Jules Bordet
Service de Médecine Interne
et Laboratoire d'Investigation Clinique H.J. Tagnon
Centre des Tumeurs de l'Université Libre de Bruxelles
1, rue Héger-Bordet
B-1000 Brussels
Belgium

Henry Wagner, MD
Thoracic Oncology Program and
Division of Radiation Oncology
H. Lee Moffitt Cancer Center
12902 Magnolia Drive
Tampa, FL 33612-9416
USA

Florian Wuerschmidt, MD
Hermann-Holthusen-Institut für Strahlentherapie
Allgemeines Krankenhaus St. Georg
Lohmühlenstrasse 5
D-20099 Hamburg
Germany

Alba Zappala, MD
Department of Medicine
Institut Gustave Roussy
39, rue Camille Desmoulins
F-94805 Villejuif
France

Medical Radiology

Diagnostic Imaging and Radiation Oncology

Titles in the series already published

Radiation Oncology

Interventional Radiation Therapy Techniques - Brachytherapy
Edited by R. Sauer

Radiopathology of Organs and Tissues
Edited by E. Scherer, C. Streffer, and K.-R. Trott

Concomitant Continuous Infusion Chemotherapy and Radiation
Edited by M. Rotman and C.J. Rosenthal

Intraoperative Radiotherapy – Clinical Experiences and Results
Edited by F.A. Calvo, M. Santos, and L.W. Brady

Radiotherapy of Intraocular and Orbital Tumors
Edited by W.E. Alberti and R.H. Sagerman

Interstitial and Intracavitary Thermoradiotherapy
Edited by M.H. Seegenschmiedt and R. Sauer

Non-Disseminated Breast Cancer
Controversial Issues in Management
Edited by G.H. Fletcher and S.H. Levitt

Current Topics in Clinical Radiobiology of Tumors
Edited by H.-P. Beck-Bornholdt

Practical Approaches to Cancer Invasion and Metastases
A Compendium of Radiation Oncologists' Responses to 40 Histories
Edited by A.R. Kagan with the Assistance of R.J. Steckel

Radiation Therapy in Pediatric Oncology
Edited by J.R. Cassady

Radiation Therapy Physics
Edited by A.R. Smith

Late Sequelae in Oncology
Edited by J. Dunst and R. Sauer

Mediastinal Tumors. Update 1995
Edited by D.E. Wood and C.R. Thomas, Jr.

Thermoradiotherapy and Thermochemotherapy
Volume 1:
Biology, Physiology, and Physics
Volume 2:
Clinical Applications
Edited by M.H. Seegenschmiedt, P. Fessenden, and C.C. Vernon

Carcinoma of the Prostate
Innovations in Management
Edited by Z. Petrovich, L. Baert, and L.W. Brady

Radiation Oncology of Gynecological Cancers
Edited by H.W. Vahrson

Carcinoma of the Bladder
Innovations in Management
Edited by Z. Petrovich, L. Baert, and L.W. Brady

Blood Perfusion and Microenvironment of Human Tumors
Implications for Clinical Radiooncology
Edited by M. Molls and P. Vaupel

Radiation Therapy of Benign Diseases. A Clinical Guide
2nd revised edition
S.E. Order and S.S. Donaldson

Carcinoma of the Kidney and Testis, and Rare Urologic Malignancies
Innovations in Management
Edited by Z. Petrovich, L. Baert, and L.W. Brady

Progress and Perspectives in the Treatment of Lung Cancer
Edited by P. Van Houtte, J. Klastersky, and P. Rocmans

MEDICAL RADIOLOGY
Diagnostic Imaging and Radiation Oncology

Titles in the series already published

DIAGNOSTIC IMAGING

Innovations in Diagnostic Imaging
Edited by J.H. Anderson

Radiology of the Upper Urinary Tract
Edited by E.K. Lang

The Thymus - Diagnostic Imaging, Functions, and Pathologic Anatomy
Edited by E. Walter, E. Willich, and W.R. Webb

Interventional Neuroradiology
Edited by A. Valavanis

Radiology of the Pancreas
Edited by A.L. Baert, co-edited by G. Delorme

Radiology of the Lower Urinary Tract
Edited by E.K. Lang

Magnetic Resonance Angiography
Edited by I.P. Arlart, G.M. Bongartz, and G. Marchal

Contrast-Enhanced MRI of the Breast
S. Heywang-Köbrunner and R. Beck

Spiral CT of the Chest
Edited by M. Rémy-Jardin and J. Rémy

Radiological Diagnosis of Breast Diseases
Edited by M. Friedrich and E.A. Sickles

Radiology of the Trauma
Edited by M. Heller and A. Fink

Biliary Tract Radiology
Edited by P. Rossi

Radiological Imaging of Sports Injuries
Edited by C. Masciocchi

Modern Imaging of the Alimentary Tube
Edited by A. R. Margulis

Diagnosis and Therapy of Spinal Tumors
Edited by P. R. Algra, J. Valk, and J. J. Heimans

Interventional Magnetic Resonance Imaging
Edited by J. F. Debatin and G. Adam

Abdominal and Pelvic MRI
Edited by A. Heuck and M. Reiser

Orthopedic Imaging
Techniques and Applications
Edited by A.M. Davies and H. Pettersson

Radiology of the Female Pelvic Organs
Edited by E.K.Lang

Magnetic Resonance of the Heart and Great Vessels
Clinical Applications
Edited by J. Bogaert, A. J. Duerinckx, and F. E. Rademakers

Modern Head and Neck Imaging
Edited by S. K. Mukherji and J. A. Castelijns

Radiology Imaging of Endocrine Diseases
Edited by J. N. Bruneton in collaboration with B. Padovani and M.-Y. Mourou

Trends in Contrast Media
Edited by H. S. Thomsen, R. N. Muller, and R. F. Mattrey

Functional MRI
Edited by C. T. W. Moonen and P. A. Bandettini

RADIATION ONCOLOGY

Lung Cancer
Edited by C.W. Scarantino

Innovations in Radiation Oncology
Edited by H.R. Withers and L.J. Peters

Radiation Therapy of Head and Neck Cancer
Edited by G.E. Laramore

Gastrointestinal Cancer – Radiation Therapy
Edited by R.R. Dobelbower, Jr.

Radiation Exposure and Occupational Risks
Edited by E. Scherer, C. Streffer, and K.-R. Trott

Radiation Therapy of Benign Diseases - A Clinical Guide
S.E. Order and S.S. Donaldson

Printing and binding: Druckerei Triltsch, Würzburg